DUKE RADIOLOGY CASE REVIEW

Imaging, Differential Diagnosis, and Discussion

JAMES M. PROVENZALE, M.D.
Associate Professor of Radiology
Director, Neuroradiology
Duke University Medical Center
Durham, North Carolina

RENDON C. NELSON, M.D.
Professor of Radiology
Director, Abdominal Imaging
Duke University Medical Center
Durham, North Carolina

Editors

with 64 contributors

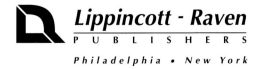

Lippincott - Raven
P U B L I S H E R S
Philadelphia • New York

Acquisitions Editor: James Ryan
Developmental Editor: Brian Brown
Manufacturing Manager: Dennis Teston
Associate Managing Editor: Kathleen Bubbeo
Production Editor: Elizabeth Willingham, Silverchair Science + Communications
Cover Designer: Karen Quigley
Indexer: Elizabeth Willingham, Silverchair Science + Communications
Compositor: Jake Zarnegar, Silverchair Science + Communications
Printer: Courier Westford

Printed in the United States of America

9 8 7 6 5 4 3 2 1

Library of Congress Cataloging-in-Publication Data

Duke radiology case review : inaging, differential diagnosis, and
   discussion / James M. Provenzale, Rendon C. Nelson, editors ; with
   62 contributors.
       p.   cm.
   Includes bibliographical references and index.
   ISBN 0–397–51613–4
   1. Diagnostic imaging--case studies. I. Provenzale, James M.
II. Nelson, Rendon C. III. Duke University. Medical Center. Dept.
of Radiology.
   [DNLM: 1. Radiology--case studies. WN 100 D877 1998]
RC78.7.D53D85   1998
616.07'54--DC21
DNLM/DLC
for Library of Congress   97–34795
                                                  CIP

To our wives, Dawn and Heidi,
and our children, Kate and Curran,
and in memory of our deceased colleagues,
Andrew Yeates, Michael Brothers, and Reed Rice

CONTENTS

CONTRIBUTORS

Sheri L. Albers, M.D.
Associate
Department of Radiology
Duke University Medical Center
Durham, North Carolina

Jeffrey B. Betts, M.D.
Northeast Radiology, Inc.
Cincinnati, Ohio

George S. Bisset III, M.D.
Vice Chairman and Professor of Radiology
Duke University Medical Center
Durham, North Carolina

Salvador Borges-Neto, M.D.
Assistant Professor of Radiology
Duke University Medical Center
Durham, North Carolina

James D. Bowie, M.D.
Professor of Radiology
Duke University Medical Center
Durham, North Carolina

D. Lawrence Burk, M.D.
Associate Professor of Radiology
Duke University Medical Center
Durham, North Carolina

Barbara A. Carroll, M.D.
Professor of Radiology
Duke University Medical Center
Durham, North Carolina

James T.T. Chen, M.D.
Professor of Radiology
Duke University Medical Center
Durham, North Carolina

R. Edward Coleman, M.D.
Professor of Radiology
Duke University Medical Center
Durham, North Carolina

Andrew J. Collins, M.D.
Assistant Professor of Radiology
Duke University Medical Center
Durham, North Carolina

Joseph B. Cornett, M.D.
Associate
Department of Radiology
Duke University Medical Center
Durham, North Carolina

Charles B. Donovan, M.D.
Radiological Consultant Associates
Methodist Medical Center
Dallas, Texas

David S. Enterline, M.D.
Assistant Professor of Radiology
Duke University Medical Center
Durham, North Carolina

Jeremy J. Erasmus, M.D.
Assistant Professor of Radiology
Duke University Medical Center
Durham, North Carolina

Anthony M. Foti, M.D.
Windsong Radiology
Williamsville, New York

M. Gena Frederick, M.D.
Delaney Radiologists Group, P.A.
Wilmington, North Carolina

Kelly S. Freed, M.D.
Assistant Professor of Radiology
Duke University Medical Center
Durham, North Carolina

Donald P. Frush, M.D.
Assistant Professor of Radiology
Duke University Medical Center
Durham, North Carolina

R. Chapman Gilkeson, M.D.
Assistant Professor of Radiology
University Hospitals of Cleveland
Cleveland, Ohio

Katrina Glazebrook, M.D.
Consultant Radiologist
Auckland Hospital
Auckland, New Zealand

Philip C. Goodman, M.D.
Professor of Radiology
Duke University Medical Center
Durham, North Carolina

Herman Grossman, M.D.
Professor of Radiology
Duke University Medical Center
Durham, North Carolina

Rosalie J. Hagge, M.D.
Resident
Department of Radiology
Duke University Medical Center
Durham, North Carolina

Bruce P. Hall, M.D.
Department of Radiology
Children's Hospital of Buffalo
Buffalo, New York

Michael W. Hanson, M.D.
Assistant Professor of Radiology
Duke University Medical Center
Durham, North Carolina

E. Ralph Heinz, M.D.
Professor of Radiology
Duke University Medical Center
Durham, North Carolina

Barbara S. Hertzberg, M.D.
Associate Professor of Radiology
Duke University Medical Center
Durham, North Carolina

David M. Hough, M.D.
Consultant Radiologist
Auckland Hospital
Auckland, New Zealand

Michael J. Kelley, M.D.
Clinical Associate of Radiology
Duke University Medical Center
Durham, North Carolina
and
Department of Radiology
Carolinas Medical Center
Charlotte, North Carolina

Mary T. Keogan, M.D.
Assistant Professor of Radiology
Duke University Medical Center
Durham, North Carolina

Michael L. Kerner, M.D.
Department of Radiology
Kaiser Permanente
Raleigh, North Carolina

Mark A. Kliewer, M.D.
Associate Professor of Radiology
Duke University Medical Center
Durham, North Carolina

Phyllis J. Kornguth, M.D.
Associate Professor of Radiology
Duke University Medical Center
Durham, North Carolina

Jeremy A.L. Lawrance, M.B.ChB(UCT), M.R.C.P.(UK)
Doctor of Diagnostic Radiology
Christie Hospital
Manchester, United Kingdom

Richard A. Leder, M.D.
Associate Professor of Radiology
Duke University Medical Center
Durham, North Carolina

Vincent H.S. Low, M.D.
Assistant Professor of Radiology
Duke University Medical Center
Durham, North Carolina

Salutario J. Martinez, M.D.
Professor of Radiology
Duke University Medical Center
Durham, North Carolina

H. Page McAdams, M.D.
Assistant Professor of Radiology
Duke University Medical Center
Durham, North Carolina

Philip T. McAndrew, M.D.
Department of Radiology
Eastbourne District Hospital
Eastbourne, United Kingdom

Vincent G. McDermott, M.D.
Assistant Professor of Radiology
Duke University Medical Center
Durham, North Carolina

Joseph W. Melamed, M.D.
Attending Radiologist
Wake Medical Center
Raleigh, North Carolina

Cindy R. Miller, M.D.
Assistant Professor of Radiology
Duke University Medical Center
Durham, North Carolina

John G. Murray, M.D.
Consultant Radiologist
Department of Radiology
Mater Misericordiae Hospital
Dublin, Ireland

Rendon C. Nelson, M.D.
Professor of Radiology
Director, Abdominal Imaging
Duke University Medical Center
Durham, North Carolina

Glenn E. Newman, M.D.
Associate Professor of Radiology
Duke University Medical Center
Durham, North Carolina

Sara M. O'Hara, M.D.
Assistant Professor of Radiology
Duke University Medical Center
Durham, North Carolina

Edward F. Patz, Jr., M.D.
Associate Professor of Radiology
Duke University Medical Center
Durham, North Carolina

Erik K. Paulson, M.D.
Associate Professor of Radiology
Duke University Medical Center
Durham, North Carolina

Cynthia S. Payne, M.D.
Assistant Professor of Radiology
Duke University Medical Center
Durham, North Carolina

James M. Provenzale, M.D.
Associate Professor of Radiology
Director, Neuroradiology
Duke University Medical Center
Durham, North Carolina

Carl E. Ravin, M.D.
Professor and Chairman
Department of Radiology
Duke University Medical Center
Durham, North Carolina

Robert R. Reiman, Jr., M.D.
Formerly of the Department of Radiology
Duke University Medical Center
Durham, North Carolina

Jeffrey T. Seabourn, M.D.
Department of Radiology
St. Alphonsus Regional Medical Center
Boise, Idaho

Douglas H. Sheafor, M.D.
Clinical Associate
Department of Radiology
Duke University Medical Center
Durham, North Carolina

Tony P. Smith, M.D.
Professor of Radiology
Duke University Medical Center
Durham, North Carolina

Mary Scott Soo, M.D.
Assistant Professor of Radiology
Duke University Medical Center
Durham, North Carolina

Charles E. Spritzer, M.D.
Associate Professor of Radiology
Duke University Medical Center
Durham, North Carolina

Daniel J. Stackhouse, M.D.
Department of Radiology
Carolinas Medical Center
Charlotte, North Carolina

John A. Stahl, M.D.
Department of Radiology
Fairfax Hospital
Falls Church, Virginia

Paul V. Suhocki, M.D.
Assistant Professor of Radiology
Duke University Medical Center
Durham, North Carolina

Robert D. Tien, M.D.
Department of Diagnostic Imaging
Tan Tock Seng Hospital
Singapore

Robert M. Vandemark, M.D.
Associate Clinical Professor
Department of Radiology
Duke University Medical Center
Durham, North Carolina

Ruth Walsh, M.D.
Assistant Clinical Professor
Department of Radiology
Duke University Medical Center
Durham, North Carolina

Robert H. Wilkinson, Jr., M.D.
Associate Professor of Radiology
Duke University Medical Center
Durham, North Carolina

Margaret E. Williford, M.D.
Assistant Clinical Professor
Department of Radiology
Duke University Medical Center
Durham, North Carolina

Fernando M. Zalduondo, M.D.
Department of Radiology
Hospital Auxilio Mutuo
Hato Rey, Puerto Rico

PREFACE

The intent of this book is to provide a radiology review that simulates the way radiology residents are generally taught. The teaching of radiology residents and fellows is typically performed using the case discussion technique, wherein trainees are presented with images and clinical history but not the diagnosis (so-called unknown cases). In this standard format, the discussant is required to determine pertinent imaging findings on imaging studies, generate a reasonable differential diagnosis based on the imaging findings and clinical history, and, by the process of elimination, decide on the most likely diagnosis. Because this book is intended for trainees in radiology, we thought it best to present the information in case discussion format. Surprisingly, this format is used in very few radiology books, even those designed for resident use.

Teachers of radiology often emphasize to radiology residents that the way one reaches the correct diagnosis is as important as actually producing the correct answer. Providing reasonable arguments for exclusion of incorrect diagnoses is an important part of this process. Most radiology teaching file books (to which this book bears the closest resemblance) simply state the correct diagnosis. Implicit in our approach is the belief that understanding why a false diagnosis is incorrect is as important as understanding why a true diagnosis is correct. Throughout this book, therefore, readers will find explanations of why particular incorrect diagnoses should be discounted.

We designed the cases in this book to represent the spectrum of knowledge expected of a radiologist at the end of residency training. No doubt arguments could be made that some important cases have been excluded. Nonetheless, we believe that a resident who can discuss all the cases in this book in the systematic way we have

outlined them is indeed well trained. The collection of cases is divided into the ten major subsections of radiology. Each subsection can serve as an independent body of material for review during a radiology residency rotation or as a means of review for examinations. To familiarize the reader with various imaging techniques, we have provided different images of the same entity obtained with different techniques, whenever possible, correlating the findings. For each case discussion, the clinical history, imaging findings, and, where space allows, differential diagnoses are presented on the left-side page. In reading each case, the reader should direct attention to that page, which will allow the case to be approached as an unknown diagnosis. After reaching a diagnosis, the reader should then direct attention to the right-side page for the correct diagnosis as well as key clinical and radiologic facts. These facts are not intended to be all-encompassing but should serve as the fundamental framework on which one can add information from more comprehensive texts. Each case is followed by a concise list of particularly relevant references for the reader seeking a deeper understanding of the entity under consideration.

The cases in this book can be likened to the scales that musicians repetitively practice before playing an instrument. Musical scales serve as useful exercises for beginners and seasoned musicians alike. We anticipate that the cases in this book will provide challenging exercises for radiologists at all levels of training.

James M. Provenzale
Rendon C. Nelson

ACKNOWLEDGMENTS

We acknowledge the contributions of the entire faculty of the Duke Department of Radiology and the support of the chairman, Carl E. Ravin, M.D. We also acknowledge Mitzi K. Daniels, Kathy Thompson, and Patricia Jordon for clerical support.

DUKE RADIOLOGY
CASE REVIEW

Imaging, Differential Diagnosis, and Discussion

CHAPTER 1

CHEST IMAGING

H. Page McAdams, *chapter editor*

Jeremy J. Erasmus, R. Chapman Gilkeson,
Philip C. Goodman, H. Page McAdams,
John G. Murray, and Edward F. Patz, Jr.

CASE 1

Edward F. Patz, Jr.

HISTORY

A 26-year-old woman with malaise and night sweats.

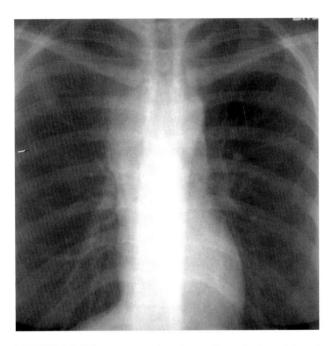

FIGURE 1-1A Posteroanterior chest radiograph shows bilateral (right > left) mediastinal widening.

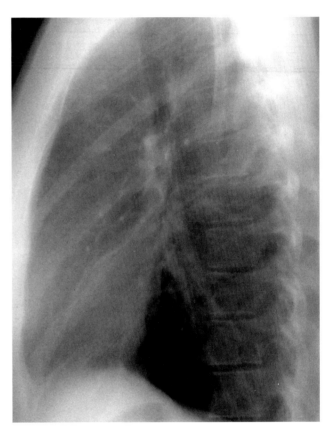

FIGURE 1-1B Left lateral chest radiograph shows increased soft-tissue density in the anterior superior mediastinum.

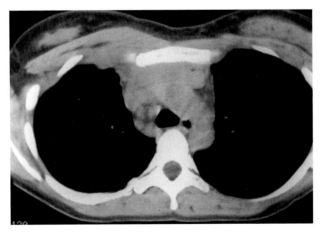

FIGURE 1-1C Noncontrast chest CT (mediastinal window) reveals a lobulated, homogeneous, soft-tissue attenuation mass in the anterior mediastinum. Multiple 8–10 mm right paratracheal lymph nodes are also present.

◆ DIFFERENTIAL DIAGNOSIS

- **Lymphoma:** This is the most likely diagnosis given the age of the patient, appearance of the mass, and associated paratracheal adenopathy.
- **Thymoma:** This is less likely because these lesions usually occur in older patients, are typically more focal and unilateral, and are not associated with right paratracheal adenopathy.
- **Germ cell tumor:** A primary germ cell tumor of the mediastinum cannot be definitively excluded on the basis of age or radiologic appearance. However, associated adenopathy makes lymphoma more likely. Radiologic features that suggest germ cell tumors are fat and calcification.
- **Metastatic disease:** Although the mediastinum is a common site of metastatic disease from testicular germ cell tumors, renal cell carcinoma, or melanoma, the middle mediastinum is preferentially involved.

◆ DIAGNOSIS: Hodgkin's lymphoma.

◆ KEY FACTS

CLINICAL

- At least 50% of patients with Hodgkin's lymphoma have intrathoracic lymph node disease.

- At least 90% of those with intrathoracic disease have an anterior mediastinal mass.
- Pleural disease is unusual at presentation.

RADIOLOGIC

- Hodgkin's lymphoma typically manifests as a lobulated, anterior mediastinal mass that most likely represents matted lymph nodes. Associated mediastinal lymphadenopathy is common and is a *key* differentiating feature from thymoma and germ cell tumor.
- Intratumoral calcification is rare in patients with untreated lymphoma.
- Lung parenchymal involvement in the absence of hilar or mediastinal adenopathy is rare before therapy.

◆ SUGGESTED READING

Fraser RG, Pare JAP. Diagnosis of Diseases of the Chest (2nd ed). Philadelphia: Saunders, 1979.

Heitzman ER. The Mediastinum: Radiologic Correlations with Anatomy and Pathology. St. Louis: Mosby, 1977.

North LB, Libshitz HI, Lorigan JG. Thoracic lymphoma. Radiol Clin North Am 1990;4:745–762.

Tecce PM, Fishman EK, Kuhlman JE. CT evaluation of the anterior mediastinum: Spectrum of disease. Radiographics 1994;14:973–990.

Edward F. Patz, Jr.

HISTORY

Asymptomatic 45-year-old woman with a history of breast carcinoma.

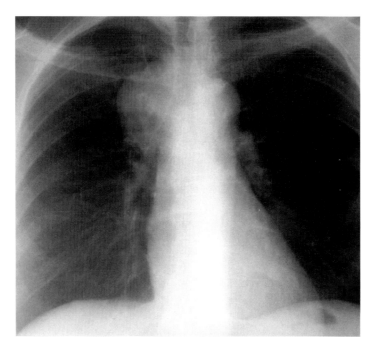

FIGURE 1-2A Posteroanterior chest radiograph. There is a right-sided, smoothly marginated mediastinal mass.

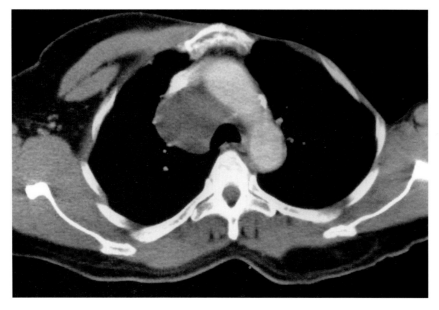

FIGURE 1-2B Contrast-enhanced chest CT (mediastinal window) reveals a homogeneous, low-attenuation mass in the right paratracheal region. The patient is status post left mastectomy.

◆ DIFFERENTIAL DIAGNOSIS

- **Metastatic breast carcinoma:** Isolated metastatic disease to the right paratracheal nodes is an unusual manifestation of breast carcinoma. Biopsy is required, however, as metastatic disease cannot be definitively excluded.
- **Bronchogenic cyst:** The most likely diagnosis given the location and predominantly cystic appearance.
- **Lymphadenopathy:** Low-attenuation paratracheal adenopathy can result from central necrosis due to tumor or infection (mycobacterial, fungal). Necrotic nodes are typically more heterogeneous and may have an enhancing rim.

◆ DIAGNOSIS: Bronchogenic cyst.

◆ KEY FACTS

CLINICAL

- Bronchogenic cysts, also known as *foregut malformations*, are congenital anomalies caused by abnormal budding of the tracheobronchial tree.
- They are typically lined by bronchial and respiratory mucosa but can contain gastric mucosa as well. They are filled with variable amounts of mucus, protein, and cellular debris.
- They can be associated with esophageal duplication cysts and sequestrations.
- Bronchogenic cysts are usually asymptomatic but can enlarge and produce symptoms by compression of adjacent mediastinal structures.
- No treatment is necessary unless the patient becomes symptomatic.

RADIOLOGIC

- Bronchogenic cysts most commonly occur in the subcarinal and right paratracheal regions.
- They usually manifest as smooth, well-marginated mediastinal masses on chest radiographs and CT.
- They are typically homogeneous on CT. Fifty percent are of water attenuation, and 50% are of soft-tissue attenuation due to intracystic hemorrhage or proteinaceous debris.
- On MRI, they are usually of high signal intensity on T2-weighted images. Signal intensity on T1-weighted images is variable depending on the presence of hemorrhage or protein (high signal intensity).
- Air-fluid levels are rare and are usually due to infection or instrumentation.

◆ SUGGESTED READING

Fraser RG, Pare JAP. Diagnosis of Diseases of the Chest (2nd ed). Philadelphia: Saunders, 1979.

Heitzman ER. The Mediastinum: Radiologic Correlations with Anatomy and Pathology. St. Louis: Mosby, 1977.

Naidich DP, Rumancik WM, Ettenger NA, et al. Congenital anomalies of the lungs in adults. AJR Am J Roentgenol 1988;151: 13–19.

Patel SR, Meeker DP, Biscotti CV, et al. Presentation and management of bronchogenic cysts in the adult. Chest 1994;105:79–85.

St. Georges R, Deslauriers J, Duranceau A, et al. Clinical spectrum of bronchogenic cysts of the mediastinum and lung in the adult. Ann Thorac Surg 1991;52:6–13.

CASE 3

Edward F. Patz, Jr.

HISTORY

A 33-year-old woman with mild upper back pain.

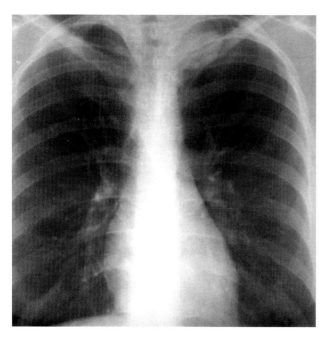

FIGURE 1-3A Posteroanterior chest radiograph. There is a left-sided, smooth, sharply marginated mass in the superior mediastinum. Note that the mass is seen above the clavicles.

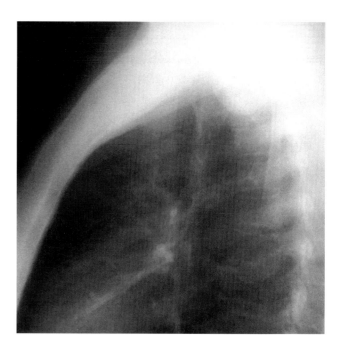

FIGURE 1-3B Left lateral chest radiograph confirms the posterior location of the mass.

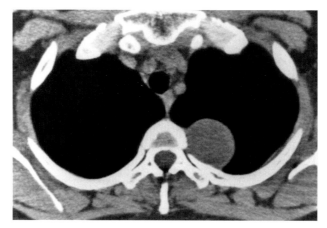

FIGURE 1-3C Noncontrast chest CT (mediastinal window) reveals a homogeneous, sharply marginated left paraspinal mass.

◆ DIFFERENTIAL DIAGNOSIS

◆ **Neurogenic tumor:** A neurogenic tumor is the most common cause of a posterior mediastinal or paravertebral mass.

◆ **Neuroenteric cyst:** This is unlikely since there are no vertebral body anomalies.

◆ **Paraspinal abscess:** This is unlikely in a minimally symptomatic patient without radiologic evidence of vertebral body destruction or disk space narrowing.

◆ **Localized fibrous tumor of pleura:** This is a rare pleural tumor that can manifest as a paraspinal mass. These tumors are often pedunculated and can be quite large. They are typically of heterogeneous attenuation on CT.

◆ **Extramedullary hematopoiesis:** This usually manifests with bilateral, lobulated paraspinal masses in a patient with severe anemia.

◆ **Lymphoma:** Isolated paraspinal disease is an uncommon manifestation of thoracic lymphoma.

◆ **Metastatic disease:** Isolated metastatic disease to the pleura or mediastinum is less likely than a neurogenic tumor given the minimal symptomatology and no history of a primary malignancy.

◆ DIAGNOSIS: Neurofibroma.

◆ KEY FACTS

CLINICAL

◆ There are three groups of neurogenic tumors of varying malignant potential: peripheral nerve tumors (schwannomas, neurofibromas, malignant nerve sheath tumors), sympathetic ganglia tumors (neuroblastomas, ganglioneuroblastomas, ganglioneuromas), and paragangliomas.

◆ Schwannomas and neurofibromas are the most common neurogenic tumors of the posterior mediastinum.

◆ Malignant degeneration (malignant nerve sheath tumor) is rare.

◆ Patients with schwannomas or neurofibromas can be asymptomatic or present with back pain.

◆ Multiple peripheral nerve tumors are usually associated with neurofibromatosis.

RADIOLOGIC

◆ The peripheral nerve tumors (schwannomas and neurofibromas) manifest as round, paravertebral masses that span two vertebral bodies or less. They may invade the neural canal. Rib erosion is common. They manifest as homogeneous, soft-tissue attenuation masses on CT.

◆ The tumors of the sympathetic ganglia manifest as elongated paraspinal masses, spanning multiple vertebral levels. Intratumoral calcification is common in these tumors.

◆ SUGGESTED READING

Fraser RG, Pare JAP. Diagnosis of Diseases of the Chest (2nd ed). Philadelphia: Saunders, 1979.

Heitzman ER. The Mediastinum: Radiologic Correlations with Anatomy and Pathology. St. Louis: Mosby, 1977.

Reed JC, Hallett KK, Feigin DS. Neural tumors of the thorax: Subject review from the AFIP. Radiology 1978;126:9–17.

CASE 4

Edward F. Patz, Jr.

HISTORY

A 61-year-old man presents with progressive shortness of breath.

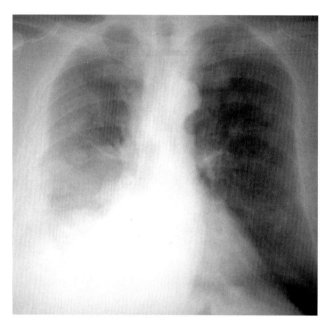

FIGURE 1-4A Posteroanterior chest radiograph. There is a lobulated, soft-tissue mass surrounding the right hemithorax with slight ipsilateral shift of the mediastinum. Several poorly defined opacities project over the left hemithorax.

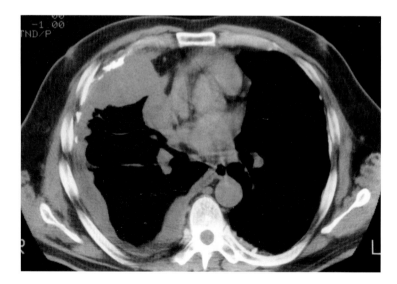

FIGURE 1-4B Noncontrast chest CT (mediastinal window) demonstrates a lobulated pleural mass encasing the right lung. Several calcified pleural plaques are seen in the left hemithorax.

◆ DIFFERENTIAL DIAGNOSIS

- **Pleural metastatic disease:** Metastatic disease is the most common malignancy of the pleura. However, the appearance of diffuse pleural thickening and a tumor rind is more suggestive of mesothelioma than metastases.
- **Malignant pleural mesothelioma (MPM):** This is the most likely diagnosis given the age of the patient, the radiologic appearance of the mass, and the evidence of prior asbestos exposure (pleural plaques).
- **Loculated empyema:** This patient had no signs and symptoms of empyema. The degree of pleural thickening argues for a long-standing process.

◆ DIAGNOSIS: Malignant pleural mesothelioma.

◆ KEY FACTS

CLINICAL

- MPM is rare. There are approximately 1,500 new cases in the United States each year.
- Patients usually present with increasing dyspnea in the sixth to seventh decade of life.
- There is a 5 to 1 male-female ratio.
- Treatment options are limited, and the prognosis is dismal, with a median survival of 12 months.
- There is a high association with prior asbestos exposure.
- There is no relationship with smoking.

RADIOLOGIC

- MPM manifests as a unilateral pleural mass, which can be focal or diffuse, surrounding the hemithorax.
- MPM is often associated with a pleural effusion.
- Contralateral pleural plaques from prior asbestos exposure may be identified.
- Local invasion of the chest wall, mediastinum, or diaphragm is common.
- Lymphadenopathy occurs with more extensive tumor and in the later stages of disease.
- Intra-abdominal extension and contralateral lung or brain metastases are unusual features.

◆ SUGGESTED READING

Achatzy R, Beba W, Ritschler R, et al. The diagnosis, therapy and prognosis of diffuse malignant pleural mesothelioma. Eur J Cardiothorac Surg 1989;3:445–448.

Legha SS, Muggia F. Pleural mesothelioma: Clinical features and therapeutic implications. Ann Intern Med 1977;87:613–621.

Patz EF, Shaffer K, Piwnicka-Worms DR, et al. Malignant pleural mesothelioma: Value of CT and MR imaging in predicting resectability. AJR Am J Roentgenol 1992;159:961–966.

CASE 5

Edward F. Patz, Jr.

HISTORY

A 63-year-old asymptomatic man.

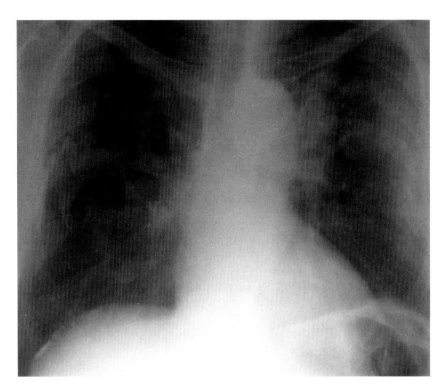

FIGURE 1-5 Posteroanterior chest radiograph. Scattered peripheral opacities project over both lungs. Calcified diaphragmatic and lateral chest wall plaques are also identified.

◈ DIFFERENTIAL DIAGNOSIS

◆ **Calcified hemothorax:** This is unlikely because a calcified hemothorax is usually focal and unilateral.

◆ **Old empyema:** These are also typically focal and unilateral. A calcified empyema is usually due to prior tuberculosis (TB).

◆ **Asbestos-related pleural disease:** This is the most likely diagnosis given bilateral calcified pleural plaques.

◈ DIAGNOSIS: Asbestos-related pleural disease.

◈ KEY FACTS

CLINICAL

◆ Patients with plaque disease are usually asymptomatic. Dyspnea can result from very extensive pleural disease (diffuse pleural fibrosis) or be associated with interstitial fibrosis (asbestosis).

◆ Patients with asbestos-related pleural disease are at increased risk for malignant pleural mesothelioma and lung cancer.

◆ Plaques usually arise from the parietal pleura. The visceral pleura is uncommonly involved.

◆ The frequency and number of plaques is thought to be a dose-dependent phenomenon.

◆ Pleural plaques are usually seen 20 years after asbestos exposure.

RADIOLOGIC

◆ Bilateral calcified pleural plaques are virtually pathognomonic for asbestos-related pleural disease. The plaques are usually larger and more numerous in the mid- and lower hemithoraces.

◆ They can be associated with rounded atelectasis, malignant pleural mesothelioma, and bronchogenic carcinoma.

◆ Plaques often calcify, although this may not be evident on plain radiographs.

◈ SUGGESTED READING

Fraser RG, Pare JAP. Diagnosis of Diseases of the Chest (2nd ed). Philadelphia: Saunders, 1979.

Goodman PC. Asbestos-Related Lung and Pleural Disease. In AR Margulis, CA Gooding (eds), Diagnostic Radiology. St. Louis: Mosby, 1985;155–164.

Greenberg SD. Asbestos lung disease. Semin Respir Med 1982;4:130–137.

CASE 6

Edward F. Patz, Jr.

HISTORY

A 35-year-old woman status post bilateral lung transplantation for pulmonary hypertension.

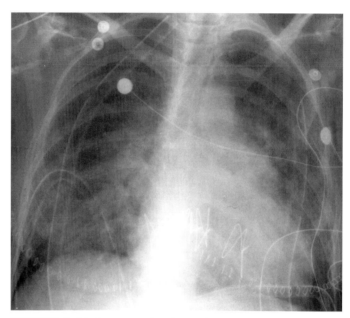

FIGURE 1-6A Anteroposterior chest radiograph 2 days after transplantation shows bilateral, perihilar airspace opacities and cardiomegaly.

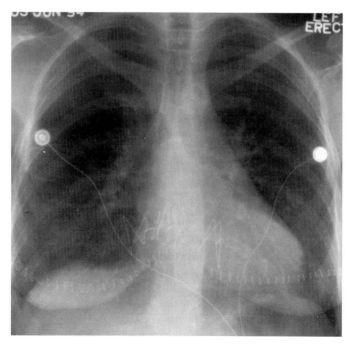

FIGURE 1-6B Posteroanterior chest radiograph 1 week after transplantation shows interval resolution of airspace opacities, small bilateral pleural effusions, and a diminished cardiac silhouette.

◆DIFFERENTIAL DIAGNOSIS

◆ **Infection:** This is less likely because graft infection is uncommon in the first week after transplantation.

◆ **Reimplantation response:** This is the most likely cause of diffuse airspace opacities occurring in the first few days after transplantation and resolving within a week.

◆ **Acute rejection:** This is less likely because the radiographic manifestations of rejection are uncommon in the first week after transplantation.

◆DIAGNOSIS: Reimplantation response to lung transplantation.

◆KEY FACTS

CLINICAL

◆ Possible causes of the reimplantation response include graft ischemia, lymphatic or vascular disruption at the time of surgery, or graft denervation.

◆ It is a diagnosis of exclusion.

◆ Other complications, such as acute rejection and infection, are usually not seen until 5 to 10 days post-transplantation.

◆ Most graft infections in the first month post-transplant are bacterial. Thereafter, cytomegalovirus pneumonia and fungal pneumonia are more common.

RADIOLOGIC

◆ Radiographically, the reimplantation response usually begins within 2 days of surgery, peaks at 4 days, and resolves within a week.

◆ The radiographic appearance varies from subtle, perihilar linear opacities to diffuse consolidation. Pleural effusions are common.

◆SUGGESTED READING

Herman SJ, Rappaport DC, Weisbrod GL, et al. Single lung transplantation: Imaging features. Radiology 1989;170:89–93.

Herman SJ. Radiologic assessment after lung transplantation. Clin Chest Med 1990;11:333–346.

Medina LS, Siegel MJ, Glazer HS, et al. Diagnosis of pulmonary complications associated with lung transplantation in children: Value of CT vs. histopathologic studies. AJR Am J Roentgenol 1994;162:969–974.

O'Donovan PB. Imaging of complications of lung transplantation. Radiographics 1993;13:787–796.

CASE 7

H. Page McAdams

HISTORY

A 25-year-old man and a 60-year-old woman with cough, fever, and chest pain. Both have a history of recurrent pneumonia in the same pulmonary segment.

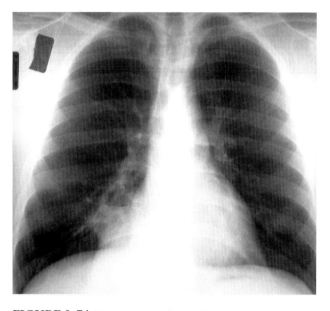

FIGURE 1-7A Posteroanterior chest radiograph (patient 1) reveals consolidation in the posterior basilar segment of the right lower lobe. Note the air-fluid level.

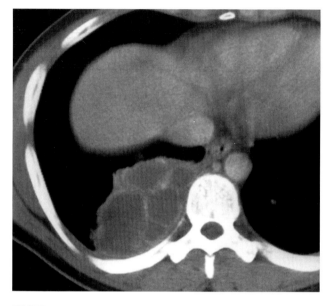

FIGURE 1-7B Contrast-enhanced chest CT (mediastinal window) (patient 1) reveals multiple, well-circumscribed, low attenuation areas within the consolidated segment. Note also the thin, enhancing septae.

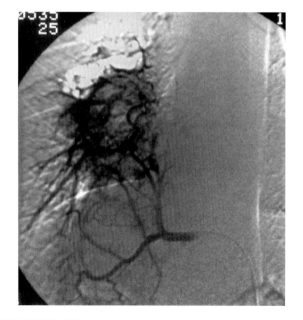

FIGURE 1-7C Digital subtraction arteriogram (patient 1) demonstrates a systemic vascular supply to the lesion. Delayed images (not shown) revealed pulmonary venous drainage.

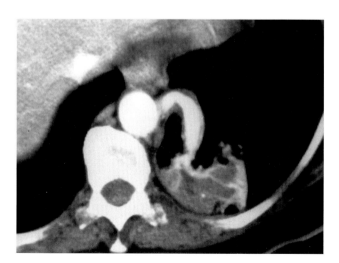

FIGURE 1-7D Contrast-enhanced spiral CT (mediastinal window) (patient 2) demonstrates an anomalous vessel arising from the distal thoracic aorta to supply the chronically consolidated segment in the left lower lobe.

◆ DIFFERENTIAL DIAGNOSIS

◆ **Infected bronchogenic cyst:** The multilocular nature of the opacity argues against an intraparenchymal bronchogenic cyst.

◆ **Congenital cystic adenomatoid malformation (CCAM):** Although the location and appearance of the lesion is consistent with this diagnosis, CCAM is very rare in adults.

◆ **Intralobar sequestration (ILS):** This is the most likely diagnosis given the history of recurrent pneumonia and the radiologic demonstration of a systemic vascular supply to the infected segment.

◆ DIAGNOSIS: Intralobar sequestration.

◆ KEY FACTS

CLINICAL

◆ ILS typically manifests in young patients with signs and symptoms of recurrent pneumonia.

◆ ILS usually occurs in the posterior or medial basilar segments of the lower lobes.

◆ ILS is more common on the left than the right (6 to 4).

RADIOLOGIC

◆ On chest radiographs, ILS commonly manifests as a focal, parenchymal consolidation. Air-fluid levels are also common.

◆ Other, less common, manifestations include a focal mass or a hyperlucent segment (sometimes with a central mucus plug).

◆ By CT, MRI, or ultrasound, ILS usually manifests as a unilocular or multilocular cystic mass. Solid masses are sometimes seen.

◆ ILS is usually supplied by a systemic artery arising from the abdominal or thoracic aorta, lumbar arteries, or celiac axis. Venous drainage is usually via the pulmonary veins. Inferior vena cava or azygous venous drainage is less common.

◆ Diagnosis of ILS is made by radiologic demonstration of systemic vascular supply. This can be accomplished with angiography, contrast-enhanced CT (spiral CT is best), or MRI.

◆ SUGGESTED READING

Felson B. Pulmonary sequestration revisited. Medical Radiography Photography 1988;64:1–27.

Naidich DP, Rumancik WM, Ettenger NA, et al. Congenital anomalies of the lungs in adults: MR diagnosis. AJR Am J Roentgenol 1988;151:13–19.

Panicek DM, Heitzman ER, Randall PA, et al. The continuum of pulmonary developmental anomalies. Radiographics 1987;7:747–772.

HISTORY

A 50-year-old man with cough and hemoptysis.

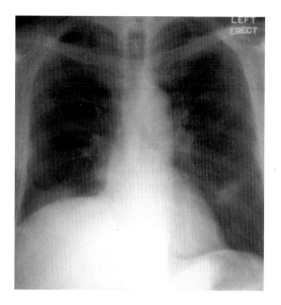

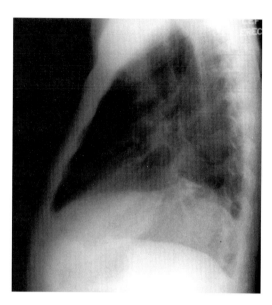

A

B

FIGURES 1-8A and 1-8B Posteroanterior chest radiograph (**A**) and lateral chest radiograph (**B**). There is a right hilar mass, right middle and lower lobe atelectasis, and a sclerotic metastasis to the left fifth rib anteriorly.

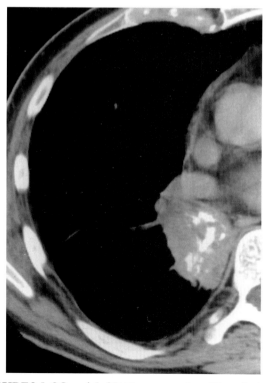

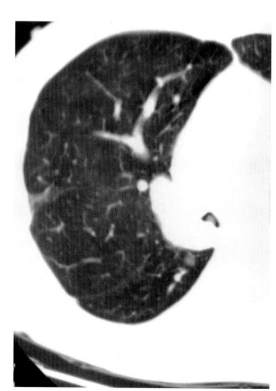

C

D

FIGURES 1-8C and 1-8D Noncontrast chest CT mediastinal window (**C**) and lung window (**D**) demonstrate a large soft-tissue mass in the right lower lobe with central, chunky calcifications. Lung window shows a small endobronchial component within the bronchus intermedius.

◆ DIFFERENTIAL DIAGNOSIS

- **Bronchial carcinoid tumor:** This is the best single diagnosis given the radiologic appearance of the mass and the sclerotic rib metastasis.
- **Lung cancer:** Although lung cancer cannot be excluded, the central calcification and sclerotic metastasis are more suggestive of bronchial carcinoid.
- **Lymphoma:** Lobar atelectasis is a very uncommon manifestation of lymphoma. Central calcification also argues against this diagnosis.
- **Metastatic osteosarcoma:** This could account for the radiologic findings but is less common than carcinoid.
- **Fibrosing mediastinitis:** This can result in lobar atelectasis but would not explain the sclerotic metastasis. Also, fibrosing mediastinitis usually manifests as a calcified, infiltrative process, not a focal mass.

◆ DIAGNOSIS: Metastatic bronchial carcinoid tumor.

◆ KEY FACTS

CLINICAL

- Eighty-five percent of carcinoid tumors occur within the central bronchi (central carcinoid); 15% arise distal to segmental bronchi (peripheral carcinoid).
- Peripheral tumors manifest as asymptomatic pulmonary nodules.
- Central tumors manifest with symptoms of bronchial obstruction such as hemoptysis, chest pain, or recurrent pneumonia.
- Bronchial carcinoid tumors are rarely associated with paraneoplastic syndromes such as carcinoid syndrome, Cushing's syndrome, or acromegaly.

- Carcinoids are histologically divided into two types: typical (75% to 90%) and atypical (10% to 25%).
- The prognosis for typical carcinoid tumors is excellent. The prognosis for atypical carcinoid tumors is less favorable.

RADIOLOGIC

- Peripheral tumors manifest as solitary, well-circumscribed pulmonary nodules.
- Central lesions manifest as hilar masses with or without obstructive atelectasis or pneumonia.
- In some cases, a small endobronchial component is associated with a larger exobronchial component. This is termed the "iceberg" phenomenon.
- Calcifications, central and chunk-like, are seen by CT in up to 26% of cases.
- On T2-weighted MR images, bronchial carcinoid tumors have a very high signal intensity.
- Uptake by I^{131} metaiodobenzylguanidine (MIBG) or indium^{111} pentetreotide can also be seen.
- A typical carcinoid manifests as a small mass (<2.5 cm in diameter) with no associated adenopathy.
- An atypical carcinoid manifests as a larger mass (>2.5 cm) with localized adenopathy.

◆ SUGGESTED READING

Forster BB, Muller NL, Miller RR, et al. Neuroendocrine carcinomas of the lung: Clinical, radiologic and pathologic correlation. Radiology 1989;170:440–445.

Muller NL, Miller RR. Neuroendocrine carcinomas of the lung. Semin Roentgenol 1990;25:96–104.

Zwiebel BR, Austin JHM, Grimes MM. Bronchial carcinoid tumors: Assessment of location and intratumoral calcification in thirty-one patients. Radiology 1991;279:483–486.

HISTORY

A 65-year-old man with a long history of sinus disease presents with cough, fever, and hemoptysis.

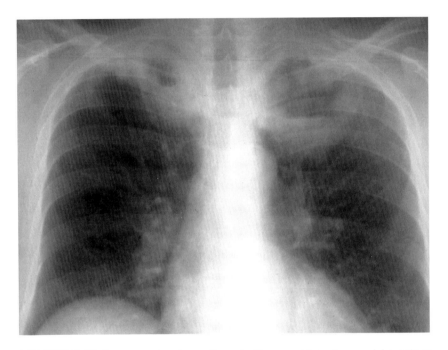

FIGURE 1-9A Posteroanterior chest radiograph. There are bilateral, upper lobe cavitary masses with thick irregular walls and air-fluid levels.

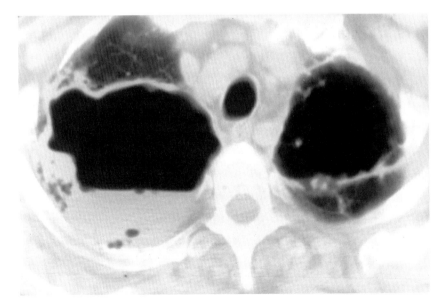

FIGURE 1-9B Chest CT (lung window) performed 3 months later demonstrates progressive thinning of the cavity walls. An air-fluid level is noted within the inferior aspect of the right upper cavity.

◆ DIFFERENTIAL DIAGNOSIS

◆ **Infection:** Likely organisms include postprimary tuberculosis (TB), chronic progressive fungal infection, nocardia, and possibly anaerobic abscesses. Given the radiologic findings, postprimary TB must be strongly considered.

◆ **Neoplasm:** Potential neoplastic etiologies include synchronous primary lung cancers (squamous cell carcinoma), metastatic disease, or less likely, cavitary parenchymal lymphoma (Hodgkin's disease). Potential primary tumors metastatic to the lung include squamous cell carcinoma of the head and neck, squamous cell carcinoma of the cervix, and metastatic sarcoma. However, apical predominance is uncommon in pulmonary metastatic disease.

◆ **Vasculitis:** Potential vasculitic etiologies include Wegener's granulomatosis and, less likely, cavitary rheumatoid nodules. The historic clue of chronic sinus disease makes Wegener's granulomatosis a likely diagnosis.

◆ DIAGNOSIS: Wegener's granulomatosis.

◆ KEY FACTS

CLINICAL

◆ Wegener's granulomatosis is a multisystem granulomatous vasculitis.

◆ Major sites of involvement include the sinonasal cavity, lungs, and kidneys.

◆ Elevated c-ANCA (antineutrophil cytoplasm antibody) titers are sensitive and specific for active Wegener's granulomatosis.

◆ Wegener's granulomatosis has a good prognosis with aggressive medical management.

RADIOLOGIC

◆ Patients typically present with multiple pulmonary nodules or masses. One-third to one-half of nodules cavitate.

◆ The disease can also manifest as focal or diffuse parenchymal consolidation. Diffuse pulmonary hemorrhage is the presenting manifestation in up to 10% of cases.

◆ Involvement of the trachea and bronchi is uncommon and can result in lobar atelectasis and bronchial stenoses.

◆ Pleural effusions are uncommon and adenopathy is rare.

◆ New pulmonary opacities in a patient being treated for known Wegener's granulomatosis suggest opportunistic infection, either fungal or *Pneumocystis carinii* pneumonia.

◆ SUGGESTED READING

Aberle DR, Gamsu G, Lynch D. Thoracic manifestations of Wegener granulomatosis: Diagnosis and course. Radiology 1990;174: 703–709.

Warren J, Pitchenik AE, Saldana MJ. Granulomatous vasculitides of the lung: A clinicopathologic approach to diagnosis and treatment. South Med J 1989;82:481–491.

Weisbrod GL. Pulmonary angiitis and granulomatosis: A review. Can Assoc Radiol J 1989;40:127–134.

H. Page McAdams

HISTORY

A 25-year-old woman with progressive dyspnea.

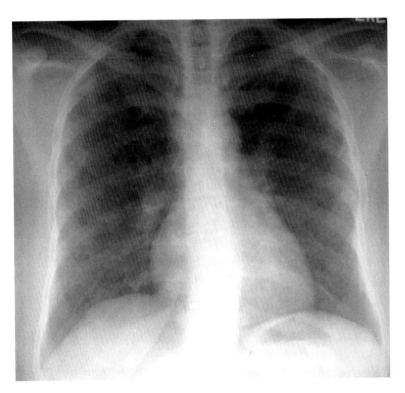

FIGURE 1-10A Posteroanterior chest radiograph shows bilateral 3- to 5-mm nodular opacities. There is a slight reticular component and a definite upper lobe predominance. The lung volumes are preserved. The right paratracheal stripe is full, but there is no other evidence of adenopathy.

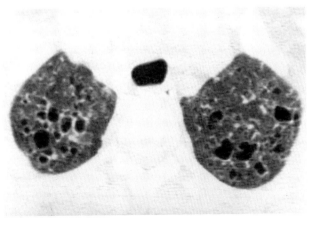

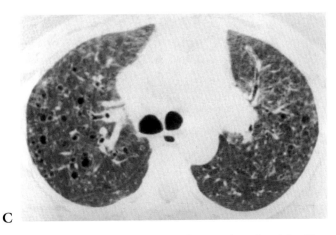

B   C

FIGURES 1-10B and 1-10C High-resolution CT (lung window) shows multiple upper lobe "air cysts" and scattered, small nodules. Note that the cysts in the left upper lobe have coalesced to form unusual shapes.

◆ DIFFERENTIAL DIAGNOSIS

- **Chest radiograph:** Differential diagnosis based on the chest radiograph includes sarcoidosis, pulmonary histiocytosis X (PHX), tuberculosis (TB), pneumoconiosis, and hypersensitivity pneumonitis.
- **High-resolution CT (HRCT)—nodules:** Differential diagnosis for nodules on HRCT includes sarcoidosis, PHX, hypersensitivity pneumonitis, pneumoconiosis, TB, and various forms of bronchiolitis.
- **HRCT—air cysts:** Differential diagnosis for air cysts on HRCT includes lymphangioleiomyomatosis, PHX, *Pneumocystis carinii* pneumonia, bronchiectasis, and "honeycomb" lung (idiopathic pulmonary fibrosis).
- The combination of nodules and air cysts on HRCT makes PHX the most likely diagnosis.

◆ DIAGNOSIS: Pulmonary histiocytosis X.

◆ KEY FACTS

CLINICAL

- Also known as Langerhans's cell histiocytosis or eosinophilic granuloma of lung.
- Patients are typically young to middle aged, with a higher incidence in men.
- Patients typically present with cough and dyspnea. Twenty percent present with a spontaneous pneumothorax.
- At least 90% of patients with PHX are cigarette smokers.

RADIOLOGIC

- Typical radiographic manifestations include nodular or reticulonodular opacities in the mid- and upper lung zones. Lung volumes are typically normal or increased. Adenopathy and pleural effusion are uncommon.
- Typical HRCT findings include thick- or thin-walled air cysts and 3- to 5-mm centrilobular nodules. The cysts may coalesce into unusual shapes. Both cysts and nodules are more common in the mid- to upper lung zones, typically sparing the costophrenic angles.
- The combination of air cysts and 3- to 5-mm nodules is highly suggestive of the diagnosis.

◆ SUGGESTED READING

Brauner MW, Grenier P, Mouelhi MM, et al. Pulmonary histiocytosis X: Evaluation with high resolution CT. Radiology 1989;172:255–258.

Lacronique J, Roth C, Battesti JP, et al. Chest radiologic features of pulmonary histiocytosis X: A report based on 50 adult cases. Thorax 1982;37:104–109.

Webb WR, Muller NL, Naidich DP. High Resolution CT of the Lung. New York: Raven, 1992;111–133.

CASE 11

H. Page McAdams

HISTORY

A 65-year-old man with progressive dyspnea and dry cough.

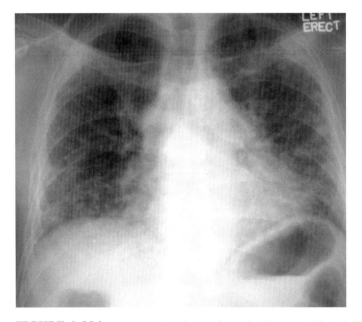

FIGURE 1-11A Posteroanterior chest radiograph. There are bilateral irregular linear opacities and loss of lung volume. There is no evidence of adenopathy or of pleural effusions.

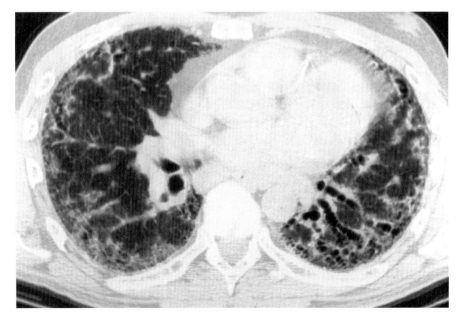

FIGURE 1-11B High-resolution CT of the chest (lung window) shows peripheral, irregular linear opacities, traction bronchiectasis, and honeycomb cyst formation. There are also peripheral ground-glass opacities.

◆ DIFFERENTIAL DIAGNOSIS

- **Usual interstitial pneumonia (UIP):** This is the most likely diagnosis because of the pattern of irregular linear opacities, ground-glass opacities, traction bronchiectasis, and honeycomb cysts in a peripheral distribution.
- **Rheumatoid lung:** In most cases, rheumatoid lung cannot be differentiated radiologically from UIP. *Key* radiologic clues to this diagnosis include pleural effusion or rheumatoid nodules.
- **Scleroderma lung:** In most cases, scleroderma lung cannot be differentiated radiologically from UIP. *Key* radiologic clues to this diagnosis include soft-tissue calcifications or a dilated, air-filled esophagus.
- **Chronic hypersensitivity pneumonitis (CHP):** In many cases, CHP cannot be differentiated radiologically from UIP. *Key* radiologic clues to this diagnosis include small nodules or an upper lobe predominance.
- **Asbestosis:** In most cases, asbestosis cannot be differentiated radiologically from UIP. *Key* radiologic clues to this diagnosis include pleural effusion or pleural plaques.
- **Pulmonary drug toxicity (nitrofurantoin, methotrexate, bleomycin):** In most cases, fibrosis from drug toxicity cannot be differentiated radiologically from UIP.

◆ DIAGNOSIS: Usual interstitial pneumonia.

◆ KEY FACTS

CLINICAL

- UIP typically manifests in middle-aged to elderly adults with progressive dyspnea and dry cough.
- As many as 30% have a positive rheumatoid factor or antinuclear antibodies without clinical signs of collagen vascular disease.
- Twenty percent have associated collagen vascular disease.
- UIP is a progressive, fatal illness with a median survival of 4 years.
- Corticosteroid and cytotoxic therapy is of limited benefit. Lung transplantation is a viable option in appropriate candidates.

RADIOLOGIC

- Typical chest radiographic manifestations of UIP include bibasilar irregular linear opacities, honeycombing, and volume loss.
- Adenopathy and pleural effusions are rare.
- There is poor correlation between radiologic abnormality and clinical or functional derangement.
- On high-resolution CT, UIP manifests with irregular linear opacities, ground-glass opacities, traction bronchiectasis, and honeycomb cysts in a peripheral distribution. This pattern of parenchymal involvement is virtually diagnostic of UIP.
- It should be noted that fibrosis due to collagen vascular disease, drug toxicity, and end-stage hypersensitivity pneumonitis cannot be distinguished radiologically from UIP.

◆ SUGGESTED READING

Carrington CB, Gaensler EA, Couto RE, et al. The natural history and treated course of usual and desquamative interstitial pneumonia. N Engl J Med 1978;298:801–809.

Staples CA, Muller NL, Vedal S, et al. Usual interstitial pneumonia: Correlation of CT with clinical, functional, and radiologic findings. Radiology 1987;162:377–381.

Webb WR, Muller NL, Naidich DP. High Resolution CT of the Lung. New York: Raven, 1992;111–133.

CASE *12*

H. Page McAdams

HISTORY

A 53-year-old woman with progressive dyspnea, cough, and low-grade fever over the past 8 weeks.

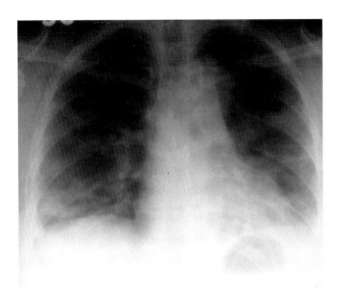

FIGURE 1-12A Posteroanterior chest radiograph. There are bilateral, scattered air space opacities with slightly diminished lung volumes. There is no evidence of adenopathy or of pleural effusions.

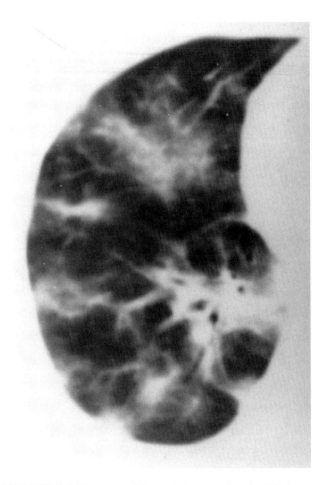

FIGURE 1-12B Chest CT (lung window, coned to the right lower lobe) shows peripheral ground-glass opacities and consolidations. There are no discrete nodules. There is also no evidence of fibrosis (honeycomb cysts, architectural distortion, traction bronchiectasis).

◆ DIFFERENTIAL DIAGNOSIS

- **Bronchiolitis obliterans organizing pneumonia (BOOP):** This is the most likely diagnosis given the radiologic and clinical findings.
- **Atypical pneumonia:** Resolving mycoplasma pneumonia is a less likely consideration.
- **Eosinophilic pneumonia:** Although eosinophilic pneumonia should be considered, it usually manifests with peripheral, upper lobe consolidation.
- **Multifocal bronchioalveolar carcinoma (BAC):** Although the radiologic appearance is consistent with BAC, the clinical history makes BOOP more likely.
- **Pulmonary lymphoma:** Again, although the radiologic appearance is consistent with lymphoma, the clinical history makes BOOP more likely.
- **Alveolar proteinosis:** This usually manifests with more diffuse, basilar opacities.
- **Alveolar sarcoidosis:** The age of the patient, the clinical signs and symptoms, and the lack of adenopathy argue against sarcoidosis.

◆ DIAGNOSIS: Bronchiolitis obliterans organizing pneumonia.

◆ KEY FACTS

CLINICAL

- Fifty percent of cases are idiopathic; the remainder are associated with collagen vascular disease, drug toxicity, toxic fume exposure, infection, or recurrent aspiration.
- Idiopathic BOOP is also known as *cryptogenic organizing pneumonia*. It manifests as a subacute illness with cough, dyspnea, and low-grade fever.
- Restrictive abnormalities on pulmonary function testing are common.
- Idiopathic BOOP responds well to steroids and has a good prognosis.

RADIOLOGIC

- BOOP manifests with scattered air space consolidations or ground-glass opacities. These are typically peripheral and subpleural in distribution.
- Less common manifestations include nodules or irregular linear opacities.
- Bronchial wall thickening or bronchiectasis is common.
- Pleural effusions are seen in up to 20% of cases.

◆ SUGGESTED READING

Bellomo R, Finlay M, McLaughlin P, Tai E. Clinical spectrum of cryptogenic organizing pneumonia. Thorax 1991;41:554–559.

Epler GR, Colby TV, McLoud TC, et al. Bronchiolitis obliterans organizing pneumonia. N Engl J Med 1985;312:152–158.

Lee KS, Kullnig P, Hartman TE, Muller NL. Cryptogenic organizing pneumonia: CT findings in 43 patients. AJR Am J Roentgenol 1994;162:543–546.

CASE 13

John G. Murray

HISTORY

A 35-year-old man with acute shortness of breath and a history of drug abuse.

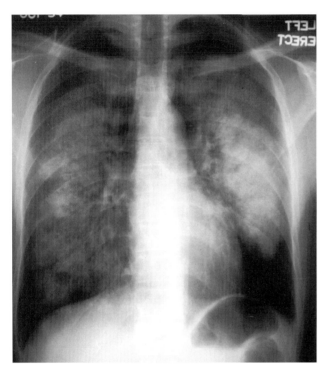

FIGURE 1-13A Posteroanterior chest radiograph in the emergency room. There is bilateral, predominantly perihilar consolidation. The cardiomediastinal silhouette is normal, and there are no pleural effusions.

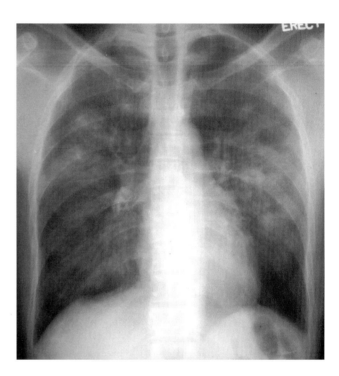

FIGURE 1-13B Posteroanterior chest radiograph 12 hours later shows marked interval improvement.

◆ DIFFERENTIAL DIAGNOSIS

- *Pneumocystis carinii* **pneumonia (PCP):** This is a possibility, particularly if the patient has acquired immunodeficiency syndrome (AIDS) and a CD4 count <400 mm³. The absence of adenopathy or pleural effusion is consistent with this diagnosis. However, rapid clearance is very atypical for PCP.
- **Diffuse pulmonary hemorrhage (DPH):** DPH cannot be excluded radiographically. It can be associated with drug abuse (inhaled or intravenous).
- **Hydrostatic edema:** The "bat's wing" distribution and rapid clearance is consistent with this diagnosis. Hydrostatic edema with normal heart size is seen in patients with acute (first) myocardial infarction or cardiac arrythmia.
- **Permeability edema:** This is the single best diagnosis given the normal heart size and rapid clearance. Potential etiologies in this patient include inhaled or intravenous opiate abuse or inhalation of noxious gases (solvents).

◆ DIAGNOSIS: Pulmonary edema due to inhaled "crack" cocaine.

◆ KEY FACTS

CLINICAL

- Patients usually present with acute shortness of breath following intravenous administration or inhalation of crack cocaine.

- The mechanism of pulmonary edema is unclear. Possible explanations include a direct effect on the central nervous system leading to neurogenic pulmonary edema, direct drug toxicity to the alveolar capillary membrane, or an allergic response.

RADIOLOGIC

- Up to one-third of patients with opiate overdose develop pulmonary edema.
- Rapid clearance is typical.
- Pneumomediastinum or pneumothorax is occasionally seen.

◆ SUGGESTED READING

Forrester JM, Steele AW, Waldron JA, Parsons PE. Crack lung: An acute pulmonary syndrome with a spectrum of clinical and histopathologic findings. Am Rev Respir Dis 1990;142:462–467.

Frand UI, Shim CS, Williams MK. Methadone induced pulmonary edema. Intern Med 1972;76:975–979.

Smith WR, Wells ID, Glauser FL, et al. Immunological abnormalities in heroin lung. Chest 1975;68:651–653.

Steinberg AD, Karliner JS. The clinical spectrum of heroin pulmonary edema. Arch Intern Med 1968;122:122–127.

HISTORY

A 40-year-old woman with a history of cigarette smoking and progressive dyspnea.

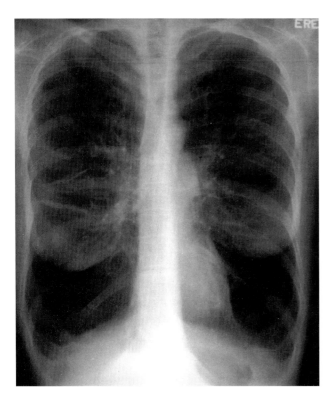

FIGURE 1-14A Posteroanterior chest radiograph. There is marked hyperinflation with decreased lung vascularity bilaterally. Findings are most marked at the bases, where there are several large bullae.

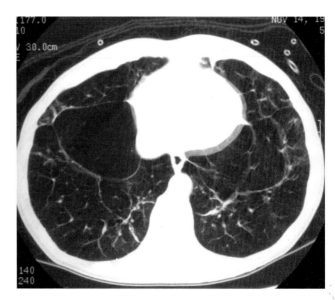

FIGURE 1-14B High-resolution chest CT scan of the lung bases reveals uniform destruction of the pulmonary lobules, with widespread areas of decreased lung attenuation. A large bulla is seen on the right.

◆ DIFFERENTIAL DIAGNOSIS

- **Pulmonary histiocytosis X (PHX):** This is unlikely because the air "cysts" of PHX have well-defined walls and are usually more numerous in the apices than the bases.
- **Lymphangiolieomyomatosis (LAM):** This is unlikely because the air "cysts" of LAM have well-defined walls. Also, the intervening lung parenchyma is normal in LAM.
- **Centrilobular (CL) emphysema:** This is not the best diagnosis since CL emphysema affects the apices preferentially. CL emphysema initially manifests as focal (2 to 10 mm) lucencies without walls surrounding the core lobular artery. These lucencies may later coalesce into larger regions of decreased lung attenuation.
- **Panlobular (PL) emphysema:** This is the best diagnosis since the bases are affected preferentially, the lucencies have no walls, and there is no evidence of CL emphysema. Although PL emphysema can be idiopathic, many cases are related to alpha-1-antiprotease deficiency (A1AD) and smoking.

◆ DIAGNOSIS: Panlobular emphysema due to alpha-1-antiprotease deficiency.

◆ KEY FACTS

CLINICAL

- Alpha-1-antiprotease (A1A) inhibits proteolytic enzymes such as trypsin, elastase, and collagenase that can cause emphysema. Patients with low levels of A1A are at risk for early-onset of emphysema, and the risk is increased in smokers.

- A1AD is an autosomal recessive disease. Homozygotes have 10% to 15% of the normal A1A levels, and heterozygotes have 60%.
- Almost all homozygotes develop early-onset emphysema (age 35 to 50 years). Smokers present 10 years earlier. Heterozygotes can develop emphysema in the presence of other risk factors.
- Histologically the emphysema is panlobular in type.
- There is an association with neonatal hepatitis and cirrhosis.

RADIOLOGIC

- Radiographic evidence of panlobular emphysema is seen in up to 80% of homozygous A1AD patients.
- PL emphysema is distinguished from air "cysts" by the absence of perceptible walls. It typically manifests with regional or generalized decreased lung attenuation. The lung bases are preferentially affected.
- In A1AD, the lower lungs are affected in 98% of cases and are the only site of disease in 24%.
- Bullae are an uncommon feature of A1AD.

◆ SUGGESTED READING

Bergin CJ, Muller NL, Miller RR. CT in the qualitative assessment of emphysema. J Thorac Imaging 1986;1:94–103.

Hepper NG, Mulm JR, Sheehan WC, et al. Roentgenographic study of chronic obstructive pulmonary disease by alpha-1-antitrypsin phenotype. Mayo Clin Proc 1978;53:166–172.

Rosen RA, Dalinka MK, Gralino BJ, et al. The roentgenographic findings in alpha-1-antitrypsin deficency. Radiology 1970;95:25–28.

Webb WR, Muller NL, Naidich DP. Diseases Characterized by Primarily Cystic Abnormalities, Lung Destruction, or Decreased Lung Opacity. In High-Resolution CT of the Lung. New York: Raven, 1992;111–133.

CASE 15

John G. Murray

HISTORY

A 23-year-old woman with sinusitis and recurrent respiratory infection.

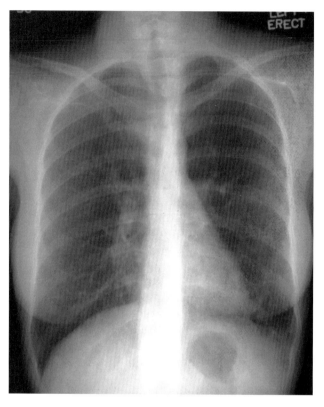

FIGURE 1-15A Posteroanterior chest radiograph. There are linear opacities that radiate from both hili and numerous small, basal nodular opacities. There is no evidence of intrathoracic adenopathy or pleural disease.

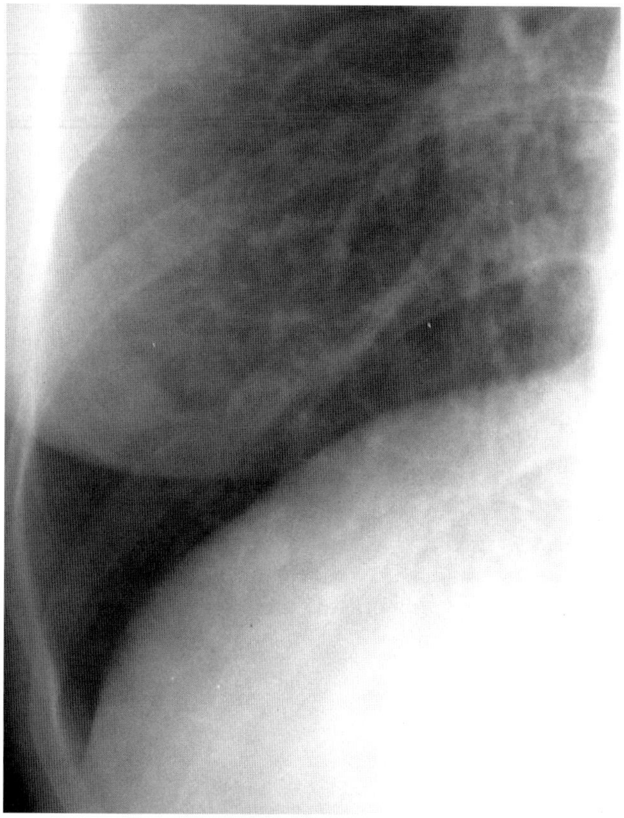

FIGURE 1-15B Posteroanterior chest radiograph (coned down view of right lower lobe). A branching mucus plug is seen in the right lower lobe.

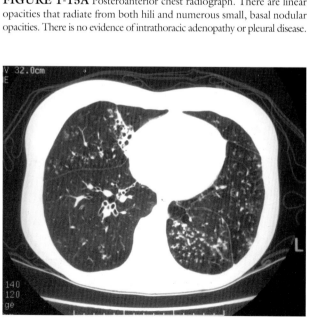

FIGURE 1-15C Chest CT (lung window) of the lung bases reveals extensive cylindrical bronchiectasis that is most pronounced in the right middle and lower lobes. Mucoid impactions are seen in the left lower lobe.

◆ DIFFERENTIAL DIAGNOSIS

- **Cystic fibrosis (CF):** Not the most likely diagnosis since bronchiectasis due to CF involves the upper lobes to a greater extent than the lower lobes.
- **Allergic bronchopulmonary aspergillosis (ABPA):** Also not the most likely diagnosis since ABPA typically manifests with cylindrical or saccular central (not peripheral) bronchiectasis. Also, ABPA preferentially involves the upper lobe bronchi.
- **Postinfectious bronchiectasis:** Childhood viral pneumonia (adenovirus, measles), repeated aspiration, or prior necrotizing pneumonias can also result in basilar bronchiectasis. This is not the most likely diagnosis given the clinical history.
- **Primary ciliary dyskinesia (PCD):** The clinical history and radiologic findings of basilar bronchiectasis and mucoid impaction make this the most likely diagnosis.

◆ DIAGNOSIS: Primary ciliary dyskinesia.

◆ KEY FACTS

CLINICAL

- Symptoms of bronchiectasis include chronic cough, excess sputum production, and recurrent pulmonary infection.
- Hemoptysis occurs in 50% of patients, usually due to bronchial artery hypertophy.

- Aggressive medical therapy has largely obviated the need for surgical resection of affected lobes.
- PCD is characterized by recurrent sinusitis, bronchiectasis, and infertility. It results from a genetic defect in the dynein arms of the cilia.
- Fifty percent of patients with PCD have situs inversus (Kartagener's syndrome).

RADIOLOGIC

- Radiographic findings of bronchiectasis include parallel lines (tram tracks), ring shadows, and mucus plugs.
- CT, especially high-resolution CT (HRCT), is more sensitive than chest radiography in the detection of bronchiectasis. HRCT has also replaced bronchography for this purpose.
- CT findings of bronchiectasis include bronchial wall thickening and the signet ring sign. Visible bronchi in the outer one-third of the lung are abnormal.
- CT can also suggest an etiology. Central bronchiectasis suggests ABPA. Upper lobe bronchiectasis suggests mycobacterial infection or cystic fibrosis. Basilar disease suggests postinfection bronchiectasis, immune deficiencies, or PCD.

◆ SUGGESTED READING

Barker AF, Bardana EJ. Bronchiectasis: Update of an orphan disease. Am Rev Respir Disease 1988;137:969–978.

Schidow D. Primary ciliary dyskinesia. Ann Allergy 1994;73:457–468.

Westcott JL. Bronchiectasis. Radiol Clin North Am 1991;29: 1031–1042.

HISTORY

A 57-year-old woman with cough, progressive dyspnea, and fever of several months' duration.

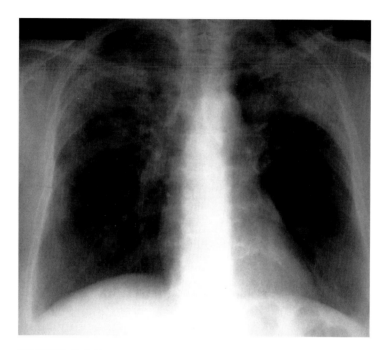

FIGURE 1-16A Posteroanterior chest radiograph. There are peripheral air space consolidations in both upper lobes. There is no evidence of intrathoracic adenopathy or of pleural effusions.

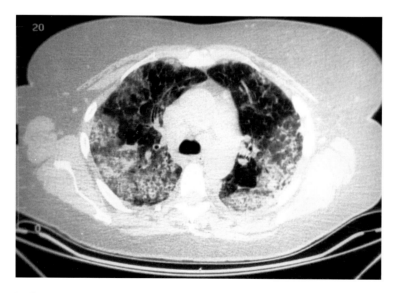

FIGURE 1-16B Chest CT (lung window) through the lung apices confirms the peripheral nature of the opacities.

◆ DIFFERENTIAL DIAGNOSIS

- **Bacterial pneumonia:** The radiologic pattern is unusual for bacterial pneumonia.
- **Eosinophilic pneumonia (EP):** The clinical history and distribution (peripheral and upper lobe) of opacities makes this the most likely diagnosis.
- **Postprimary tuberculosis (TB):** TB must be strongly considered given the radiologic and clinical findings. However, the absence of cavitation makes TB less likely than EP.
- **Bronchiolitis obliterans organizing pneumonia (BOOP):** Because of the distinct upper lobe predominance, EP is more likely than BOOP in this case.
- **Pulmonary infarct (septic or bland):** Although infarcts are typically peripheral, they are usually wedge-shaped and more numerous in the lung bases. Septic infarcts also cavitate.

◆ DIAGNOSIS: Chronic eosinophilic pneumonia.

◆ KEY FACTS

CLINICAL

- EP results from alveolar and interstitial infiltration by eosinophils and other inflammatory cells.
- Known etiologies include parasitic infestation, allergic bronchopulmonary aspergillosis, drug reactions, and pulmonary vasculitis (Churg-Strauss syndrome).

- Idiopathic EP is divided into acute and chronic forms depending on the severity and duration of symptoms.
- Chronic eosinophilic pneumonia (CEP) usually occurs in middle-aged women who present with several months of cough, dyspnea, and fever. Two-thirds have blood eosinophilia.

RADIOLOGIC

- CEP typically manifests with progressive air space consolidation on chest radiographs. The opacities are usually peripheral and upper lobe in distribution. The classic "reverse pulmonary edema" pattern is seen in fewer than half of cases.
- CT can be useful for demonstrating the peripheral nature of the opacities.
- CEP is a remarkably steroid-responsive disease. Symptoms and radiographic opacities usually resolve within days. However, as many as 80% of patients relapse following steroid withdrawal.

◆ SUGGESTED READING

Carrington CB, Addington WM, et al. Chronic eosinophilic pneumonia. N Engl J Med 1969;280:787–788.

Dothager DW, Kollat MH. Peripheral infiltrates in a post partum woman. Chest 1993;99:463–464.

Jederlinc PJ, Sicilian L, Gamsha EA. Chronic eosinophilic pneumonia: 19 cases and a review of the literature. Medicine 1988;154:62–69.

HISTORY

Previously healthy 27-year-old woman presents with weight loss, malaise, and non-productive cough.

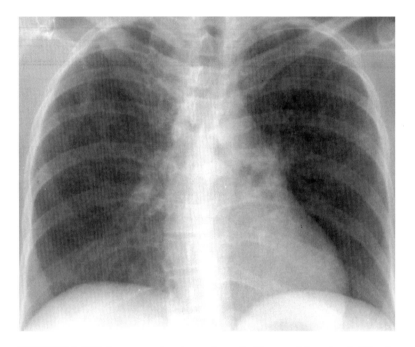

FIGURE 1-17A Posteroanterior chest radiograph. There are bilateral and diffuse 1- to 3-mm pulmonary nodules. There is no consolidation, cavitation, or pleural effusion. Paratracheal adenopathy is present.

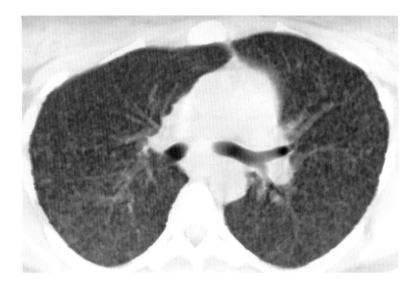

FIGURE 1-17B Chest CT (lung window) confirms the radiographic finding of innumerable 1- to 3-mm pulmonary nodules.

◈ DIFFERENTIAL DIAGNOSIS

- **Sarcoidosis:** The absence of significant intrathoracic adenopathy makes this a less likely diagnosis.
- **Metastatic disease:** Metastatic nodules are usually more variable in size. Possible primaries include thyroid, breast, and pancreatic carcinoma as well as melanoma.
- **Disseminated (miliary) tuberculosis (TB):** The clinical and radiologic findings are most consistent with this diagnosis.
- **Disseminated fungus:** Although the radiologic findings are also consistent with disseminated histoplasmosis, coccidioidomycosis, blastomycosis, or cryptococcosis, disseminated fungal infection most commonly occurs in immunocompromised patients.
- *Pneumocystis carinii* **pneumonia:** This pattern would be a less common manifestation in AIDS patients.

◈ DIAGNOSIS: Miliary tuberculosis.

◈ KEY FACTS

CLINICAL
- Symptomatic hematogenous dissemination occurs in 1% to 7% of patients with TB.
- Miliary TB is more frequent in young children (<2 years), the elderly, and immunocompromised patients.
- Miliary dissemination usually occurs within 6 months of the primary infection.

RADIOLOGIC
- The chest radiograph is usually normal at the onset of clinical symptoms.
- Miliary TB usually manifests with diffuse, evenly distributed 1- to 3-mm nodules. However, they may not be visible until 6 weeks after dissemination.
- In 15% of patients, the distribution is asymmetric.
- The nodules usually have a perivascular and periseptal distribution on CT.
- Intrathoracic adenopathy is seen in 95% of children and 12% of adults.
- Associated consolidation is seen in 42% of children and 12% of adults.
- Response to appropriate antituberculous therapy is typically rapid, with radiographic resolution within 4 to 6 weeks.

◈ SUGGESTED READING

McAdams HP, Erasmus JJ, Winter J. The radiographic manifestations of pulmonary tuberculosis. Radiol Clin North Am 1995;33:655–678.

Miller WT, Miller WT Jr. Tuberculosis in the normal host: Radiologic findings. Semin Roentgenol 1993;28:109–118.

Webb WR, Müller NL, Naidich DP. High-Resolution CT of the Lung. New York: Raven, 1992.

Woodring JW, Vandiviere HM, Fried AM, et al. Update: The radiographic features of tuberculosis. AJR Am J Roentgenol 1986; 148:497–506.

CASE 18

Jeremy J. Erasmus

HISTORY

A 56-year-old man presents with fever, weight loss, and productive cough.

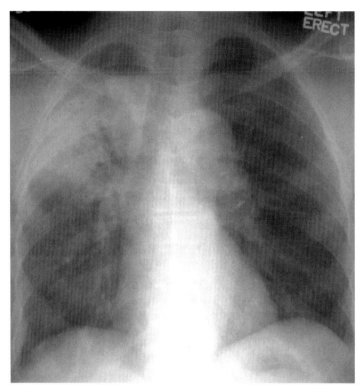

FIGURE 1-18A Posteroanterior chest radiograph. There is extensive right upper lobe consolidation with focal cavitation. Small, poorly defined nodular opacities are present in the right lower lobe and mid aspect of the left lung.

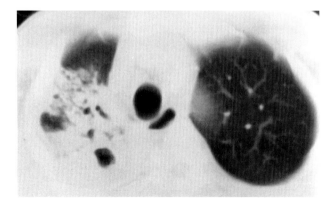

FIGURE 1-18B Chest CT (lung windows) through the upper lobes shows cavitary consolidation of the right upper lobe.

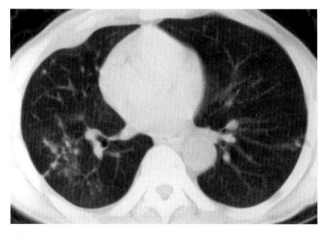

FIGURE 1-18C Chest CT (lung window) through the midportion of the lungs. There are small, poorly marginated nodules in the superior segments of both lower lobes. This finding suggests endobronchial spread of infection.

◆ DIFFERENTIAL DIAGNOSIS

◆ **Aspiration:** This commonly causes bilateral, multilobar, poorly defined consolidation in dependent pulmonary segments.

◆ **Pulmonary malignancy:** Postobstructive cavitary consolidation can occur secondary to an endobronchial neoplasm. A further possibility is bronchioalveolar carcinoma.

◆ **Wegener's granulomatosis:** The most common radiographic findings are nodular opacities with a high propensity for cavitation. Pulmonary consolidation, which may be scattered and heterogeneous, or homogeneous and lobar, occurs in approximately 30% of patients.

◆ **Pneumonia:** Lobar consolidation is usually bacterial in origin. The bacteria that commonly cause cavitation are *Staphylococcus aureus, Klebsiella, Pseudomonas, Proteus,* and anaerobic organisms. Mycobacteria tuberculosis (TB) is increasingly a cause of consolidation and cavitation.

◆ DIAGNOSIS: Postprimary tuberculosis.

◆ KEY FACTS

CLINICAL

◆ The highest incidence of postprimary TB is in patients >65 years of age.

◆ Postprimary TB usually occurs due to reactivation of dormant bacilli, although some cases may be due to reinfection of a previously sensitized host.

◆ Reactivation occurs in 55% to 15% of patients, usually in the secondary foci in the apical/posterior segments of the upper lobes and superior segments of the lower lobes.

◆ Because of host hypersensitivity acquired from primary infection, progressive disease with caseous necrosis occurs and can rapidly destroy the lung.

◆ Most patients have a delayed cutaneous response to the intradermal injection of purified protein derivative.

RADIOLOGIC

◆ The earliest findings are heterogeneous, poorly marginated opacities in the apical or posterior segments of the upper lobes or in the superior segments of the lower lobes.

◆ The initial opacities usually evolve into more well-defined reticular and nodular opacities.

◆ The infection may occasionally progress to lobar or complete lung consolidation.

◆ Cavitation is common (40% to 87%) and typically occurs within areas of consolidation.

◆ A complication of cavitation is endobronchial spread of infection.

◆ Endobronchial dissemination results in 5- to 10-mm, poorly defined peribronchiolar and centrilobular nodules.

◆ Miliary TB occurs less commonly in postprimary than in primary TB, and the classic radiographic findings are diffuse, small (1 to 3 mm), well-defined nodules.

◆ Pleural effusions are uncommon (6% to 18%) and usually small.

◆ Hilar and mediastinal adenopathy is rare with postprimary TB.

◆ Healing may be associated with scarring, cicatricial atelectasis, traction bronchiectasis, residual nodules, and parenchymal calcification.

◆ SUGGESTED READING
Armstrong P, Wilson AG, Dee P, Hansell DM. Imaging of Diseases of the Chest (2nd ed). St. Louis: Mosby, 1995.

Fraser RG, Pare JAP, Pare PD, et al. Diagnosis of Diseases of the Chest (3rd ed). Philadelphia: Saunders, 1991;882–939.

McAdams HP, Erasmus JJ, Winter JA. Radiologic manifestations of pulmonary tuberculosis. Radiol Clin North Am 1995;33: 655–678.

Miller WT, Miller WT Jr. Tuberculosis in the normal host: Radiologic findings. Semin Roentgenol 1993;28:109–118.

Woodring JW, Vandiviere HM, Fried AM, et al. Update: The radiographic features of pulmonary tuberculosis. AJR Am J Roentgenol 1986;148:497–506.

HISTORY

A 75-year-old woman with mild dyspnea, chronic weight loss, and no history of fever.

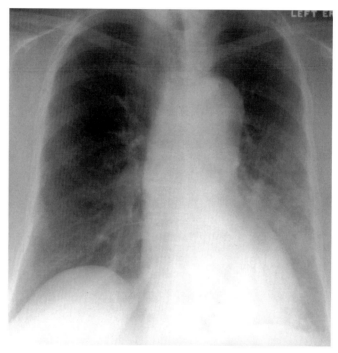

FIGURE 1-19A Posteroanterior chest radiograph. There is diffuse, homogeneous consolidation in the left lower lobe, and poorly defined, nodular, and heterogeneous opacities in the left upper lobe. No hilar or mediastinal adenopathy is present.

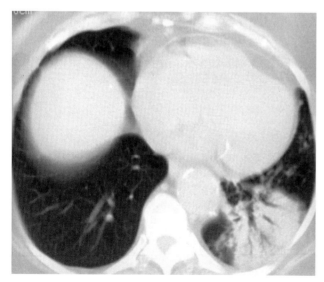

FIGURE 1-19B Chest CT (lung window) through the lower lung fields. There is diffuse, homogeneous consolidation without cavitation in the left lower lobe.

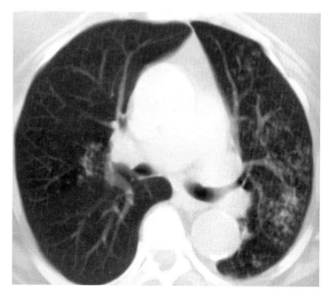

FIGURE 1-19C Chest CT (lung window) through the mid lung fields. Numerous small, poorly defined nodules are present in the left lung.

◆ DIFFERENTIAL DIAGNOSIS

◆ **Pneumonia:** Lobar consolidation is usually caused by bacterial infection. Organisms include *Streptococcus pneumoniae, Staphylococcus aureus, Legionella pneumophila,* gram-negative bacteria, and *Mycobacterium tuberculosis.* A bacterial infection is unlikely with a history of chronic weight loss and no fever, although tuberculosis (TB) can have a subacute presentation.

◆ **Aspiration pneumonia:** Aspiration of gram-negative or anaerobic bacteria may cause lobar consolidation. Aspiration commonly causes scattered, poorly defined consolidation in the dependent segments. Involvement of the anterior portions of the lungs in this patient makes this diagnosis unlikely.

◆ **Wegener's granulomatosis:** Although the disease can be indolent, presentation is usually acute, with upper airway involvement (sinusitis, rhinitis, otitis) and functional renal impairment. Nodular opacities, which frequently cavitate, are the most common presentation. Lobar consolidation and numerous, small nodular opacities occur in 30% of patients.

◆ **Primary lymphoma of lung:** This rare non-Hodgkin's lymphoma is usually low grade, and patients are often asymptomatic. Consolidation with air bronchograms and poorly defined margins is the most common presentation. Mass-like and reticulonodular opacities are less frequent.

◆ **Bronchioalveolar cell carcinoma (BAC):** The clinical presentation and homogeneous consolidation with nodules could be due to the diffuse form of BAC.

◆ DIAGNOSIS: Bronchioalveolar cell carcinoma.

◆ KEY FACTS

CLINICAL

◆ BAC constitutes 1.5% to 10.0% of all lung cancers.
◆ It is a subtype of adenocarcinoma and can be localized or multifocal. The localized form can, after an indolent period of local growth, progress rapidly to diffuse tho-racic metastases. The biologic behavior of BAC is, however, controversial, and a further possibility is that the two presentations are distinct, with the localized form rarely evolving into diffuse BAC.

◆ Clinical features that distinguish BAC from other lung cancers are (1) younger age at presentation, (2) equal distribution of men and women, (3) copious watery sputum (bronchorrhea), and (4) higher incidence in nonsmokers.

RADIOLOGIC

◆ The most common finding is a well-circumscribed, solitary nodule (60%).
◆ The nodule may remain unchanged in size over many years.
◆ The solitary nodule is usually peripheral in location.
◆ Pseudocavitation, the presence of small, low-attenuation regions within or surrounding the nodule, is more common with this malignancy than other non–small cell carcinomas.
◆ The diffuse form may present as (1) multiple pulmonary nodules of varying size; (2) focal, poorly defined opacities resembling pneumonia; (3) reticulonodular opacities resembling interstitial lung disease; (4) other radiographic findings associated with parenchymal disease include hilar and mediastinal adenopathy (18%), pleural effusions (1% to 10%), and atelectasis (3%).

◆ SUGGESTED READING

Erasmus JJ, Patz EF. Diagnostic Imaging of Bronchogenic Carcinoma. In C Chiles, C Putnam (eds), Pulmonary and Cardiac Imaging. New York: Marcel Dekker, 1997.

Hill CA. Bronchioloalveolar carcinoma: A review. Radiology 1984;150:15–20.

Kuhlman JE, Fishman EK, Kuhajda FP, et al. Solitary bronchioloalveolar carcinoma: CT criteria. Radiology 1988;167: 379–382.

Miller WT, Husted J, Freiman D, et al. Bronchioloalveolar carcinoma: Two clinical entities with one pathologic diagnosis. AJR Am J Roentgenol 1978;130:905–912.

HISTORY

Asymptomatic 71-year-old man undergoes a routine annual chest radiograph.

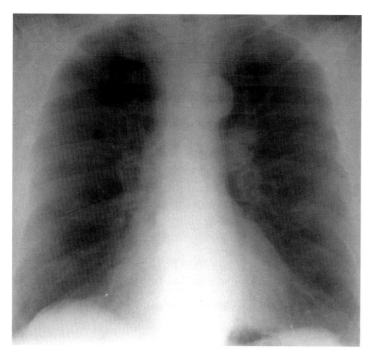

FIGURE 1-20A Posteroanterior chest radiograph. There is a well-circumscribed 3-cm nodule in the mid-aspect of the left lung superimposed over the left hilum.

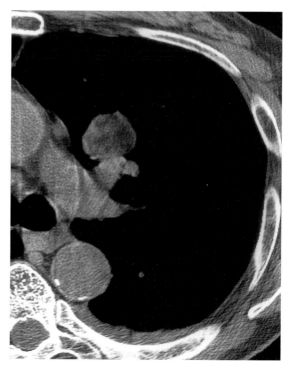

FIGURE 1-20B Noncontrast chest CT (mediastinal window). There is a left upper lobe mass anterior to the left pulmonary artery. The mass is heterogeneous with small areas of fat attenuation (−41 HU).

◆ DIFFERENTIAL DIAGNOSIS

◆ **Malignancy:** A primary pulmonary cancer and a single, isolated metastatic nodule would be considerations on the chest radiograph.

◆ **Tuberculomas:** Persistent mass-like opacities are an uncommon manifestation of parenchymal tuberculosis (TB). They are usually encountered in asymptomatic adults. The majority (75%) occur in the upper lobes, and they are usually <3 cm in size. Smaller satellite lesions are seen in as many as 80%.

◆ **Hamartoma:** This is the best diagnosis because of the focal collections of fat (CT attenuation between −40 and −120 Hounsfield units [HU]).

◆ **Arteriovenous malformations:** These are single in about two-thirds of cases. They are usually round, sharply defined, and most often in the medial third of the lung. Size ranges from one to several centimeters in diameter. Identification of feeding and draining vessels, which are essential to the diagnosis, may be difficult to visualize on plain radiographs.

◆ DIAGNOSIS: Hamartoma.

◆ KEY FACTS

CLINICAL

◆ A hamartoma is a developmental malformation of disorganized tissues that normally constitute the organ in which the tumor occurs.

◆ It has been proposed that they are best regarded as benign neoplasms.

◆ Peak incidence is in the sixth decade, and they are uncommon in patients <30 years of age.

◆ They most often occur in males (3 to 1).

◆ Hamartomas are usually solitary, although multiple pulmonary hamartomas can occur rarely in the multiple hamartoma syndrome (Cowden's disease), which is characterized by multiple mucocutaneous lesions and gastrointestinal hamartomatous polyps.

◆ Carney's triad: (1) pulmonary chondroma (often multiple), (2) gastric leiomyosarcoma, and (3) extra-adrenal paraganglioma, has been described. This occurs mostly in women <35 years of age.

RADIOLOGIC

◆ Hamartomas characteristically are well-defined solitary nodules that are usually <4 cm in diameter.

◆ The majority are located peripherally (90%), although occasionally they may arise in the central bronchi.

◆ Calcification occurs in up to 50% and typically resembles popcorn.

◆ The nodule may increase slowly over time; although rapid growth can occur, it is rare.

◆ Cavitation is extremely rare.

◆ The presence of fat attenuation within the mass, best demonstrated on CT, is a diagnostic feature. Fat may be identified by CT numbers in the range of −80 to −120 HU.

◆ Fat may not be present in the hamartomatous nodule in approximately one-third of cases.

◆ In the small percentage of centrally occuring hamartomas, atelectasis and obstructive pneumonia may occur.

◆ SUGGESTED READING

Armstrong P, Wilson AG, Dee P, Hansell DM. Imaging of Diseases of the Chest (2nd ed). St. Louis: Mosby, 1990;296–297.

Fraser RG, Pare JAP, Pare PD, et al. Diagnosis of Diseases of the Chest (3rd ed). Philadelphia: Saunders, 1991;882–939.

Poirier TJ, Van Ordstrand HS, et al. Pulmonary chondromatous hamartoma: Report of seventeen cases and review of the literature. Chest 1971;59:50–55.

Siegelman SS, Khouri NF, Scott WW, et al. Pulmonary hamartoma: CT findings. Radiology 1986;160:313–317.

CASE 21

Jeremy J. Erasmus

HISTORY

A 52-year-old man presenting with a cerebral stroke.

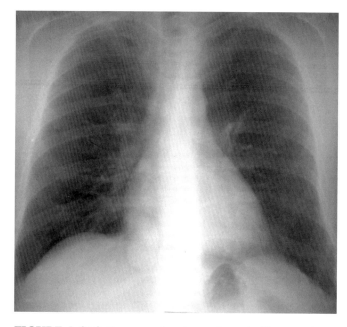

FIGURE 1-21A Posteroanterior chest radiograph. There is a large, lobulated right lower lobe mass without cavitation or calcification. There is no hilar or mediastinal adenopathy.

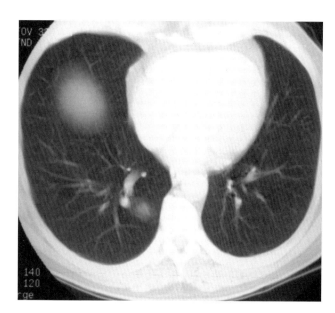

FIGURE 1-21B Chest CT (lung window) through the lung bases. Well-defined, lobulated mass with enlarged feeding artery and draining vein.

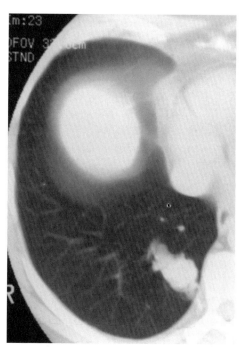

FIGURE 1-21C Chest CT (lung window) through the right lung base. Coned down view of the right lower lobe mass.

◆ DIFFERENTIAL DIAGNOSIS

- **Non–small cell carcinoma:** The large size of the mass and the age of the patient would favor this diagnosis on the chest radiograph. The presence of enlarged vessels, however, excludes the diagnosis.
- **Metastatic lung disease:** The solitary nature, large size, and absence of a history of primary extrathoracic malignancy would make this diagnosis unlikely.
- **Arteriovenous malformation (AVM):** The well-defined, lobulated contour, medial location, and identification of feeding and draining vessel would be characteristic for this diagnosis.
- **Tuberculoma:** This is usually in the upper lobes (75%) and <3 cm in size.

◆ DIAGNOSIS: Arteriovenous malformation.

◆ KEY FACTS

CLINICAL
- Ten percent of cases are identified in infancy or childhood, although the vast majority are not recognized until the third and fourth decade of life.
- They are twice as frequent in women as in men.
- Patients commonly present with hemoptysis or dyspnea on exertion or occasionally with cerebral embolism.
- Of all pulmonary AVMs, 40% to 65% are associated with Osler-Weber-Rendu disease (hereditary hemorrhagic telangiectasia). This is an autosomal dominant disorder that manifests clinically in adult life. Many of these patients have arteriovenous communications elsewhere, including the skin, mucous membranes, and other organs.

RADIOLOGIC
- The typical finding is a round, lobulated, well-defined mass, most often in the medial third of the lung.
- About 33% of cases will have multiple pulmonary AVMs.
- The size of the AVMs is less than one to several centimeters in diameter.
- The feeding artery and draining vein are often enlarged and identifiable on the chest radiograph.
- The vascular nature of the radiographic opacities can be demonstrated by an increase in size during a Mueller maneuver and a decrease during a Valsalva maneuver.
- A change in size may also be visible when erect (smaller) and supine (larger) radiographs are compared.
- Pulmonary angiography remains the standard imaging technique and is performed to confirm the presence of pulmonary AVMs, detect synchronous malformations, and delineate the anatomy of the feeding and draining vessels.
- CT is a sensitive, noninvasive means of establishing the diagnosis and eliminates the need for angiography when treatment is not being contemplated.
- Embolization is now the preferred treatment for this condition and is performed with detachable balloons or steel coils.

◆ SUGGESTED READING
Allison DJ, Pinet F, Allison HJ. Interventional Techniques in the Thorax. In EJ Potchen, RG Grainger, R Greens (eds), Pulmonary Radiology—By Members of The Fleischner Society. Philadelphia: Saunders, 1993;340–360.

Fraser RG, Pare JAP, Pare PD, et al. Diagnosis of Diseases of the Chest (3rd ed). Philadelphia: Saunders, 1991;882–939.

Remy-Jardin M, Wattinne L, Deffontaines C. Pulmonary arteriovenous malformations: Evaluation with CT of the chest before and after treatment. Radiology 1992;182:809–816.

CASE 22

R. Chapman Gilkeson

HISTORY

A 60-year-old man who is a foundry worker presents with progressive dyspnea.

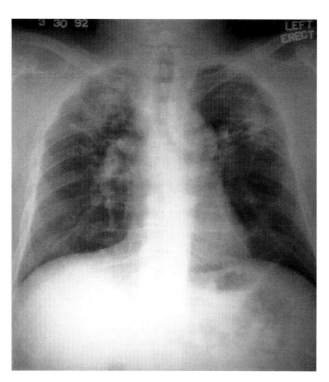

FIGURE 1-22A Posteroanterior chest radiograph. There are bilateral, symmetric upper lobe opacities with sharp lateral margins and multiple calcified hilar lymph nodes. There is no significant pleural disease.

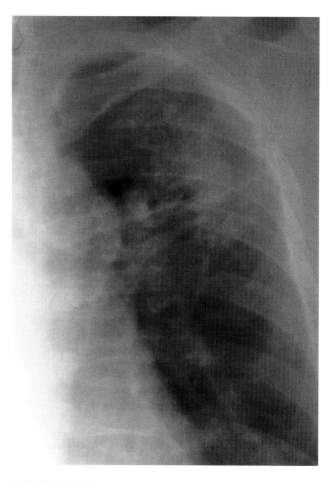

FIGURE 1-22B Coned down view of the mediastinum on a posteroanterior chest radiograph confirms the presence of "eggshell" calcification in the hilar lymph nodes.

◆ DIFFERENTIAL DIAGNOSIS

- **Silicosis:** This is the best diagnosis given the eggshell calcifications and conglomerate masses. Coal worker's pneumoconiosis is indistinguishable radiographically from silicosis and should be included in the differential diagnosis.
- **Sarcoidosis:** Both eggshell calcifications and conglomerate masses can also be seen in sarcoidosis. However, the symmetry and sharp lateral borders of the opacities, along with the clinical history, makes silicosis more likely.
- **Tuberculosis (TB)/histoplasmosis:** Eggshell calcifications and conglomerate masses can result from pulmonary infection by TB or histoplasmosis. However, the symmetry and sharp lateral borders of the opacities, along with the clinical history, makes silicosis more likely.
- **Lymphoma:** Treated lymphoma can result in eggshell calcification of hilar or mediastinal nodes. The parenchymal findings and clinical history make silicosis more likely.

◆ DIAGNOSIS: Silicosis with conglomerate masses.

◆ KEY FACTS

CLINICAL

- Silicosis is a chronic, nodular, and fibrotic disease caused by long-term exposure to silica.
- Typical occupational histories include hard-rock mining, foundry work, and sandblasting.
- Clinical symptoms and radiographic findings usually require 10 to 20 years of exposure.
- There is an acute form known as acute silicoproteinosis. It is associated with heavy exposure and can occur over a period of several months. Its clinical and radiographic course resembles alveolar proteinosis.

- Silicosis increases the risk of TB, particularly in patients with conglomerate masses. Culture of the organism is difficult in these patients.

RADIOLOGIC

- Simple silicosis is characterized by multiple 1- to 10-mm nodules that predominate in the upper lobes; 20% of nodules calcify.
- Complicated silicosis is characterized by coalescence of the nodules into conglomerate masses >1 cm in diameter. These masses can reach 10 cm in size and typically migrate toward the hila with time. Paracicatricial emphysema is common.
- The conglomerate masses can cavitate due to ischemic necrosis. Development of TB in these cavities (silicotuberculosis) is common. Other signs of TB in patients with silicosis include apical pleural thickening and rapid progression of nodules.
- Caplan's syndrome (cavitary rheumatoid nodules in patients with coal worker's pneumoconiosis) can closely resemble complicated silicosis.
- CT is superior to plain chest radiographs in the detection of early silicosis and in identifying other conditions that cause dyspnea, such as emphysema. It can also be *key* for the diagnosis of superimposed TB and lung cancer.

◆ SUGGESTED READING

Begin R, Bergeron D, Samson L, et al. CT assessment of silicosis in exposed workers. AJR Am J Roentgenol 1987;148:509–514.

Dee P, Suratt P, Winn W. The radiographic findings in acute silicosis. Radiology 1978;126;359–363.

McLoud TC, Gamsu G. Pneumoconiosis: Radiology and High-Resolution Computed Tomography. In EJ Potchen, RG Grainger, R Greene (eds), Pulmonary Radiology. Philadelphia: Saunders, 1993;81–93.

CASE 23

Philip C. Goodman

HISTORY

A 23-year-old man presents with an acute onset of productive cough, fever, and chills. The patient is otherwise healthy and has no prior illnesses.

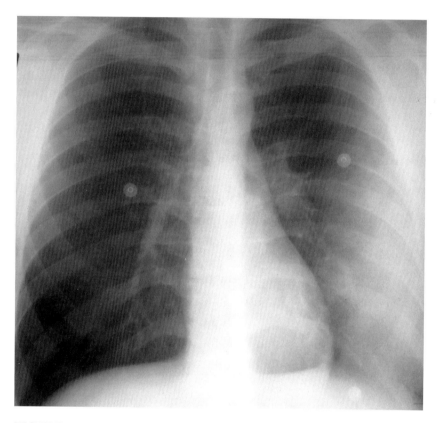

FIGURE 1-23 Posteroanterior chest radiograph reveals a homogeneous opacity overlying the left lateral hemithorax. The medial margins are indistinct, and the lateral aspect abuts the pleura. There is no definite evidence of hilar or mediastinal adenopathy or of a pleural effusion.

◆ DIFFERENTIAL DIAGNOSIS

◆ **Community-acquired bacterial pneumonia:** The acute onset of symptoms and the radiographic findings suggest a community-acquired pneumonia such as that caused by *Streptococcus pneumoniae* or *Haemophilus influenzae*.

◆ **Pneumonia due to other organisms:** Less common causes of pneumonia that can mimic the more common bacterial varieties include primary tuberculosis (TB), Legionnaires' pneumonia, actinomycosis, and coccidioidomycosis or blastomycosis pneumonias in endemic regions.

◆ **Noninfectious entities:** Pulmonary embolism, eosinophilic pneumonia, contusion or hemorrhage, and bronchitis obliterans organizing pneumonia (BOOP) should also be considered as they can manifest with peripheral consolidation.

◆ DIAGNOSIS: Pneumococcal pneumonia.

◆ KEY FACTS

CLINICAL

◆ The diagnosis of community-acquired pneumonia may be difficult since the pathogens are not identified in as many as 50% of patients. Nevertheless, *S. pneumoniae* is the most frequent cause. Other pathogens include *Mycoplasma pneumoniae*, respiratory viruses, *Chlamydia* pneumonia, and *Haemophilus influenzae*.

◆ *S. pneumoniae* can occur in healthy people but is frequently found in noncritically ill patients who require hospitalization. These patients are usually >65 years of age or have coexisting illness such as diabetes mellitus, chronic renal failure, congestive heart failure, or chronic obstructive pulmonary disease.

◆ Mortality rates range from 5% to 25%, with death usually occurring in the first 7 days of hospitalization.

◆ Severe pneumonia with mortality rates as high as 50% is recognized when certain conditions exist. These conditions include a respiratory rate >30, low urine output, shock, or chest radiographs revealing multiple lobe involvement or significant increase in opacity within 2 days of admission.

◆ While *S. pneumoniae* is particularly sensitive to penicillin, some clinicians direct therapy at a broader group of organisms and may include antibiotics such as erythromycin, third-generation cephalosporins, or trimethaprim-sulfamethoxazole. Many recommend immunization with pneumococcal vaccines.

RADIOLOGIC

◆ Pneumococcal pneumonia usually manifests as a homogeneous parenchymal opacity that begins at the periphery and spreads to involve the entire segment or lobe.

◆ Air bronchograms are common.

◆ Lymphadenopathy is rare; cavitation occurs with some serotypes of *S. pneumoniae*.

◆ Pleural fluid or parapneumonic effusions can be seen in as many as 50% of patients.

◆ With appropriate antibiotic therapy, some radiologic evidence of improvement is usually seen within a few days, and complete resolution may be seen in approximately 2 weeks. In some cases, complete resolution requires up to 6 weeks.

◆ Failure of clinical or radiographic response to ordinary antibiotics should suggest the possibility of another infectious agent, an obstructing lesion, or an insensitive organism.

◆ SUGGESTED READING

Chien S, Pichotta P, Seipman N, Chan CK. Treatment of community-acquired pneumonia. Chest 1993;103:697–701.

Frame PT. Acute infectious pneumonia in the adult. ATS News 1982;18–25.

Niederman MS, Bass JB Jr, Campbell GD, et al. Guidelines for the initial management of adults with community-acquired pneumonia: Diagnosis, assessment of severity, and initial antimicrobial therapy. Am Rev Respir Dis 1993;148:1418–1426.

Ostergaard L, Andersen PL. Etiology of community-acquired pneumonia. Chest 1993;104:1400–1407.

CASE 24 *Philip C. Goodman*

HISTORY

A 25-year-old woman presents with pleuritic chest pain, high fever, nonproductive cough, and a history of intravenous drug abuse.

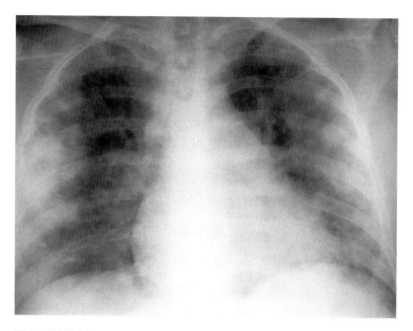

FIGURE 1-24A Anteroposterior chest radiograph shows bilateral, peripheral, homogeneous opacities. There are poorly defined, 1.0- to 1.5-cm nodules at the superior margins of the consolidations.

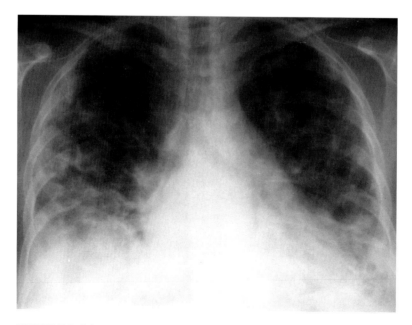

FIGURE 1-24B Anteroposterior chest radiograph 1 week later shows multiple lung cavities with both thin and thick walls. There is a moderate right pleural effusion.

◆ DIFFERENTIAL DIAGNOSIS

- **Eosinophilic pneumonia–chronic eosinophilic pneumonia (EP-CEP):** This disorder typically manifests with bilateral peripheral opacities as in this case. However, cavitation is rarely, if ever, seen in eosinophilic pneumonia.
- **Bacterial pneumonia:** Bacterial pneumonia usually begins in the periphery of the lung and can be multilobar. However, the symmetry shown in this case is unusual for this diagnosis.
- **Pulmonary infarction:** Pulmonary infarcts can manifest as peripheral consolidation (Hampton's hump). However, multifocal pulmonary cavitation is not a typical feature of pulmonary embolism with infarction.
- **Septic pulmonary embolism:** Septic emboli usually manifest as peripheral, poorly defined nodular opacities. In severe cases, the nodules can coalesce into larger areas of consolidation. Cavitation is common.
- **Bronchitis obliterans organizing pneumonia (BOOP):** Although BOOP usually manifests with scattered peripheral consolidation, cavitation virtually excludes this diagnosis.
- **Trauma:** Pulmonary contusion or hemorrhage often occurs in the lung periphery, and lung cysts or cavitation can also occur after thoracic trauma. However, the number of lesions seen in this case makes this diagnosis less likely.
- **Metastatic disease:** Multiple cavities can result from metastatic disease to the lung, particularly from squamous cell carcinomas. Metastases are generally discreet and do not coalesce, as seen in this case.
- **Collagen vascular disease:** Entities such as Wegener's granulomatosis and rheumatoid lung disease can result in cavitary nodules, but the number and close proximity of the cavities to one another, as seen in this case, are not typical features of these disorders.

◆ DIAGNOSIS: Septic emboli.

◆ KEY FACTS

CLINICAL

- Septic pulmonary emboli usually result from tricuspid valve endocarditis due to intravenous drug abuse, head and neck infections with pharyngeal or internal jugular vein phlebitis, or phlebitis from an indwelling catheter or an infected arteriovenous fistula.
- Symptoms include high fever, cough, dyspnea, chest pain, and occasional hemoptysis.
- Typical organisms include *Staphylococcus aureus* and anaerobes.
- Antibiotic therapy is usually successful, although clinical improvement can take several weeks.

RADIOLOGIC

- Septic emboli manifest as poorly defined nodules (usually 1 to 2 cm in diameter) in the lung periphery. They are usually more numerous in cases of tricuspid endocarditis than from other sources.
- In the first few days after initiation of therapy, new nodules may appear.
- Cavitation is seen in approximately 50% of nodules. The walls are moderately thick and irregular.
- Healing of these nodules or cavities is noted by a decrease in size and eventual resolution. Occasionally, a peripheral linear scar remains.
- Hilar and mediastinal lymphadenopathy has been reported rarely.
- Pleural effusion(s) are not uncommon.
- CT is generally not indicated but, as in other situations, can reveal a greater extent of involvement than chest radiographs. On CT, a vessel leading into the nodule is a suggestive, but nonspecific, finding.

◆ SUGGESTED READING

Gumbs RV, McCauley DI. Hilar and mediastinal adenopathy in septic pulmonary embolic disease. Radiology 1982;142:313–315.

Hadlock FP, Wallace RJ Jr, Rivera M. Pulmonary septic emboli secondary to parapharyngeal abscess: Postanginal sepsis. Radiology 1979;130:29–33.

Jaffe RB, Koschmann EB. Septic pulmonary emboli. Radiology 1970;96:527–532.

Kuhlman JE, Fishman EK, Teigen C. Pulmonary septic emboli: Diagnosis with CT. Radiology 1990;174:211–213.

CASE 25

Philip C. Goodman

HISTORY

A 21-year-old man presents with fever, cough, and dyspnea. On physical examination, a severe vesicular skin rash is discovered.

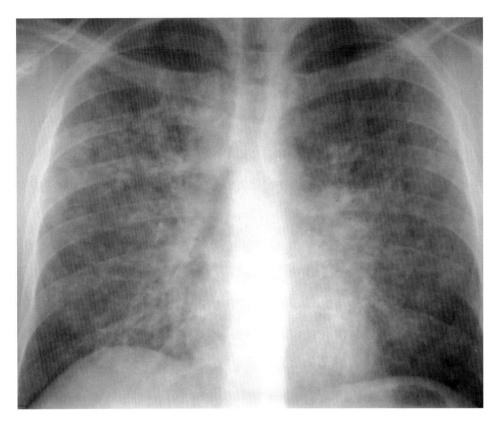

FIGURE 1-25 Posteroanterior chest radiograph demonstrates bilateral, symmetric, coarse, poorly defined nodular opacities. There is evidence of left hilar and right paratracheal adenopathy, but there are no pleural effusions.

◆ DIFFERENTIAL DIAGNOSIS

◆ **Primary lung neoplasm:** Multiple, poorly defined nodules can be seen in both bronchoalveolar cell carcinoma and lymphoma. With alveolar cell carcinoma and lymphoma, larger areas of consolidation are frequently seen. With lymphoma, lymphadenopathy and pleural fluid are frequent.

◆ **Kaposi's sarcoma:** The poorly defined nodules of Kaposi's sarcoma are generally less numerous and larger than those seen in this case.

◆ **Metastases:** Metastatic disease from a variety of primary sources could account for this radiographic pattern.

◆ **Disseminated fungal infection:** In disseminated fungal infection, the nodules are usually more discrete than seen in this case. However, in cases of overwhelming infection, the nodules can sometimes be poorly defined and coalescent. Severe primary histoplasmosis can also manifest with multiple, poorly defined nodules, but the degree of coalescence noted in this case is unusual.

◆ **Miliary tuberculosis:** This is unlikely because the size of nodules in this case is larger than the usual 1- to 3-mm opacities seen in classic miliary infections.

◆ **Collagen vascular disease:** Entities such as Wegener's granulomatosis and rheumatoid lung disease can manifest with multiple nodules, but generally they are larger, less numerous, and more discrete than the ones noted in this case. Cavitation is frequently seen in these entities.

◆ **Varicella pneumonia:** The vesicular skin rash associated with diffuse poorly defined pulmonary nodules and lymphadenopathy make this the most likely diagnosis.

◆ DIAGNOSIS: Varicella pneumonia.

◆ KEY FACTS

CLINICAL

◆ Pneumonia usually develops 2 to 3 days after the appearance of the vesicular eruption. The incubation time postexposure is 3 to 21 days.

◆ The rash is particularly severe at the onset of pneumonia.

◆ Presenting symptoms include cough, dyspnea, hemoptysis, tachypnea, chest pain, and high fever.

◆ Pneumonia without fever or new skin lesions is rare.

◆ The incidence of pneumonia ranges from 10% to 50%, with a greater frequency in cigarette smokers.

◆ Twenty-five percent of the fatalities related to varicella pneumonia occur in adults, although only 2% of the 3 to 4 million annual cases of varicella occur in adults.

◆ Untreated adult varicella pneumonia has a 10% fatality rate; a fatality rate of 40% is seen in pregnant or postpartum women and in cancer and bone marrow transplant patients. Therapy with acyclovir may be effective in shortening the course of cutaneous disease, as well as in preventing pneumonia. Patients treated with acyclovir also have a lower mortality rate.

◆ Varicella vaccines may provide protection in approximately 70% of adults and 90% of children.

RADIOLOGIC

◆ Varicella pneumonia typically manifests with poorly defined nodular opacities that are distributed diffusely throughout both lungs. The nodules are usually 5 to 10 mm in diameter. Coalescence is frequent as the nodules enlarge.

◆ Hilar lymph node enlargement may be seen in some cases. The nodes do not usually calcify.

◆ Resolution occurs in 3 to 5 days in mild cases; however, radiographic abnormalities can persist for weeks in severe disease.

◆ Healing can result in small calcific opacities throughout the lungs. These are usually smaller and less uniform than the calcifications seen with prior histoplasmosis. Less than 2% of affected patients have residual pulmonary calcification.

◆ Pleural effusions are rare.

◆ SUGGESTED READING

Feldman S. Varicella-zoster virus pneumonitis. Chest 1994; 106:22S–27S.

Fraser RG, Pare JAP, Pare PD, et al. Diagnosis of Diseases of the Chest. Philadelphia: Saunders, 1989;1062–1068.

Sargent EN, Carson MJ, Reilly ED. Roentgenographic manifestations of varicella pneumonia with postmortem correlation. Radiology 1966;98:305–317.

CASE 26   *Philip C. Goodman*

HISTORY

A 47-year-old man presents with a 3-week history of low-grade fevers, night sweats, and a 10-pound weight loss. The patient is an alcoholic. Periodontal disease is observed on physical examination.

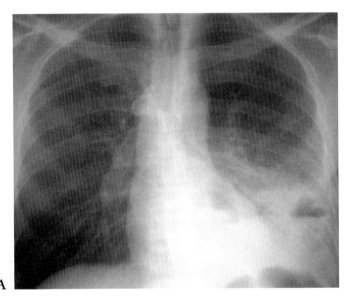

A

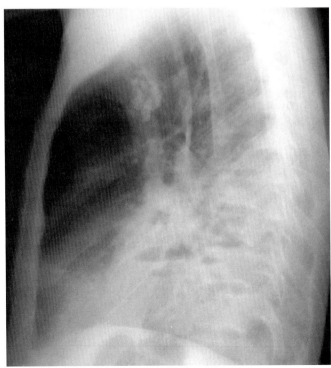

B

FIGURES 1-26A and 1-26B Posteroanterior (A) and lateral (B) chest radiographs show a left lower lobe consolidation with multiple areas of cavitation and air-fluid levels. There is also calcified right paratracheal adenopathy consistent with prior histoplasmosis or tuberculosis.

◆ DIFFERENTIAL DIAGNOSIS

◆ **Postprimary tuberculosis (TB):** Postprimary TB usually manifests as cavitary disease in the superior segment of the lower lobe or the posterior segment of the upper lobe.

◆ **Bronchogenic carcinoma:** A cavitating neoplasm such as squamous cell carcinoma should be considered but is less likely due to the extent of the consolidation and multifocal cavitation.

◆ **Trauma:** Pulmonary contusion with traumatic lung cysts would also be a consideration in the proper clinical setting.

◆ **Pneumonia with lung abscess:** Pneumonias due to *Klebsiella pneumoniae*, other gram-negative organisms, or certain serotypes of *Streptococcus pneumoniae* can result in necrosis and abscess formation. The indolent clinical symptoms, however, do not favor these diagnoses.

◆ **Anaerobic pneumonia:** These usually occur in the dependent portions of the lungs following aspiration and may pursue an indolent clinical course, as in this case. Cavitation is common.

◆ DIAGNOSIS: Anaerobic pneumonia from aspiration.

◆ KEY FACTS

CLINICAL

◆ Patients with a history of unconsciousness, alcoholism, seizure disorder, severe trauma, or recent anesthesia are at risk for aspiration and anaerobic pneumonia.

◆ Clinical features of fever, cough, and white blood cell count elevation can be seen within 12 hours after aspiration but are more typical in the first 48 hours.

◆ Symptoms can be minimal, with a more indolent course of nonproductive cough, low-grade fever, and weight loss. With cavitation, expectoration increases and hemoptysis can occur.

◆ Periodontal disease may be observed, although this is not necessary as poor endobronchial clearance alone may contribute to the development of anaerobic infection.

◆ The foul odor of anaerobic bacteria is fairly specific and can suggest the diagnosis.

RADIOLOGIC

◆ Aspiration pneumonia occurs almost exclusively in the superior segment of the lower lobes, posterior segment of the upper lobes, and posterior basal segment of the lower lobes. The remainder of the upper lobes, the lingula, and the right middle lobe are rarely involved.

◆ Initially, a heterogeneous opacity is noted within 2 days of aspiration. Within a week, more homogeneous consolidation develops, sometimes with cavitation.

◆ Over the next few weeks, chronic low-grade infection can develop and manifest as a thick-walled cavity. At this point, the clinical features and radiographic appearance can mimic postprimary TB.

◆ Air-fluid levels are common.

◆ Associated empyema is common. Approximately 50% of patients have pleural fluid alone or in combination with lung disease.

◆ Lymphadenopathy is uncommon.

◆ Healing of large abscess cavities is slow and is recognized by a decrease in the diameter of the cavity. The size of the air-fluid level within the cavity reflects the patency of communication with an airway and does not correlate with either clinical worsening or improvement.

◆ SUGGESTED READING

Bartlett JG. Anaerobic bacterial pneumonitis. Am Rev Respir Dis 1979;119:19–23.

Bartlett JG. Anaerobic bacterial infections of the lung. Chest 1987;91:901–909.

Landay MJ, Christensen EE, Bynum LJ, Goodman PC. Anaerobic pleural and pulmonary infections. AJR Am J Roentgenol 1980;134:233–240.

CASE 27

Philip C. Goodman

HISTORY

A 54-year-old man was hospitalized for an orthopedic surgical procedure. The pre-operative chest film was normal. Two days into hospitalization, the patient developed a fever, cough, and elevated white blood cell count. His chest film abnormalities and clinical symptoms were similar to those seen in four other patients in the hospital within a period of 3 weeks.

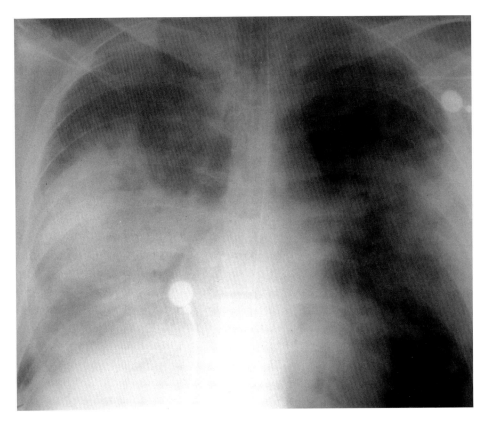

FIGURE 1-27 Anteroposterior supine chest radiograph demonstrates bilateral homogeneous consolidations involving large, almost mass-like areas of lung parenchyma. There is a right pleural effusion.

◆ DIFFERENTIAL DIAGNOSIS

- **Neoplasm:** Neoplasm is unlikely given the rapid onset of symptoms and radiographic appearance of the lungs.
- **Gram-negative pneumonia:** Pneumonia caused by nosocomial gram-negative organisms should be considered. However, the homogeneity of this opacity and the mass-like appearance are somewhat peculiar. Gram-negative organisms hematogenously disseminated tend to cause more peripheral amorphous and heterogeneous opacity. They also have a strong tendency to cavitate and may induce a parapneumonic effusion.
- **Community-acquired pneumonia:** The coincidental development of community-acquired pneumonia such as pneumococcal pneumonia should be considered. If there is a failure to respond to ordinary antibiotics, however, other considerations need to be raised. Among these are the possibility of primary TB, fungal infections such as blastomycosis or coccidioidomycosis, or unusual organisms such as nocardia or actinomycosis.
- *Legionella* **pneumonia:** The outbreak of similar cases in other patients in the hospital supports a diagnosis of hospital contamination with *Legionella pneumophila*.

◆ DIAGNOSIS: Legionnaires' disease.

◆ KEY FACTS

CLINICAL

- Legionnaires' disease is caused by *L. pneumophila*, a pleomorphic gram-negative bacillus recognized in 1976 during an outbreak in Philadelphia. Other epidemics have occurred in nursing homes and hospitals and generally arise from contaminated water sources.
- Patients usually present with gradual onset of fever, chills, cough, and dyspnea. Headaches, gastrointestinal symptoms, and pleuritic pain have also been reported.

Hyponatremia is more frequent in early legionellosis than in other pneumonias.

- Direct fluorescent antibody staining of sputum provides rapid diagnosis but is less sensitive than culture.
- Treatment with erythromycin generally results in a successful outcome.

RADIOLOGIC

- Legionnaires' disease usually begins with a focal area of homogeneous opacity that may manifest as a large, poorly marginated mass.
- Progression to bilateral lung involvement occurs in 70% of patients, typically within the first few days. Progression of radiographic findings is rapid and may continue after institution of therapy.
- Lymphadenopathy is rare. Pleural fluid has been reported in 30% to 60% of patients with Legionnaires' disease.
- Cavitation is uncommon but has been reported primarily in patients who are immunosuppressed.
- Resolution is usually rapid but on occasion is quite prolonged.

◆ SUGGESTED READING

Dietrich PA, Johnson RD, Fairbank JT, Walke JS. The chest radiograph in Legionnaires' disease. Radiology 1978;127:577–582.

Edelstein PH. Legionnaires' disease. Clin Infect Dis 1993;16:741–749.

MacFarlane JT, Miller AC, Smith WHR, et al. Comparative radiographic features of community acquired Legionnaires' disease, pneumococcal pneumonia, mycoplasma pneumonia, and psittacosis. Thorax 1994;39:28–33.

Meenhorst PL, Mulder JD. The chest X-ray in Legionella pneumonia (Legionnaires' disease). Eur J Radiol 1983;3:180–186.

Moore EH, Webb WR, Gamsu G, Golden JA. Legionnaires' disease in the renal transplant patient: Clinical presentation and radiographic progression. Radiology 1984;153:589–593.

Roig J, Domingo C, Morera J. Legionnaires' disease. Chest 1994;105:1817–1825.

CASE 28

Philip C. Goodman

HISTORY

A 32-year-old homosexual man who tested positive for the human immunodeficiency virus (HIV) 3 years earlier now presents with gradual onset of shortness of breath and slight fever.

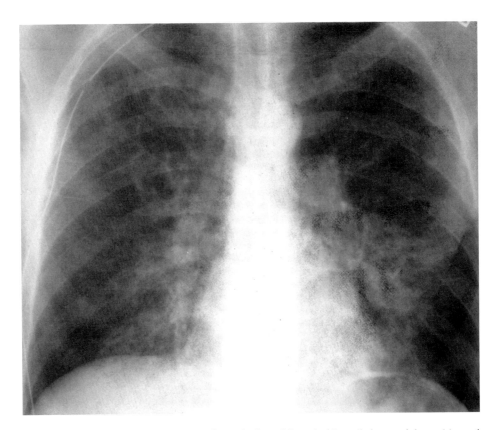

FIGURE 1-28 Posteroanterior chest radiograph shows bilateral, thin-walled upper lobe cavities and perihilar heterogeneous parenchymal opacities. A right-sided pleural chest tube was placed for evacuation of a spontaneous pneumothorax.

◆ DIFFERENTIAL DIAGNOSIS

◆ **Bronchiectasis:** The size and type of cavitation is occasionally seen in severe bronchiectasis, although there is no other evidence of peribronchial thickening nor is there a history of a chronic productive cough.

◆ **Pneumatoceles:** Those due to trauma, staphylococcal pneumonia, or hydrocarbon inhalation are usually localized to a single lobe rather than disseminated throughout the lungs. However, pneumatoceles due to *Pneumocystis carinii* pneumonia can be diffuse.

◆ **Coccidioidomycosis:** Chronic coccidioidomycosis can result in thin-walled cavities, but the extent of involvement in this patient is unusual for coccidioidomycosis, particularly given the mild symptoms.

◆ **Cavitary metastases:** Although cavitary metastases can be this thin-walled, there is usually more irregularity to the walls. Also, the presence of noncavitary nodules would have been more suggestive of this diagnosis.

◆ **Collagen vascular disease:** Wegener's granulomatosis and rheumatoid lung disease can manifest with cavitary nodules/masses. However, the walls are generally not this thin, nor are the nodules this numerous.

◆ DIAGNOSIS: *Pneumocystis carinii* pneumonia with pneumatoceles.

◆ KEY FACTS

CLINICAL

◆ *P. carinii* was initially considered a trypanosome, was then reclassified as a protozoan, but is phylogenetically more closely related to fungi.

◆ In the United States, asymptomatic infection with *P. carinii* occurs mainly in early childhood. Clinically identifiable disease manifests in severely immunocompromised patients.

◆ Symptoms are generally nonspecific, including fever, dyspnea, nonproductive cough, fatigue, and weight loss.

◆ Prophylaxis with aerosolized pentamidine or periodic trimethoprim-sulfamethoxasole therapy has been effective in decreasing the number of patients presenting with *P. carinii* pneumonia.

◆ The diagnosis is made by observing organisms on induced sputum, bronchoalveolar lavage, or transbronchial lung biopsy specimens.

◆ Treatment is generally with trimethoprim-sulfamethoxazole or pentamidine. Steroids, dapsone, or clindamycin-primaquine have also been used.

◆ Response to therapy is generally excellent. Clinical improvement is typically seen within several days. Nevertheless, some patients will procede to respiratory failure, requiring stringent therapeutic supportive measures.

◆ Pneumatoceles observed in PCP are the result of the organism and not a result of aerosolized pentamidine therapy.

RADIOLOGIC

◆ PCP typically manifests with diffuse, bilateral, fine to medium reticulonodular opacities.

◆ Unusual appearances include focal homogeneous opacities and larger (1 to 2 cm) nodules with or without cavitation.

◆ Pneumatoceles are seen in approximately 10% of patients with PCP. Although their size may fluctuate daily, pneumatoceles are usually stable for several days to weeks. They typically resolve within 6 months. Fluid levels in pneumatoceles are extremely rare. Spontaneous pneumothorax occurs in 5% to 6% of patients with PCP.

◆ Lymphadenopathy and pleural effusions are extremely rare in patients with PCP.

◆ With appropriate therapy, resolution of abnormalities can be complete after 10 days. Occasionally, residual fibrosis is observed.

◆ SUGGESTED READING

Goodman PC, Daley C, Minagi H. Spontaneous pneumothorax in AIDS patients with *Pneumocystis carinii* pneumonia. AJR Am J Roentgenol 1985;147:29–31.

Goodman PC. AIDS. In IM Freundlich, DG Bragg (eds), A Radiologic Approach to Diseases of the Chest. Baltimore: Williams & Wilkins, 1992.

Hopewell PC, Masur H. *Pneumocystis carinii* Pneumonia: Current Concepts. In MA Sande, PA Volberding (eds), The Medical Management of AIDS (4th ed). Philadelphia: Saunders, 1995.

Sandhu JS, Goodman PC. Pulmonary cysts associated with *Pneumocystis carinii* pneumonia in patients with AIDS. Radiology 1989;173:33–35.

CHAPTER 2

BREAST IMAGING

Mary Scott Soo, *chapter editor*

Phyllis J. Kornguth, Mary Scott Soo,
Ruth Walsh, and Margaret E. Williford

CASE 1

Margaret E. Williford

HISTORY

Screening mammogram in a 44-year-old woman.

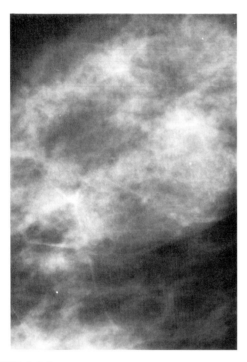

FIGURE 2-1A Photographically enlarged craniocaudal mammogram of posterior right breast. Multiple smudge-like densities are present. No calcifications were identified in other regions of the breast.

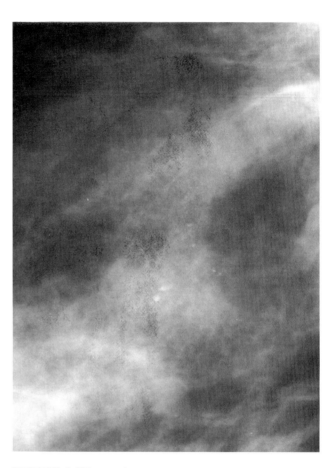

FIGURE 2-1B Magnified mediolateral oblique mammogram of the right breast, imaging the same region seen in Figure 2-1A. Smudge-like densities are seen more prominently and have calcium density.

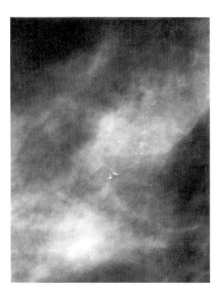

FIGURE 2-1C Magnified true lateral mammogram of the right breast in the same region seen in Figures 2-1A and 2-1B. The calcifications are denser and assume a teacup or meniscus appearance as they layer dependently.

◆ DIFFERENTIAL DIAGNOSIS

◆ **Milk of calcium:** This is the best diagnosis because milk of calcium has different appearances depending on the mammographic projection obtained. The calcifications are often smudge-like or indistinct on the craniocaudal views but have a teacup or meniscus appearance on horizontal beam radiographs.

◆ **Fat necrosis:** The calcifications associated with fat necrosis often vary in density and shape and can be indistinguishable from carcinoma. Many of the calcifications evolve over time to a more coarse configuration, or may have an eggshell appearance, as seen in oil cysts. However, the appearance of fat necrosis does not usually vary on the different projections, making this an unlikely diagnosis in this case.

◆ DIAGNOSIS: Milk of calcium.

◆ KEY FACTS

CLINICAL

◆ Milk of calcium represents calcified debris that is sedimented in the dependent portions of microcysts or cystically dilated acini of cystic lobular hyperplasia.

◆ Benign milk of calcium calcifications are seen in 4% to 6% of women undergoing mammography.

◆ Milk of calcium is usually seen in multiple areas of the breast and is usually bilateral. It can be a diagnostic problem when it appears as a unilateral focus. It is important to recognize milk of calcium so that an inappropriate biopsy is not recommended.

◆ Milk of calcium calcifications are benign and do not require a biopsy, but carcinomas can occur adjacent to such microcystic calcifications. Therefore, each group of calcifications must be inspected carefully.

RADIOLOGIC

◆ The shape of milk of calcium calcifications has been described as meniscus, crescent, teacup, or semilunar.

The meniscus or crescent shape is best seen on an erect 90-degree lateral projection since the x-ray beam is horizontal and therefore tangential to the fluid calcium interface in the microcyst.

◆ On the 90-degree lateral view, the tops of the calcifications will be oriented parallel to one another along the horizontal axis. The upper border of the calcification may be less distinct than the lower border where the sedimented calcified debris is sharply bounded by the wall of the microcyst.

◆ The characteristic meniscus or crescent shape is not as well seen on the 45-degree mediolateral oblique view.

◆ On the craniocaudal projection, the calcifications are seen en face since the x-ray beam is vertical and therefore perpendicular to the fluid calcium interface in the microcyst.

◆ On the craniocaudal projection, the calcifications are amorphous, round, or ovoid smudges. They can be so faint that they are invisible.

◆ The dramatic difference in the appearance of the calcifications on the craniocaudal, mediolateral, and 90-degree lateral projections is a characteristic feature of benign milk of calcium.

◆ When milk of calcium calcifications are suspected, a magnification view in the 90-degree lateral projection should be performed.

◆ SUGGESTED READING

Hamer MJ, Cooper AG, Pile-Spellman ER. Milk of calcium in breast microcysts: Manifestation as a solitary focal disease. AJR Am J Roentgenol 1988;150:789.

Linden SS, Sickles EA. Sedimented calcium in benign breast cysts. AJR Am J Roentgenol 1989;152:957.

Sickles EA, Abele JS. Milk of calcium within tiny benign breast cysts. Radiology 1981;141:655.

CASE 2

Ruth Walsh

HISTORY

A 45-year-old asymptomatic woman presenting for a screening mammogram. A breast ultrasound was subsequently performed.

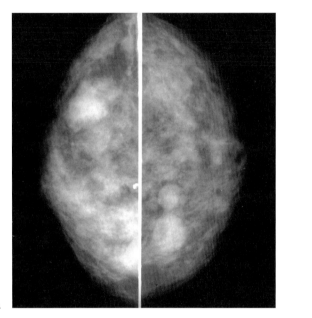

A

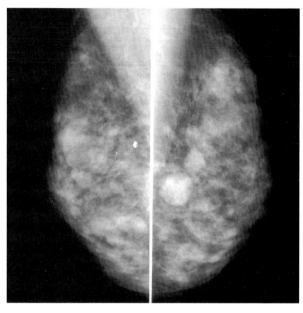

B

FIGURES 2-2A and 2-2B Craniocaudal (**A**) and mediolateral oblique (**B**) mammograms of both breasts. Multiple, bilateral, predominantly well-circumscribed oval and round masses are present.

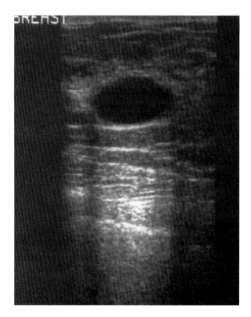

FIGURE 2-2C Longitudinal sonographic image of the medial left breast, 10:00 position. Sonography of one of the masses shows an anechoic, well-circumscribed oval mass with posterior acoustic enhancement. This appearance was typical of the remainder of the masses.

◆ DIFFERENTIAL DIAGNOSIS

◆ **Cysts:** As seen in this case, cysts are anechoic, well-circumscribed masses that have posterior acoustic enhancement. Cysts are the most commonly encountered breast masses, which cannot be differentiated from other circumscribed masses at mammography unless they contain milk of calcium. Sonography can differentiate cysts from solid breast masses accurately.

◆ **Fibroadenomas:** Fibroadenomas can be multiple or bilateral in 15% of cases and are the most common palpable breast masses in adolescents and young women. Although noncalcified fibroadenomas cannot be differentiated at mammography from other circumscribed masses, fibroadenomas appear solid at sonography, unlike the lesions in this case. Large, coarse, popcorn-like calcifications are pathognomonic mammographic findings of degenerating fibroadenomas.

◆ **Metastases:** The sonographic appearance of metastases is that of a solid mass, differing from the lesions seen in this case. Metastatic disease to the breast from an extramammary primary malignancy is rare (0.5% to 1.3% of breast malignancies) and most often has the mammographic appearance of single or multiple circumscribed masses. A clinical history of extramammary malignancy should be present to suspect this diagnosis.

◆ **Papillomas:** Papillomas are rarely visible at mammography. They are usually <1 cm in size and are typically located in the subareolar region. At sonography, papillomas are often solid, lobulated masses. These features make this diagnosis unlikely in the case illustrated. A papilloma can also present as a solid nodule within a cyst, for which biopsy is indicated to exclude a malignant lesion.

◆ **Lymph nodes:** Intramammary lymph nodes are typically <1 cm in size, often demonstrate a fatty hilus at mammography, and are usually located in the upper outer quadrants of the breasts. At sonography, lymph nodes are usually hypoechoic with an echogenic fatty hilus. All these features make this an unlikely diagnosis in this case.

◆ DIAGNOSIS: Bilateral simple cysts confirmed by ultrasound.

◆ KEY FACTS

CLINICAL

◆ Cysts can be seen in all age groups but are more common in women 30 to 50 years of age.

◆ Cysts arise in the terminal-duct lobular units. They can be grossly visible at mammography or seen only microscopically.

◆ Autopsy studies report grossly visible cysts in 20% to 50% of women.

◆ Cysts cannot be differentiated reliably from solid palpable masses on physical examination. Therefore, sonography or needle aspiration is necessary to confirm the diagnosis.

RADIOLOGIC

◆ Cysts are typically round, oval, or lobular in shape and often multiple and bilateral.

◆ Cyst margins are usually well defined on mammography if not obscured by adjacent fibroglandular tissue. Occasionally, the margins can be indistinct.

◆ Because cysts cannot be differentiated from other circumscribed masses at mammography, sonography is often performed to establish the diagnosis.

◆ Strict sonographic criteria for a simple cyst include anechoic appearance, smooth, well-defined margins, and posterior acoustic enhancement.

◆ When multiple, bilateral, well-circumscribed masses are present on a baseline screening mammogram, sonography can be performed to determine if the masses are cystic or solid. A 12-month follow-up mammogram is usually recommended for cystic or solid masses if there are no suspicious features, dominant mass, or history of an extramammary malignancy.

◆ SUGGESTED READING

Adler DD. Mammographic Evaluation of Masses. In DB Kopans (ed), Syllabus: A Categorical Course in Breast Imaging. Oak Brook, IL: RSNA, 1995;107–116.

Bohman LG, Bassett LW, Gold RH, Volt R. Breast metastases from extramammary malignancies. Radiology 1982;144:309–312.

Jackson VP. Circumscribed Microlobulated Noncalcified Mass. In BA Siegel (ed), Breast Disease Test and Syllabus (2nd series). Reston, VA: American College of Radiology, 1993;89–99.

Kopans DB (ed). Breast Imaging. Philadelphia: Lippincott, 1989.

CASE 3

Phyllis J. Kornguth

HISTORY

Screening mammogram in a 63-year-old woman.

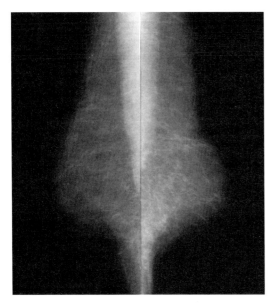

FIGURE 2-3A Mediolateral oblique mammograms of both breasts show no mammographic abnormality in fatty replaced breasts.

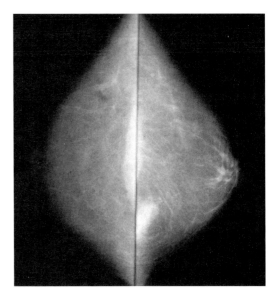

FIGURE 2-3B Craniocaudal mammograms of both breasts demonstrate an incompletely imaged, well-defined mass posteriorly and medially in the left breast.

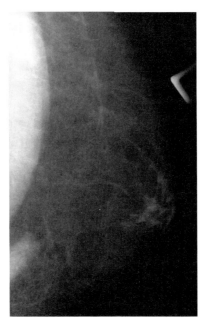

FIGURE 2-3C Medially exaggerated craniocaudal mammogram of the left breast better defines the mass. However, it cannot be completely imaged even on exaggerated views.

◆ DIFFERENTIAL DIAGNOSIS

- **Sternalis muscle:** This is the typical mammographic appearance and correct anatomic location for the sternalis muscle, making this the best diagnosis.
- **Fibroadenoma:** Fibroadenomas result from stromal overgrowth of the lobules and are typically seen more anteriorly in the breast. The inability to image the lesion on the mediolateral oblique view makes this diagnosis less likely.
- **Carcinoma:** Because carcinomas can occur at any location in the breast, this diagnosis was considered and prompted biopsy in this case.

◆ DIAGNOSIS: Sternalis muscle.

◆ KEY FACTS

CLINICAL

- The sternalis muscle is a normal variant of chest wall musculature.
- It lies anterior to the pectoralis muscle along the edge of the sternum, extending from the inferior clavicle to the caudal sternum.
- This muscle is uncommon, occurring in <u>8%</u> of men and women, and <u>occurs unilaterally twice as often</u> as bilaterally.

RADIOLOGIC

- The sternalis muscle appears as a small asymmetric density of varying shapes that projects into the medial breast posteriorly.
- The sternalis muscle should be differentiated from the pectoralis muscle, which is seen as a long convex bulge along the chest wall on 30% of craniocaudal mammograms.
- The sternalis muscle is seen on the craniocaudal mammogram only and not on the mediolateral oblique mammogram.
- In the case illustrated here, the mass could not be localized in two views; therefore needle localization was performed using stereotactic guidance.
- Awareness of this entity prevents needless biopsies. If necessary, this finding can be confirmed to be sternalis muscle using CT or MRI.

◆ SUGGESTED READING

Bradley FM, Hoover HC, Hulka CA, et al. The sternalis muscle: An unusual normal finding seen on mammography. AJR Am J Roentgenol 1996;166:33–36.

Kopans DB. Pathologic, Mammographic, and Sonographic Correlation. In DB Kopans (ed), Breast Imaging. Philadelphia: Lippincott, 1989;262–265.

CASE 4

Phyllis J. Kornguth

HISTORY

Screening mammogram in a 73-year-old woman. Past medical history is significant for abdominal surgery 1 year ago with chronic wound dehiscence.

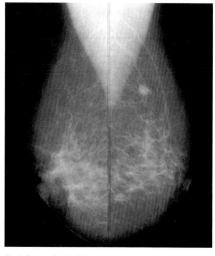

A

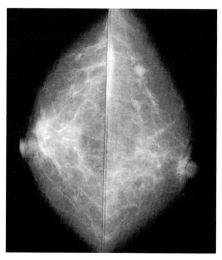

B

FIGURES 2-4A and 2-4B Mediolateral oblique (**A**) and craniocaudal (**B**) mammograms of both breasts. A well-circumscribed, solitary 8-mm nodule is located in the upper outer quadrant of the left breast.

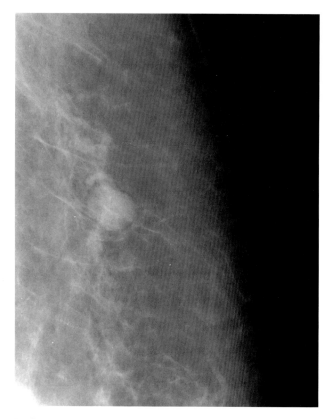

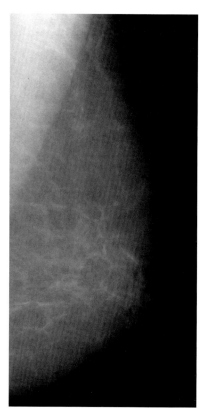

FIGURE 2-4C Magnification craniocaudal mammogram of the left breast shows the well-defined margins of the mass and a small lucent area posteriorly, suggestive of fatty hilum in a lymph node.

FIGURE 2-4D Mediolateral oblique mammogram of left breast from 1 year prior to the current study shows that the nodule is an intra-mammary lymph node, which was smaller on the previous examination.

◆ DIFFERENTIAL DIAGNOSIS

- **Metastatic breast carcinoma:** This diagnosis is considered unlikely because no evidence for primary breast carcinoma is seen within the fatty replaced breast.
- **Metastasis from an extramammary carcinoma:** If the patient's abdominal surgery was for resection of ovarian or colon carcinoma, the diagnosis of metastatic carcinoma should be considered, although metastases to the breast are very rare. Without a history of metastases elsewhere from an extramammary primary, this diagnosis should be considered very unlikely.
- **Reactive lymph node:** In a patient with the clinical history of chronic abdominal wound infection, a reactive intramammary lymph node should be considered likely if no other abnormalities are identified throughout the ipsilateral breast.

◆ DIAGNOSIS: Reactive enlargement of an intramammary lymph node.

◆ KEY FACTS

CLINICAL

- Intramammary lymph nodes can enlarge secondary to infections located on the chest, in the breast, in the abdomen and upper extremity, or due to dermatologic abnormalities such as psoriasis.

- Physical examination to search for inciting infectious or dermatologic abnormalities is essential in correctly diagnosing correctly reactive lymph nodes within the breast.

RADIOLOGIC

- Magnification views are often useful in evaluating a suspected intramammary lymph node because they may better demonstrate the fatty hilum.
- The management of enlarged intramammary lymph nodes that occur without other mammographic abnormality requires mammographic follow-up after treatment of the infectious or dermatologic abnormality to assure that the lymph node returns to normal size and density.

◆ SUGGESTED READING

Kopans DB. Mammography. In DB Kopans (ed), Breast Imaging. Philadelphia: Lippincott, 1989;34–226.

Kopans DB, Meyer JE. Benign lymph nodes associated with dermatitis presenting as breast masses. Radiology 1980;137:15–19.

Lindfors KK, Kopans DB, McCarthy KA, et al. Breast metastasis to intramammary lymph nodes. AJR Am J Roentgenol 1986;146: 133–136.

Meyers JE, Kopans DB, Lawrence WD. Normal intramammary lymph nodes presenting as occult breast masses. Breast 1982;8:30–32.

Svane G, Franzen S. Radiologic appearance of nonpalpable intramammary lymph nodes. Acta Radiol 1993;34:577–580.

HISTORY

A 43-year-old woman with a palpable lump in the upper outer quadrant of the right breast presents for diagnostic mammography. There is no past surgical history.

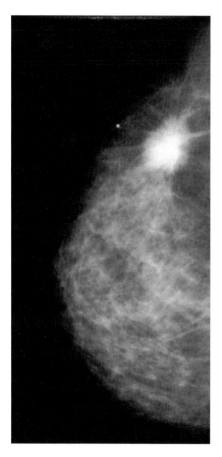

A

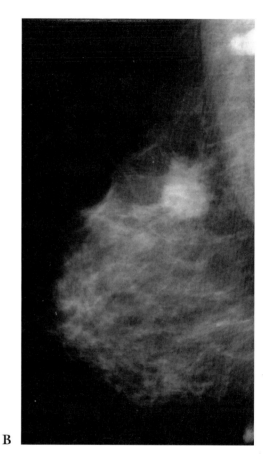

B

FIGURES 2-5A and 2-5B Exaggerated lateral craniocaudal view of the right breast with cutaneous BB marking the palpable lump (**A**), and mediolateral oblique view of the right breast (**B**). A 3-cm irregular mass with spiculated margins is present in the upper outer quadrant of the right breast. Several faint punctate microcalcifications are present within the mass. A rounded, dense 1.5-cm lymph node is present in the right axilla.

◆ DIFFERENTIAL DIAGNOSIS

◆ **Carcinoma:** A mass with spiculated margins is almost pathognomonic of malignancy. The abnormal axillary lymph node is suggestive of metastatic disease. These features make carcinoma the most likely diagnosis. Although a few benign processes can present as spiculated lesions, biopsy is indicated to exclude malignancy.

◆ **Post-traumatic scarring and fat necrosis:** There is no history of prior trauma or breast surgery, making this diagnosis unlikely. A postoperative scar can appear as an area of architectural distortion or a spiculated mass that should either decrease in size and density or remain stable over time. Any increase in size should prompt biopsy. To confirm the diagnosis of a surgical scar, the site of the spiculated lesion must match the location of the patient's cutaneous scar and the location of the biopsied lesion on preoperative or needle localization mammograms (if available).

◆ **Radial scar/complex sclerosing lesion:** Radial scars are spiculated masses or regions of architectural distortion that typically have long, thin spicules radiating outward from a radiolucent center. However, occasionally they can appear dense centrally and contain microcalcifications. The large central mass in this case makes the diagnosis of radial scar unlikely. The term *radial scar* is used when the lesion measures <1 cm and *complex sclerosing lesion* is used when the lesion measures >1 cm. These benign proliferative lesions of unknown etiology are usually nonpalpable and cannot be differentiated reliably from carcinoma without biopsy.

◆ **Abscess:** Because there is no history of pain, swelling, or erythema, this is an unlikely diagnosis. Abscesses tend to occur in the subareolar region and often are associated with mammographic changes of mastitis, such as diffuse skin thickening and increased trabecular density.

◆ **Granular cell tumor:** These benign tumors have a spiculated appearance at mammography but are very rare, making this diagnosis less likely. Biopsy is indicated to differentiate these lesions from carcinoma.

◆ **Extra-abdominal desmoid tumor:** These are locally invasive tumors that do not metastasize. Their mammographic appearance mimics that of an invasive breast cancer, requiring biopsy for diagnosis. These, too, are rare, making the diagnosis unlikely in the case illustrated.

◆ DIAGNOSIS: Infiltrating ductal carcinoma with metastatic carcinoma to axillary lymph nodes.

◆ KEY FACTS

CLINICAL

◆ Breast cancer is the most common malignancy in American women, excluding skin cancers. After lung cancer, it is the second leading cause of cancer death among women.

◆ According to current estimates, breast cancer will be diagnosed in approximately 1 in 8 women in their lifetime.

◆ Invasive ductal carcinoma, not otherwise specified, comprises 65% to 80% of invasive breast cancers. The second most common type is invasive lobular carcinoma, accounting for 3% to 14% of cases. Other, less common specific forms of ductal carcinoma include medullary, mucinous, papillary, and tubular carcinoma.

RADIOLOGIC

◆ A spiculated mass, characterized by lines radiating outward from a central mass, is the most common mammographic appearance for invasive ductal carcinoma.

◆ Spiculated margins usually signify invasion.

◆ Spiculated projections result from (1) a desmoplastic response (connective tissue proliferation) that distorts the adjacent tissue, (2) tumor infiltrating into the surrounding tissue, or (3) both conditions.

◆ A spectrum of mammographic appearances can be seen with invasive ductal carcinoma, including: (1) masses with either spiculated, microlobulated, indistinct, and circumscribed margins; (2) architectural distortion; and (3) focal asymmetric or developing densities.

◆ SUGGESTED READING

Adler DD. Mammographic Evaluation of Masses. In DB Kopans (ed), Syllabus: A Categorical Course in Breast Imaging. Oak Brook, IL: RSNA, 1995;107–116.

De Paredes ES. Atlas of Film-Screen Mammography. Baltimore: Williams & Wilkins, 1992.

Feig SA. Breast masses: Mammographic and sonographic evaluation. Radiol Clin North Am 1992;30:67–92.

Smith RA. The Epidemiology of Breast Cancer. In DB Kopans (ed), Syllabus: A Categorical Course in Breast Imaging. Oak Brook, IL: RSNA, 1995;7–20.

CASE 6

Margaret E. Williford

HISTORY

Screening mammogram in a 70-year-old woman, status post right lumpectomy and radiation therapy for treatment of carcinoma.

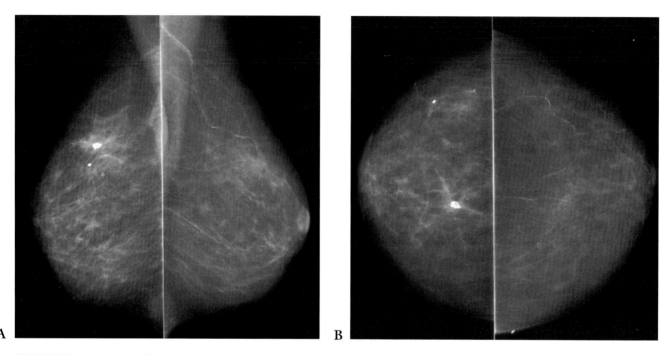

FIGURES 2-6A and 2-6B Mediolateral oblique (**A**) and craniocaudal (**B**) mammograms of right and left breasts. Right breast shows diffuse, increased asymmetric density and focal distortion with coarse dystrophic calcification in the superior medial quadrant.

◆DIFFERENTIAL DIAGNOSIS

◆ **Postoperative and postradiation changes of right breast**: This is the best diagnosis given the history.
◆ **Edema:** This diagnosis is less likely because edema is commonly bilateral, with no associated mass or focal distortion. Correlation with physical exam is helpful.
◆ **Inflammatory carcinoma:** Inflammatory carcinoma has prominent, diffuse asymmetric density and skin thickening. In its pure form, there is no focal mass or distortion, but in many cases, there is a focal mass-like density. Clinical presentation and physical exam are important correlates, which demonstrate an erythematous, nontender breast with peau d'orange appearance of the skin. This diagnosis is considered less likely due to the history of radiation therapy. Inflammatory carcinoma also would not be expected to be associated with dystrophic calcifications.
◆ **Mastitis:** Mastitis presents with a clinical history of tenderness and fever, not present in this case. Physical exam reveals cutaneous inflammatory changes and tenderness. Focal mass is usually not present unless there is an abscess. Biopsy is indicated if there is incomplete resolution with antibiotic therapy.

◆ DIAGNOSIS: Postoperative and postradiation changes following lumpectomy and radiation therapy.

◆KEY FACTS

CLINICAL

◆ Lumpectomy creates focal distortion of normal breast parenchyma at the site of the tumor. Radiation causes fibrosis throughout the breast and can enhance the distortion created by the surgical excision.
◆ Skin thickening and asymmetry in breast size may be evident on clinical exam.

RADIOLOGIC

◆ Diagnosis of postoperative distortion can be confirmed by correlating post-therapy films with preoperative films showing the site of the tumor and needle localization done before the surgical excision.
◆ Postoperative distortion and asymmetric increased density due to surgery and radiation are most prominent on the first post-therapy film done 6 to 12 months after therapy.
◆ Distortion and asymmetric density gradually stabilize or resolve over time, usually 2.5 to 3.0 years following therapy.
◆ Dystrophic calcifications are a commonly associated finding, particularly at the lumpectomy site. Radiation and surgery can also cause benign fat necrosis calcifications.
◆ Recurrent tumor can occur at the site of the primary tumor. Increased mass, distortion, or malignant-appearing calcifications are signs that may indicate recurrence. These findings should prompt biopsy.

◆SUGGESTED READING

Mendelson EB. Evaluation of the post-operative breast. Radiol Clin North Am 1992;30:107–138.

HISTORY

Diagnostic mammogram in a 33-year-old woman with pain in her left breast. Sixteen years ago she underwent breast augmentation with silicone implants; the right implant was ruptured and replaced 3 years before the mammogram.

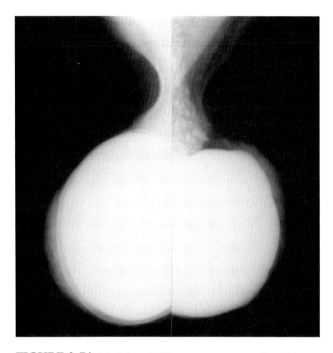

FIGURE 2-7A Mediolateral oblique mammograms of both breasts. Bilateral subglandular implants are present. On the left, the contour of the single-lumen silicone implant is lobulated, and multiple high-density nodules are seen in the left axilla. On the right, a double-lumen implant is present with the outer saline lumen intact.

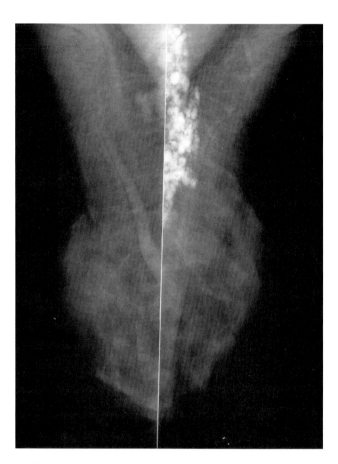

FIGURE 2-7B Repeat mediolateral oblique mammograms of both breasts 1 year after explantation of the prostheses. The prostheses have been removed. There are persistent high-density nodules within the left axilla. No mammographic abnormality is seen within either breast.

◆ DIFFERENTIAL DIAGNOSIS

◆ **Ruptured silicone implant with free silicone extravasation into the left axilla:** This is the best diagnosis because the high-density nodules in the axilla are equal in density to the silicone prosthesis, resulting from migration of free silicone away from the ruptured prosthesis. The lobulated contour of the prosthesis is not specific for implant rupture if seen as an isolated finding but should raise the question of rupture and prompt further evaluation.

◆ **Breast carcinoma metastatic to axillary lymph nodes:** This diagnosis is unlikely because the density of the nodules in the axilla is equal to silicone, higher even than expected for nodes involved with metastatic disease. In addition, there are no breast lesions that are suspicious for carcinoma.

◆ **Sarcoidosis:** Axillary lymph nodes can be seen at mammography in patients with sarcoidosis. However, the process is usually bilateral, and nodes are usually enlarged. Abnormal lymph nodes associated with sarcoidosis are denser than normal fatty-replaced lymph nodes but do not have density as high as silicone, making this an unlikely diagnosis in this case.

◆ DIAGNOSIS: Ruptured silicone prosthesis on the left, with residual free silicone seen 1 year later.

◆ KEY FACTS

CLINICAL

◆ Rupture of prostheses (intracapsular or extracapsular) is considered a major complication of prosthesis placement, which necessitates surgical explantation of the ruptured implant.

◆ Intracapsular rupture occurs when the gel escaping from a ruptured implant is contained within the surrounding fibrous capsule.

◆ Extracapsular rupture occurs when free silicone from a ruptured implant extends outside of the fibrous capsule. This free silicone is difficult to remove completely at surgery and can stimulate a granulomatous reaction within the breast.

◆ Silicone granulomas can cause a palpable mass which is difficult to differentiate from carcinoma.

RADIOLOGIC

◆ When extracapsular free silicone is present, the diagnosis of rupture can often be made mammographically because the density of the free silicone within the breast tissue is higher than that of other structures.

◆ The presence of extracapsular silicone is often diagnostic of implant rupture. However, sometimes prior films are needed to document the source of the rupture. For instance, in a patient in whom a previously ruptured implant has been replaced, prior films would be needed to determine which implant was the source of the extracapsular silicone.

◆ Ruptures that occur posteriorly or ruptures in which only a small amount of silicone escapes into the breast parenchyma may not be detected mammographically because they are either not included on the image or the dense prosthesis obscures visualization of the free silicone. In these situations, other imaging studies, such as MRI or sonography, are necessary to make the diagnosis.

◆ Mammography cannot detect intracapsular rupture reliably. MRI has the highest sensitivity and specificity for diagnosing intracapsular rupture.

◆ SUGGESTED READING

Berg WA, Caskey CI, Hamper UM, et al. Diagnosing breast implant rupture with MR imaging, US, and mammography. Radiographics 1993;13:1323–1336.

Berg WA, Caskey CI, Hamper UM, et al. Single- and double-lumen silicone breast implant integrity: Prospective evaluation of MR and US criteria. Radiology 1995;197:45–52.

Destouet JM, Monsees BS, Oser RF, et al. Screening mammography in 350 women with breast implants: Prevalence and findings of implant complications. AJR Am J Roentgenol 1992;159: 973–987.

Everson LI, Parantainen H, Detlie T, et al. Diagnosis of breast implant rupture: Imaging findings and relative efficacies of imaging techniques. AJR Am J Roentgenol 1994;163:57–60.

Gorczyca DP, Sinha S, Ahn CY, et al. Silicone breast implants in vivo: MR imaging. Radiology 1992;185:407–410.

CASE 8

Ruth Walsh

HISTORY

Diagnostic mammogram in a 52-year-old female, status post left mastectomy for breast cancer and right subcutaneous mastectomy with reconstruction.

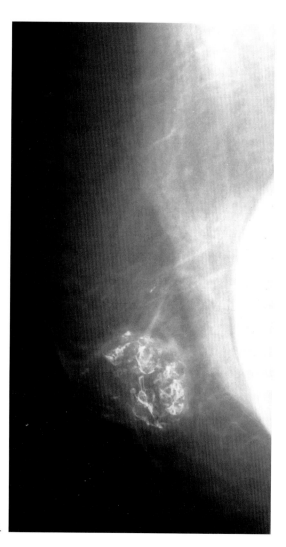

A

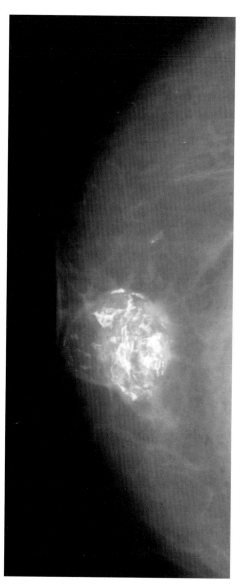

B

FIGURES 2-8A and 2-8B Routine mediolateral oblique (**A**) and craniocaudal "exclusion" or "push-back" (**B**) mammograms of the right breast. Minimal residual fibroglandular tissue remains in the breast status post subcutaneous mastectomy. A 3-cm radiolucent mass with associated rim-like and dystrophic calcifications is present in the subareolar region. A submuscular silicone implant is partially visualized on the mediolateral oblique view.

◆ DIFFERENTIAL DIAGNOSIS

◆ **Fat necrosis:** Low-density (fatty) masses in the breast are almost always benign. A low-density mass associated with dystrophic (bizarre, irregular, and plaque-like) calcifications, as is seen in this case, is most consistent with fat necrosis. Dystrophic calcifications can be seen with fat necrosis secondary to trauma, surgery, or radiation therapy.

◆ **Carcinoma:** Malignant calcifications are usually <0.5 mm in size, ranging from minute up to 3 mm. Many of the calcifications in the case illustrated are >2 to 3 mm in size and have benign rim and plaque-like shapes, making carcinoma an unlikely diagnosis.

◆ **Fibroadenoma:** Although fibroadenomas can contain large, bizarre, irregular calcifications, as seen in this case, involuting fibroadenomas typically contain coarse or "popcorn-like" calcifications. The mass in this case is not consistent with a fibroadenoma because it has low density, as opposed to fibroadenomas, which are water-density masses.

◆ **Secondary hyperparathyroidism with metastatic calcifications:** Patients with hypercalcemia can develop coarse amorphous calcifications within the breast. However, calcifications would not be expected to be rim-like or associated with a radiolucent mass, making this diagnosis unlikely.

◆ DIAGNOSIS: Fat necrosis secondary to prior surgery.

◆ KEY FACTS

CLINICAL

◆ Fat necrosis is an inflammatory response that is usually due to trauma or surgery but can be idiopathic.

◆ Fat necrosis can be difficult to distinguish from carcinoma on both physical examination and mammography.

◆ Clinically, fat necrosis can present as a hard painless mass that is ill-defined and poorly mobile. Skin thickening or retraction may also be identified, increasing the clinical suspicion of carcinoma.

◆ In some cases, the traumatic event leading to fat necrosis is forgotten or unknown.

RADIOLOGIC

◆ At mammography, fat necrosis has a wide spectrum of appearances, ranging from well-defined oil cysts to spiculated masses that simulate carcinoma.

◆ Calcifications are commonly associated with fat necrosis. When calcifications first appear they can be small and pleomorphic, mimicking malignant calcifications. However, they usually evolve into larger, coarse, plaque-like calcifications that have a more benign appearance.

◆ Early dystrophic calcifications can be difficult to distinguish from malignancy. Magnification mammography and close (4 to 6 months) mammographic follow-up are often indicated in patients with suspected fat necrosis. Occasionally biopsy is necessary to exclude malignancy.

◆ SUGGESTED READING

De Paredes ES. Atlas of Film-Screen Mammography. Baltimore: Williams & Wilkins, 1992.

Feig SA. Mammographic Evaluation of Calcifications. In DB Kopans, EB Mendelson (eds), Syllabus: A Categorical Course in Breast Imaging. Oak Brook, IL: RSNA, 1995.

Mendelson EB. Evaluation of the post operative breast. Radiol Clin North Am 1992;30:107–138.

Morrow M. Breast Trauma, Hematoma, and Fat Necrosis. In JR Harris, S Hellman, IC Henderson, DW Kinne (eds), Breast Disease. Philadelphia: Lippincott, 1991.

CASE 9

Phyllis J. Kornguth

HISTORY

Screening mammogram in a 36-year-old woman. The family history is significant for a sister with premenopausal breast carcinoma.

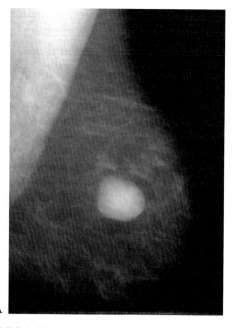

A

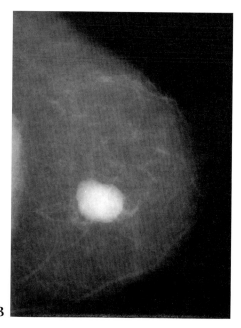

B

FIGURES 2-9A and 2-9B Mediolateral oblique (**A**) and craniocaudal (**B**) mammograms of the left breast show a large, well-circumscribed, solitary noncalcified mass located centrally in a predominantly fatty-replaced breast. The mass was new compared to the prior exam.

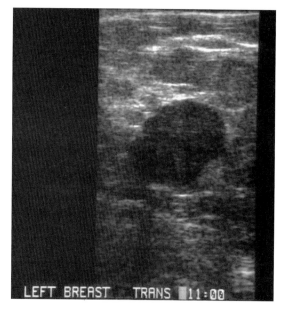

FIGURE 2-9C Sonogram of the mass seen in Figures 2-9A and 2-9B shows a well-defined, solid hypoechoic mass with no posterior acoustic enhancement or shadowing.

◆DIFFERENTIAL DIAGNOSIS

- **Fibroadenoma:** The mammographic and sonographic features of this lesion, as well as the young age of the patient, are typical of a fibroadenoma.
- **Carcinoma:** Some well-defined carcinomas (medullary, mucinous, papillary) can have these mammographic and sonographic features. However, these tumors are uncommon tumors, making this diagnosis less likely.
- **Phyllodes tumor:** At mammography, phyllodes tumors are well-circumscribed, often large masses indistinguishable from fibroadenomas or other tumors. The sonographic appearance of a phyllodes tumor can be identical to the lesion in the case illustrated. However, many phyllodes tumors contain cystic spaces, producing a more heterogeneous sonographic appearance.
- **Cyst:** The mammographic features of a cyst can be identical to the appearance of the mass in this case. However, the sonogram reveals a solid mass, not a simple cyst.

◆DIAGNOSIS: Fibroadenoma.

◆KEY FACTS

CLINICAL

- Fibroadenomas are common benign breast lesions that occur in premenopausal and perimenopausal age groups.
- On physical examination, the mass is usually firm, well-defined, and mobile.
- Growth of fibroadenomas is stimulated by hormonal influence.
- Fibroadenomas can be multiple and bilateral. Multiplicity and bilaterality are more common in black women.

RADIOLOGIC

- The management of a probably benign mass involves close mammographic follow-up at 6-month intervals. Mammographic follow-up is less expensive and less invasive than surgical biopsy. Only a small proportion (~1.5%) of well-circumscribed masses are found to be malignant tumors.
- In the small proportion of masses that prove to be malignant tumors, the delay in diagnosis due to mammographic follow-up does not alter the prognosis when compared to diagnosing the cancer at the time of initial screening.
- In the case illustrated, the mass was considered probably benign by mammographic and sonographic features. However, biopsy was performed because the mass was new and the patient had a strong family history for premenopausal breast carcinoma.
- Stereotactic biopsy is often useful in these cases to make the diagnosis because it is less invasive and less expensive than open surgical biopsy.

◆SUGGESTED READING

Liberman L, Bonaccio E, Hamele-Bena D, et al. Benign and malignant phyllodes tumors: Mammographic and sonographic findings. Radiology 1996;198:122–124.

Sickles EA. Nonpalpable, circumscribed, noncalcified solid breast masses: Likelihood of malignancy based on lesion size and age of patient. Radiology 1994;192:439–442.

Smith BL. Fibroadenomas. In JR Harris, S Hellman, IC Henderson, DW Kinne (eds), Breast Diseases. Philadelphia: Lippincott, 1991;34–37.

HISTORY

Screening mammogram in a 64-year-old women. A true lateral mammogram was performed because of a questionable area of distortion anteriorly on the right that did not persist. A sonogram of the superior right breast was subsequently performed.

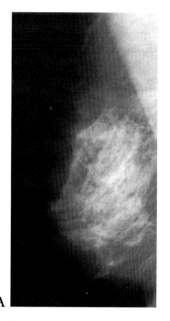

A

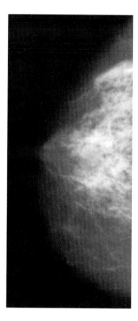

B

FIGURES 2-10A and 2-10B Mediolateral oblique (**A**) and craniocaudal (**B**) mammograms of the right breast show dense fibroglandular tissue with no mammographic abnormality.

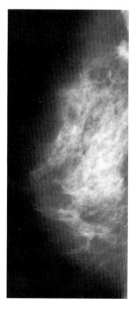

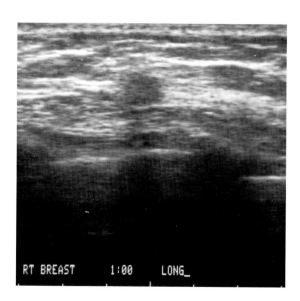

FIGURE 2-10C A true lateral mammogram of the right breast demonstrates a spiculated 1-cm mass superiorly in the right breast. Multiple repeated craniocaudal images failed to demonstrate its location.

FIGURE 2-10D Sonogram of the superior portion of the right breast demonstrates a 1-cm hypoechoic mass with posterior acoustic shadowing at the 1:00 position corresponding to the nodule seen mammographically.

◆ DIFFERENTIAL DIAGNOSIS

◆ **Breast carcinoma:** This diagnosis should be considered until proved otherwise. After the lesion is seen initially on the true lateral image, every effort should be made to confirm the location of the lesion, including exaggerated craniocaudal views, sonography, or even stereotactic localization if necessary.

◆ **Summation artifact:** Summation artifact can sometimes produce an apparent focal density on one view. However, this diagnosis was proved incorrect when sonography showed a solid mass was present.

◆ DIAGNOSIS: Infiltrating ductal carcinoma.

◆ KEY FACTS

CLINICAL

◆ Carcinomas can occur in areas of the breast that are not routinely imaged at screening or are difficult to localize on diagnostic exams. This is one reason for the 7% to 10% false-negative rate of screening mammography in detecting carcinoma. Therefore, a patient should not be considered completely screened until evaluated with both physical exam and mammography.

RADIOLOGIC: EVALUATING A LESION SEEN IN ONE VIEW

◆ Attempts must be made to ensure that the region of abnormality is included on the orthogonal view (as in this case, repeated exaggerated craniocaudal views attempted to localize the lesion).

◆ If the abnormality is not seen in the two views, summation artifact is a consideration. However, other modalities may be necessary to confirm this diagnosis.

◆ If a lesion is seen on the screening mediolateral oblique mammogram only, a true lateral will be useful in determining how the lesion moves in relation to the central axis of the breast. Lateral lesions move lower in the breast on the true lateral view, while medial lesions move up in the breast.

◆ If a lesion is seen on the screening craniocaudal mammogram only, a roll craniocaudal view or a craniocaudal mammogram at 5-degrees tube angulation can be performed. If the superior part of the breast is rolled laterally and the lesion moves laterally, then it can be determined to be in the superior portion of the breast. Likewise, if the lesion moves medially when the superior breast is rolled laterally, the lesion can be shown to be inferior in the breast.

◆ Sonography and physical examination are often useful in localizing lesions seen in only one view, as in this case.

◆ If necessary, the finding can be confirmed to be a true mass using stereotactic localization. CT or MRI can also be used to localize a lesion seen in one view.

◆ SUGGESTED READING

Kopans DB, Waitzkin ED, Linetsky L, et al. Localization of breast lesions identified on only one mammographic view. AJR Am J Roentgenol 1987;149:39–41.

Sickles EA. Practical solutions to common mammographic problems: Tailoring the examination. AJR Am J Roentgenol 1988;151:31–39.

Swann CA, Kopans DB, McCarthy KA, et al. Localization of occult breast lesions: Practical solutions to problems of triangulation. Radiology 1987;163:577–578.

CASE 11

Margaret E. Williford

HISTORY

Screening mammogram in a 49-year-old premenopausal woman. She had no palpable abnormality or history of surgery.

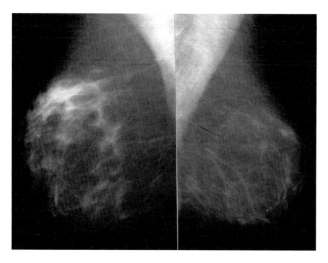

FIGURE 2-11A Mediolateral oblique mammograms of right and left breasts show asymmetric density in the superior right breast.

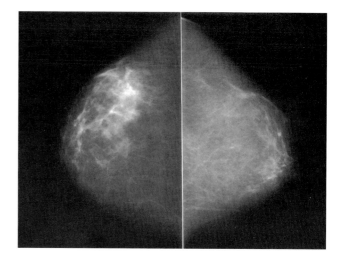

FIGURE 2-11B Craniocaudal mammograms of right and left breasts show asymmetric density in the outer right breast.

◆ DIFFERENTIAL DIAGNOSIS

- **Asymmetric breast tissue:** This is the best diagnosis because the density has the appearance of normal parenchyma with no underlying suspicious characteristics. No corresponding palpable mass was identified to raise the suspicion for other processes.
- **Postoperative change with removal of breast tissue from the contralateral breast:** This diagnosis is unlikely because there is no history of prior breast surgery.
- **Carcinoma:** Although carcinoma may present as an asymmetric density, there is no associated palpable mass or associated suspicious mammographic feature to suggest malignancy.

◆ DIAGNOSIS: Asymmetric breast tissue.

◆ KEY FACTS

CLINICAL

- Asymmetric breast tissue density has been described as a secondary sign of malignancy, but this is unlikely unless there is a corresponding palpable abnormality.
- The area of asymmetry should be evaluated with a careful physical breast examination. If there is a palpable abnormality or palpable asymmetry, biopsy should be recommended.

- A clinical history of prior breast surgery is important. For instance, asymmetry can be due to removal of tissue during biopsy of the contralateral breast.

RADIOLOGIC

- At least 3% of women have asymmetric breast tissue that appears as increased volume or density relative to the contralateral breast. This is most commonly seen in the upper outer quadrants. It reflects normal asymmetric development or variable response to hormonal stimulation.
- Additional mammographic views, including focal compression and magnification, may be necessary to evaluate the asymmetric density for mass, architectural distortion, or microcalcifications.
- Asymmetric density represents a normal variant if the glandular structures and fat are normally dispersed in the area with no mass, distortion, or microcalcifications, and no corresponding palpable abnormality.
- Comparison with prior films or close interval mammographic follow-up can be recommended to document the stability of the pattern.

◆ SUGGESTED READING

Kopans DB (ed). Breast Imaging. Philadelphia: Lippincott, 1989.

Kopans DB, Swann CA, White CA, et al. Asymmetric breast tissue. Radiology 1989;171:639–643.

CASE *12*   *Ruth Walsh*

HISTORY

A 43-year-old asymptomatic woman presenting for a screening mammogram.

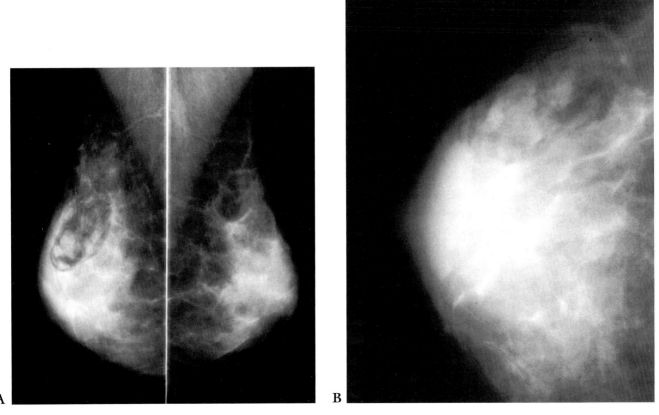

FIGURES 2-12A and 2-12B Mediolateral oblique (**A**) and craniocaudal (**B**) mammograms of both breasts show a circumscribed 3- × 2-cm mass present in the upper outer quadrant of the right breast. This mass contains both radiolucent regions and regions that are isodense to parenchyma.

◆ DIFFERENTIAL DIAGNOSIS

◆ **Hamartoma (fibroadenolipoma):** The encapsulated, well-circumscribed mass with internal fat and fibroglandular tissue in disorganized array is typical of a hamartoma. These findings make this the best diagnosis.

◆ **Intramammary lymph node:** Normal intramammary lymph nodes are typically round, oval, or lobulated isodense masses that measure <1 cm in size and usually contain a central fatty hilum. The size of the lesion presented here and the haphazardly arranged fatty and soft-tissue components make lymph node an unlikely diagnosis.

◆ **Galactocele:** Galactoceles are milk-containing cysts that appear as a radiolucent or mixed-density circumscribed mass that can have a mottled appearance, mimicking a hamartoma. A fat-fluid level can be seen on horizontal beam radiograph, which is not present in this case. This diagnosis is also unlikely in the present case because there is no history of current or recent lactation.

◆ **Lipoma:** Lipomas are circumscribed, fat-containing masses that are radiolucent on mammograms. However, in addition to radiolucent regions, the lesion presented here has regions that are isodense with breast parenchyma. This finding would not be found in a pure lipoma and makes this diagnosis unlikely.

◆ **Oil cyst:** Oil cysts would also be a consideration in a lesion that was predominantly radiolucent. Again, the mixed density arranged in a haphazard pattern argues against this diagnosis in the case illustrated.

◆ DIAGNOSIS: Hamartoma.

◆ KEY FACTS

CLINICAL

◆ Hamartomas are uncommon, benign breast tumors containing ducts, lobules, adipose tissue, and fibrous tissue in varying proportions. Smooth muscle can also be present.

◆ Hamartomas can be discovered incidentally on screening mammography or present clinically as a painless breast lump or enlarging breast.

◆ When palpable, hamartomas are usually firm, smooth, and mobile.

◆ Hamartomas usually grow slowly but can reach a large size, producing marked asymmetry of the breast.

RADIOLOGIC

◆ The characteristic mammographic appearance of a hamartoma is a circumscribed oval or round mass composed of mixed radiolucent and radiodense areas. This classic appearance is pathognomonic for a hamartoma, obviating the need for surgical excision.

◆ Not all hamartomas have a classic mammographic appearance. The mass can vary from relatively radiolucent to very dense, depending on the proportions of fibrous and fatty tissue. Sometimes the mass can be uniformly dense with obscured margins. In these cases, the appearance is nonspecific, and biopsy may be required for diagnosis.

◆ The mass displaces adjacent fibroglandular tissue, often leaving a thin intervening radiolucent zone. It usually has a well-defined margin and can appear encapsulated.

◆ If small or in a dense breast, hamartomas can be inapparent at mammography.

◆ SUGGESTED READING

Dean D, Trus T, D'souza TJ, et al. Hamartoma of the breast, an underrecognized breast lesion. Am J Clin Pathol 1995;103:685–689.

Harris JR, Hellman S, Henderson IC, Kinne DW (eds). Breast Diseases. Philadelphia: Lippincott, 1991.

Helvie MA, Adler DD, Rebner M, Oberman HA. Breast hamartomas: Variable mammographic appearance. Radiology 1989;170:417–421.

Kopans DB (ed). Breast Imaging. Philadelphia: Lippincott, 1989.

McGuire LI, Cohn D. Hamartoma of the breast. Aust N Z J Surg 1991;61:713–716.

HISTORY

Screening mammogram in a 36-year-old asymptomatic woman with no past surgical history. She has no palpable breast masses.

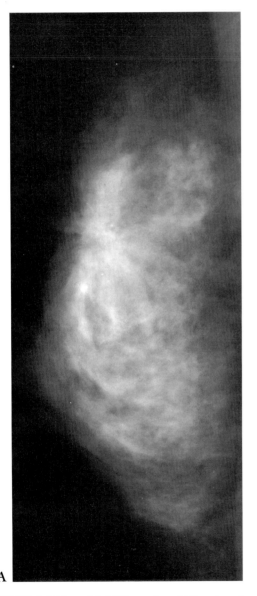

A

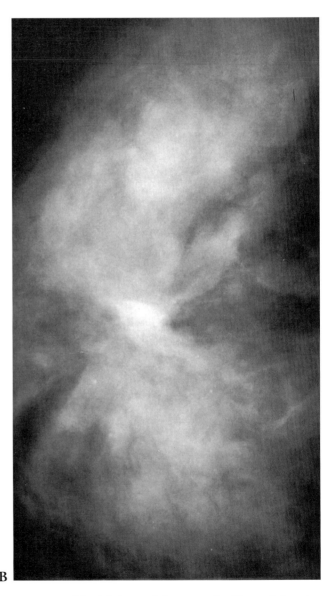

B

FIGURES 2-13A and 2-13B True lateral (**A**) and craniocaudal (**B**) mammograms of the right breast. A 3-cm area of architectural distortion is present in the upper central right breast. Numerous calcifications are associated with the distortion.

◆ DIFFERENTIAL DIAGNOSIS

- **Infiltrating ductal carcinoma:** The mammographic finding of a large area of architectural distortion associated with pleomorphic microcalcifications is consistent with infiltrating carcinoma and is an indication for biopsy. However, the absence of a palpable mass in this large area of distortion raised the possibility of another diagnosis.
- **Complex sclerosing lesion/radial scar:** Because this lesion is not palpable, a complex sclerosing lesion is a diagnostic consideration. A complex sclerosing lesion often appears at mammography as an area of architectural distortion or a spiculated mass with a lucent center. However, any area of distortion that does not correspond to a surgical scar must be biopsied to exclude malignancy.
- **Postsurgical scar:** Surgical scars often appear as an area of architectural distortion that may appear somewhat mass-like in one view but elongated in another view. Although the mammographic appearance of a surgical scar can be similar to the findings in this case, this diagnosis is not possible because there is no history of surgical biopsy.

◆ DIAGNOSIS: Complex sclerosing lesion.

◆ KEY FACTS

CLINICAL

- The term *complex sclerosing lesion* refers to a lesion that measures >10 mm. Similar lesions measuring <10 mm are termed *radial scar, infiltrating epitheliosis, elastosis,* or *indurative mastopathy.*
- Complex sclerosing lesions are not usually palpable. They are most often detected at mammography.
- Histologically, complex sclerosing lesions are characterized by a central area of elastosis surrounded by a disorganized array of tubules. They can also contain papillomas, apocrine change, and sclerosing adenosis.

- Radial scars and complex sclerosing lesions were previously thought to have an association with tubular carcinoma. This has been refuted because those cases in question have proved to represent tubular carcinomas misdiagnosed histologically, not radial scars.
- Excisional biopsy is necessary to differentiate complex sclerosing lesions from malignant lesions. They can be difficult to differentiate histologically from tubular carcinoma on core biopsies. Therefore, excisional biopsy is preferred over stereotactic biopsy when this diagnosis is considered.

RADIOLOGIC

- Complex sclerosing lesions often present as focal areas of architectural distortion or a spiculated mass with central density.
- Associated microcalcifications have been reported in 14% to 40% of cases.
- Central lucency can be evident, but this does not differentiate this lesion from malignant lesions reliably.
- The length of spiculations cannot differentiate these lesions from malignant lesions reliably.

◆ SUGGESTED READING

American College of Radiology (ACR). Breast Imaging Reporting and Data System (BI-RADS). Reston, VA: American College of Radiology, 1993.

Ciatto S, Morrone D, Catarzi S, et al. Radial scars of the breast: Review of 38 consecutive mammographic diagnoses. Radiology 1993;187:757–760.

Franquet T, DeMiguel C, Cozcolleula R, Donoso L. Spiculated lesions of the breast: Mammographic–pathologic correlation. Radiographics 1993;13:841–852.

Kopans DB. Specific, Non-Specific, and Supporting Signs of Malignancy. In DB Kopans (ed), Breast Imaging. Philadelphia: Lippincott, 1989;115–133.

Mendelson EB. Evaluation of the post-operative breast. Radiol Clin North Am 1992;30:107–138.

Orel SC, Evers K, Yeh I-T, Troupin RH. Radial scar with microcalcifications: Radiologic–pathologic correlation. Radiology 1992;183:479–482.

CASE 14

Mary Scott Soo

HISTORY

A 45-year-old woman presenting for screening mammography 2 years after lumpectomy and radiation therapy to the upper inner quadrant of the right breast for carcinoma.

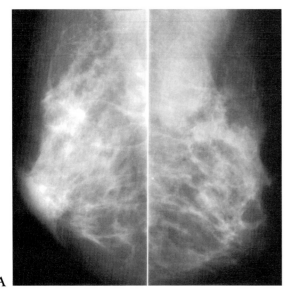

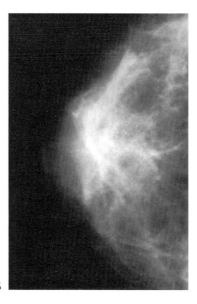

A

B

FIGURES 2-14A and 2-14B Mediolateral oblique mammograms of both breasts (**A**) and craniocaudal mammogram of the right breast (**B**). In the upper outer quadrant of the right breast, there is a cluster of pleomorphic microcalcifications. These are lateral to the lumpectomy site.

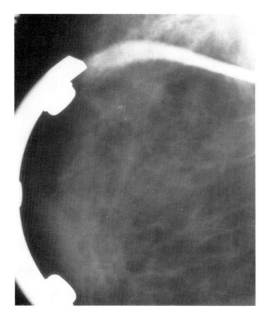

FIGURE 2-14C Mediolateral oblique magnification mammogram of the right breast. The magnification view demonstrates variation in the appearance of the calcifications, some having a linear or branching morphology, while others are more punctate in appearance. A large number of calcifications are clustered in a small area.

◆ DIFFERENTIAL DIAGNOSIS

◆ **Sclerosing adenosis:** Sclerosing adenosis is a benign lobular proliferation that results in enlargement and distortion of the lobules. Sclerosing adenosis can have many mammographic appearances. However, the associated calcifications are usually seen diffusely throughout the breast, characterized by uniformly dense and round or amorphous intralobular calcifications, unlike the calcifications in this case. Sclerosing adenosis sometimes forms an isolated cluster of calcifications that may require biopsy to differentiate them from malignant lesions.

◆ **Comedo carcinoma:** This is the best diagnosis because the calcifications in this case vary in size and density and have irregular, linear, and branching shapes, all of which are typical of comedo carcinoma in situ.

◆ **Plasma cell mastitis:** In plasma cell mastitis, calcific deposits occur in areas of extruded cellular debris surrounding inflamed ducts. Unlike the pleomorphic calcifications in this case, secretory calcifications associated with plasma cell mastitis are usually large (>0.5 mm) and rod shaped, with uniform density, making this diagnosis unlikely.

◆ **Dystrophic calcifications from fat necrosis following surgery and radiation therapy:** Calcifications associated with fat necrosis can sometimes mimic malignant calcifications. When they first appear, they can vary in size and density and have irregular, pleomorphic shapes. These calcifications are often clustered, being localized to the site of traumatic insult. Dystrophic calcifications usually evolve over time to coarser, plaque-like forms that have a more benign appearance. In the case illustrated, the cluster of calcifications is in the outer quadrant, lateral to the lumpectomy site, making fat necrosis an unlikely diagnosis.

◆ DIAGNOSIS: Comedo carcinoma in situ.

◆ KEY FACTS

CLINICAL

◆ Comedo carcinoma is one of several forms of ductal carcinoma in situ characterized histologically by central necrosis within the involved ducts. Calcification of the necrotic tissue is common. Tumor cells often demonstrate nuclear pleomorphism, and mitotic cells are frequently seen.

◆ Comedo carcinoma in situ can be present alone or associated with invasive ductal carcinoma.

◆ Comedo carcinoma has a higher recurrence rate than low-grade forms of carcinoma in situ.

RADIOLOGIC

◆ A cluster of microcalcifications is considered suspicious if it contains five or more indeterminate calcifications localized to a 1-cm³ area. However, the specificity of this finding is low, as carcinoma may be identified in only 10% to 35% of cases with this mammographic appearance.

◆ Comedo carcinoma most commonly presents mammographically as clustered microcalcifications.

◆ Calcifications associated with comedo carcinoma vary in size, shape, and density. Fine linear or branching calcifications due to necrotic debris within the central portion of the ducts are seen frequently and may be associated with rounded or granular calcifications.

◆ The finding of new microcalcifications at the lumpectomy site is the most common mammographic feature of early recurrence. For this reason, magnification images of lumpectomy sites are performed routinely in the follow-up of patients who have undergone lumpectomy and radiation therapy for carcinoma.

◆ SUGGESTED READING

Kopans DB. Specific, Non-Specific, and Supporting Signs of Malignancy. In DB Kopans (ed), Breast Imaging. Philadelphia: Lippincott, 1989;115–133.

Page DL, Anderson TJ. Adenosis. In DL Page, TJ Anderson (eds), Diagnostic Histopathology of the Breast. New York: Churchill Livingstone, 1987;51–56.

Page DL, Anderson TJ, Rogers LW. Carcinoma in Situ. In DL Page, TJ Anderson (eds), Diagnostic Histopathology of the Breast. New York: Churchill Livingstone, 1987;157–192.

Stomper PC, Margolin FR. Ductal carcinoma in situ: The mammographer's perspective. AJR Am J Roentgenol 1994;162:585–591.

CASE 15 *Ruth Walsh*

HISTORY

Diagnostic mammogram in a 58-year-old woman with a palpable lump in the right central breast and a clinical history of melanoma. There were no prior mammograms for comparison.

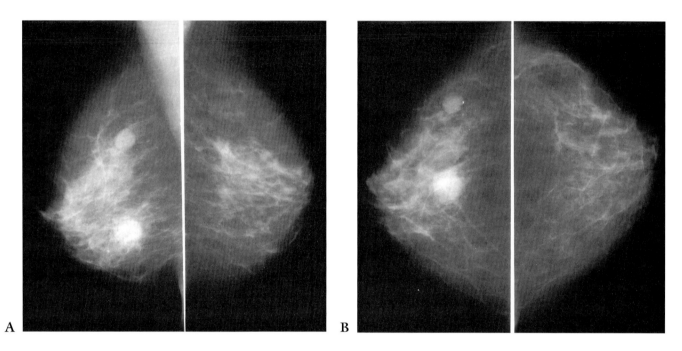

A

B

FIGURES 2-15A and 2-15B Mediolateral oblique (**A**) and craniocaudal (**B**) mammograms of both breasts. Two round masses are present in the right breast. The smaller mass in the 10:00 position is well-circumscribed, measuring 10 mm; the larger mass in the central breast is partly obscured.

◆DIFFERENTIAL DIAGNOSIS

◆ **Cysts:** Cysts are commonly detected, well-circumscribed breast masses that are often multiple and bilateral and can fluctuate in size or resolve over time. This diagnosis would be a good consideration in this case. However, cysts cannot be confirmed by mammography alone. Sonography or needle aspiration would be necessary to complete the evaluation. These lesions proved solid at sonography, making this an incorrect diagnosis.

◆ **Fibroadenomas:** Fibroadenomas are also common breast masses that cannot be differentiated from cysts or other solid circumscribed masses by mammography unless they contain characteristic coarse, "popcorn-like" calcifications. Fibroadenomas are often oval or lobulated in shape and tend to be oriented toward the nipple. This diagnosis should be considered in this case but cannot be confirmed by this mammographic appearance.

◆ **Metastases:** Metastases to the breast are usually well-circumscribed round masses that cannot be differentiated from cysts or fibroadenomas by mammography alone. Knowledge of a history of an extramammary malignancy is necessary for the diagnosis of metastases to be considered, and biopsy is necessary to confirm the diagnosis.

◆ **Lymph nodes:** The masses in this case are not consistent with benign intramammary lymph nodes because benign lymph nodes are typically oval or reniform in shape and have a hilar notch or lucent center. Intramammary nodes tend to be <1 cm in size. Enlarged reactive or metastatic nodes could have this appearance.

◆ **Multifocal or multicentric breast cancer:** Multifocal breast cancer usually presents at mammography as multiple, ill-defined or spiculated masses or multiple clusters of microcalcifications, making this diagnosis unlikely in this case. However, primary breast cancers rarely present as multiple, unilateral, well-circumscribed masses (for example, an invasive papillary carcinoma with satellite nodules).

◆DIAGNOSIS: Metastatic melanoma of the right breast.

◆KEY FACTS

CLINICAL

◆ Melanoma is the eighth most prevalent malignancy in the United States, with approximately 32,000 new cases in the United States each year.

◆ The most common sites for metastases from melanoma are skin, subcutaneous tissue, lymph nodes, lungs, bone, central nervous system, and liver.

◆ Although the breast is an unusual site for melanoma metastases, melanoma is the most common source of metastases to the breast. Lymphoma and lung carcinoma are also common causes of metastases to the breast.

◆ When metastases to the breast are considered in a patient with appropriate history and physical examination, mammograms are necessary to exclude primary breast carcinoma, support the clinical suspicion of metastases, and monitor any therapeutic response following treatment.

RADIOLOGIC

◆ Metastatic disease to the breast from an extramammary malignancy can present as a solitary circumscribed mass, multiple circumscribed masses, or much less commonly as diffuse involvement of skin and parenchyma. Associated microcalcifications are very rarely identified.

◆ Management of multiple, unilateral, well-circumscribed masses: Sonography should be used to differentiate cystic from solid masses. If simple cysts are identified, routine follow-up is recommended. If masses are solid and there is no history of malignancy, short-term mammographic follow-up would be recommended (every 6 months for 1 year, then every 12 months). In patients with a history of extramammary malignancy, solid masses should be compared with prior films to determine stability and biopsied if stability cannot be established.

◆SUGGESTED READING

Bohman LG, Bassett LW, Gold DRH, Volt R. Breast metastases from extramammary malignancies. Radiology 1982;144: 309–312.

Feig SA. Breast masses: Mammographic and sonographic evaluation. Radiol Clin North Am 1992;30:67–92.

Paulus DD, Libshitz HI. Metastases to the breast. Radiol Clin North Am 1982;20:561–568.

Runkle GP, Zaloznik AJ. Malignant melanoma. Am Fam Physician 1994;49:91–98.

Soo MS, Williford ME, Walsh R, et al. Papillary carcinoma of the breast: Imaging findings. AJR Am J Roentgenol 1995;164: 321–326.

Tucker AT (ed). Textbook of Mammography. New York: Churchill Livingstone, 1993.

CASE 16

Margaret E. Williford

HISTORY

A 73-year-old asymptomatic woman presenting for a screening mammogram who had begun hormone replacement therapy 1 year previously. She had no family history of breast cancer.

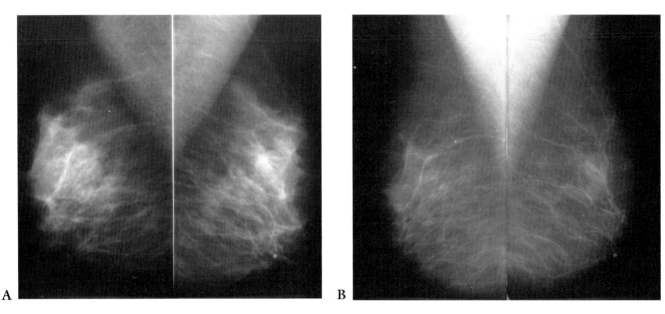

FIGURES 2-16A and 2-16B Mediolateral oblique mammograms of right and left breasts (**A**) and mediolateral oblique mammograms of right and left breasts from 18 months earlier (**B**). Diffuse bilateral increased parenchymal density is present relative to the prior mammogram (**B**).

◆ DIFFERENTIAL DIAGNOSIS

- **Glandular stimulation from hormone replacement therapy:** This is the best diagnosis because the change has occurred diffusely and bilaterally, without other associated suspicious features. The clinical history is also consistent with this diagnosis.
- **Edema:** This diagnosis is less likely because the change predominantly involves the breast parenchyma, without skin or trabecular thickening, which is commonly associated with edema.
- **Mastitis:** This diagnosis is unlikely because the change is bilateral. Mastitis can present as a segmental area of increased density and can be associated with abscess. The clinical history is also inconsistent with mastitis, as the patient was asymptomatic.
- **Carcinoma:** Although locally advanced breast carcinoma can present as a diffuse increase in density, the bilateral change makes this unlikely. Other features such as skin and trabecular thickening often seen with inflammatory carcinoma are not present, and the breasts do not appear smaller and contracted compared with the prior study.

◆ DIAGNOSIS: Glandular stimulation from hormone replacement therapy.

◆ KEY FACTS

CLINICAL

- Hormone replacement therapy is relatively common among postmenopausal women due to the beneficial result of decreasing cardiovascular disease and osteoporosis.
- Estrogen promotes growth of ducts and stimulates surrounding connective tissue. Progesterone promotes growth of lobuloalveolar structures and differentiation of ductal cells.

- Treatment with estrogen promotes enlargement of cysts and fibroadenomas. Treatment with a combination of estrogen and progesterone is associated with diffuse increase in fibroglandular tissue.
- A number of studies have evaluated the risk of breast cancer for women on hormone replacement therapy. The results are conflicting, but there appears to be a slight increase in risk based on the duration of use.

RADIOLOGIC

- Effects of hormone replacement therapy that can be apparent on mammograms include symmetric or asymmetric increase in breast density, increase in size of fibroadenomas, and development or increase in size of cysts.
- Mammographic changes develop in 24% of postmenopausal women undergoing hormone replacement therapy.
- Mammographic changes are more common in women treated with the combination of estrogen and progesterone than in women treated with estrogen alone.
- Asymmetric or focal increase in breast density is more problematic. It may be interpreted as a developing density. Further evaluation may include breast ultrasound, physical correlation, mammographic follow-up with or without cessation of hormones, or even biopsy to exclude malignancy.

◆ SUGGESTED READING

Berkowitz JE, Gatewood OMB, Goldblum LE, Gayler BM. Hormonal replacement therapy: Mammographic manifestations. Radiology 1990;174:199–201.

Cyrlak D, Wang CH. Mammographic changes in post-menopausal women undergoing hormonal replacement therapy. AJR Am J Roentgenol 1993;161:1177–1183.

Stamper DC, Von Voorhis BJ, Ravnikar VA, Meyer JE. Mammographic changes associated with post-menopausal hormone replacement therapy: A longitudinal study. Radiology 1990;174:487–490.

CASE 17

Margaret E. Williford

HISTORY

Screening mammogram in a 42-year-old woman.

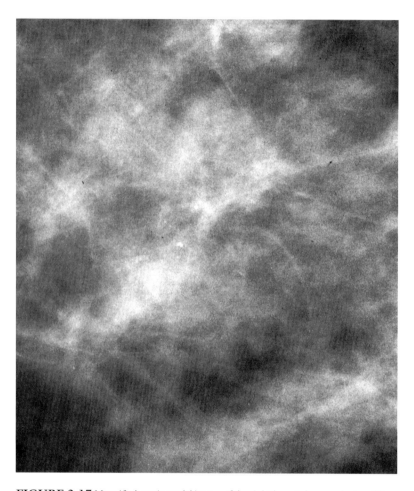

FIGURE 2-17 Magnified craniocaudal image of the right breast shows a cluster of four punctate calcifications. There is no associated mass, asymmetric density, or distortion.

◆ DIFFERENTIAL DIAGNOSIS

- **Benign calcifications:** This is the best diagnosis due to microcalcification number and morphology. Stability should be established by follow-up mammography.
- **Cutaneous calcifications:** Cutaneous calcifications are usually located along the periphery of the breast and are round with lucent centers, unlike the calcifications in this case.
- **Calcifications highly suspicious for malignancy:** This diagnosis is less likely because the calcifications in this case are few in number and morphology of the cluster is uniform, not linear, branching, or pleomorphic.

◆ DIAGNOSIS: Probably benign calcifications.

◆ KEY FACTS

CLINICAL

- The calcifications described in this case form from benign processes such as focal sclerosing adenosis, focal fibrosis, and occasionally, early manifestations of fat necrosis.

RADIOLOGIC

- Isolated clusters of calcifications can display features that indicate a low probability of malignancy. They are as follows:

1. Such calcifications are round or punctate and are uniform in shape and density, allowing for variation in size.
2. The number of calcifications within the isolated cluster is five or less.
3. Calcifications are not associated with any other mammographic abnormality such as a mass, distortion, or focal asymmetry.

- Spot compression magnified images are necessary for initial evaluation of number and morphology. Spot compression magnified images are also used in follow-up examinations.
- Such indeterminate calcifications are usually managed with close interval mammographic follow-up. Calcifications are reimaged at 6, 12, and 24 months. Any change in the number or morphology should be viewed as suspicious for possible malignancy, and biopsy may be indicated. Stability over a 24-month period is generally considered as an indication of a benign process. After this period of close follow-up, a routine screening schedule is resumed.

◆ SUGGESTED READING

Feig SA. Mammographic evaluation of calcifications. RSNA Categorical Course in Breast Imaging 1995;93–105.

Sickles EA. Breast calcifications: Mammographic evaluation. Radiology 1986;160:289–293.

CASE 18

Phyllis J. Kornguth

HISTORY

Diagnostic mammogram in a 72-year-old woman who presented with a 2-cm palpable mass in the upper inner quadrant of the right breast. The family history was significant for a sister with postmenopausal breast carcinoma.

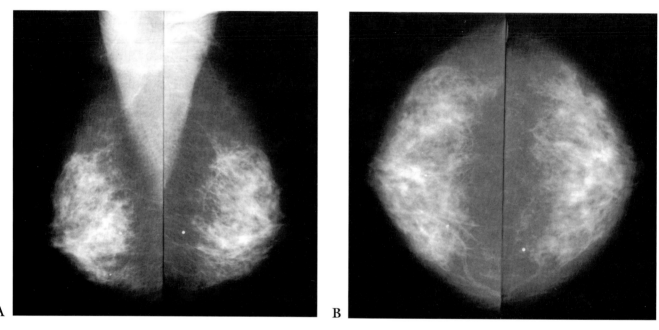

A   B

FIGURES 2-18A and 2-18B Mediolateral oblique (**A**) and craniocaudal (**B**) mammograms of both breasts. Figures show moderately dense fibroglandular tissue throughout both breasts with no suspicious lesions identified.

◆ REASONS FOR A FALSE-NEGATIVE MAMMOGRAM

◆ **Poor-quality study:** In this case, positioning and technical factors are optimal, making this an unlikely reason for a false-negative mammogram. The radiologist is responsible for assuring high-quality mammography.

◆ **The lesion is not imaged:** Breast tissue can occur in areas not covered on a routine mammogram. In this case, the lesion was close to the areola and should have been included on both images. A cutaneous marker should be placed at the site of the mass and images repeated to confirm mass location has been included on the films.

◆ **Error of interpretation:** In reviewing this case, no mammographic abnormality was identified, even in retrospect.

◆ **Mass obscured by dense breast tissue:** In breasts with very dense breast tissue, even a well-defined mass can be completely obscured by breast tissue, making this the most common cause of a false-negative mammogram.

◆ **Infiltrating lobular carcinoma:** Unlike infiltrating ductal carcinoma, infiltrating lobular carcinoma does not form a discrete mass. The malignant cells invade the surrounding breast tissue in a single-file fashion and often cannot be distinguished from surrounding breast parenchyma at mammography.

◆ DIAGNOSIS: Infiltrating lobular carcinoma.

◆ KEY FACTS

CLINICAL

◆ Infiltrating lobular carcinoma feels like an area of thickening rather than a discrete lump on physical examination.

◆ At the cellular level, it invades the surrounding breast tissue in a linear, single-file fashion.

◆ Metastases to axillary lymph nodes are common at the time of diagnosis.

RADIOLOGIC

◆ Infiltrating lobular carcinoma can appear as a slowly developing asymmetric density or an area of mild architectural distortion, but it often is not seen on mammograms.

◆ Infiltrating lobular carcinoma has a variety of sonographic appearances, but no findings or only a nonspecific region of posterior acoustic shadowing may be present.

◆ SUGGESTED READING

Krecke KN, Gisvold JJ. Invasive lobular carcinoma of the breast: Mammographic findings and extent of disease at diagnosis in 184 patients. AJR Am J Roentgenol 1993;161:957–960.

Paramagul CP, Helvie MA, Adler DD. Invasive lobular carcinoma: Sonographic appearance and role of sonography in improving diagnostic sensitivity. Radiology 1995;195:231–234.

Rosen, PP. The Pathology of Invasive Breast Carcinoma. In JR Harris, S Hellman, IC Henderson, DW Kinne (eds), Breast Diseases. Philadelphia: Lippincott, 1991;272–276.

CASE 19

Phyllis J. Kornguth

HISTORY

Screening mammogram in a 73-year-old female. Family history is significant for a sister with postmenopausal breast carcinoma. There is no past surgical history or history of hormone replacement therapy.

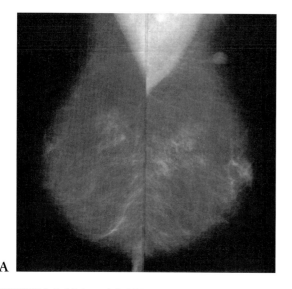 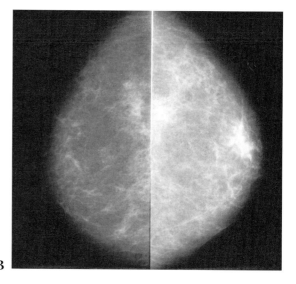

FIGURES 2-19A and 2-19B Mediolateral oblique (**A**) and craniocaudal (**B**) mammograms of both breasts. Figures show an asymmetric density in the retroareolar region of the left breast and a 10-mm, well-circumscribed, solitary nodule in the upper outer quadrant of the left breast.

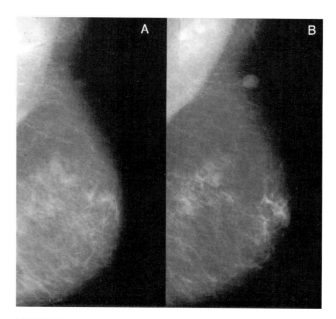

FIGURE 2-19C Mediolateral oblique mammogram of the left breast 1 year ago (**A**) and mediolateral oblique left mammogram from the current study (**B**). The asymmetric density is new compared to the prior study. The nodule previously represented an intramammary lymph node and has enlarged compared to the prior exam.

◆DIFFERENTIAL DIAGNOSIS

◆ **Breast carcinoma with metastatic disease to an intramammary lymph node:** A developing asymmetric density within the breast must be viewed with suspicion because this is one mammographic presentation of breast carcinoma. The associated enlargement and increased density of the intramammary lymph node increases the suspicion for carcinoma with metastatic disease, making this the best diagnosis.

◆ **Mastitis with reactive lymph node:** Mastitis can be seen at mammography as a localized asymmetric density, and intramammary lymph nodes can enlarge as a result of infections of the breast. However, the patient in this case was asymptomatic and had no physical signs of infection, making this diagnosis unlikely.

◆ **Focal glandular stimulation from hormone replacement therapy:** This process could cause a developing density within the breast, with enlargement of nodules corresponding to cyst formation. However, the patient in the case illustrated has no history of hormone replacement therapy, and the nodule seen in this case was previously shown to represent an intramammary lymph node.

◆ **Normal asymmetric breast parenchyma:** The mammographic appearance of the asymmetric density in this case could be consistent with asymmetric glandular tissue. However, glandular tissue would not be expected to increase over time without hormonal stimulation, and the enlargement of the intramammary lymph node could not be explained with this diagnosis.

◆DIAGNOSIS: Infiltrating ductal carcinoma with 1/34 positive lymph nodes.

◆KEY FACTS

CLINICAL

◆ Infiltrating ductal carcinoma can be metastatic to intramammary lymph nodes.

◆ Intramammary lymph nodes with metastatic involvement are often palpable, located in the upper outer quadrant of the breast. Careful physical examination in this breast proved this node to be palpable.

RADIOLOGIC

◆ Infiltrating ductal carcinoma can present infrequently as a developing asymmetric density. Any change in the mammogram from one year to the next must be explained.

◆ When an asymmetric density is identified on the mammogram, additional focal compression images and physical examination to evaluate for a palpable mass are essential to complete the evaluation.

◆ When intramammary lymph nodes enlarge over time, the breast must be inspected carefully for evidence of primary breast carcinoma. Considerations in the differential diagnosis of enlarged intramammary nodes include metastatic disease from breast primary, metastatic disease from extramammary malignancies, and reactive change from inflammatory processes.

◆SUGGESTED READING

Kopans DB. Mammography. In DB Kopans (ed), Breast Imaging. Philadelphia: Lippincott, 1989;34–226.

Kopans DB, Meyer JE. Benign lymph nodes associated with dermatitis presenting as breast masses. Radiology 1980;137:15–19.

Lindfors KK, Kopans DB, McCarthy KA, et al. Breast metastasis to intramammary lymph nodes. AJR Am J Roentgenol 1986;146: 133–136.

Meyers JE, Kopans DB, Lawrence WD. Normal intramammary lymph nodes presenting as occult breast masses. Breast 1982;8:30–32.

Svane G, Franzen S. Radiologic appearance of nonpalpable intramammary lymph nodes. Acta Radiol 1993;34:577–580.

CASE 20

Phyllis J. Kornguth

HISTORY

Diagnostic mammogram in a 70-year-old woman who presented with a painless, swollen erythematous right breast. There was no significant past medical history.

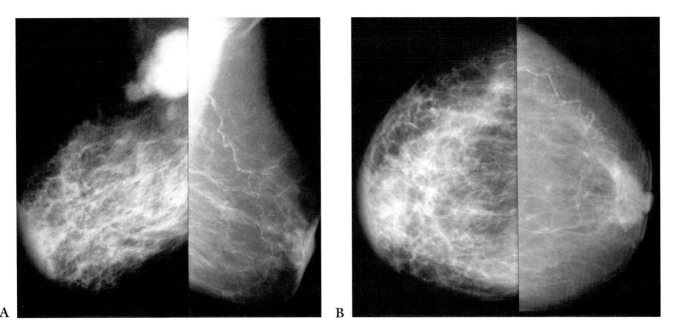

FIGURES 2-20A and 2-20B Mediolateral oblique (**A**) and craniocaudal (**B**) mammograms of both breasts show diffuse increased density throughout the right breast, with marked thickening of the skin and trabeculae. A large lobulated mass is seen in the right axilla.

◆ DIFFERENTIAL DIAGNOSIS

- **Inflammatory carcinoma:** The clinical presentation of a painless, swollen, erythematous breast and the mammographic findings of thickening of the skin and trabeculae in association with a mass make this the most likely diagnosis.
- **Axillary mass obstructing the lymphatics:** The mammographic findings of the large axillary mass and trabecular and skin thickening make this a reasonable choice. However, this diagnosis would be ruled out based on the physical examination because obstructed lymphatics would not result in an inflamed, erythematous appearance of the breast.
- **Radiation therapy:** Radiation therapy often results in skin and trabecular thickening. However, there was no history of radiation therapy in this case.
- **Mastitis:** Mammographic changes of skin and trabecular thickening are often seen in cases of mastitis or cellulitis, and the large axillary mass could represent reactive lymph node(s) due to infection. In cases of mastitis, however, skin and trabecular thickening are usually localized to one segment or region, not spread diffusely throughout the breast. Furthermore, the clinical history of "painless" swelling of the breast is not consistent with mastitis.
- **Congestive heart failure:** Congestive heart failure can result in unilateral skin and trabecular thickening in the dependent breast if the patient lies on one side. However, the mass in the right axilla makes this diagnosis unlikely.

◆ DIAGNOSIS: Inflammatory breast carcinoma.

◆ KEY FACTS

CLINICAL

- Inflammatory breast carcinoma is a diffuse carcinoma involving all portions of the breast, including the dermal lymphatics.
- On physical examination, the patient has a painless, red, hot, swollen breast with a peau d'orange appearance of the skin.
- Antibiotics (used if mastitis is considered in the differential diagnosis) can result in clinical regression of symptoms of inflammatory carcinoma. Biopsy is often necessary to make the diagnosis.
- The diagnosis can be made by a punch biopsy of the skin to determine the presence of carcinoma in the dermal lymphatics.

RADIOLOGIC

- The involved breast is asymmetrically dense compared to the contralateral breast.
- Thickening of the skin and trabeculae are typically present throughout the involved breast.
- An underlying dominant mass may or may not be present.

◆ SUGGESTED READING

Kopans DB. Pathologic, Mammographic, and Sonographic Correlation. In DB Kopans (ed), Breast Imaging. Philadelphia: Lippincott, 1989;299–301.

Rosen, PP. The Pathology of Invasive Breast Carcinoma. In JR Harris, S Hellman, IC Henderson, DW Kinne (eds), Breast Diseases. Philadelphia: Lippincott, 1991;278–279.

CASE 21

Margaret E. Williford

HISTORY

Diagnostic mammogram in a 60-year-old woman who is status post lumpectomy for infiltrating ductal carcinoma in the inferior portion of the right breast.

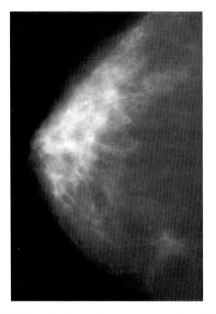

FIGURE 2-21A Craniocaudal mammogram of the right breast. A spiculated lesion is present in the medial portion of the breast.

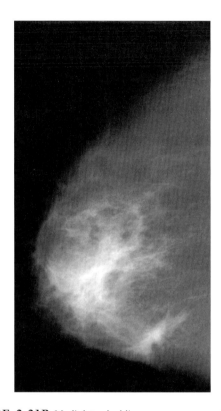

FIGURE 2-21B Mediolateral oblique mammogram of the right breast. A spiculated lesion lies inferior and is associated with skin thickening.

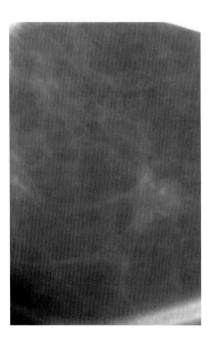

FIGURE 2-21C Focal compression magnified image. A stellate lesion with long spicules is present without a central mass or density. The central portion of the lesion is lucent.

◆ DIFFERENTIAL DIAGNOSIS

- **Spiculated carcinoma:** Carcinoma often presents as a mass with spiculated margins or an area of architectural distortion. The lesion in the case illustrated has no central mass and corresponds to the site of prior biopsy, making carcinoma a less likely diagnosis.
- **Postsurgical or post-traumatic scar:** A postsurgical scar often appears as an area of architectural distortion or a spiculated mass that decreases in size over time. The site of the spiculated lesion must match the location of the patient's cutaneous scar and the location of the biopsied lesion on preoperative or needle localization mammograms (if available). The lesion in the case illustrated corresponds to the site of prior biopsy, making this a likely diagnosis.
- **Radial scar:** Radial scars typically appear as lesions with long, thin spicules radiating outward from a radiolucent center. The lesion in the case illustrated has some of the mammographic features of a radial scar. However, a radial scar would not be expected to occur at a site of prior biopsy, making this diagnosis less likely.
- **Granular cell tumor:** These benign tumors have a spiculated appearance at mammography but are very rare and would not be expected to occur at biopsy sites, making this diagnosis unlikely.
- **Extra-abdominal desmoid tumor:** These are locally invasive tumors that do not metastasize. Their mammographic appearance mimics that of an invasive breast cancer, requiring biopsy for diagnosis. These lesions are rare, and location at a site of prior biopsy would be unlikely.

◆ DIAGNOSIS: Postsurgical scar.

◆ KEY FACTS

CLINICAL

- Fibrosis and fat necrosis at a surgical site (or site of trauma) can cause a spiculated mass or architectural distortion simulating the appearance of tumor.

- On palpation, scars feel like an area of thickening, whereas carcinomas feel more discrete and larger than an associated abnormality seen on mammogram.
- History of surgery at the site of the mammographic abnormality is helpful. The cutaneous surgical scar may not always correlate with the parenchymal scar since the surgeon may make the skin incision at some distance from the lesion to be removed.

RADIOLOGIC

- Postsurgical or post-traumatic scars frequently present as a spiculated mass or area of architectural distortion on mammogram, which is often identical to the appearance of carcinoma.
- Scars do not have a central mass or density after initial postoperative seroma has resolved; central lucency is commonly seen within the scar.
- The preoperative and needle localization mammograms and specimen radiograph can be used to confirm that the suspected scar correlates with the surgical site.
- If prior mammograms are not available but the density is strongly suspected to be a scar, it can be further evaluated with close-interval mammographic follow-up.
- A scar should decrease in density and distortion or remain stable during follow-up.
- Any increase in size or density of a suspected scar warrants biopsy.

◆ SUGGESTED READING

Peters ME. The Benign Post Surgical Breast. In ME Peters (ed), Handbook of Breast Imaging. New York: Churchill Livingstone, New York, 1989.

Sickles FA, Herzog KA. Intrammary scar tissue: A mimic of the mammographic appearance of carcinoma. AJR Am J Roentgenol 1980;135:349–352.

Stigers KB, King JG, Dowey DD, Stelling CB. Abnormalities of the breast caused by biopsy: Spectrum of mammographic findings. AJR Am J Roentgenol 1991;156:287–291.

CASE 22 *Mary Scott Soo*

HISTORY

Diagnostic mammogram in a 62-year-old woman with pain in her left breast. She had a right-sided modified radical mastectomy for carcinoma and a left-sided subcutaneous mastectomy, with breast reconstruction bilaterally using silicone prostheses. Subsequent sonogram and MRI of the left breast were performed.

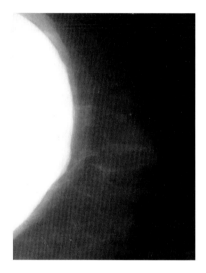

FIGURE 2-22A Craniocaudal mammogram of the left breast. Mild contour irregularity of the anterior margin of the subpectoral silicone implant is seen. No outer saline lumen is identified. No abnormalities are seen within the breast tissue.

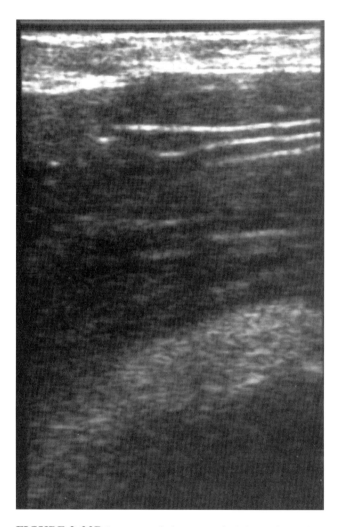

FIGURE 2-22B Sonogram of a breast prosthesis in another patient with the same diagnosis. Multiple, parallel echogenic lines are present within the silicone implant ("stepladder" sign).

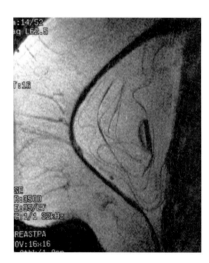

FIGURE 2-22C Sagittal T2-weighted, fast spin-echo water suppression MRI of the left breast. A hyperintense silicone prosthesis is present, surrounded by a hypointense fibrous capsule. Curvilinear hypointense lines ("linguine" sign) are present within the silicone, and the valve of this double-lumen implant is displaced anteriorly from its normal position along the posterior aspect of the fibrous capsule. No saline remains in the collapsed outer lumen.

◈ DIFFERENTIAL DIAGNOSIS

◆ **Intracapsular implant rupture:** This is the best diagnosis because MRI demonstrates numerous curvilinear hypointense lines within the hyperintense silicone gel, corresponding to the ruptured and collapsed shell of the prosthesis ("linguine" sign). No silicone is seen outside of the fibrous capsule.

◆ **Extracapsular implant rupture:** The mild contour abnormality of the implant on the mammogram is a nonspecific finding, but in conjunction with the clinical symptoms, raised the question of implant rupture, prompting further investigation using MRI. Neither the mammogram nor MRI show signs of free silicone within the breast parenchyma, making extracapsular rupture unlikely. The breast parenchyma should be studied carefully on all MRI images obtained to search for free silicone, particularly when intracapsular implant rupture is identified.

◆ **Intact implant with radial folds:** Radial folds are infoldings of the intact silicone shell, generally seen on MRI as straight, hypointense, double thickness lines, originating at the fibrous capsule and ending blindly in the silicone gel. Occasionally they appear angular or curvilinear. The lines seen centrally in the case illustrated do not correspond to radial folds, making this diagnosis unlikely.

◆ **Breast carcinoma:** Localized breast pain is only very infrequently associated with breast carcinoma. However, on any breast imaging examination (whether the study is indicated for screening or for prosthesis evaluation), the breast parenchyma must be evaluated carefully for signs of occult carcinoma. Large silicone implants are identified by both modalities in this case, which can obscure lesions at mammography. Carcinoma is unlikely in this case because no mass or other parenchymal abnormality is identified.

◈ DIAGNOSIS: Intracapsular rupture of the silicone breast prosthesis.

◈ KEY FACTS

CLINICAL

◆ Implantable silicone prostheses have been in use since 1962 for breast augmentation or breast reconstruction following subcutaneous or modified radical mastectomy.

◆ Silicone, saline, or double-lumen silicone and saline implants have been used most commonly and can be placed in subglandular or submuscular positions.

◆ Early complications of silicone prostheses include hemorrhage or infection in the postoperative period. Sonography is useful for detecting these periprosthetic fluid collections. CT and MRI are less frequently used for this purpose.

◆ Late complications of breast prostheses include capsular contracture, rupture, migration, and rarely, extrusion of the implant.

◆ Silicone implants were initially implicated in causing autoimmune diseases, prompting the Food and Drug Administration to limit their use. Subsequent studies have not confirmed an association between silicone and autoimmune diseases.

◆ Most of the late complications of silicone prostheses are best evaluated by physical examination. However, imaging studies are often necessary to detect implant rupture.

RADIOLOGIC

◆ Mammography: Mammograms have high specificity in evaluating implant integrity, but sensitivity is low because intracapsular rupture is frequently not detected by mammography.

◆ Reliable signs of implant rupture at mammography include free silicone within the breast parenchyma, irregular or large smooth protrusions of the silicone implant, and streaming of silicone away from the body of the implant.

◆ Sonography: Sonographic findings of implant rupture include the "snowstorm" sign (an echodense column located at the site of extracapsular silicone that obscures underlying structures), the "stepladder" sign (echogenic parallel lines resembling a stepladder within the implant, corresponding to the collapsed silicone shell), and the presence of anechoic nodules with echogenic back wall and echogenic reverberation, corresponding to free silicone globules in the breast parenchyma.

◆ MRI: Intracapsular rupture (ruptured implant with silicone contained within the surrounding fibrous capsule) is best detected by MRI, where the "linguine" sign corresponds to the collapsed silicone shell. Extracapsular silicone (gel extravasation into the breast tissue) can also be detected by MRI as parenchymal masses that have signal intensities paralleling those of the implant on T2-weighted fast spin-echo images (with and without water suppression) and on T1-weighted images. These sequences allow differentiation between silicone and other breast masses.

◈ SUGGESTED READING

DeBruhl ND, Gorczyca DP, Ahn CY, et al. Silicone breast implants: US evaluation. Radiology 1993;189:95–98.

Everson LI, Parantainen H, Detlie T, et al. Diagnosis of breast implant rupture: Imaging findings and relative efficacies of imaging techniques. AJR Am J Roentgenol 1994;163:57–60.

Gorczyca DP, Sinha S, Ahn CY, et al. Silicone breast implants in vivo: MR imaging. Radiology 1992;185:407–410.

Harris KM, Ganott MA, Shestak KC, et al. Silicone implant rupture: Detection with US. Radiology 1993;187:761–768.

Steinbach BG, Hardt NS, Abbitt PL. Mammography: Breast implants—types, complications and adjacent breast pathology. Curr Probl Diagn Radiol 1993; 22:39–86.

CHAPTER 3

GASTRO-INTESTINAL IMAGING

Vincent H.S. Low, *chapter editor*

Kelly S. Freed, David M. Hough,
Mary T. Keogan, Michael L. Kerner,
Vincent H.S. Low, Philip T. McAndrew,
Rendon C. Nelson, Erik K. Paulson,
Jeffrey T. Seabourn, and Paul V. Suhocki

CASE 1

Vincent H.S. Low

HISTORY

A 28-year-old man presents with odynophagia.

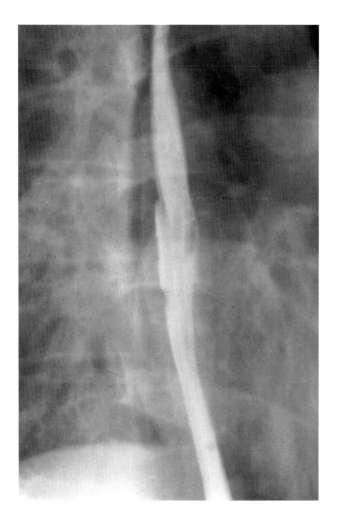

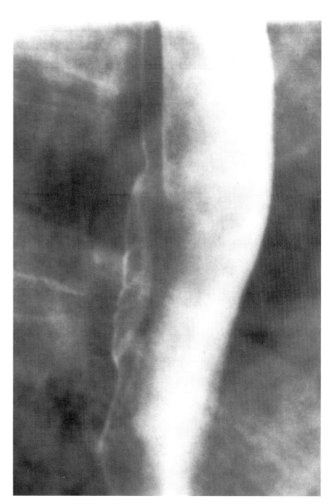

FIGURE 3-1A Barium swallow: mucosal relief view of the mid to distal esophagus. There is a large (3-cm), shallow ulcer, sometimes given the term "giant" ulcer in the mid to distal esophagus. The floor of the ulcer appears clean and smooth. There is no evidence of mass, mucosal irregularity, infiltration, or rigidity.

FIGURE 3-1B Barium swallow: detail distended view of the lesion at the junction of the mid to distal esophagus. The ulcer has a well-defined lucent rim, suggesting that it is benign.

◆ DIFFERENTIAL DIAGNOSIS

◆ **Gastroesophageal reflux disease:** This is the most common cause of esophageal ulceration, and such a large proximal ulcer raises the possibility of Barrett's change.

◆ **Infectious esophagitis:** Cytomegalovirus (CMV) should be suspected in the immunocompromised patient. The human immunodeficiency virus (HIV) itself can also result in giant esophageal ulcers.

◆ **Medication-induced esophagitis:** A history of recent ingestion of certain medications (particularly tetracycline antibiotics) would be relevant.

◆ **Radiation esophagitis:** Close anatomic relationship of the area of ulceration to the portal of radiation therapy would be relevant.

◆ DIAGNOSIS: Cytomegalovirus esophagitis.

◆ KEY FACTS

CLINICAL

◆ CMV is a member of the herpesvirus group. It causes opportunistic esophagitis in patients with acquired immunodeficiency syndrome (AIDS) and only rarely in other immunocompromised patients.

◆ Patients usually present with odynophagia, which may be severe. On endoscopy, ulcerative esophagitis is seen with lesions that may be shallow or deep. It is impossible to differentiate this disorder from other viral esophagitides, including involvement by the HIV itself.

◆ Diagnosis is made from endoscopic brushings or biopsy specimens from the base of ulcers, by detection of characteristic intranuclear inclusion bodies in endothe-lial cells or fibroblasts, or by positive viral cultures. Histologic findings are required to differentiate CMV from herpetic esophagitis. HIV ulcers may respond to the administration of steroids, but CMV esophagitis requires antiviral agents such as ganciclovir.

RADIOLOGIC

◆ CMV esophagitis may appear as discrete, small, superficial ulcers similar to those of herpes. Occasionally, a nonspecific esophagitis with nodular thickened folds only is seen, which may simulate reflux esophagitis.

◆ Giant, flat, single or multiple ulcers, often with a thin radiolucent rim of edematous mucosa, are very suggestive of CMV esophagitis. These ulcers may be several centimeters in length and appear ovoid because of the limited diameter of the esophagus.

◆ HIV ulcers may have an identical radiologic appearance, requiring endoscopy and biopsy for culture and histologic examination to make a definitive diagnosis before appropriate treatment can commence.

◆ *Candida* esophagitis is characterized by longitudinally orientated, small, plaque-like filling defects. Severe disease appears as extensive, confluent, large plaques, giving the mucosa a "shaggy" pattern. These patterns are not typical for CMV, allowing radiologic differentiation.

◆ SUGGESTED READING

Balthazar EJ, Megibow AJ, Hulnick D, et al. Cytomegalovirus esophagitis in AIDS: Radiographic features in 16 patients. AJR Am J Roentgenol 1987;149:919–923.

Sor S, Levine MS, Kowalski TE, et al. Giant ulcers of the esophagus in patients with human immunodeficiency virus: Clinical, radiographic and pathologic findings. Radiology 1995;194:447–451.

CASE 2

David M. Hough

HISTORY

A 55-year-old man presents with dysphagia.

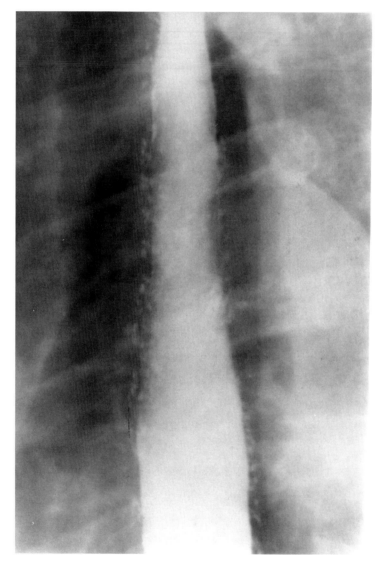

FIGURE 3-2 Barium swallow: spot film of the upper esophagus in single contrast. There are multiple, small, flask-shaped outpouchings from the esophageal lumen. Where visible, the necks are very narrow.

◆ DIFFERENTIAL DIAGNOSIS

◆ **Intramural pseudodiverticulosis:** The finding of multiple flask-shaped collections of barium, oriented almost perpendicular to the long axis of the esophagus, is characteristic of this condition. Not all of the pseudo-diverticula show a clear communication with the esophageal lumen.

◆ **Esophagitis:** Features may include fold thickening, mucosal nodularity, an irregular mucosal contour, and focal erosions or ulcers. Ulcers can usually be seen to communicate clearly with the esophageal lumen, whereas in this case, some of the barium collections do not communicate. There are no plaque like filling defects, as may be seen with *Candida* and other causes of esophagitis.

◆ **True esophageal diverticula:** These are larger and less numerous than pseudodiverticula.

◆ DIAGNOSIS: Esophageal intramural pseudo-diverticula.

◆ KEY FACTS

CLINICAL

◆ Esophageal intramural pseudodiverticula is caused by dilated excretory ducts of the deep esophageal mucous glands, due to chronic inflammation. It is usually a sequela of chronic reflux esophagitis. Secondary infection with *Candida* is a common associated finding, but it is not considered a causal factor.

◆ Esophageal intramural pseudodiverticula most commonly occurs in elderly patients, with a slight male predominance. In as many as 90% of cases, there is an associated stricture. The most common presenting symptom is dysphagia, due to the associated stricture, and management is directed at treating the stricture.

◆ Esophageal intramural pseudodiverticula occurs in approximately 0.1% of patients undergoing barium esophagography, with an increased prevalence in patients with esophageal cancer (4.5%).

RADIOLOGIC

◆ Single-contrast barium examination with low-density barium, which more readily enters the gland ducts, is more sensitive than a double-contrast technique with high-density barium for detecting intramural pseudodiverticula. Endoscopy is relatively insensitive because it is difficult to visualize the tiny duct orifices.

◆ The characteristic appearance is that of numerous small (1 to 4 mm), flask-shaped outpouchings from the esophagus. The tiny necks may not fill completely, resulting in an apparent lack of communication with the esophageal lumen.

◆ Distribution is more often segmental than diffuse. Pseudodiverticula may occur at, above, or below the level of a stricture.

◆ Strictures associated with intramural pseudodiverticula should be evaluated carefully for evidence of malignancy.

◆ SUGGESTED READING

Levine MS, Moolten DN, Herlinger H, et al. Esophageal intramural pseudodiverticulosis: A re-evaluation. AJR Am J Roentgenol 1986;147:1165–1170.

Plavsic BN, Chen MYM, Gelfand DW, et al. Intramural pseudodiverticulosis of the esophagus detected on barium esophagograms: Increased prevalence in patients with esophageal carcinoma. AJR Am J Roentgenol 1995;165:1381–1385.

Sabanathan S, Salama FD, Morgan WE. Esophageal intramural pseudodiverticulosis. Thorax 1985;40:849–857.

CASE 3

Erik K. Paulson

HISTORY

A 57-year-old man presents with a long history of heartburn and gradual onset of dysphagia.

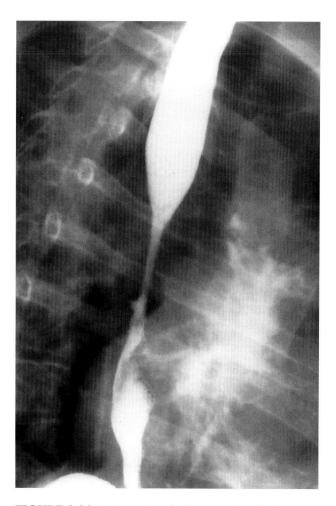

FIGURE 3-3A Barium swallow, single-contrast view. Single-contrast esophagram shows a smooth stricture in the mid esophagus with a small ulcer crater filled with barium.

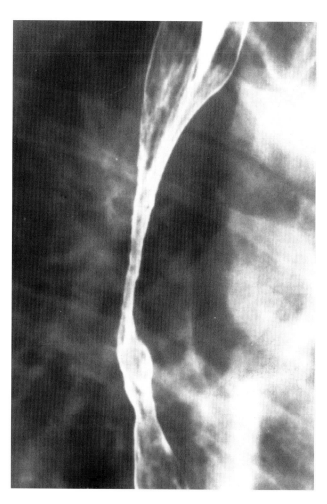

FIGURE 3-3B Barium swallow, double-contrast view, shows smooth mucosa within the stricture.

◈ DIFFERENTIAL DIAGNOSIS

◆ **Peptic stricture:** Peptic strictures are nearly always located in the distal esophagus, making this diagnosis unlikely. There is, however, an overlap in the appearance of peptic strictures and Barrett's esophagus.

◆ **Caustic ingestion:** A caustic stricture could have this appearance. In this scenario, clinical history would be the key to the diagnosis.

◆ **Mediastinal radiation:** While radiation strictures may be long and smooth, as in this case, clinical history and port-limited changes should be apparent in the mediastinum and pulmonary parenchyma. With radiation strictures, there is often displacement of both walls of the esophagus.

◆ **Barrett's esophagus:** This is the most likely diagnosis given the ulcer and the length and mid-esophageal location of the stricture.

◆ **Esophageal carcinoma:** It is uncommon for esophageal carcinoma to present with a smooth stricture.

◈ DIAGNOSIS: Barrett's esophagus with a stricture and esophageal ulcer.

◈ KEY FACTS

CLINICAL

◆ Barrett's esophagus represents columnar metaplasia of the squamous mucosa of the esophagus, associated with gastroesophageal reflux and esophagitis.

◆ Barrett's is a premalignant condition, placing the patient at risk for esophageal carcinoma. Prevalence of adenocarcinoma in this population is approximately 15%.

◆ Of patients with Barrett's esophagus, 20% to 40% are asymptomatic.

◆ Approximately 10% of patients with chronic reflux esophagitis also have Barrett's esophagus.

RADIOLOGIC

◆ The classic findings of Barrett's esophagus include a high esophageal stricture with or without an associated ulcer. However, the classic findings are relatively uncommon. Patients with Barrett's esophagus may have an unremarkable esophagram or may have a stricture in the distal esophagus, giving the appearance of a peptic stricture.

◆ As in this case, the stricture may be long and smooth or web-like.

◆ On double-contrast esophagography, a reticular pattern may be present in the region of the columnar metaplasia that may resemble the area gastricae found in the stomach.

◆ Radiographic findings are neither sensitive nor specific for this condition. Therefore, endoscopy and biopsy are the procedures of choice to diagnose and follow these patients.

◈ SUGGESTED READING

Levine MS. Gastroesophageal Reflux Disease. In RM Gore, MS Levine, I Laufer (eds), Textbook of Gastrointestinal Radiology. Philadelphia: Saunders, 1994;360–384.

Levine MS, Caroline DF, Thompson JJ, et al. Adenocarcinoma of the esophagus: Relationship to Barrett mucosa. Radiology 1984;150:305–309.

Levine MS, Kressel HY, Caroline DF, et al. Barrett's esophagus: Reticular pattern of the mucosa. Radiology 1983;147:663–667.

CASE 4

Vincent H.S. Low

HISTORY

A 47-year-old woman complains of dysphagia with solid food.

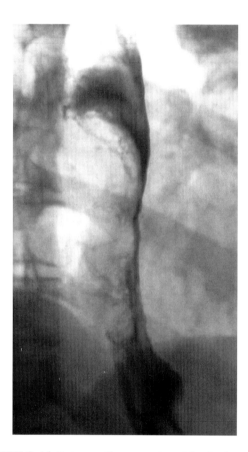

FIGURE 3-4A Barium swallow: spot view of the distal esophagus. There is a large, elongated polypoid mass arising from the esophageal wall, filling and expanding the lumen. The surface of the lesion appears lobulated.

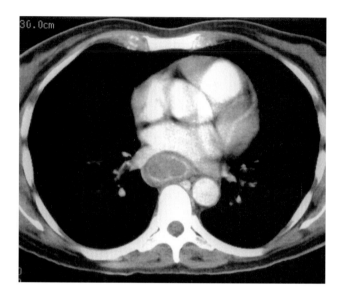

FIGURE 3-4B CT scan at the level of the right atrium following oral and intravenous contrast material. A polypoid mass distends the esophageal lumen, which is outlined by a thin rim of oral contrast material. The lesion itself is of soft tissue attenuation. The esophageal wall is thickened.

◆ DIFFERENTIAL DIAGNOSIS

- **Primary esophageal carcinoma:** This is the most common cause of an intrinsic esophageal mass lesion.
- **Leiomyosarcoma:** Leiomyosarcomas may be large tumors, but they tend to be predominantly intramural.
- **Lymphoma:** The absence of significant mediastinal lymphadenopathy makes esophageal lymphoma unusual.
- **Spindle cell carcinoma:** This rare tumor, commonly known as *carcinosarcoma*, usually manifests as a large polypoid tumor in the distal esophagus.
- **Intramural hematoma:** A history of bleeding, coagulation disorder, or anticoagulant therapy would be relevant to this diagnosis.

◆ DIAGNOSIS: Esophageal lymphoma.

◆ KEY FACTS

CLINICAL

- Esophageal lymphoma is a rare condition, seen in only 1% to 2% of cases of gastrointestinal lymphoma.
- It usually occurs in the presence of disseminated disease, particularly lymphomatous mediastinal node involvement. Patients usually present with dysphagia due to esophageal narrowing or obstruction by a mass. It is frequently asymptomatic and occasionally presents with bleeding.

- Endoscopic biopsy is frequently negative due to the submucosal location of the tumor.
- The tumor may be complicated by perforation into the mediastinum, a bronchus, or the trachea.

RADIOLOGIC

- Intrinsic lymphoma of the esophagus may have a variable, but malignant appearance, including a polypoid, ulcerative, or infiltrative mass.
- Less frequent manifestations include numerous submucosal nodules mimicking multiple leiomyomas or esophageal varices if confluent.
- Lymphoma arising in mediastinal lymph nodes and involving the esophagus appears initially as smooth extrinsic indentation, but with progression and invasion, will result in irregularity of the esophageal contour and eventual narrowing.
- Gastric lymphoma invading up into the esophagus may result in an achalasia-like picture, and careful examination of the gastric cardia is required to detect the mass lesion.

◆ SUGGESTED READING

Doki T, Hamada S, Murayama H, et al. Primary malignant lymphoma of the esophagus. Endoscopy 1984;16:189–192.

Levine MS, Sunshine AG, Reynolds JC, et al. Diffuse nodularity in esophageal lymphoma. AJR Am J Roentgenol 1985;145: 1218–1220.

Zornoza J, Dodd GD. Lymphoma of the gastrointestinal tract. Semin Roentgenol 1980;15:272–287.

CASE 5

Jeffrey T. Seabourn

HISTORY

A 22-year-old woman presents with a several-month history of dysphagia and a 25-pound weight loss.

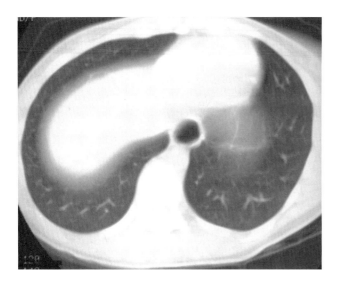

FIGURE 3-5A Chest CT (lung window) at the level of the gastroesophageal junction. There is marked dilatation of the distal esophagus with an air-fluid level. Neither mural thickening nor a mass at the gastroesophageal junction is present. The lung bases are normal.

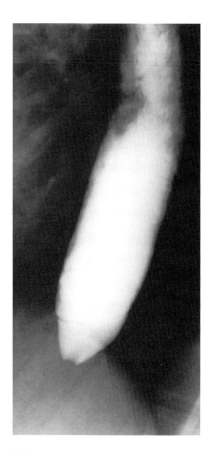

FIGURE 3-5B Barium swallow, single-contrast view. The esophagus is dilated, with smoothly marginated tapering at the gastroesophageal junction. Mucus and debris remain in the proximal esophagus. Primary peristaltic activity was absent fluoroscopically.

◆ DIFFERENTIAL DIAGNOSIS

- **Peptic stricture:** Although peptic strictures typically cause narrowing of the distal esophagus, they are usually smoothly marginated and relatively fixed.
- **Primary achalasia:** Lack of primary peristaltic activity with smooth tapering at the gastroesophageal (GE) junction and intermittent opening of the lower esophageal sphincter (LES) argue for a primary motor disorder of the esophagus. The age of the patient and lack of an obstructing or infiltrating mass favors primary achalasia.
- **Secondary achalasia due to an intrinsic or extrinsic neoplasm:** The age of the patient, duration of symptoms, and lack of a mass on imaging studies rules this entity out.
- **Complicated scleroderma:** Narrowing of the distal esophagus in complicated scleroderma is the result of a patulous LES with free GE reflux, eventually causing a peptic stricture. The chest CT usually reveals normal lung bases.
- **Chagas disease:** This protozoal infection, which involves the myenteric plexus, results in a motor disorder of the esophagus similar to achalasia.

◆ DIAGNOSIS: Primary achalasia.

◆ KEY FACTS

CLINICAL

- Achalasia is a primary motility disorder of the esophagus characterized by aperistalsis in the distal two-thirds of the esophagus and failure of the LES to relax.
- The etiology is unknown, but it is thought to be neurogenic in origin. Pathologic specimens reveal a decrease in the number of ganglion cells in Auerbach's myenteric plexus.
- Primary achalasia results in a slowly progressive dysphagia with both solids and liquids that may develop over many months or years. The patient may be able to modify dietary needs with smaller, frequent meals and, as a result, present without any weight loss despite severe dysphagia.
- Odynophagia and chest pain are much less common symptoms.
- Regurgitation may lead to choking and coughing and even to aspiration and pneumonitis.

RADIOLOGIC

- Fluoroscopic examination of esophageal motility will identify characteristic absence of the primary peristaltic wave in the distal two-thirds of the esophagus.
- The esophagus eventually dilates, with distal tapering (bird-beak or rat-tail appearance) at the GE junction.
- An important cause of this radiologic appearance is pseudoachalasia due to malignancy. This typically occurs in an older age group (>50 years) with a shorter duration (<6 months) of dysphagia. This is most commonly due to a carcinoma of the gastric cardia or fundus with invasion of the distal esophagus. This may also be due to actual infiltration of the myenteric plexus or to high-grade obstruction at the GE junction.

◆ SUGGESTED READING

Kahrilas PJ, Kishk SM, Helm JF, et al. Comparison of pseudoachalasia and achalasia. Am J Med 1987;82:439–446.

Laufer I. Motor Disorders of the Esophagus. In MS Levine (ed), Radiology of the Esophagus. Philadelphia: Saunders, 1989;229–246.

HISTORY

A 34-year-old man presents with crampy abdominal pain and diarrhea.

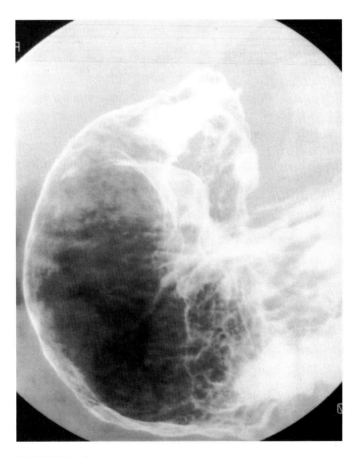

FIGURE 3-6 Double-contrast upper gastrointestinal series: spot film of the distal stomach and proximal duodenum. There is narrowing of the gastric antrum with multiple punctate collections of barium and surrounding halos of edema (aphthous lesions). The duodenal bulb is not distended, and there are ulcerations in the bulb and second portion of the duodenum.

◆ DIFFERENTIAL DIAGNOSIS

- **Erosive gastritis:** Varioliform erosions may result from ingestion of alcohol, aspirin, and nonsteroidal anti-inflammatory drugs. Other causes include ischemia, stress, and trauma. Duodenal involvement would be unusual.
- **Infectious gastritis:** *Helicobacter pylori* is important in antral gastritis. Features include fold thickening, ulceration, and sometimes antral narrowing and duodenal ulceration. CMV infection occurs in AIDS and other immunocompromised patients. Nonspecific findings include fold thickening, erosions or ulcers, and antral narrowing. *Pneumocystis carinii* pneumonia, herpesvirus, toxoplasmosis, and cryptosporidiosis may also have similar findings.
- **Granulomatous disease:** Gastroduodenal Crohn's disease typically has antral aphthous lesions, duodenal ulcers, and tapering of the antrum and pylorus, resulting in a "ram's horn" configuration. Sarcoidosis, tuberculosis (TB), and syphilis may have similar features, with antral ulcers progressing to fibrosis and scarring.
- **Zollinger-Ellison syndrome (ZES):** Although the presence of postbulbar ulcers suggests ZES, there should also be gastric fold thickening and increased fluid.
- **Eosinophilic gastritis:** Although eosinophilic gastritis typically involves the gastric antrum and proximal small bowel, nodularity and fold thickening are more common features. Gastric erosions are atypical, and duodenal ulcers are rare.
- **Scirrhous carcinoma:** This entity typically causes a smooth, funnel-shaped narrowing of the antrum. Irregular fold thickening and ulceration may also occur. It is unlikely to cross the pylorus.

◆ DIAGNOSIS: Gastroduodenal Crohn's disease.

◆ KEY FACTS

CLINICAL

- Gastroduodenal Crohn's is almost always associated with concomitant ileocecal disease but rarely may occur before the development of more distal disease.
- Although it may be asymptomatic in the early stages, pain, nausea, vomiting, and weight loss are common in advanced stages. Gastric outlet obstruction may even occur.

RADIOLOGIC

- Gastric Crohn's disease typically involves the antrum and sometimes the body, but fundal involvement is uncommon. Duodenal disease usually occurs in association with antral involvement, but isolated duodenal disease is possible.
- Aphthous lesions may appear as punctate or slit-like collections of barium with a lucent halo, indistinguishable from varioliform ulcers of erosive gastritis. Larger ulcers, mucosal effacement, or cobblestoning may also occur.
- Fibrosis may result in a funnel-shaped or ram's horn antrum. A pseudo-Billroth I sign is due to scarring of the antrum and duodenum with obliteration of the pylorus.
- Duodenal ulcers may be single or multiple. Duodenal strictures are usually postbulbar, smoothly tapering, and may be multiple. Skip lesions may occur.
- Asymmetric or eccentric scarring in the duodenum may result in pseudodiverticula.

◆ SUGGESTED READING

Farman J, Faegenburg D, Dallemand S, et al. Crohn's disease of the stomach: The "rams-horn" sign. AJR Am J Roentgenol 1975; 123:242–251.

Levine M. Crohn's disease of the upper gastrointestinal tract. Radiol Clin North Am 1987;25:79–91.

Nelson SW. Some interesting and unusual manifestations of Crohn's disease of the stomach, duodenum and small intestine. AJR Am J Roentgenol 1969;107:86–101.

CASE 7

Vincent H.S. Low

HISTORY

A 40-year-old man presents with dyspepsia. He is taking nonsteroidal anti-inflammatory agents for arthritis.

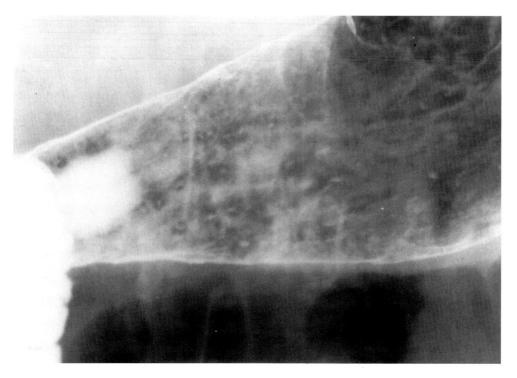

FIGURE 3-7 Double-contrast upper examination: view of distal body and antrum of the stomach. Numerous dense specks are seen along the gastric antrum, predominantly toward the greater curvature. Some of these appear longitudinally oriented, and most demonstrate a lucent surrounding halo, representing edema.

◆ DIFFERENTIAL DIAGNOSIS

- **Erosive gastritis:** This is the most likely diagnosis given the history and distribution of lesions.
- **Crohn's disease:** Gastric involvement usually occurs in the presence of advanced disease elsewhere, particularly the terminal ileum.
- **Viral infection:** This type of gastritis usually occurs in patients with immunodeficiency.
- **Ulcerated submucosal masses:** With these masses, the central ulcer, as well as the surrounding mass, tends to be larger than in this case.
- **Barium precipitates:** These artifacts do not have a radiolucent halo and will move when the patient is repositioned, either by the effect of gravity or the flowing pool of liquid barium.

◆ DIAGNOSIS: Erosive gastritis.

◆ KEY FACTS

CLINICAL

- These erosions are superficial epithelial defects that do not extend beyond the muscularis mucosa.
- Drugs are an identifiable cause of erosive gastritis, including aspirin, nonsteroidal anti-inflammatory drugs, steroids, and alcohol.
- In half the cases, no cause is identified. These cases are probably a manifestation of peptic disease.

- Other causes of gastric erosions include Crohn's disease, viral infection, and iatrogenic trauma (gastric catheters and endoscopic therapy).

RADIOLOGIC

- Erosions appear as very shallow collections of barium. These are always small and may have a variety of shapes, including round, polygonal, linear, and punctate.
- There is associated nodular thickening of the rugal folds, and the erosions are aligned along the crest of these folds. On barium studies, the abnormal folds are often more easily visualized than the erosions themselves, and they may persist after the erosions have healed.
- Because the lesions are shallow, the changes are subtle. Disease on the more dependent posterior wall is visualized more readily by manipulating a thin film of barium into the region to opacify the erosions and the spaces between the folds. Disease on the anterior wall is visualized best in the prone position using compression.

◆ SUGGESTED READING

Catalano D, Pagliari U. Gastroduodenal erosions: Radiological findings. Gastrointest Radiol 1982;7:235–240.

Laufer I, Hamilton J, Mullens JE. Demonstration of superficial gastric erosions by double contrast radiography. Gastroenterology 1975;68:387–391.

CASE 8

Vincent H.S. Low

HISTORY

A 50-year-old woman presents with epigastric pain for several months.

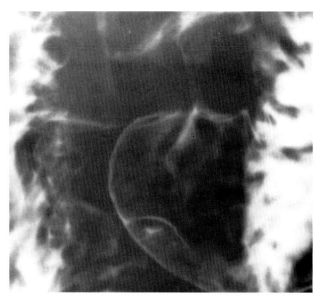

FIGURE 3-8A Double-contrast upper gastrointestinal barium examination: view of the distal gastric antrum in the left posterior oblique position. There is elevation of the mucosa measuring 2.5 cm in diameter along the greater curvature, just proximal to the pylorus. A central small collection of barium is seen within this lesion. The margins of the lesion appear smooth.

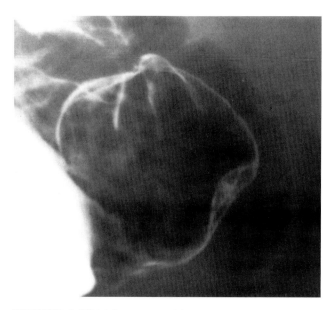

FIGURE 3-8B Right posterior oblique position view of the distal gastric antrum. Rotation of the patient into the right posterior oblique position brings the lesion into profile, further demonstrating the smooth outline of the lesion and the central (5 mm deep) niche of barium.

◆ DIFFERENTIAL DIAGNOSIS

◆ **Gastric ulcer:** An ulcer would have a central niche of barium and a surrounding mound of edema. However, such mounds usually have peripheral indistinct or fading borders, in contrast to the sharp outline of this lesion.

◆ **Leiomyoma:** This uncommon benign tumor could have this appearance, as would other benign mesenchymal tumors.

◆ **Ectopic pancreatic rest:** This is the most likely diagnosis by virtue of its benign submucosal appearance with central umbilication, as well as its location which is typical.

◆ **"Bull's eye" metastases:** These can appear with metastatic melanoma, lymphoma, or Kaposi's sarcoma. However, they are almost always multiple and occur in the context of disseminated disease elsewhere.

◆ DIAGNOSIS: Ectopic pancreatic rest.

◆ KEY FACTS

CLINICAL

◆ Ectopic pancreas occurs due to an anomaly in embryologic development where a fragment of migrating pancreatic precursor becomes implanted in the intestinal wall. Histologically, all normal pancreatic elements are present but show a disorganized arrangement.

◆ The majority of pancreatic rests occur in the stomach (80%). They are also found in the duodenum and proximal jejunum. They have also been reported in the gallbladder, bile ducts, liver, spleen, appendix, Meckel's diverticulum, omentum, mesentery, and mediastinum.

◆ These lesions are usually asymptomatic and discovery of such should not be accepted as the cause of a patient's symptoms.

◆ Rarely, enzyme production results in epigastric pain and intestinal bleeding. These lesions have also been reported to cause gastric outlet obstruction due to their strategic position near the pylorus.

RADIOLOGIC

◆ The lesion appears as a smooth, broad-based, solitary, submucosal mass.

◆ The most common location is along the distal greater curvature of the stomach, several centimeters from the pylorus.

◆ The central umbilication or dimple is thought to represent the orifice of the duct in this rest. It usually measures 1 to 5 mm in diameter and 5 to 10 mm in depth. Rarely, a rudimentary ductal system is sufficiently filled by contrast material to be visualized.

◆ SUGGESTED READING

Levine MS. Benign Tumors of the Stomach and Duodenum. In RM Gore, MS Levine, I Laufer (eds), Textbook of Gastrointestinal Radiology. Philadelphia: Saunders, 1994:649–651.

Thoeni RF, Gedgaudas RK. Ectopic pancreas: Usual and unusual features. Gastrointest Radiol 1980;5:37–42.

CASE 9

Jeffrey T. Seabourn

HISTORY

A 44-year-old woman with stage IV breast carcinoma is status post bone marrow transplant and high-dose chemotherapy.

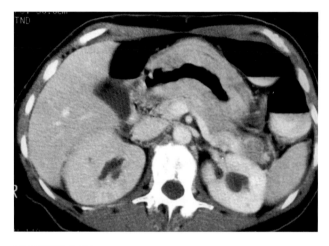

FIGURE 3-9A CT of the abdomen at the level of the superior mesenteric artery following intravenous contrast material. The gastric wall is diffusely thickened. No oral contrast was administered, but the stomach contains air. There is also bilateral pelviectasis with a delayed nephrogram on the right.

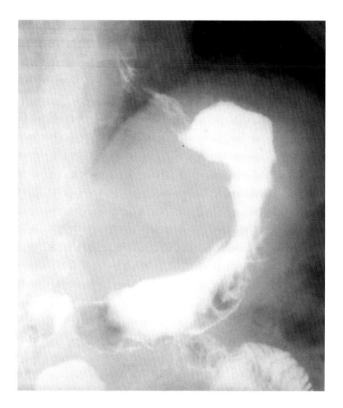

FIGURE 3-9B Double-contrast upper gastrointestinal barium examination: anteroposterior view of the stomach shows diffuse gastric narrowing, which is somewhat more pronounced in the region of the fundus and proximal body. The stomach was poorly distensible at fluoroscopy.

◆ DIFFERENTIAL DIAGNOSIS

- **Diffusely infiltrating (scirrhous) adenocarcinoma of the stomach:** The radiographic appearance of diffuse gastric wall thickening in a poorly distensible stomach is radiographically indistinguishable from diffusely infiltrating metastatic disease.
- **Diffusely infiltrating metastatic disease:** Given the patient's clinical history, this is the most likely diagnosis.
- **Lymphoma:** Diffuse gastric involvement with lymphoma may give this appearance. There is no regional abdominal or retroperitoneal lymphadenopathy. The spleen is normal size. When there is gastric involvement of lymphoma, it may cross the pylorus to involve the duodenum. The duodenum is normal in this patient.
- **Infectious/inflammatory gastritis:** Crohn's disease, chronic gastric ulcer disease with spasm, eosinophilic gastritis, sarcoidosis, tuberculosis (TB), and brucellosis are other causes of gastric wall thickening and luminal narrowing. These more typically involve the gastric antrum.
- **Physical/chemical gastritis:** Corrosive gastritis, postradiation injury, and hepatic arterial chemoinfusion are other less common causes of this appearance.

◆ DIAGNOSIS: Diffusely infiltrating metastatic breast carcinoma to the stomach (linitis plastica appearance).

◆ KEY FACTS

CLINICAL

- Metastatic disease to the stomach is not uncommon. The most common organs of origin include malignant melanoma, breast, lung, colon, prostate, leukemia, and secondary lymphoma.
- The pattern of gastric involvement is variable. Solitary mass: 50%; multiple nodules: 30%; and linitis plastica (diffusely infiltrating): 20%. The diffusely infiltrating variety is most commonly seen in breast carcinoma.
- Patients often present with early satiety, nausea, and vomiting. This patient could not tolerate oral contrast material due to severe nausea and vomiting.

RADIOLOGIC

- The differential diagnosis for diffuse gastric wall thickening with a poorly distensible lumen is fairly extensive. Malignant causes head the list and are most commonly due to the diffusely infiltrating variety of adenocarcinoma of the stomach, metastatic disease, or non-Hodgkin's lymphoma.
- Other causes of this radiographic appearance include inflammation secondary to chronic gastritis, Crohn's disease giving a pseudo-Billroth I appearance, eosinophilic gastritis, and sarcoidosis.
- Infectious etiologies include TB and brucellosis. TB may be radiographically indistinguishable from Crohn's disease as a cause of antral narrowing.
- Physical/chemical causes are most commonly due to corrosive gastritis and radiation therapy.

◆ SUGGESTED READING

Eisenberg RL. Gastrointestinal Radiology: A Pattern Approach (2nd ed). Philadelphia: Lippincott, 1990;205–222.

Jaffe M. Metastatic involvement of the stomach secondary to breast carcinoma. AJR Am J Roentgenol 1975;123:512–521.

Levine MS, Kong V, Rubesin SE, et al. Scirrhous carcinoma of the stomach: Radiologic and endoscopic diagnosis. Radiology 1990;175:151–154.

Levine MS, Megibow AJ. Stomach and Duodenum: Carcinoma. In RM Gore, MS Levine, I Laufer (eds), Textbook of Gastrointestinal Radiology (vol.1). Philadelphia: Saunders, 1994;660–683.

CASE 10

David M. Hough

HISTORY

A 38-year-old woman presents with nausea, vomiting, abdominal pain, and weight loss. Her serum amylase and lipase levels were elevated.

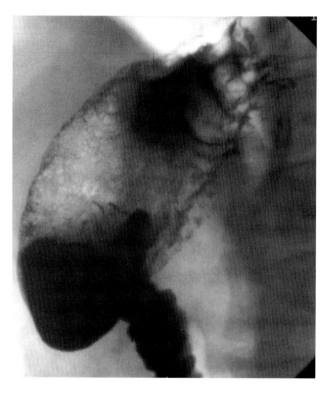

FIGURE 3-10A Double-contrast upper gastrointestinal barium examination: spot film of the stomach and duodenum. There is lobulated fold thickening in the gastric fundus.

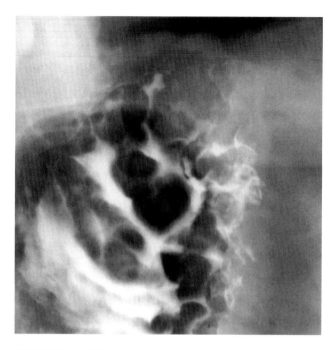

FIGURE 3-10B Spot film of the gastric fundus from the same examination. Gastric fold thickening is again seen, although the mucosa appears intact. The esophagus (not shown) was normal in appearance.

◆ DIFFERENTIAL DIAGNOSIS

◆ **Hypertrophic gastritis:** This is a condition characterized by glandular hyperplasia and increased acid secretion, with thickened folds predominantly in the fundus and body of the stomach. The majority of cases have an associated peptic ulcer. The focal nature of fold thickening in this case makes the diagnosis unlikely.

◆ **Ménétriers disease:** The gastric folds are usually more thickened than in hypertrophic gastritis, and there is relative sparing of the antrum. There may be mass-like fold thickening, although the abnormality is unlikely to be as focal as in this case. The folds in Ménétriers disease also tend to follow the distribution of normal rugae, and there are increased secretions.

◆ **Lymphoma:** Gastric lymphoma may cause irregular or lobulated fold thickening due to submucosal infiltration or multiple submucosal masses. Submucosal infiltration by carcinoma may also cause this appearance.

◆ **Varices:** Gastric varices typically appear as multiple, smooth, lobulated, filling defects that tend to change in size and shape on fluoroscopy. The serpentine appearance of the folds in this case favors this diagnosis.

◆ DIAGNOSIS: Isolated gastric varices.

◆ KEY FACTS

CLINICAL

◆ Gastric varices are less likely to bleed than esophageal varices. However, they may present with low-grade bleeding or massive hematemesis.

◆ Gastric varices are usually associated with esophageal varices and are secondary to cirrhosis with portal hypertension.

◆ Isolated gastric varices may be caused by splenic vein thrombosis, resulting in shunting of blood from the spleen through the short gastric veins to the fundus, where they anastomose with branches of the coronary vein and esophageal plexus. With normal portal venous pressure, the blood can drain via the coronary vein into the portal vein without producing esophageal varices.

RADIOLOGIC

◆ Gastric varices are characteristically multiple, lobulated, serpentine masses, but they may produce a single polypoid mass in the fundus.

◆ Gastric varices may be obscured on barium studies by the normal overlying gastric rugae. Gastric varices are seen radiographically in <50% of patients with uphill esophageal varices.

◆ It is important to examine the distal esophagus in patients with gastric varices for identification of esophageal varices.

◆ A double-contrast barium technique is considered more reliable than a single-contrast technique for identification of varices.

◆ The isolated gastric varices in this patient were due to splenic vein occlusion secondary to pancreatitis. Because portal hypertension is much more common than splenic vein occlusion, most patients with isolated gastric varices are found to have portal hypertension as the underlying cause.

◆ SUGGESTED READING

Evans JA, Delany F. Gastric varices. Radiology 1953;60:46–51.

Levine MS, Kieu K, Rubesin SE, et al. Isolated gastric varices: Splenic vein obstruction or portal hypertension? Gastrointest Radiol 1990;15:188–192.

Muhletaler C, Gerlock J, Goncharenko V, et al. Gastric varices secondary to splenic vein occlusion: Radiographic diagnosis and clinical significance. Radiology 1979;132:593–598.

CASE 11

Vincent H.S. Low

HISTORY

A 33-year-old man presents with dyspepsia. He has had many hospital admissions since childhood for recurrent pulmonary infections.

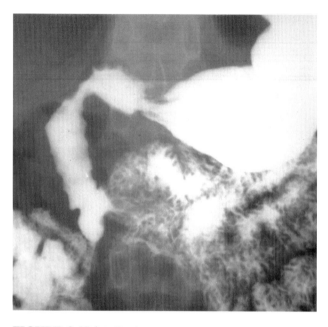

FIGURE 3-11A Full-column, single-contrast upper gastrointestinal barium examination: view of the duodenum. There are nodular indentations in the duodenal walls.

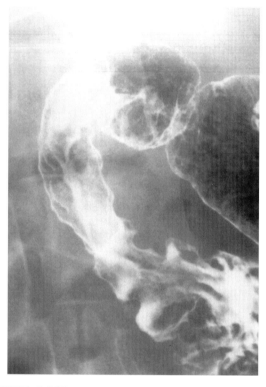

FIGURE 3-11B Double-contrast upper gastrointestinal barium examination: view of the duodenum. The duodenal folds appear flattened, smudged, and poorly defined.

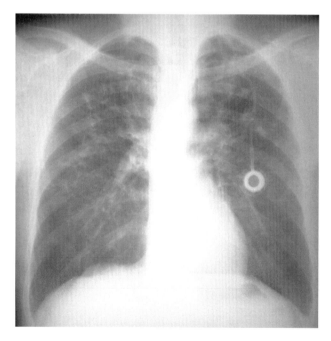

FIGURE 3-11C Frontal chest radiograph. There is fibrosis and bronchiectasis with a predominant upper lobe distribution.

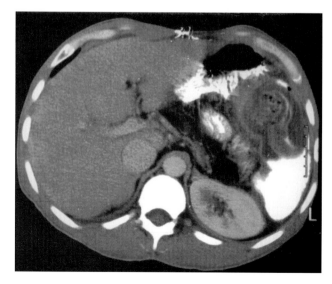

FIGURE 3-11D Contrast-enhanced CT of the upper abdomen. The pancreatic parenchyma has been replaced completely by fat.

◆ DIFFERENTIAL DIAGNOSIS

◆ **Peptic duodenitis:** This is a common condition that may coexist with other pathologic conditions causing the pulmonary changes, or may have occurred due to steroid or other medication therapy used to treat the lung condition.

◆ **Cystic fibrosis:** This is the most likely diagnosis as it would explain both the pulmonary and duodenal changes. The patient's age, however, is rather advanced for this condition.

◆ **Scleroderma:** Intestinal fibrosis from scleroderma may produce this duodenal pattern and may also be associated with pulmonary fibrosis.

◆ **Tuberculosis (TB):** TB would explain the upper lobe fibrotic changes. Duodenal involvement, however, is rare and usually results in strictures and fistulae.

◆ **Pancreatitis and other periduodenal inflammatory processes:** These conditions may cause the nonspecific duodenal changes but do not adequately explain the pulmonary abnormalities.

◆ DIAGNOSIS: Cystic fibrosis.

◆ KEY FACTS

CLINICAL

◆ Cystic fibrosis occurs in 1 in 2,000 births, predominantly in whites. Clinical and radiologic manifestations occur due to viscous secretions.

◆ The diagnosis is usually made clinically in infancy, but in about 2% of patients, symptoms may not manifest until after 18 years of age. Older patients present with hepatobiliary or gastrointestinal tract symptoms.

◆ With improvements in pulmonary care, increasing numbers of cystic fibrosis patients are surviving into adulthood.

◆ A majority (85%) of patients will have malabsorption due to impaired exocrine pancreatic secretions. These secretions are viscous, low in bicarbonates, and low in enzymes.

RADIOLOGIC

◆ Duodenal changes are seen in 60% to 80% of patients and consist of fold thickening, mucosal nodularity, fold flattening, luminal dilatation, smudging, and poor definition of the mucosal fold pattern. These changes are usually confined to the first and second portions of the duodenum and occur without ulcerations.

◆ In the small bowel, blobs of mucous result in a network pattern of curved lines, predominantly involving the distal small bowel.

◆ Intestinal obstruction and impaction can occur during and after childhood.

◆ Pancreatic calcification may be evident on plain radiographs.

◆ SUGGESTED READING

Phelan MS, Fine DR, Zentler-Munro L, et al. Radiographic abnormalities of the duodenum in cystic fibrosis. Clin Radiol 1983;34:573–577.

Taussig LM, Saldino RM, di Sant'Agnese PA. Radiographic abnormalities of the duodenum and small bowel in cystic fibrosis of the pancreas (mucoviscidosis). Pediatr Radiol 1973;106:369–376.

CASE 12

Vincent H.S. Low

HISTORY

A 35-year-old man presents with several months of intermittent vomiting.

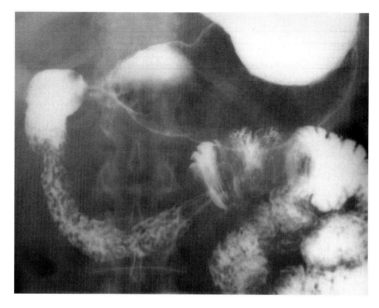

FIGURE 3-12A Double-contrast upper gastrointestinal barium examination: anteroposterior view. There is a short segment of narrowing in the distal duodenum with paradoxical dilatation of the adjacent proximal jejunum.

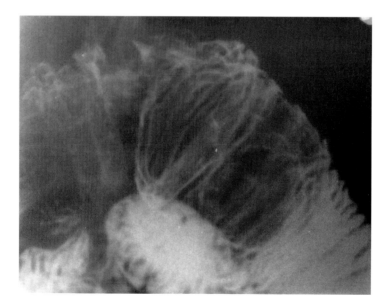

FIGURE 3-12B Double-contrast upper gastrointestinal barium examination: spot view of the distal duodenum. The proximal jejunum is dilated with resultant transverse stretching of the mucosal fold pattern. The mucosal folds otherwise appear normal. There is lucency within the lumen of the dilated jejunum, indicating a large filling defect, and the lumen of the narrowed distal duodenum appears to pass centrally through this filling defect.

◆ DIFFERENTIAL DIAGNOSIS

- **Benign duodenal polyp with intussusception:** A solitary duodenal polyp is usually hyperplastic or adenomatous.
- **Polyposis syndrome:** These polyps are either adenomas or hamartomas. Characteristically, there will be other polyps throughout the intestinal tract.
- **Benign mesenchymal tumor:** Leiomyoma and lipoma are the most common of this group. These tumors are usually submucosal but may demonstrate central ulceration.
- **Leiomyosarcoma:** This usually occurs as a large, lobulated, submucosal mass, and ulceration or cavitation is common.
- **Duodenal carcinoma:** This may present as a polypoid mass but usually has more aggressive features, such as infiltration and annular narrowing.

◆ DIAGNOSIS: Leiomyosarcoma with intussusception.

◆ KEY FACTS

CLINICAL

- Leiomyosarcomas represent about 10% of duodenal malignant tumors. These tumors are typically slow growing; therefore patients may remain asymptomatic for a long period of time. Clinical presentations include gastrointestinal bleeding and anemia, abdominal pain, epigastric mass, weight loss, and jaundice.
- These tumors are of smooth muscle origin, and they vary in clinical and histologic degrees of aggression from nearly benign to highly invasive.
- The tumor spreads by direct invasion of adjacent structures and metastases to the liver.
- Aggressive resection is indicated in surgical candidates.

RADIOLOGIC

- The majority of duodenal leiomyosarcomas (80%) occur in the descending (D2) and transverse segments (D3).
- On barium studies, they usually appear as submucosal masses, usually with ulceration or even cavitation. They may enlarge to several centimeters in diameter but still remain nonobstructive.
- Some tumors have a predominantly exoenteric growth pattern. These will appear on barium studies as extrinsic lesions, more suggestive of a mass arising from an adjacent structure, such as the pancreas. The full extent of such tumors is assessed best by CT.
- Areas of necrosis result in low attenuation on CT, usually within the central portion of the tumor.

◆ SUGGESTED READING

Kanematsu M, Imada T, Iianuluma G, et al. Leiomyosarcoma of the duodenum. Gastrointest Radiol 1991;16:109–112.

Pujari BD, Deadhare SG. Leiomyosarcoma of the duodenum. Int Surg 1976;61:237–238.

CASE 13

Vincent H.S. Low

HISTORY

A 75-year-old man has persistent nausea and vomiting since an abdominal aortic aneurysm repair 1 month previously.

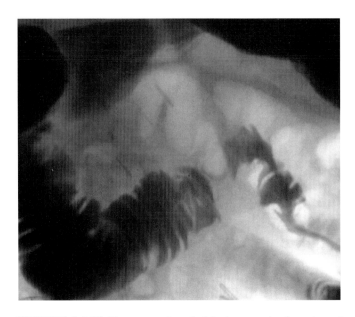

FIGURE 3-13A Upper gastrointestinal barium examination: view of the distal duodenum. There is a tight stricture of the distal duodenum just proximal to the ligament of Trietz.

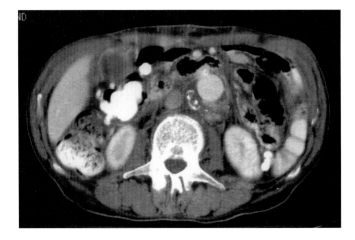

FIGURE 3-13B CT scan of the abdomen at the level of the proximal aortic anastomosis following intravenous and oral contrast material. The distal duodenum is the gas-filled structure immediately anterior to the aorta, just to the left of midline. The enhancing longtitudinal, tubular structures immediately anterior to the duodenum are the superior mesenteric artery and vein. There is no soft-tissue mass or abnormal fluid collection in the vicinity.

◆ DIFFERENTIAL DIAGNOSIS

- **Mesenteric root syndrome:** This is the appropriate clinical scenario for this condition, and the point of narrowing does appear to correspond to the location at which the duodenum passes between the superior mesenteric artery and the aorta.
- **Duodenal obstruction by adhesions:** The transverse duodenum lies in close proximity to the site of major surgery in this case. Extensive dissection of the retroperitoneal tissues is required for this procedure, and a dense inflammatory reaction may result in adhesions and duodenal obstruction.
- **Intramural hematoma:** Hemorrhage should always be considered in the postoperative patient. The absence of a para-aortic or paraduodenal soft tissue mass or fluid collection excludes this possibility.
- **Duodenal malignancy:** Duodenal carcinoma or invasion of the duodenum from carcinoma of an adjacent organ may present as a partially obstructing stricture. The absence of a soft-tissue mass on CT scan excludes this diagnosis.

◆ DIAGNOSIS: Duodenal obstruction by adhesions after abdominal aortic aneurysm repair.

◆ KEY FACTS

CLINICAL

- Complications involving the gastrointestinal tract following abdominal aortic aneurysm repair have been reported in up to 30% of cases. Some of these complications carry a very high mortality.
- Complications specifically involving the duodenum include aortoduodenal fistula and resultant massive hemorrhage, hematoma, retroperitoneal abscess, fibrosis and adhesion, ischemic stricture, and mesenteric root syndrome.

- Major aortic and retroperitoneal surgery is complicated frequently by postoperative ileus, which may be quite prolonged.
- An aortoduodenal fistula may present with massive intestinal hemorrhage. An abscess would typically present with fever and leukocytosis. The various complications of mechanical obstruction and paralytic ileus usually present with nonspecific nausea and vomiting.

RADIOLOGIC

- The location of the stricture in this case illustrates the importance of continuing an examination of the upper gastrointestinal tract to the level of the jejunum.
- Cross-sectional imaging techniques such as CT and ultrasound are useful in the evaluation of duodenal strictures, particularly for detecting a mass arising from the duodenum or one involving the duodenum from an adjacent structure. A soft-tissue duodenal mass raises the possibility of duodenal carcinoma or leiomyosarcoma. Carcinoma of the pancreas, because of its close proximity, may also involve the duodenum. Paraduodenal fluid collections (cysts, abscess, hematoma, pancreatic pseudocyst) would be seen as low attenuation on CT and hypoechoic on ultrasound.
- CT scanning is useful in this clinical scenario for demonstrating the close proximity of the point of duodenal obstruction to the site of surgery, as well as to demonstrate dense, adjacent inflammatory changes in the retroperitoneum.

◆ SUGGESTED READING

Budorick NE, Love L. Duodenal obstruction after repair of abdominal aortic aneurysm. Radiology 1988;169:421–422.

Eisenberg RL. Miscellaneous Abnormalities of the Stomach and Duodenum—Duodenal Obstruction. In RM Gore, MS Levine, I Laufer (eds), Textbook of Gastrointestinal Radiology. Philadelphia: Saunders, 1994;724–726.

CASE 14

Kelly S. Freed

HISTORY

A 35-year-old man presents with a 6-month history of diarrhea.

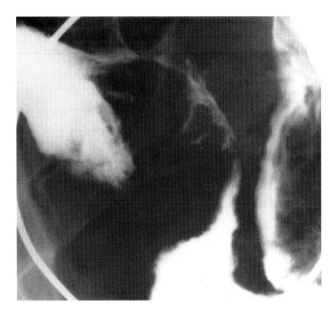

FIGURE 3-14A Small-bowel follow-through barium examination: spot film of the terminal ileum. The terminal ileum demonstrates luminal narrowing, known as the "string sign." There is also involvement of an adjacent loop of ileum. The intervening section of small bowel, which is relatively dilated, is less involved by the disease process. Linear ulceration is seen along the mesenteric border of the terminal ileum. At least two fistulae are seen along the antimesenteric border.

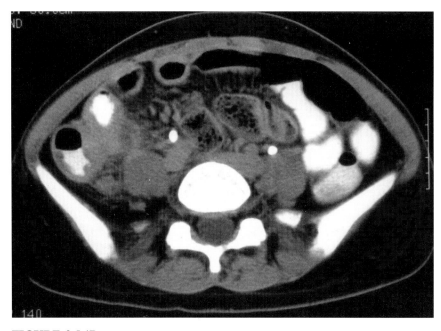

FIGURE 3-14B CT scan of the pelvis following intravenous and oral contrast material. The terminal ileum and cecum demonstrate bowel wall thickening with inflammatory change in the adjacent mesenteric fat.

◆ DIFFERENTIAL DIAGNOSIS

◆ **Crohn's disease:** Involvement of the terminal ileum and distal ileum, discontinuous segments of disease, stricture, and fistulae formation are characteristic of Crohn's disease. The CT appearance is also typical, with the marked mural thickening and inflammatory change in the mesenteric fat.

◆ **Ulcerative colitis:** Ulcerative colitis can involve the terminal ileum by backwash ileitis, but the discontinuous involvement makes this diagnosis less likely. Additionally, the fistula formation and inflammatory change in the adjacent mesenteric fat are unusual.

◆ **Ischemia:** The distribution of disease makes a vascular etiology lower in the differential. Ischemic insult to bowel more commonly involves the left colon than the right colon, and small bowel involvement is less common.

◆ **Neoplasms:** Adenocarcinoma more commonly involves the duodenum and proximal jejunum. Lymphoma usually presents as polyps or large excavating lesions.

◆ **Infection:** Tuberculosis (TB) is rare in developed countries. Features that suggest TB rather than Crohn's disease include greater involvement of the cecum than the terminal ileum. The ulcers tend to be larger than in Crohn's disease. *Yersinia* ileitis may also have an appearance similar to Crohn's disease, but the disease is self-limited and the radiographic changes would return to normal in time.

◆ **Other perienteric inflammatory conditions:** Appendicitis or endometriosis are differential considerations. The involvement of a loop of distal ileum in addition to the cecum and terminal ileum makes appendicitis less likely. Endometriosis may cause serosal abnormality of bowel, but not the strictures and fistulas seen in this patient. Additionally, endometriosis more commonly affects the sigmoid and transverse mesocolon.

◆ DIAGNOSIS: Crohn's disease.

◆ KEY FACTS
CLINICAL
◆ Crohn's disease is an inflammatory bowel disease of unknown etiology. There is a family history in approximately 40% of cases. The overall incidence is approximately 5 in 100,000. The age of onset is usually in adolescence or young adulthood.

◆ Early Crohn's disease is a mucosal disorder characterized by aphthous erosions or ulcers, which can be detected by a barium examination or endoscopy. The disease progresses to the submucosa and eventually becomes transmural. Any portion of the gastrointesti-

nal tract can be involved, although the terminal ileum is the most common site of disease. Extraintestinal involvement includes uveitis, arthritis, and erythema nodosum. The treatment includes medical suppression of the inflammatory reaction and surgical resection. The disease often recurs following surgical resection, often at the anastomotic site.

RADIOLOGIC
◆ The radiologic diagnosis is typically made by a contrast examination such as an upper gastrointestinal examination, small-bowel follow-through, enteroclysis, or barium enema. The earliest changes of Crohn's disease are aphthous lesions or erosions, which appear as a central fleck of barium surrounded by a translucent halo. These initial changes occur in the mucosal lymphoid tissue. The appearance is nonspecific and can be seen in other inflammatory diseases.

◆ With progression of disease, mural thickening occurs, often >1 cm. The bowel wall thickening in Crohn's disease is usually greater than that seen in ulcerative colitis. Asymmetric or discontinuous involvement of the gastrointestinal tract is characteristic, as opposed to the continuous involvement by ulcerative colitis. A typical nodular, cobblestone appearance is seen consisting of longitudinally oriented ulcerations.

◆ The terminal ileum is the most common site of involvement. Techniques to delineate the terminal ileum include enteroclysis, peroral pneumocolon, and a prone-angled compression view on SBFT. Strictures, fistulae, and abscess formation are more commonly seen in Crohn's disease than in ulcerative colitis.

◆ CT demonstrates the extraluminal extent of disease. The most common CT finding in Crohn's disease is bowel wall thickening. Another common finding is inflammatory change in the adjacent mesenteric fat. This mesenteric change is seen in Crohn's disease rather than ulcerative colitis as the former is a transmural process and the latter is limited to the mucosa. Fibrofatty proliferation of the mesentery and enlarged mesenteric lymph nodes are also seen in Crohn's disease. CT is also helpful in the diagnosis of abscess formation.

◆ SUGGESTED READING
Hizawa K, Iida M, et al. Crohn's disease: Early recognition and progress of aphthous lesions. Radiology 1994;190:451–454.

Nanakawa S, Takahashi M, et al. The role of computed tomography in management of patients with Crohn's disease. Clin Imag 1993;17:193–198.

Yue NC, Jones B. Crohn's disease: Prone-angled compression view in radiographic evaluation. Radiology 1993;187:577–580.

CASE 15

Vincent H.S. Low

HISTORY

A 61-year-old woman has frequent and severe episodes of abdominal pain and distention.

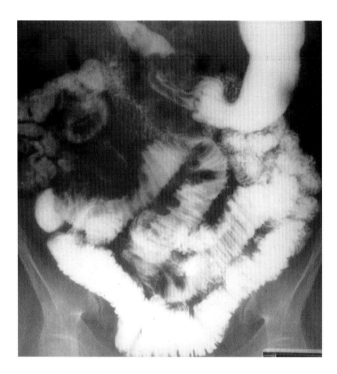

FIGURE 3-15A Barium small-bowel follow-through: 60-minute frontal overview. There is a large area of mass effect in the right mid abdomen, displacing loops of bowel. Caliber change is seen, with dilatation of proximal small bowel. Abnormal separation of loops of small bowel is present in the lower abdomen. The margins of small bowel loops adjacent to these areas of separation and mass effect show spiculation.

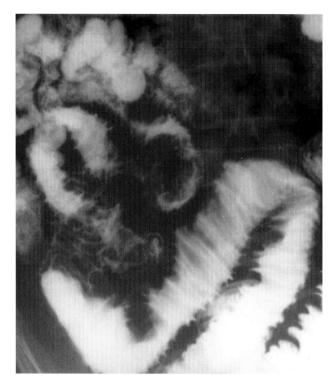

FIGURE 3-15B Barium small-bowel follow-through: spot view of the right lower quadrant. The mucosal folds are thickened, smooth in some areas and nodular in others. No specific intraluminal mass is seen.

◆ DIFFERENTIAL DIAGNOSIS

◆ **Mesenteric metastatic disease:** Marked desmoplastic reaction may be seen with certain metastatic tumors, such as scirrhous gastrointestinal tract cancers and breast cancer.

◆ **Carcinoid tumor:** This would explain the region of mass effect, which may be due to the tumor itself together with surrounding fibrosis. Similarly, small-bowel loop separation represents mesenteric infiltration, and the spiculation is due to the tumor's desmoplastic response.

◆ **Endometriosis:** This entity is unlikely, as the patient is postmenopausal.

◆ **Crohn's disease:** This disorder could provide an explanation for the inflammatory mass and mesenteric inflammation. However, the lack of fistula formation and terminal ileal disease makes this diagnosis unlikely.

◆ **Hemorrhage:** Mesenteric and intramural hemorrhage may occur with bleeding disorders or anticoagulant therapy.

◆ DIAGNOSIS: Carcinoid tumor.

◆ KEY FACTS

CLINICAL

◆ Carcinoid tumors account for one-fourth of small-bowel tumors, and the ileum is the most common site for malignant carcinoids.

◆ Carcinoids arise from enterochromaffin cells and are slow growing, but essentially all are potentially malignant. The jejunum may remain asymptomatic for many years. Later, symptoms suggestive of a small-bowel lesion may occur, such as intermittent obstruction, diarrhea, and blood loss.

◆ The tumor produces active hormones such as 5-hydroxytryptamine, histamine, and serotonin. These result in the carcinoid syndrome (cutaneous flushing, diarrhea, and bronchospasm) in the presence of metastases to the liver.

RADIOLOGIC

◆ Early tumors (<2 cm in diameter) are usually found in the distal or terminal ileum as nonspecific smooth, round mucosal, or submucosal masses.

◆ When the tumor invades through the muscularis, serotonin is released, resulting in an intense desmoplastic reaction. This produces fibrosis with tethering, angulation, and spiculation of adjacent loops of bowel. This phenomenon may be well in excess of the extent of the tumor mass itself. Actual extension of tumor beyond the bowel will be seen as a soft-tissue mass displacing and surrounding adjacent bowel loops. The tumor will also spread through the mesentery.

◆ On CT, a carcinoid tumor is seen as a mesenteric mass with soft-tissue strands extending through the mesentery toward adjacent bowel loops. Liver metastases are usually well defined and hypervascular. They tend to be iso- to hypoattenuating precontrast, hyperattenuating in the hepatic arterial dominant phase, and hypo- to isoattenuating in the portal venous dominant phase.

◆ SUGGESTED READING

Balthazar EJ. Carcinoid tumors of the elementary tract: Radiographic diagnosis. Gastrointest Radiol 1978;3:47–56.

Herlinger H, Maglinte DDT. Tumors of the Small Intestine. In H Herlinger, DDT Maglinte (eds), Clinical Radiology of the Small Intestine. Philadelphia: Saunders, 1989;406–409.

HISTORY

A 49-year-old woman presents with crampy abdominal pain, steatorrhea, and weight loss.

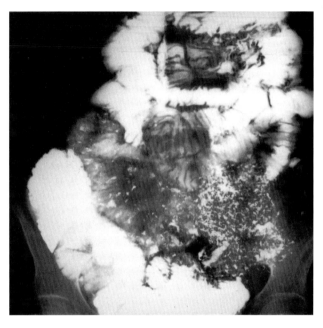

FIGURE 3-16A Barium small-bowel follow-through examination: 2 hours frontal overview. There is diffuse small-bowel dilatation, flocculation of the barium column, and reversal of the small-bowel fold pattern (jejunization of the ileum).

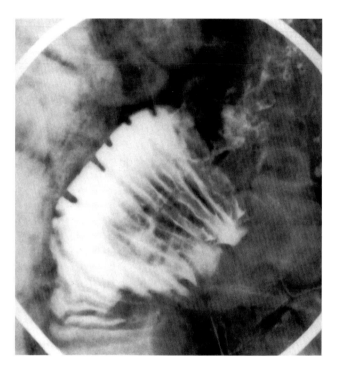

FIGURE 3-16B Barium small-bowel follow-through examination: spot film of an ileal loop. There is an intussuscepting mass in the right lower quadrant that was transient.

◆ DIFFERENTIAL DIAGNOSIS

◆ **Sprue, tropical or nontropical (celiac disease):** The hallmark is small-bowel dilatation with segmentation of the barium column, flocculation, fragmentation, jejunization of ileal loops, transient nonobstructive intussusceptions, and the "moulage sign" (50%).

◆ **Lymphoma of small bowel:** Lymphoma does not have signs of hypersecretion or jejunization but can present as a diffuse small-bowel disease with nodular fold thickening. Lymphoma can also be associated with intussusceptions.

◆ **Crohn's disease:** This disorder typically involves the terminal ileum and is characterized by skip areas, transmural disease with fistula formation, and involves the jejunum-ileum in 15% to 55% of cases. However, Crohn's is not associated with intussusceptions.

◆ DIAGNOSIS: Nontropical sprue (celiac disease).

◆ KEY FACTS

CLINICAL

◆ Sprue is manifested by diarrhea and steatorrhea, as well as fatigue, weight loss, anemia, neuropathy, stomatitis, osteomalacia, and depression.

◆ Nontropical sprue responds to a gluten-free diet, and tropical sprue responds to antibiotics.

◆ The diagnosis is made by duodenal or jejunal biopsy showing total or subtotal villous atrophy and a clinical and histologic response to a gluten-free diet or antibiotic regimen.

RADIOLOGIC

◆ The classic radiographic findings in patients with sprue are small-bowel dilatation, segmentation and flocculation of barium, hypersecretion, and the "moulage sign."

◆ Jejunization of the ileum is the result of atrophy of jejunal mucosal folds with an increase in ileal folds as an adaptive response to increase functional surface area.

◆ Intussusceptions are seen on small-bowel series in approximately 20% of celiac patients. Intussusceptions can be transient and asymptomatic and are diagnosed when there is a localized filling defect with a "coiled-spring" appearance.

◆ SUGGESTED READING

Cohen MD, Lintott DJ. Transient small bowel intussusception in adult celiac disease. Clin Radiol 1978;29:529–534.

Eisenberg RL. Gastrointestinal Radiology. Philadelphia: Lippincott, 1983;448–451.

Rubesin SE, Herlinger H, Saul SH, et al. Adult celiac disease and its complications. Radiographics 1989;9:1045–1065.

HISTORY

A 57-year-old woman presents with sudden onset of watery diarrhea, fever, and abdominal tenderness.

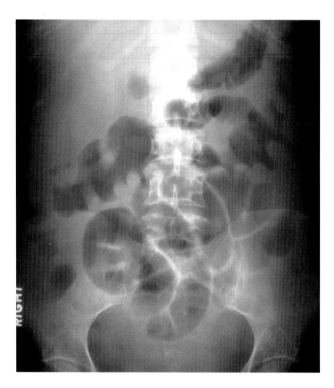

FIGURE 3-17A Supine abdominal radiograph. Nodular haustral fold thickening is seen in the transverse colon. There is also small-bowel dilatation indicating ileus.

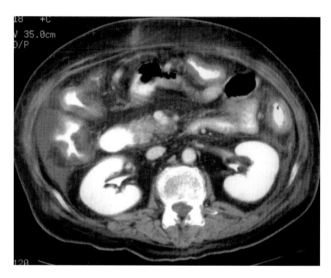

FIGURE 3-17B CT scan of the mid abdomen following intravenous and oral contrast material. There is extensive nodular thickening of the wall of the colon. Ascites is present in the paracolic gutters.

◆ DIFFERENTIAL DIAGNOSIS

◆ **Pseudomembranous colitis:** This is the best diagnosis because of widespread thumbprinting in the colon, ascites, and small bowel ileus.

◆ **Infectious colitis:** Colitis with thumbprinting can be seen with bacteria, including *Salmonella* and *Escherichia coli*, and parasites, including *Anisakis* and *Amoebae*.

◆ **Ischemic colitis:** The distribution is atypical for ischemia since the watershed region is located toward the splenic flexure. However, ischemia due to a vasculitis may not follow such vascular territories.

◆ **Intramural hemorrhage:** A history of trauma, bleeding disorder, or anticoagulant therapy would be contributory.

◆ **Inflammatory bowel disease:** This is unlikely because Crohn's disease is usually segmental, and ulcerative colitis of this severity would tend to show toxic dilatation as well.

◆ **Lymphoma:** This is unlikely because there is usually a large cavitary mass, most often localized to the right colon. Diffuse changes may be seen in advanced disseminated lymphoma, although lymphadenopathy would be expected.

◆ DIAGNOSIS: Pseudomembranous colitis.

◆ KEY FACTS

CLINICAL

◆ Pseudomembranous colitis occurs due to toxins (A and B) liberated by *Clostridium difficile*, a gram-positive organism in patients with recent exposure to either antibiotics (most commonly clindamycin, ampicillin, or cephalosporins, but almost all antibiotics have been implicated) or chemotherapy (usually methotrexate or fluorouracil). Onset is usually within 2 days to 2 weeks after introduction of the treatment but may be as late as 8 weeks.

◆ Clinical illness ranges from mild diarrhea to fulminant colitis with toxic megacolon and death. Fever, leukocytosis, and abdominal pain may also occur.

◆ Characteristic pseudomembranes may be seen endoscopically. However, the distal colon may appear normal in up to 50% of patients. Visible pseudomembranes may not have developed early in the course of the illness, and colitis may be limited to the right colon and remain undetected unless full colonoscopy is performed.

◆ The diagnosis is established by detection of the specific toxins in the stool, but this takes 2 days to complete.

◆ Specific treatment is comprised of oral vancomycin or metronidazole.

RADIOLOGIC

◆ The plain abdominal radiograph is normal in >60% of patients with pseudomembranous colitis. When abnormal, thumbprinting due to mucosal edema is visible in over half the cases. Other manifestations include colonic or small bowel ileus and ascites.

◆ Abdominal CT is more sensitive to the detection of colonic or other manifestations of the disease, but up to 40% of patients have normal scans. CT has the advantage of visualizing the colonic wall directly without having to rely on the presence of luminal gas to render the mucosal surface radiographically visible. Additional signs include pericolonic stranding and ascites.

◆ SUGGESTED READING

Boland GW, Lee MJ, Cats A, et al. Antibiotic-induced diarrhea: Specificity of abdominal CT for the diagnosis of *Clostridium difficile* disease. Radiology 1994;191:103–106.

Boland GW, Lee MJ, Cats A, Mueller PR. Pseudomembranous colitis: Diagnostic sensitivity of the abdominal plain radiograph. Clin Radiol 1994;49:473–475.

Fishman EK, Kavaru M, Jones B, et al. Pseudomembranous colitis: CT evaluation of 26 cases. Radiology 1991;180:57–60.

Glick SN. Other Inflammatory Conditions. In RM Gore, MS Levine, I Laufer (eds), Textbook of Gastrointestinal Radiology. Philadelphia: Saunders, 1994;1156–1157.

CASE 18

Jeffrey T. Seabourn

HISTORY

A 56-year-old woman has fevers, left-lower quadrant tenderness, and an elevated white blood cell count.

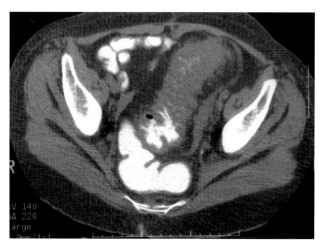

FIGURE 3-18A CT of the pelvis following rectal contrast material administration. There is mild soft-tissue stranding in the fat surrounding the sigmoid colon, with fluid and focal thickening at the root of the sigmoid mesocolon. There is also a long segment of irregular luminal narrowing secondary to circumferential wall thickening and an air-containing diverticulum.

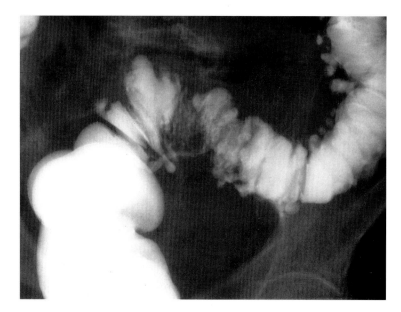

FIGURE 3-18B Barium enema 3 weeks later: spot view of the sigmoid colon. The sigmoid colon is narrowed and markedly distorted. An intramural track of barium extends inferiorly from the center of this diseased segment. Numerous diverticula are seen in the descending colon.

◆ DIFFERENTIAL DIAGNOSIS

- **Diverticulitis:** The CT findings and clinical history make this the most likely diagnosis. The lack of extensive diverticular changes should not discourage one from making this diagnosis.
- **Perforated colon cancer:** Circumferential tumor infiltration can be difficult to distinguish from diverticulitis. A longer segment of colonic involvement argues against colon cancer. The saw-tooth appearance of the lumen also favors diverticulitis.
- **Crohn's disease:** Mural thickening and pericolic inflammatory changes may also be seen in Crohn's disease. Crohn's disease typically has eccentric mural thickening as well as skip areas of colonic and small bowel involvement.
- **Radiation colitis:** There is no clinical history to support this diagnosis. Radiation therapy to the pelvis would likely involve the rectum as well.
- **Ischemic colitis:** Isolated ischemia of the sigmoid colon would be unusual.

◆ DIAGNOSIS: Sigmoid diverticulitis.

◆ KEY FACTS

CLINICAL

- Classic clinical features are left-lower quadrant pain, tenderness, fever, and leukocytosis. Of patients with diverticulosis, 15% to 30% will develop diverticulitis.
- Clinical management includes antibiotics for mild disease and surgery for more severe cases. Percutaneous abscess drainage and antibiotics can help convert colonic surgery into a single- rather than a two-stage procedure.
- Complications of diverticulitis include perforation, muscular hypertrophy and obstruction, pericolic

abscess, and vesicocolic fistula. Most inflammatory complications are secondary to a ruptured diverticulum and occur in a pericolic location.
- The sigmoid colon is involved in 95%, and the cecum in 5% of cases.

RADIOLOGIC

- Contrast enema (CE) depicts the bowel lumen, spasm, and muscle hypertrophy, but the pericolic inflammatory changes can only be inferred indirectly. A CE underestimates the degree of pericolic inflammatory changes that are the hallmark of acute diverticulitis. However, CE is often valuable in differentiating diverticulitis from colon cancer.
- The CT hallmark of acute diverticulitis is the presence of inflammatory changes in the pericolic fat. Induration and thickening of the root of the sigmoid mesocolon is not pathognomonic but highly suggestive of sigmoid diverticulitis.
- On CT, associated diverticuli are seen in 84%, thickened colonic wall in 79%, and pericolic fluid collections/abscess in approximately 35% of cases.
- CT is not able to distinguish colon cancer from diverticulitis in approximately 10% of cases.
- CT should be the primary method of radiologic diagnosis as well as the method for evaluation and staging of complicated diverticulitis.

◆ SUGGESTED READING

Birnbaum BA, Balthazar EJ. CT of appendicitis and diverticulitis. Radiol Clin North Am 1994;32:885–898.

Johnson CD, Baker ME, Rice RP, et al. Diagnosis of acute colonic diverticulitis: Comparison of barium enema and CT. AJR Am J Roentgenol 1987;148:541–546.

Neff CC, vanSonnenberg E. CT of diverticulitis: Diagnosis and treatment. Radiol Clin North Am 1989;27:743–752.

Pohlman T. Diverticulitis. Gastroenterol Clin North Am 1988;17:357–358.

CASE *19*   *Vincent H.S. Low*

HISTORY

A 55-year-old man has a 2-month history of anorexia, nausea and vomiting, and guaiac-positive stool.

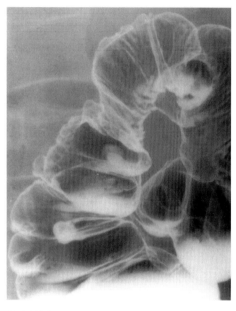

FIGURE 3-19A Double-contrast barium enema: spot view of the hepatic flexure. There is a short segment of circumferential narrowing. The mucosa here is slightly puckered but otherwise normal, with no nodularity, ulceration, or fold thickening.

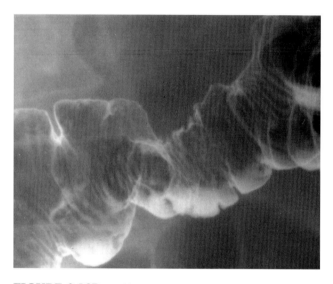

FIGURE 3-19B Double-contrast barium enema: spot view of the transverse colon. An extrinsic mass-like impression indents the superior border of the transverse colon. The mucosal contour is spiculated, but the mucosal folds are otherwise normal.

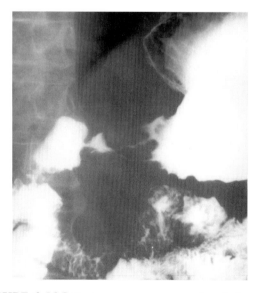

FIGURE 3-19C Single-contrast upper gastrointestinal examination: left posterior oblique view. An area of gross abnormality involves the gastric antrum, where there is luminal narrowing, impaired distensibility, and course lobulation of the mucosal folds.

◆ DIFFERENTIAL DIAGNOSIS

- **Cancer:** Primary malignancy, including the possibility of synchronous tumors, must be considered in the presence of malignant-appearing mass lesions and strictures.
- **Crohn's disease:** This disease is typified by multiple skip and asymmetric lesions involving predominantly distal small bowel and colon but may also involve other segments of the gastrointestinal tract.
- **Serosal implants from disseminated peritoneal disease:** The colon may be involved by disseminated malignancy (e.g., ovarian cancer), paraneoplastic processes (e.g., endometriosis), and inflammatory conditions (e.g., peritoneal abscesses).
- **Mesenteric metastases involving the colon:** This is the most likely diagnosis, with the gastric antral abnormality representing the primary malignancy.

◆ DIAGNOSIS: Mesenteric metastases to colon.

◆ KEY FACTS

CLINICAL

- The colon is not uncommonly involved by metastases, and indeed symptoms produced by such lesions may be the initial manifestation of disseminated disease. The colon may be involved by malignant spread via a number of pathways, including direct invasion from an adjacent tumor, spread via peritoneal ligaments and mesenteries, and/or embolic hematogenous dissemination.
- Direct invasion of the colon commonly arises from the prostate, ovary, uterus, cervix, kidney, and gallbladder. The location of colonic involvement is determined by the site of the adjacent primary tumor.
- Malignancy may reach the colon through the mesentery. Carcinoma of the stomach will first involve the superior border of the transverse colon by tracking down the gastrocolic ligament. Pancreatic carcinoma may invade the transverse colon via the transverse mesocolon and will first involve the inferior border of the colon. Carcinoma of the pancreatic tail may extend along the phrenicocolic ligament to invade the splenic flexure.

- Intraperitoneal seeding most commonly occurs with ovarian carcinoma but can also occur with gastric, colon, and pancreatic malignancy. The locations of these tumors are dictated by the flow of ascitic fluid along peritoneal reflections. Tumor deposits will settle in the most dependent portions of the peritoneal cavity, which are the pouch of Douglas or rectovesicular space. Other common sites are the medial border of the cecum, superior border of the sigmoid colon, and the right paracolic gutter.
- Hematogenous metastases most commonly arise from melanoma but also from lung and breast carcinoma.

RADIOLOGIC

- Involvement of the colon by an adjacent tumor may appear as simple extrinsic mass effect displacing the colon without evidence of fixation or tethering, even if actual serosal invasion has not yet occurred.
- Serosal involvement of the colon by tumor deposits, whether by direct invasion, mesenteric spread, or intraperitoneal seeding, will have a similar appearance. The contour of the involved segment of bowel will show puckering when viewed en face and spiculation ("saw-tooth" contour) when viewed in profile. There may be subtle mass effect. The segment of bowel will be fixed and tethered.
- Serosal changes may also be created by endometriosis and inflammatory processes such as peritoneal abscess.
- Hematogenous metastases manifest as a wide variety of appearances, including bulky polyps, umbilicated or ulcerated submucosal ("target") masses, annular or eccentric strictures, or long infiltrative segments of irregular narrowing.

◆ SUGGESTED READING

Meyers MA. Intraperitoneal spread of malignancies and its effect on the bowel. Clin Radiol 1981;32:129–146.

Rubesin SE, Furth EE. Other Tumors of the Colon. In RM Gore, ES Levine, I Laufer (eds), Textbook of Gastrointestinal Radiology. Philadelphia: Saunders, 1994;1213–1222.

CASE 20   *Erik K. Paulson*

HISTORY

63-year-old woman with a palpable right upper quadrant mass.

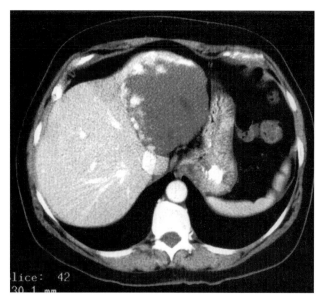

FIGURE 3-20A Dynamic contrast-enhanced CT scan of the upper abdomen. There is a large mass in the lateral segment of the left hepatic lobe with peripheral globular, "cloud-like" enhancement.

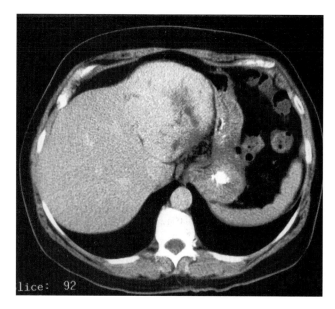

FIGURE 3-20B CT of upper abdomen 5 minutes after intravenous contrast material administration. Delayed image shows that the mass has "filled-in" with contrast material. Some hypoattenuated areas remain centrally.

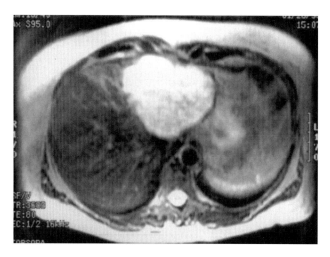

FIGURE 3-20C T2-weighted MRI of the upper abdomen (TR-3683, TE-80). MRI shows a well-circumscribed mass with uniform, homogenous, high-signal intensity.

◆ DIFFERENTIAL DIAGNOSIS

◆ **Hypervascular metastases:** Metastases to the liver from an islet cell tumor of the pancreas, thyroid carcinoma, breast carcinoma, and carcinoid tumors may be hypervascular. Because hypervascular metastases may enhance in a fashion similar to normal liver parenchyma, they may be difficult to detect during the portal venous dominant phase of enhancement. However, the peripheral globular enhancement in this case would be atypical for any hypervascular metastases. Further, while metastases are typically of high signal intensity compared to liver on T2-weighted MRI, they are not usually this "bright."

◆ **Focal nodular hyperplasia:** These tumors are hamartomas and have imaging characteristics similar to hepatic parenchyma. On dynamic contrast-enhanced CT during the hepatic arterial dominant phase, these tumors typically have early intense uniform enhancement, not present in this case. In about half of the cases, there may be a central scar that may be of low attenuation on a dynamic contrast-enhanced CT. On T2-weighted MRI, these lesions may be slightly hyperintense but often are quite subtle, with signal characteristics similar to those of normal liver.

◆ **Hepatocellular carcinoma:** These tumors are often heterogenous "ugly" masses that may invade the portal and/or hepatic veins. While they are often hypervascular, they usually have areas of central enhancement due to prominent central feeding arteries; they lack the peripheral globular enhancement shown in this lesion. Patients with hepatocellular carcinoma often have underlying cirrhosis, which is not present here.

◆ **Metastatic colon cancer:** Occasionally colon cancer may present as a solitary mass in the liver. However, colon carcinoma metastases are not hypervascular, very rarely have delayed contrast enhancement, and are of lower signal intensity on T2-weighted MRI than shown in this case.

◆ **Cavernous hemangioma:** This is the most likely diagnosis given the peripheral nodular enhancement pattern and centripetal "fill-in."

◆ DIAGNOSIS: Cavernous hemangioma of the liver.

◆ KEY FACTS

CLINICAL

◆ Second to cysts, hemangiomas are the most common benign tumor of the liver, with a reported incidence ranging from 1% to 10%. There is a female predominance of 4 to 1.

◆ Pathologically, the tumor represents numerous endothelial-lined, blood-filled spaces. Larger hemangiomas (≤20 cm) are nearly always heterogenous, with central areas of fibrosis, necrosis, and cyst formation. Calcifications are uncommon.

◆ Hemangiomas are one of the few tumors that can be confidently diagnosed using noninvasive imaging techniques, including ultrasound, dynamic contrast-enhanced CT, MRI, or a Tc[99m]-tagged red blood cell scintigraphy. Biopsy is rarely indicated unless the lesion has atypical features.

RADIOLOGIC

◆ On precontrast CT, hemangiomas are usually of uniform low attenuation with well-circumscribed, lobulated borders. On dynamic contrast-enhanced CT, hemangiomas nearly always demonstrate globular enhancement about the periphery. Over time (≤30 minutes) the tumors "fill-in" in a centripetal fashion. Large tumors may have central areas of necrosis, fibrosis, or scar that may not entirely "fill-in" with contrast material.

◆ On T1-weighted MRI, the lesions are well circumscribed and of low signal intensity compared to the hepatic parenchyma. On a dynamic contrast-enhanced MRI with a gadolinium-chelate, hemangiomas demonstrate enhancement identical to that described for dynamic CT. On T2-weighted MRI, hemangiomas typically have a very high signal intensity, similar to that of a hepatic cyst or fluid in the gallbladder or spinal canal, leading some to call hemangiomas "light bulb" lesions. Because of this characteristic appearance, MRI has proven useful in distinguishing hemangiomas from other hepatic tumors.

◆ On ultrasound, hemangiomas are well circumscribed and are uniformly hyperechoic relative to the liver parenchyma. They may demonstrate enhanced through-transmission but do not have a halo. With color Doppler ultrasound, they usually do not have central blood flow.

◆ On Tc[99m]-labeled red blood cell scintigraphy, hemangiomas will appear as a defect in the early phases of the scan that will "fill-in" on delayed scans. SPECT imaging improves the accuracy in detecting and characterizing small hemangiomas.

◆ SUGGESTED READING

Nelson RC, Chezmar JL. Diagnostic approach to hepatic hemangiomas. Radiology 1990;176:11–13.

Quinn SF, Benjamin GG. Hepatic cavernous hemangiomas: Simple diagnostic sign with dynamic bolus CT. Radiology 1992;182:545–548.

Ros PR. Benign Liver Tumors. In RM Gore, MS Levine, I Laufer (eds), Textbook of Gastrointestinal Radiology. Philadelphia: Saunders, 1994;1861–1898.

HISTORY

A 30-year-old woman presents with right-upper quadrant pain and intermittent jaundice.

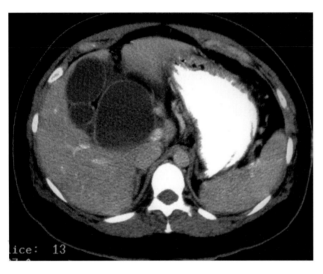

FIGURE 3-21A Contrast-enhanced CT scan of the liver. There is a low-attenuation cystic structure situated medial to the gallbladder. Adjacent scans showed the structure to extend from the porta hepatis to the pancreatic head. The wall is smooth and well defined, and the contents are of water attenuation. There is no dilatation of the intrahepatic bile ducts.

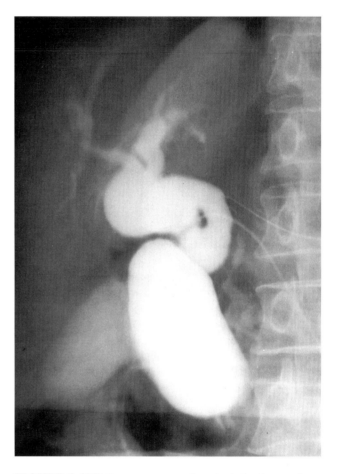

FIGURE 3-21B Percutaneous transhepatic cholangiogram shows a large tubular contrast-filled structure communicating with the gallbladder and cystic duct.

◆ DIFFERENTIAL DIAGNOSIS

- **Loculated biloma:** A biloma would be unlikely in the absence of a history of recent trauma or biliary surgery, and would not have a well-defined tubular appearance on cholangiography.
- **Enteric duplication cyst:** These cysts can be of water attenuation on CT but would be unlikely to follow the line of the common bile duct and would not communicate with the biliary tree on cholangiography.
- **Hepatic cyst:** The extrahepatic location of this structure on CT and communication with the biliary tree on cholangiography excludes this diagnosis.
- **Choledochal cyst:** This is the most likely diagnosis since on CT the cystic structure is in the expected location of the extrahepatic biliary tree, and on cholangiography the cyst is confirmed to be in continuity with the biliary tree.
- **Pancreatic pseudocyst:** A pseudocyst could have this appearance on CT, but the cholangiogram excludes this diagnosis.
- **Biliary cystadenoma:** A cystadenoma would be unlikely because of the extrahepatic location. Biliary cyst adenomas are usually intrahepatic, of low attenuation, and may have internal septa and a thick, irregular wall.

◆ DIAGNOSIS: Choledochal cyst.

◆ KEY FACTS

CLINICAL

- Choledochal cysts are an uncommon cause of biliary obstruction and are characterized as cystic dilatation of the extrahepatic or intrahepatic biliary tree, or both.
- They are three times more common in females than males. Although they may present at any age, they are typically discovered in children and young adults, with 60% presenting before the age of 10 years.
- The classic clinical triad of pain, jaundice, and abdominal mass occurs in only 30% of patients.
- The etiology is unknown, but they are thought to be related to an anomalous insertion of the common bile duct (CBD) into the pancreatic duct proximal to the ampulla, resulting in chronic reflux of pancreatic

enzymes into the biliary tree. They are associated with other biliary anomalies, including a double CBD, double gallbladder, absent gallbladder, atresia of bile ducts, sclerosing cholangitis, congenital hepatic fibrosis, and annular pancreas.
- Complications include cholangitis, biliary cirrhosis, portal hypertension, calculi, and cyst rupture. They are associated with an increased risk of carcinoma of the bile duct.

RADIOLOGIC

- The diagnosis can be made with CT and ultrasound if direct communication between the cyst and the biliary tree can be shown. Appearances depend on the extent of involvement and degree of dilatation. Scans may show mild dilatation of the extrahepatic biliary tree, or a large water attenuation mass in the porta hepatis.
- Cholangiography may be necessary to demonstrate communication with the biliary tree. Percutaneous transhepatic cholangiography (PTC) allows detailed imaging of the intrahepatic ductal anatomy in addition to imaging the cyst. Endoscopic retrograde cholangiopancreatography (ERCP) provides detailed information about the distal portion of the CBD and about the often anomalous junction with the pancreatic duct.
- Tc^{99m}-hepatobiliary scanning shows late filling of the cyst with delayed clearance, and effectively excludes all other possibilities from the differential diagnosis.
- Type I: the most common type (89% to 90%), characterized by cystic or fusiform dilatation of the CBD
- Type II (2%): diverticulum from the CBD
- Type III (1% to 5%): choledochocele; characterized by dilatation of the intraduodenal portion of the CBD
- Type IV: multiple cysts of the extrahepatic and intrahepatic bile ducts
- Type V: Caroli's disease; multiple intrahepatic duct cysts

◆ SUGGESTED READING

Crittenden SL, McKinley MJ. Choledochal cyst: Clinical features and classification. Am J Gastroenterol 1985;80:643–647.

Savedar SJ, Benenati JF, Venbrux AC, et al. Choledochal cysts: Classification and cholangiographic appearance. AJR Am J Roentgenol 1991;156:327–331.

Todani T, Watanabe Y, Narusue M. Congenital bile duct cyst. Am J Surg 1977;134:263–269.

CASE 22

Philip T. McAndrew

HISTORY

A 54-year-old white woman has had right-upper quadrant pain over a period of 1 week. Jaundice developed within the previous 48 hours. On examination she was febrile, and initial blood work revealed leukocytosis.

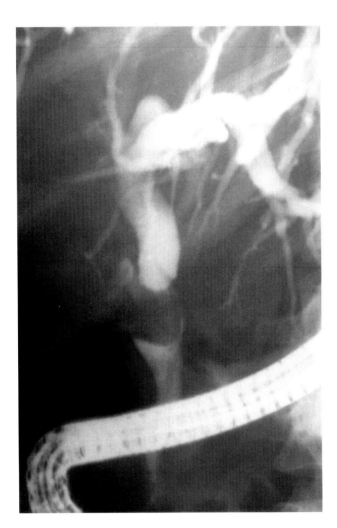

FIGURE 3-22A Endoscopic retrograde cholangiopancreatography demonstrated an eccentric filling defect in the common bile duct at the level of the cystic duct. There is proximal dilatation of the biliary system.

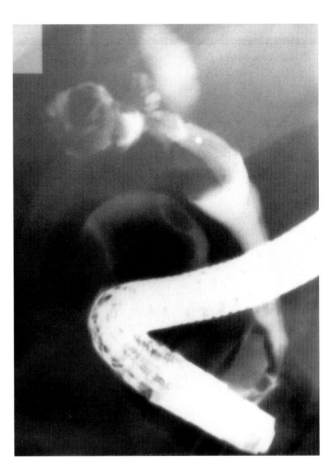

FIGURE 3-22B There is impaired filling of the gallbladder, with multiple filling defects in the neck and cystic duct suggesting calculi.

◆ DIFFERENTIAL DIAGNOSIS

- **Gallbladder carcinoma:** A malignant mass arising from the gallbladder neck and extending to the common hepatic duct may produce this cholangiographic appearance. Conversely, an aggressive cholangiocarcinoma extending to the cystic ducts needs to be considered.
- **Lymphadenopathy:** The strategic position of the common hepatic duct in the porta hepatis allows it to be compressed by lymphadenopathy and other mass lesions in this location.
- **Mirizzi's syndrome:** This is the most likely diagnosis given this constellation of clinical findings (acute cholecystitis with obstruction) and imaging findings (extrinsic-appearing obstruction of the common hepatic duct and impaired opacification of the gallbladder suggestive of partial cystic ductal obstruction).

◆ DIAGNOSIS: Mirizzi's syndrome.

◆ KEY FACTS

CLINICAL

- In Mirizzi's syndrome, there is jaundice because of obstruction of the common hepatic duct at its junction with the cystic duct, which is due to periductal inflammatory changes occurring around a calculus impacted in the distal cystic duct.
- Patients present with features of acute cholecystitis (abdominal pain and tenderness, fever, and leukocytosis) as well as jaundice. Occasionally, jaundice resolves spontaneously with conservative management of the cholecystitis.

- It is important to make this diagnosis before operative management because it is difficult to identify the various ducts coming out of the resultant inflammatory mass. As a result, the surgeon may inadvertently ligate the common hepatic duct, mistaking it for the cystic duct.
- Type I Mirizzi's syndrome occurs when there is an impacted calculus in the cystic duct. Type II is much less common and occurs when a stone erodes from the gallbladder into the bile duct.

RADIOLOGIC

- Plain radiographs may demonstrate the offending calculus if sufficiently radiodense, especially if one of the stones is seen to be separate and more medial to the main cluster of gallstones. The plain film is also useful for correlation with cholangiographic or CT studies.
- Cholangiography typically demonstrates a smooth, lateral, extrinsic narrowing of the common hepatic duct. There will be proximal biliary dilatation, and a calculus may actually be visible in the adjacent, expected position of the cystic duct.
- On CT scan, an inflammatory mass will be seen in the porta hepatis. The greater contrast resolution of CT usually allows visualization of the cystic duct calculus. The nonspecific features of acute cholecystitis and biliary dilatation may also be present.

◆ SUGGESTED READING

Toscano RL, Taylor PH, Peters J, Edgin R. Mirizzi syndrome. Am Surgeon 1994;60:889–891.

Zeman RK. Cholelithiasis and Cholecystitis. In RM Gore, MS Levine, I Laufer (eds), Textbook of Gastrointestinal Radiology. Philadelphia: Saunders, 1994;1651–1652.

CASE 23

Vincent H.S. Low

HISTORY

A 65-year-old man with jaundice and anorexia.

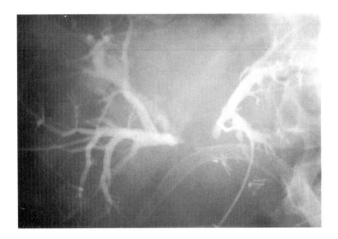

FIGURE 3-23A Percutaneous transhepatic cholangiogram with separate punctures of both the left and right ductal systems. There is dilatation and crowding of all opacified intrahepatic bile ducts, with failure of opacification of the central intrahepatic ducts at their confluence.

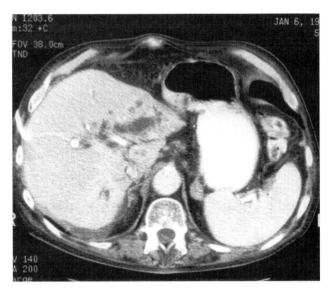

FIGURE 3-23B Contrast-enhanced CT scan at the level of porta hepatis. There is biliary ductal dilatation, but no discrete enhancing mass is identified. The liver itself shows atrophy, especially of the left hepatic lobe.

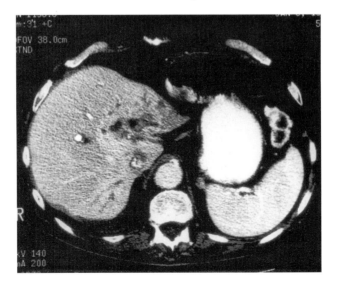

FIGURE 3-23C Contrast-enhanced CT scan at the level of porta hepatis. The same CT image viewed at a narrow "liver" window. A subtle region of altered attenuation is seen in the porta hepatis central to the dilated ducts with vague, central periductal enhancement.

◆ DIFFERENTIAL DIAGNOSIS

- **Pancreatic carcinoma:** This diagnosis is unlikely in view of the calcifications, which are rarely seen in pancreatic adenocarcinoma.
- **Cystic pancreatic neoplasm:** A microcystic adenoma of the pancreas may contain calcification, but small cysts, typically <2 cm in diameter, would also be visible.
- **Pancreatic islet cell tumor:** These tumors may calcify but typically show marked enhancement due to hypervascularity.
- **Chronic pancreatitis:** Pancreatitis often manifests as diffuse glandular enlargement, although it may present as a focal mass. Parenchymal and/or intraductal calcifications may or may not be present.

◆ DIAGNOSIS: Chronic pancreatitis.

◆ KEY FACTS

CLINICAL

- Symptoms at presentation are usually nonspecific, although patients may have either or both weight loss and upper abdominal pain.
- A history of long-term alcohol abuse is often present.
- Most patients have had a prior episode of acute pancreatitis; with each episode, there is progressive pancreatic parenchymal destruction.

RADIOLOGIC

- Endoscopic retrograde cholangiopancreatography (ERCP) is the most sensitive test for early disease, as duct strictures, side branch enlargement, and intraluminal filling defects may be seen before CT and ultrasound changes occur.
- Intraluminal filling defects in the pancreatic ducts on ERCP usually represent mucin collections, which may be detected before they calcify and thus before they are apparent on CT.
- Either CT or ultrasound may show a heterogenous gland due to the presence of fat and fibrosis. Encapsulated fluid collections or pseudocysts may also be present.
- The gland size is variable and may be involved either diffusely or focally. The gland may be normal in size, small (atrophy of the gland), or large (recent pancreatitis).
- CT may also show a focal mass with or without dilatation of the pancreatic and/or bile ducts.
- Calcifications are present in only 50% of cases, therefore a noncalcified mass can still represent chronic pancreatitis.

◆ SUGGESTED READING

Ferrucci JT, Wittenberg J, Mack EB, et al. Computed body tomography in chronic pancreatitis. Radiology 1979;130:175–182.

Luetmer PH, Stephens DH, Ward EM. Chronic pancreatitis: Reassessment with current CT. Radiology 1989;171:353–357.

CASE 25

Mary T. Keogan

HISTORY

A 27-year-old woman has upper abdominal discomfort. She had been well previously.

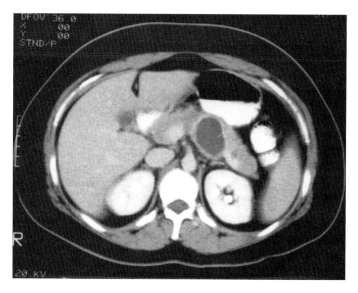

FIGURE 3-25A Contrast-enhanced CT of the upper abdomen shows a cystic mass in the body of the pancreas with a well-defined enhancing wall. Thin, incomplete septa are seen arising from the anterior wall.

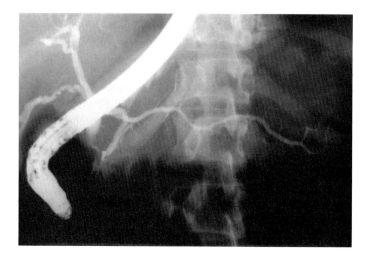

FIGURE 3-25B Endoscopic retrograde cholangiopancreatography showing a pancreatogram. The main pancreatic duct is displaced inferiorly in its mid-portion but is not narrowed or disrupted.

◆ DIFFERENTIAL DIAGNOSIS

◆ **Pancreatic pseudocyst:** The pancreatic body and tail are good locations for pseudocysts, but the patient would be expected to have a previous history of pancreatitis. Pseudocysts often communicate with the pancreatic duct at ERCP.

◆ **Mucinous cystic tumor:** This is the most likely diagnosis since these tumors typically have one or a few large cysts (>2 cm) and well-defined septations. Calcifications are uncommon.

◆ **Serous cystic tumor:** This diagnosis is unlikely as the classical features of numerous small cysts (<2 cm) with an enhancing central "scar" are not present. These tumors often show calcifications.

◆ DIAGNOSIS: Mucinous cystic tumor.

◆ KEY FACTS

CLINICAL

◆ Cystic pancreatic tumors are much less common than pancreatic ductal adenocarcinoma.

◆ They typically occur in 40- to 60-year-old patients; women are more common than men (9 to 1).

◆ Symptoms such as pain or jaundice are uncommon. The cysts are often an incidental finding.

◆ Although these tumors have malignant potential, they are slow growing and have an indolent course.

RADIOLOGIC

◆ CT or ultrasound shows a cystic mass, typically <6 cysts in number and >2 cm in size, with thin or thick intervening septa.

◆ Calcifications are seen in 14%. There is no central scar. (A central scar is typical of a serous tumor.)

◆ Communication with the pancreatic duct is uncommon at ERCP, unlike pseudocysts.

◆ Radiologically, one cannot differentiate a cystadenoma from a cystadenocarcinoma.

◆ A biopsy is indicated if there is no good history of pancreatitis to exclude pseudocyst and also to differentiate benign from malignant tumors. Histologically, the mucinous tumors almost always have some foci of malignancy.

◆ SUGGESTED READING

Friedman AC, Lichtenstein JE, Dachman AH. Cystic neoplasms of the pancreas: Radiological-pathological correlation. Radiology 1983;149:45–50.

Itai Y, Moss AA, Ohtomo K. Computed tomography of cystadenoma and cystadenocarcinoma of the pancreas. Radiology 1982;145:419–425.

HISTORY

A 61-year-old woman has weight loss and a history of peptic ulcer disease.

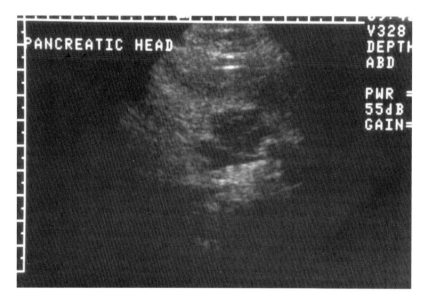

FIGURE 3-26A Ultrasound of the upper abdomen in the transverse plane. A hypoechoic mass is seen in the body of the pancreas anterior to the portal venous confluence.

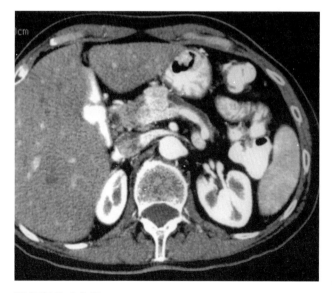

FIGURE 3-26B Contrast-enhanced CT of the upper abdomen during the arterial dominant phase. There is an enhancing mass in the pancreatic body. There is atrophy of the pancreatic tail and dilatation of the main pancreatic duct.

◆ DIFFERENTIAL DIAGNOSIS

◆ **Pancreatic islet cell tumor, nonfunctioning:** These tumors do not secrete hormones and are clinically silent. Hence, they are often of larger size at presentation than functioning tumors. They may calcify.

◆ **Pancreatic islet cell tumor, functioning:** Gastrinoma is a likely diagnosis in view of the history of peptic ulcer disease. Insulinomas are the most common functioning tumor but are usually small and not associated with peptic ulcers. Calcifications are rare in functioning tumors.

◆ **Pancreatic hypervascular metastasis (e.g., renal):** This diagnosis is unlikely since pancreatic metastases are usually not isolated.

◆ DIAGNOSIS: Gastrinoma.

◆ KEY FACTS

CLINICAL

◆ These tumors present early with symptoms of gastric hypersecretion (Zollinger-Ellison syndrome [ZES]).

◆ Peptic ulcers are often resistant to medical management and present in atypical locations—e.g., the postbulbar region. The most common location continues to be the duodenal bulb.

◆ They are associated with multiple endocrine neoplasm syndrome, type 1.

RADIOLOGIC

◆ Islet cell tumors are very vascular and, when large enough, are seen on CT as an enhancing pancreatic mass.

◆ Up to 50% of gastrinomas have metastasized to the liver at the time of presentation (typically hyperenhancing metastases); hence, CT is important for staging. By comparison, only 10% of insulinomas will have metastases at the time of presentation.

◆ Barium studies often show associated peptic ulcers, which may be multiple and/or postbulbar.

◆ Gastrinomas causing ZES usually originate in the head of the pancreas or the duodenum.

◆ SUGGESTED READING

Frucht H, Doppman JL, Norton JA, et al. Gastrinomas: Comparison of MR imaging with CT, angiography and ultrasound. Radiology 1989;171:713–717.

Semelka RC, Ascher SM. MR Imaging of the pancreas. Radiology 1993;188:593–602.

Wank SA, Doppman JL, Miller DL, et al. Prospective study of the ability of computed axial tomography to localize gastrinomas in patients with Zollinger-Ellison syndrome. Gastroenterology 1987;92:905–912.

CASE 27

Mary T. Keogan

HISTORY

A 55-year-old woman presents with progressive back pain and rapid weight loss.

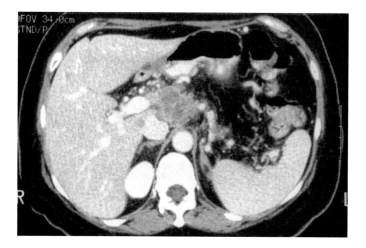

FIGURE 3-27A Contrast-enhanced CT of the pancreas. There is a low-attenuation mass in the head of the pancreas with dilatation of the pancreatic duct and associated atrophy of the gland. Note the absence of pancreatic calcifications.

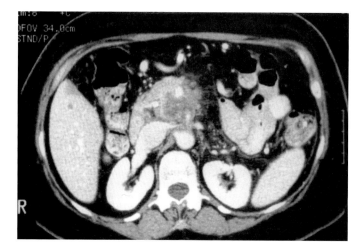

FIGURE 3-27B Contrast-enhanced CT at a more caudal level. The superior mesenteric artery is compressed and the surrounding fat planes are obliterated, indicating complete vascular encasement by tumor. This finding indicates that the patient is unresectable.

DIFFERENTIAL DIAGNOSIS

- **Pancreatic adenocarcinoma:** This patient has the classic appearance of a pancreatic carcinoma: a nonenhancing mass in the pancreatic head associated with obstruction of the pancreatic duct and atrophy of the body and tail.
- **Chronic pancreatitis:** There may be a focal mass in patients with chronic pancreatitis that, in the absence of calcifications (50%), is indistinguishable from pancreatic carcinoma. It often requires a biopsy to make this distinction.
- **Pancreatic lymphoma:** Lymphoma rarely arises in the pancreas. Involvement of peripancreatic nodes is more typical. Associated abdominal lymphadenopathy would also be expected.
- **Pancreatic metastases:** Malignancy of the lung, breast, kidneys, or gastrointestinal tract may spread hematogenously to the pancreas. This diagnosis should be considered if there is a history of a primary malignancy.

DIAGNOSIS: Pancreatic adenocarcinoma.

KEY FACTS

CLINICAL

- Pancreatic carcinoma presents late in the course of the disease, usually with liver and nodal metastases. Less than 30% are resectable at initial presentation.
- Pancreatic carcinoma is more common in males and blacks.
- There is an association between pancreatic carcinoma and smoking and familial pancreatitis. There is no association, however, with alcohol use.

RADIOLOGIC

- Typically, a focal mass is present (75% in the pancreatic head). On contrast-enhanced CT, 95% are of low attenuation. Typically the masses are nonenhancing, but they may appear isoattenuating postcontrast.
- The pancreatic duct may be dilated and the pancreatic parenchyma atrophic.
- Local extension is present in 90% of patients—i.e., either or both into the duodenum and the celiac/porta hepatis lymph nodes. Vascular encasement (superior mesenteric or celiac artery) indicates an unresectable tumor.
- CT is 95% accurate in determining unresectability, but it is only 50% accurate in determining resectability as small liver metastases and peritoneal implants may not be detected.

SUGGESTED READING

DelMaschio A, Vanzulli A, Sironi S, et al. Pancreatic cancer versus chronic pancreatitis: Diagnosis with CA 19-9 assessment, US, CT, and CT-guided fine-needle biopsy. Radiology 1991;178:95–99.

Zeiss J, Coombs RJ, Bielke D. CT presentation and staging accuracy of pancreatic adenocarcinoma. J Pancreatol 1990;7:49–53.

CASE 28

Vincent H.S. Low

HISTORY

A 30-year-old man with a history of intravenous drug abuse presents with fever and abdominal pain.

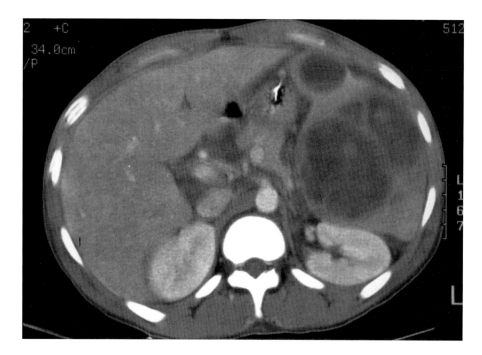

FIGURE 3-28 Contrast-enhanced CT scan of the upper abdomen. The spleen is enlarged, and there are several low-attenuation lesions. These lesions are of variable size and their contours are ill-defined. The smaller lesion anteriorly demonstrates a horizontal level, suggesting the presence of fluid or debris. Some of the other larger lesions also demonstrate central foci of high attenuation, consistent with hemorrhage or debris within a liquefied lesion.

◆ DIFFERENTIAL DIAGNOSIS

- **Pyogenic abscess:** In the immunocompetent patient, an abscess is usually due to aerobic organisms, including *Salmonella*, which develop in the setting of underlying splenic damage.
- **Opportunistic infection:** In the immunocompromised patient, unusual organisms including fungi, *Mycobacterium tuberculosis, M. avium-intracellulare*, and *Pneumocystis carinii* may infect the liver and spleen. The lesions usually appear as multiple microabscesses.
- **Lymphoma:** Diffuse histiocytic or immunoblastic types of lymphoma are seen occasionally as ill-defined, low-attenuation splenic masses on CT.
- **Hematoma:** This should be considered in the context of trauma or a coagulopathy, either due to an underlying disease state or as a result of therapy.
- **Metastases:** Apart from malignant melanoma, macroscopic metastases to the spleen are very unusual. In the immunocompromised patient, disseminated Kaposi's sarcoma may occur, although there is usually evidence of disseminated disease elsewhere.
- **Cysts:** Simple cysts are relatively uncommon and appear as round, well-defined, water attenuation lesions but become atypical in appearance if complicated by infection or hemorrhage. Hydatid cysts (*Echinococcus* infection) should be considered in patients exposed to areas where this condition is endemic.

◆ DIAGNOSIS: Splenic abscesses, *Candida*.

◆ KEY FACTS

CLINICAL

- Splenic abscesses are uncommon, but their frequency has grown because of an increasing number of immunocompromised patients. Specific diseases at risk for splenic abscess include sickle cell anemia, childhood granulomatous disease, and diabetes mellitus.
- The spleen may be infected by several routes, including metastatic hematogenous infection (e.g., bacterial endocarditis), contiguous infection (e.g., infected pancreatitis), infection of splenic infarcts, trauma, and immunodeficiency states. One-fifth of splenic abscesses have no apparent underlying source.
- The mortality rate for splenic abscess has historically been very high—up to 70%—but with earlier diagnosis by imaging, improved antibiotic therapy, image-guided diagnostic aspiration for identification of organisms, as well as for percutaneous drainage, the mortality has been reduced to <10%.
- Over half of splenic abscesses are infected by aerobic organisms, especially gram-positive cocci. Fungi are found in about one-fourth of splenic abscesses.

- The classic clinical picture of a splenic abscess is comprised of fever, chills, left-upper quadrant pain and tenderness, and splenomegaly. However, the majority of patients do not present with this classic picture early in the disease process, and signs localizing to the left upper quadrant are often absent.
- Complications of an abscess, such as rupture, subphrenic abscess, and peritonitis, will occur if the diagnosis is delayed, and these are associated with a high mortality rate.

RADIOLOGIC

- CT is the optimum diagnostic modality for the diagnosis of splenic infection, with a reported sensitivity of up to 96%. Not only will this technique localize a splenic abscess but it will also provide anatomic and diagnostic information about the perisplenic area, is useful for showing evidence of adjacent disease, and helps plan for surgical or radiologic intervention.
- A bacterial abscess appears as a low-attenuation mass lesion with an ill-defined, thick, and irregular rim. There may be slight peripheral enhancement. Occasionally, the abscess contains gas. There may be internal septa and/or fluid-debris levels.
- Fungal infections essentially occur only in immunocompromised patients. The lesions are usually small, typically <2 cm in diameter and usually <5 mm. These lesions are therefore difficult to detect on imaging. When seen, they appear as nonenhancing, low-attenuation lesions on CT. Occasionally, they may demonstrate a "bull's eye" appearance on ultrasound or CT. Tuberculosis commonly involves the spleen in its miliary form. However, the lesions are usually small, <1 cm in size, and difficult to visualize on imaging. The macronodular form of the disease (tuberculoma) is a rare manifestation, appearing as large, single or multiple, ill-defined low-attenuation masses.
- In the patient with AIDS, the spleen may be infected by *M. avium-intracellulare* or *P. carinii* organisms. The individual infected foci are usually tiny, resulting only in splenomegaly on imaging. Over time, the lesions may calcify.
- Image-guided intervention is an ideal method of sampling these lesions to allow for identification of the organism(s). Percutaneous abscess drainage is a reasonable option to surgical resection, and on occasion is completely curative.

◆ SUGGESTED READING

Freeman JL, Jafri SZ, Roberts JL, et al. CT of congenital and acquired abnormalities of the spleen. Radiographics 1993;13:597–610.

Kawashima A, Fishman EK. Benign Splenic Lesions. In RM Gore, ES Levine, I Laufer (eds), Textbook of Gastrointestinal Radiology. Philadelphia: Saunders, 1994;2251–2258.

Rendon C. Nelson

HISTORY

A 48-year-old man with fever and generalized abdominal pain.

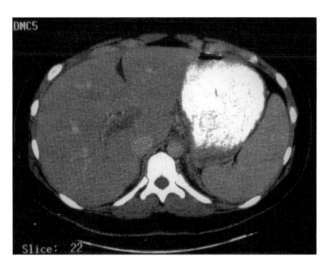

FIGURE 3-29A Dynamic contrast-enhanced CT of the upper abdomen. There is an L-shaped hypoattenuating mass in the central portion of the liver.

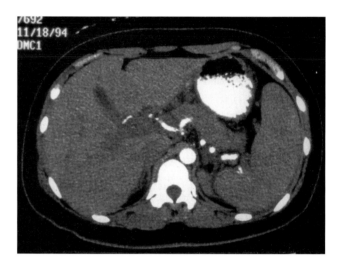

FIGURE 3-29B Dynamic contrast-enhanced CT during the hepatic arterial dominant phase obtained 6 weeks later. There is no significant enhancement in the region of the mass.

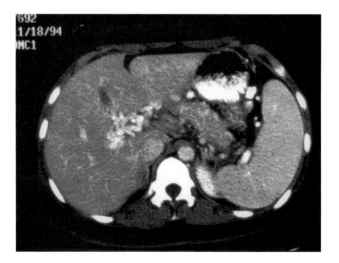

FIGURE 3-29C Dynamic contrast-enhanced CT during the portal venous dominant phase obtained 6 weeks later. The previously noted hypoattenuating mass in the central portion of the liver has been replaced by a nest of collateral vessels mostly representing veins.

◆ DIFFERENTIAL DIAGNOSIS

◆ **Hepatic metastasis:** Metastases can diminish in size or disappear after chemotherapy, although the shape of the mass favors a lesion in the portal vein. Furthermore, malignant portal vein thrombosis is more commonly associated with hepatocellular carcinoma than with metastases.

◆ **Hepatocellular carcinoma (HCC):** HCC is often associated with either portal vein or hepatic vein thrombosis. The thrombus may be bland or malignant. Furthermore, malignant thrombosis can even occur with a tumor that is remote from a major vein. This diagnosis, however, is unlikely since the mass diminished on the 6-week follow-up examination.

◆ **Traumatic laceration of the liver:** Lacerations can have an unusual, somewhat angular shape, although they usually extend to the capsular surface of the liver and are associated with perihepatic or subcapsular hemorrhage.

◆ **Portal vein thrombosis (PVT) with cavernous transformation:** This is the most likely diagnosis since there is a mass in the lumen of the portal vein that is replaced by a nest of collateral veins within a relatively short period of time (several weeks).

◆ **Hepatic infarction:** Infarcts present as wedge-shaped, hypoattenuating parenchymal defects that originate from the central portion of the liver and extend to the capsular surface. In time, bubbles may develop, and later they become more rounded and cystic in nature.

◆ DIAGNOSIS: Portal vein thrombosis with cavernous transformation.

◆ KEY FACTS

CLINICAL

◆ Pediatrics: Idiopathic PVT is the principal cause of portal hypertension. Patients present with variceal hemorrhage without elevation of liver enzymes. They often have splenomegaly, but ascites is uncommon. Other causes include neonatal septicemia, omphalitis, or umbilical vein catheterization.

◆ Adults: Causes of PVT include cirrhosis (due to either or both slow flow and intimal hyperplasia), inflammatory and neoplastic pancreatic diseases, inflammatory processes involving the gastrointestinal tract (pyothrombophlebitis is rare), pregnancy, and oral contraceptives.

◆ PVT is characterized as being extrahepatic and/or intrahepatic. In extrahepatic PVT, peribiliary venous collaterals enlarge and reconstitute the intrahepatic portal branches if patent (cavernous transformation).

RADIOLOGIC

◆ Portal venous thrombi that partially occlude the lumen may propagate proximally and/or distally, progress to complete occlusion, or diminish/resolve following anticoagulant therapy.

◆ Portal venous thrombi that totally occlude the lumen tend to be replaced by a nest of small collaterals, and this process occurs over a several-week period. The thrombus itself tends to shrink in size and is often difficult to identify. Occasionally the thrombus calcifies. Cavernous transformation is best demonstrated by a contrast-enhanced CT or an MRI with either a white-blood or black-blood technique. Although ultrasound is helpful at times, particularly using color Doppler, it tends to underestimate collateral formation.

◆ PVT can be either bland or malignant in the presence of hepatic malignancy, especially hepatocellular carcinoma. Thrombosis can develop even if the tumor is remote to the portal vein. Malignant thrombosis is suspected when enhancement is demonstrated post-contrast material, particularly when it occurs in the hepatic arterial dominant phase. The presence of arterial signal within the thrombus on Doppler ultrasound is also diagnostic. At times, a percutaneous biopsy is required to make this differentiation.

◆ PVT often develops in patients with an inflammatory process along the venous system draining the abdominal viscera. Therefore, it is prudent to look also for the presence of enteritis, inflammatory bowel disease, diverticulitis, appendicitis, or an abscess.

◆ SUGGESTED READING

Burkart DJ, Johnson CD, Morton MJ, Ehman RL. Phase-contrast cine MR-angiography in chronic liver disease. Radiology 1993;187:407–412.

Dodd GD III, Carr BI. Percutaneous biopsy of portal vein thrombosis: New staging technique for hepatocellular carcinoma. AJR Am J Roentgenol 1993;161:229–233.

Marn CS, Francis IR. CT or portal venous occlusion. AJR Am J Roentgenol 1992;159:717–726.

Pozniak MA, Baus KM. Hepatofugal arterial signal in the main portal vein: An indicator of intravascular tumor spread. Radiology 1991;180:663–666.

HISTORY

A 42-year-old woman presents with vague abdominal pain.

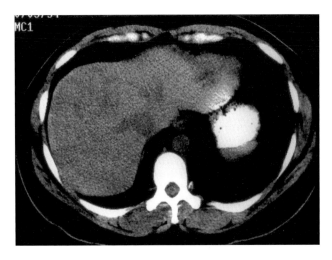

FIGURE 3-30A Noncontrast CT of the upper abdomen. There is an isoattenuating, faintly perceptible mass in the liver just under the dome of the diaphragm.

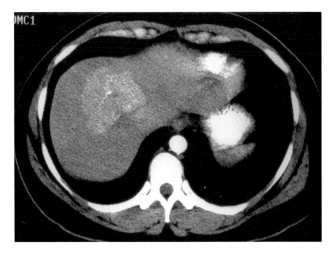

FIGURE 3-30B Dynamic contrast-enhanced CT of the liver during the hepatic arterial dominant phase. There is a hyperattenuating mass in the liver with a small hypoattenuating focus centrally.

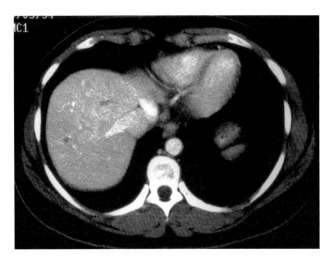

FIGURE 3-30C Dynamic contrast-enhanced CT of the liver during the portal venous dominant phase. The mass is isoattenuating to normal hepatic parenchyma. The central hypoattenuating focus continues to be apparent.

◆DIFFERENTIAL DIAGNOSIS

◆ **Hepatocellular carcinoma (HCC):** Some well-differentiated hepatomas may have these attenuation and enhancement characteristics, but when as large as this particular lesion, they are usually heterogenous.

◆ **Hepatocellular adenoma:** In the absence of internal hemorrhage, these benign tumors may have an identical appearance. A history of oral contraceptive use might suggest favoring adenoma over focal nodular hyperplasia.

◆ **Hypervascular metastasis:** Many of these metastatic implants will be visualized only in the hepatic arterial phase, although when they are this large, they are usually hypoattenuating precontrast as well as hypoattenuating in the portal venous dominant phase.

◆ **Cavernous hemangioma:** This mass has *no* enhancement features of a hemangioma. The peripheral nodular or cotton-wool enhancement pattern characteristic for these benign lesions is not present.

◆ **Focal nodular hyperplasia (FNH):** This is the most likely diagnosis since the mass has the classic features of FNH, particularly when the lesions are this large. A hepatic adenoma without internal hemorrhage, however, could have a similar appearance.

◆ **Regenerating nodule:** These masses are predominantly supplied by the portal vein, similar to normal parenchyma, and do not enhance significantly in the hepatic arterial dominant phase.

◆DIAGNOSIS: Focal nodular hyperplasia.

◆KEY FACTS

CLINICAL

◆ FHN is much more common in woman (85%); they typically present in the third to fifth decade of life.

◆ They are usually asymptomatic and therefore detected incidentally. Only 10% are symptomatic, presenting with an abdominal mass or pain.

◆ FNH are *not* associated with oral contraceptives, although there is evidence that oral contraceptives

increase the otherwise low propensity for intratumoral hemorrhage.

◆ The alpha-fetoprotein level is normal.

◆ FNH are benign tumors that do not degenerate into well-differentiated hepatocellular carcinomas.

RADIOLOGIC

◆ Histologically, FNH are composed of hepatocytes, bile ducts, and Kuppfer cells to a variable degree (there is a much higher population of Kuppfer cells compared to adenomas), laid along fibrous strands that coalesce centrally to form a scar. These features determine the imaging findings.

◆ Most FNH are solitary, but 20% are multiple.

◆ Classically, they are isoattenuating precontrast, hyperattenuating during the hepatic arterial dominant phase, and isoattenuating during the portal venous dominant phase. These differences are reflected in Tc^{99m}-sulfur colloid scintigraphy.

◆ A central hypoattenuating scar is present about 50% of the time, but this finding is not specific for FNH as it can also be seen in hepatic adenomas and hepatocellular carcinomas. On MRI, the scar tends to be of high signal intensity on T2-weighted images in FNH and of low signal intensity in HCC.

◆SUGGESTED READING

Klatskin G. Hepatic tumors: Possible relationship to the use of oral contraceptives. Gastroenterology 1977;73:386–394.

Lee MJ, Saini S, Hamm B, et al. Focal nodular hyperplasia of the liver: MR findings in 35 proven cases. AJR Am J Roentgenol 1991;156:317–320.

Park CH, Kim SM, Intenzo CM, et al. Focal nodular hyperplasia of the liver: Diagnosis by dynamic and SPECT scintigraphy. Clin Nucl Med 1993;18:701–703.

Procacci C, Fugazzola C, Cinquino M, et al. Contribution of CT to characterization of focal nodular hyperplasia of the liver. Gastrointest Radiol 1992;17:63–73.

Shamsi K, De Shepper A, Degryse H, et al. Focal nodular hyperplasia of the liver: Radiologic findings. Abdom Imag 1993;18:32–38.

CASE *31* *Paul V. Suhocki*

HISTORY

A 62-year-old man has a long-standing history of postprandial abdominal bloating. Laboratory values include a normal bilirubin level and slight elevation of alkaline phosphatase, serum glutamic-oxaloacetic transaminase, and serum glutamic-pyruvic transaminase.

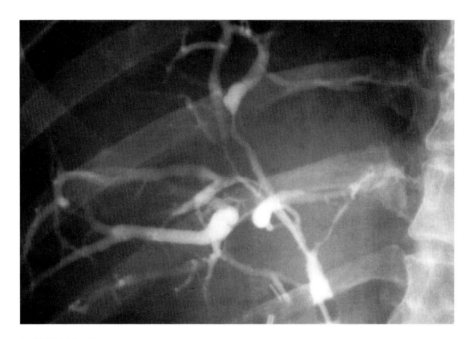

FIGURE 3-31 Balloon occlusion cholangiogram of the intrahepatic ducts during endoscopic retrograde cholangiogram. There are multiple sites of narrowing and dilatation, involving both the right and left intrahepatic bile ducts in a diffuse fashion. No intraluminal filling defects are appreciated.

◆ DIFFERENTIAL DIAGNOSIS

◆ **Bile duct carcinoma:** Bile duct carcinomas typically have the appearance of a short biliary stricture and proximal biliary obstruction. In the case illustrated here, the intrahepatic biliary system is diffusely involved. Bile duct carcinoma can rarely involve much of the biliary system in a diffuse fashion. It should be remembered that bile duct carcinoma can occur secondary to underlying primary sclerosing cholangitis, another cause of biliary duct narrowing.

◆ **Primary sclerosing cholangitis (PSC):** The appearance of multifocal strictures diffusely involving the biliary tree is typical of PSC. This is the most likely diagnosis.

◆ **Secondary sclerosing cholangitis:** This process has a radiologic appearance that simulates that of PSC. The clinical history is important in distinguishing the two entities. Secondary sclerosing cholangitis is associated with a history of recurrent biliary infections from calculus disease, a surgical stricture, or a choledochoenterostomy, all features that are absent in the case presented.

◆ DIAGNOSIS: Primary sclerosing cholangitis.

◆ KEY FACTS

CLINICAL

◆ PSC is a rare, chronic hepatobiliary disease of unknown cause. It is characterized by patchy, progressive fibrosis of either the intrahepatic or extrahepatic biliary ducts, or both.

◆ PSC is seen primarily in males, with a male-to-female ratio of 3 to 1. It typically occurs in the third to fifth decades.

◆ PSC is associated with inflammatory bowel disease. Sixty percent of patients have ulcerative colitis. On the other hand, between 1% and 4% of patients with chronic ulcerative colitis develop PSC. Five percent of patients with PSC have Crohn's disease.

◆ The HLA-B8 antigen is present in 60% to 80% of patients with PSC.

◆ PSC seems to originate in the intrahepatic ducts and progresses to involve the extrahepatic ducts. Extrahepatic ductal involvement eventually occurs in >90% of patients. Some studies indicate that intrahepatic ducts are almost always included (often to a greater degree than extrahepatic ducts).

◆ No histologic feature is pathognomonic for PSC. Typically, concentric layers of connective tissue surround the ducts, with a sparse, mixed inflammatory infiltrate.

◆ PSC can progress to biliary cirrhosis or bile duct carcinoma.

◆ The diagnosis is based on clinical features (recurrent right-upper quadrant pain and symptoms of chronic cholestasis, including jaundice and pruritus) and the appearance at cholangiography. The clinical and histologic findings overlap with those of primary biliary cirrhosis. However, the latter entity typically affects middle-aged women, does not involve the extrahepatic ducts, and is associated with high titers of antimitochondrial antibodies.

RADIOLOGIC

◆ The appearance of PSC at cholangiography is that of multifocal strictures that are diffusely distributed, usually involving both the intrahepatic and extrahepatic bile ducts.

◆ On occasion, the disease is confined to the intrahepatic or extrahepatic ducts alone.

◆ The strictures are usually short and annular, and located between normal or slightly dilated segments.

◆ SUGGESTED READING

Clement AR. The Interpretation of the Direct Cholangiogram. In RN Berk, AR Clemett (eds), Radiology of the Gallbladder and Bile Ducts. Philadelphia: Saunders, 1977;285–330.

Meyers WC, Jones RS. Primary Sclerosing Cholangitis. In WC Meyers, RS Jones (eds), Textbook of Liver and Biliary Surgery. Philadelphia: Lippincott, 1990;351–358.

CHAPTER 4

GENITO-URINARY IMAGING

Richard A. Leder, *chapter editor*

Anthony M. Foti, M. Gena Frederick,
Kelly S. Freed, Bruce P. Hall, Mary T. Keogan,
Jeremy A.L. Lawrance, Richard A. Leder,
Vincent G. McDermott, Erik K. Paulson,
Douglas H. Sheafor, and John A. Stahl

CASE 1

Kelly S. Freed

HISTORY

Patient A: a 31-year-old woman who had been in a motor vehicle accident presents with gross hematuria. Patient B: a 21-year-old woman who also had been in a motor vehicle accident presents with microscopic hematuria.

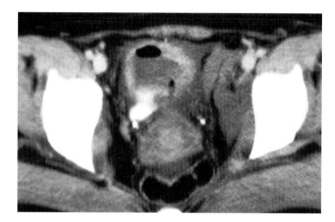

FIGURE 4-1A Patient A: Contrast-enhanced CT through the bladder. Extravasation of contrast material is seen from the right lateral aspect of the urinary bladder. The bladder is not well distended, and it is difficult to determine if the rupture is intra- or extraperitoneal. A CT cystogram or conventional cystogram could be performed to clarify this issue.

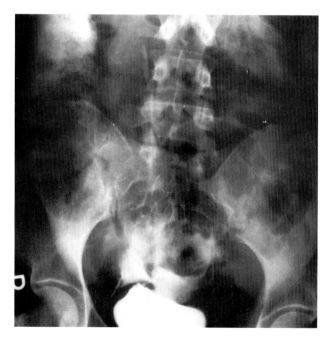

FIGURE 4-1B Patient A: Anteroposterior plain film of the abdomen performed following the contrast-enhanced CT scan. Contrast material is seen superior to the bladder, tracking up along the right paracolic gutter and adjacent to the liver.

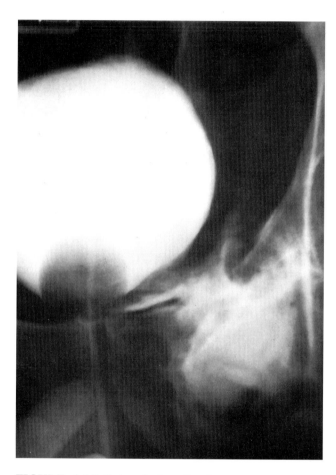

FIGURE 4-1C Patient B: Spot film from a conventional cystogram via a Foley catheter. There is a fracture of the left inferior pubic ramus. Contrast material is extravasating into the left inguinal region.

◆ DIFFERENTIAL DIAGNOSIS

◆ The differential diagnosis for both patients includes **intraperitoneal bladder rupture, extraperitoneal bladder rupture, or a combination of the two**.

◆ In patient A, **intraperitoneal rupture** is diagnosed because the contrast outlines the right paracolic gutter and liver.

◆ In patient B, **extraperitoneal rupture** is diagnosed because the contrast material does not flow into the peritoneal cavity but extends into the proximal thigh via the left inguinal region. There is an associated fracture of the inferior pubic ramus.

◆ DIAGNOSIS: Patient A: intraperitoneal bladder rupture. Patient B: extraperitoneal bladder rupture.

◆ KEY FACTS

CLINICAL

◆ Bladder rupture can be seen following blunt or penetrating trauma and may be extraperitoneal, intraperitoneal, or both.

◆ Extraperitoneal bladder rupture is more common, composing approximately 80% of cases, and is frequently associated with pelvic fractures. The rupture usually occurs at the base of the bladder. Intraperitoneal bladder rupture occurs at the dome of the bladder when the bladder is distended. Pelvic fractures are seen less commonly in intraperitoneal bladder rupture than in extraperitoneal bladder rupture.

◆ Intraperitoneal rupture is more common in children than adults.

◆ Physical findings of bladder rupture include hematuria and the inability to urinate. Significant hematuria (>50 red blood cells/high-power field) is a sensitive indicator of bladder trauma.

◆ Intraperitoneal bladder rupture requires surgery with bladder closure, whereas extraperitoneal bladder rupture can be managed with catheter drainage, antibiotics, and clinical follow-up.

RADIOLOGIC

◆ Radiologic diagnosis includes conventional cystography and CT of the abdomen and pelvis, including CT cystography.

◆ In extraperitoneal rupture, there are often associated fractures of the pubic rami or anterior pelvic ring. The extravasated contrast material can track down into the proximal thigh or scrotum. The extravasated contrast material may be ill-defined and feathery or contained.

◆ With intraperitoneal rupture, the contrast material flows freely into the peritoneum and may outline bowel loops or the paracolic gutters.

◆ CT of the abdomen and pelvis performed with the bladder only mildly or moderately distended is not as sensitive as conventional cystography for bladder injury. However, recent articles have demonstrated that CT cystography is comparably sensitive to conventional cystography. The bladder must be well distended on the CT study, either from instillation of contrast material through a Foley catheter or by using delayed images. Postdrainage CT images should also be obtained.

◆ SUGGESTED READING

Bodner DR, Selzman AA, Spirnak JP. Evaluation and treatment of bladder rupture. Semin Urol 1995;13:62–65.

Horstman WG, McClennan BL, Heiken JP. Comparison of computed tomography and conventional cystography for detection of traumatic bladder rupture. Urol Radiol 1991;12:188–193.

Rehm CG, Mure AJ, O'Malley KF, Ross SE. Blunt traumatic bladder rupture: The role of retrograde cystogram. Ann Emerg Med 1991;20:845–847.

HISTORY

A 56-year-old woman presents with a low-grade fever.

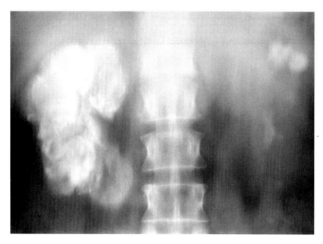

FIGURE 4-2A Noncontrast linear coronal tomogram of the renal area. Extensive calcifications are noted in the right kidney. Calcifications are also noted in the upper and lower pole calyces of the left kidney.

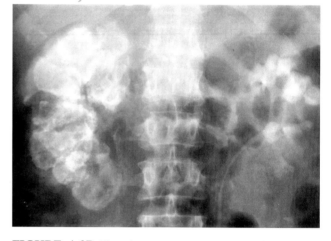

FIGURE 4-2B Five-minute anteroposterior view of the kidneys during an intravenous urogram. There is no excretion of contrast material from the right kidney. Calcifications are noted in the right proximal ureter. The left upper pole calyces are dilated, and there is no filling of the left lower pole calyces.

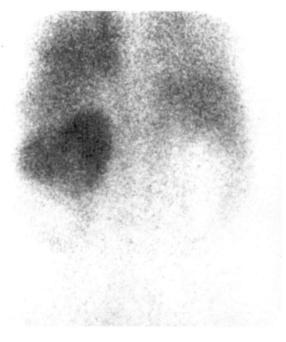

FIGURE 4-2C Tc^{99m}-diethylenetriamine penta-acetic acid scan of the renal area in the posteroanterior projection. There is marked reduction of activity in the left lower pole, with a faint rim of cortical activity. No right renal activity is seen.

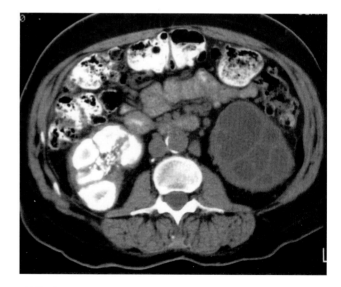

FIGURE 4-2D Noncontrast CT of the lower abdomen. There are dense calcifications in the right kidney and ureter. Low-attenuation areas are noted in the left lower pole consistent with a dilated collecting system.

◆ DIFFERENTIAL DIAGNOSIS

◆ **Renal tuberculosis (TB):** This is the best diagnosis due to extensive replacement of the nonfunctioning right kidney by calcification, producing a "putty" kidney. Calcifications in the ureter are also typical. Pyonephrosis is present in the lower pole of the left kidney.

◆ **Granulomatosis pyelonephritis:** This inflammatory process is usually related to a staghorn calculus. Calcification in the ureter is atypical.

◆ **Schistosomiasis:** This infection characteristically affects the distal ureters, causing dilation and/or stenosis. The proximal ureters and ureteropelvic junctions are rarely involved. Schistosomiasis typically causes bladder calcification, but renal calcifications are uncommon.

◆ DIAGNOSIS: Tuberculosis with right autonephrectomy and left lower pole pyonephrosis.

◆ KEY FACTS

CLINICAL

◆ Renal TB results from hematogenous spread of tuberculous bacilli to the kidneys. Ureteral involvement is secondary to bacilluria from the kidneys.

◆ Although both kidneys are usually involved, the disease process is typically more severe in one kidney.

◆ Patients are typically >40 years and present with hematuria, frequency, dysuria, or suprapubic pain.

◆ Ten percent of patients may be asymptomatic and have sterile urine.

RADIOLOGIC

◆ Radiographic findings depend on the extent of the disease process but are present in the majority of cases of renal TB.

◆ Papillary necrosis is common and may be extensive. Necrosis in renal granulomas may lead to the formation of communicating cavities.

◆ Parenchymal calcifications are present in 50% of patients. They may be amorphous in association with granulomatous masses, or dense in healed tuberculomas. Renal calculi develop in 20% of patients.

◆ Parenchymal scarring occurs in 20% of patients, either localized or involving the entire kidney. There are also associated calcifications and underlying calyceal abnormalities.

◆ Calyceal abnormalities are common, with multiple irregular strictures of the infundibula and subsequent hydrocalycosis.

◆ Renal function is impaired in 50% of patients. Antegrade or retrograde pyelography is required for evaluation.

◆ Advanced disease eventually results in a nonfunctioning kidney (autonephrectomy or "putty" kidney). These cases are associated with extensive calcifications.

◆ Failure of contrast material excretion often signifies the presence of tuberculous pyonephrosis due to stricture formation.

◆ Abnormalities of the ureters occur in 50% of cases of renal TB due to ulceration, with fibrosis, stricture, and calcification. Alternating segments of dilation and stricture produce a characteristic beaded appearance. Shortening of the ureter may also occur, producing a "pipestem" appearance.

◆ Other sites of urinary tract involvement include the prostate, epididymis, scrotum, and bladder, producing calcification with abscess formation and fistulous tracts.

◆ SUGGESTED READING

Renal Inflammatory Disease. In NR Dunnick, RW McCallum, CM Sandler (eds), Textbook of Uroradiology. Baltimore: Williams & Wilkins, 1991;135–157.

The Ureter. In NR Dunnick, RW McCallum, CM Sandler (eds), Textbook of Uroradiology. Baltimore: Williams & Wilkins, 1991;287–319.

Elkin M. Urogenital Tuberculosis. In HM Pollock, H Elkin (eds), Clinical Urography. Philadelphia: Saunders, 1990;1020–1052.

CASE 3

Mary T. Keogan

HISTORY

A 70-year-old man has a prior history of urinary tract surgery.

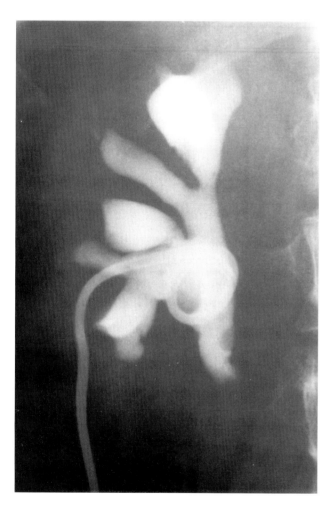

FIGURE 4-3A Anteroposterior antegrade nephrostogram of the right kidney. There are filling defects in the right renal pelvis and an abrupt obstruction to the contrast column in the right proximal ureter.

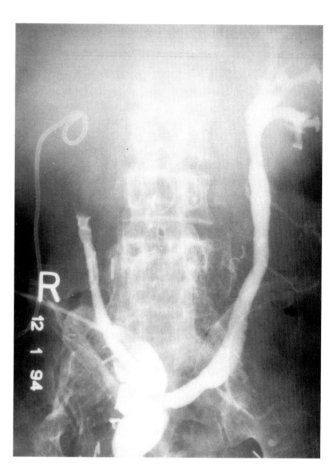

FIGURE 4-3B Retrograde loopogram that also opacifies both upper collecting systems. The left upper collecting system is normal. The right ureter is abnormal, with a "champagne glass" deformity in the mid ureter.

◆ DIFFERENTIAL DIAGNOSIS

◆ **Recurrent transitional cell tumor:** The urinary diversion procedure suggests surgery for previous carcinoma of the bladder. The mass and filling defects within the right ureter may represent either a recurrent or a metachronous transitional cell carcinoma (TCC).

◆ **Obstructing blood clot:** A blood clot could form in the right ureter, particularly since there has been recent surgery. This diagnosis would also be favored if there were a history of anticoagulation therapy.

◆ **Infectious debris (fungus ball):** A collection of thick debris, especially in the presence of infection, could cause obstruction of the ureteropelvic junction or the right ureter.

◆ DIAGNOSIS: Recurrent and obstructing transitional cell carcinoma of the right mid-ureter.

◆ KEY FACTS

CLINICAL

◆ Pain and hematuria are the most common presenting features of recurrent TCC.

◆ In a patient with a previous history of bladder carcinoma, pain and hematuria may represent recurrent tumor either within the residual bladder or in the upper tracts.

RADIOLOGIC

◆ Forty percent of patients present with a nonfunctioning kidney on intravenous urography due to long-standing ureteral obstruction.

◆ A filling defect in the lumen of the ureter is the key diagnostic finding.

◆ Multiple polypoid discrete masses within the pelvicalyceal system or ureter are a common finding.

◆ "Bergman's sign" is dilation of the ureter *distal* to a ureteral mass not associated with a renal calculus.

◆ Localized expansion of the ureter at the level of the tumor ("champagne glass" or "wine goblet" deformity) is a key finding.

◆ CT may be valuable when intravenous urography or retrograde pyelography is unsuccessful. Pre- and post-contrast CT may also be useful for distinguishing enhancing tumor from a nonopaque calculus.

◆ SUGGESTED READING

Baron RL, McClennan BL, Lee JKT, et al. Computed tomography of transitional cell carcinoma of the renal pelvis and ureter. Radiology 1982;144:125–130.

Pollack HM. Long-term follow-up of the upper urinary tract for transitional cell carcinoma: How much is enough? Radiology 1988;167:871–872.

CASE 4

M. Gena Frederick

HISTORY

A 63-year-old woman status post abdominal aortic aneurysm repair presents with abdominal pain, fever, leukocytosis.

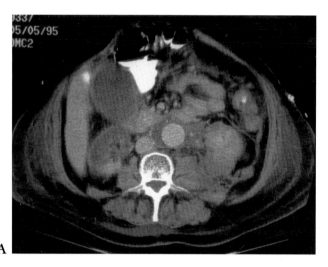
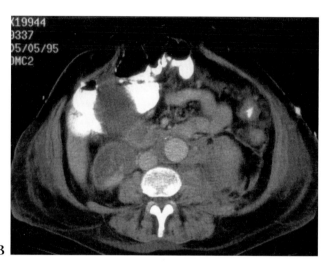

A

B

FIGURES 4-4A and 4-4B Two sequential images from a contrast-enhanced CT of the abdomen. A synthetic graft containing contrast-enhanced blood is surrounded by low-attenuation fluid within the native aneurysmal abdominal aorta. There are segmental areas of low attenuation involving the majority of the right kidney, with relative sparing of segmental portions of the posterior aspect of the right kidney. Curvilinear, peripheral subcapsular enhancement of the right kidney is also present. There is a persistent, although patchy, nephrogram in the left kidney, with perinephric inflammatory stranding, as well as low attenuation within the left psoas muscle.

◆ DIFFERENTIAL DIAGNOSIS

◆ **Renal abscess:** Renal abscesses tend to present as more focal, well-rounded areas of low attenuation producing a focal contour abnormality of the kidney. Typically, there will be enlargement of the involved kidney with perinephric inflammatory changes. The low attenuation in the left psoas muscle and adjacent left perinephric inflammatory change could be due to either a psoas abscess or postoperative hematoma.

◆ **Renal neoplasm:** A renal neoplasm may contain areas of decreased attenuation due to tumor necrosis. However, a renal neoplasm would be more mass-like, deforming the renal contour. If possible, measuring the attenuation values of a focal mass before and after contrast material administration is useful.

◆ **Renal infarction:** The segmental pattern of involvement with curvilinear renal subcapsular enhancement of the right kidney is most consistent with renal infarction. The clinical scenario of recent abdominal aortic aneurysm repair with graft placement also suggests this as the most likely diagnosis. The changes in the left kidney are most consistent with ischemia or acute tubular necrosis (ATN). The low attenuation within the left psoas muscle and left perinephric stranding may be postoperative in nature, indicative of hematoma or seroma. This appearance may also be seen with an aneurysmal leak.

◆ **Acute pyelonephritis:** The abnormal persistent nephrogram of the left kidney as well as the left perinephric inflammatory changes with low attenuation in the left psoas may be indistinguishable from severe acute pyelonephritis. However, one might expect more diffuse enlargement of the left kidney. Pyelonephritis typically has a segmental distribution, as is the case within the right kidney; however, the curvilinear enhancement in the subcapsular right renal cortex argues for renal infarction due to the presence of capsular collaterals.

◆ DIAGNOSIS: Renal infarction.

◆ KEY FACTS

CLINICAL

◆ Renal infarction typically presents with sudden onset of severe flank pain, fever, and hematuria. Nausea and vomiting are seen in 50% of patients.

◆ The clinical and laboratory findings, although consistent with renal infarction, are nonspecific and often suggest alternative diagnoses, including an acute surgical abdomen.

◆ Renal infarction may be secondary to complications of atherosclerotic disease, with resultant thrombosis or embolic occlusion of the renal artery, typically at the renal ostia. Post-traumatic dissection of the renal artery with subsequent thrombosis may also result in renal infarction.

◆ Iatrogenic causes include prolonged cross-clamp time from abdominal aneurysm repair. An aortic dissection may also extend into the abdominal aorta and involve the renal ostia. This more commonly involves the left kidney.

◆ Laboratory findings include moderate leukocytosis and albuminuria in most cases, and microscopic hematuria in 50% of cases.

RADIOLOGIC

◆ The differential diagnosis for a striated nephrogram includes acute pyelonephritis, renal contusion, renal vein thrombosis, and ureteral obstruction.

◆ The subcapsular rim sign is helpful in establishing a diagnosis of renal infarction. This sign is the result of collateral flow to the capsular plexus, which supplies the outer 2 to 4 mm of cortical rim via perforating branches.

◆ The subcapsular rim sign is not pathognomonic of renal arterial infarction, because it may also be seen in renal vein thrombosis and ATN. This pattern of subcapsular enhancement, however, serves as a crucial distinguishing feature in the differential diagnosis between infarction and pyelonephritis.

◆ The subcapsular or cortical rim sign should not be confused with the rim or shell nephrogram of hydronephrosis.

◆ SUGGESTED READING

Bankoff MS, Sarno RC, Mitcheson HD. Computed tomography differentiation of pyelonephritis and renal infarction. CT 1984;8:239–243.

Glazer GM, Francis IR, Brady TM, Teng SS. Computed tomography of renal infarction: Clinical and experimental observations. AJR Am J Roentgenol 1983;140:721–727.

Hilton S, Bosniak MA, Raghavendra BN, et al. CT findings in acute renal infarction. Urol Radiol 1984;6:158–163.

Saunders HS, Dyer RB, Shifrin RY, et al. The CT nephrogram: Implications for evaluation of urinary tract disease. Radiographics 1995;15:1069–1085.

Wong WS, Moss AA, Federle MP, et al. Renal infarction: CT diagnosis and correlation between CT findings and etiologies. Radiology 1984;150:201–205.

CASE 5

Anthony M. Foti

HISTORY

A 50-year-old man has back pain and an elevated serum creatinine.

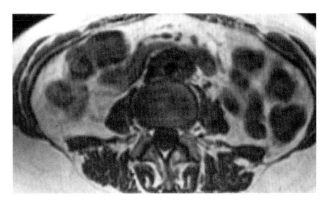

FIGURE 4-5A Axial T1-weighted MRI of the abdomen. There is a well-circumscribed mantle of soft tissue surrounding the aorta and abutting the inferior vena cava. The mass does not displace the aorta anteriorly away from the spine and is isointense to muscle.

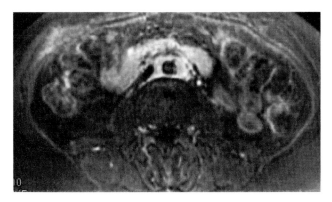

FIGURE 4-5B Axial fat-suppressed T2-weighted MRI of the abdomen. The mantle of soft tissue is mildly hyperintense and relatively homogenous.

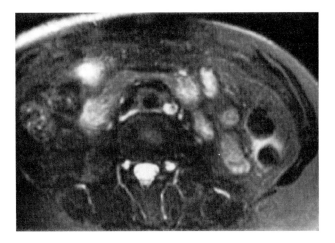

FIGURE 4-5C Axial contrast-enhanced T1-weighted MRI following the intravenous administration of a gadolinium-chelate. There is uniform enhancement of the soft tissue mass.

◆ DIFFERENTIAL DIAGNOSIS

◆ **Malignant retroperitoneal fibrosis (RPF):** Imaging cannot differentiate malignant from nonmalignant RPF reliably; however, malignant RPF tends to be more heterogeneous on T2-weighted images.

◆ **Malignant lymphadenopathy and lymphoma:** These entities tend to displace the aorta anteriorly, away from the spine.

◆ **Idiopathic RPF:** The periaortic distribution and signal characteristics are classic for this entity.

◆ DIAGNOSIS: Idiopathic (nonmalignant) retroperitoneal fibrosis.

◆ KEY FACTS

CLINICAL

◆ RPF is a rare disorder in which a fibrotic plaque encases the aorta and extends laterally to engulf the inferior vena cava (IVC) and ureters. It usually begins near the aortic bifurcation and extends cephalad to the renal hila. Occasionally, it may extend cranially into the mediastinum or anteriorly into the mesentery.

◆ At the time of diagnosis, 70% of patients are 30 to 60 years of age.

◆ Symptoms are nonspecific and include dull back pain, fatigue, and weight loss. Laboratory values include elevated serum creatinine levels and erythrocyte sedimentation rates.

◆ Two-thirds of cases are idiopathic (Ormond's disease). The presumed mechanism is autoimmune, likely a response to leakage of ceroid, an insoluble lipid, from atherosclerotic plaques into periaortic tissue. Twelve percent of cases are secondary to methysergide administration; beta blockers, hydralazine, methyldopa, and bromocriptine have also been implicated. Other causes include malignancy, hemorrhage, and aneurysms (so-called perianeurysmal fibrosis).

◆ Malignant RPF is an intense desmoplastic response to retroperitoneal metastases from a variety of primary malignancies (breast, lung, thyroid, gastrointestinal tract, genitourinary tract, and Hodgkin's lymphoma). There are only scattered malignant cells, and thus deep surgical biopsy is required to differentiate benign from malignant RPF.

◆ Histologically, perianeurysmal fibrosis (also referred to as an inflammatory aneurysm) is identical to RPF. The only difference is the caliber of the aorta.

◆ RPF usually results in ureteral dilatation by impairing peristalsis, rather than directly invading the ureter.

◆ RPF may obstruct the IVC and, rarely, the portal vein or common bile duct.

◆ Treatment consists of a combination of surgery to release the ureters (ureterolysis) and steroids.

◆ RPF has a similar histology and is associated with other systemic sclerosing diseases, including sclerosing cholangitis, orbital pseudotumor, mediastinal fibrosis, and Riedel's thyroiditis. There is also an association with other immune-mediated connective tissue disorders such as ankylosing spondylitis, Wegener's granulomatosis, systemic lupus erythematosus, Raynaud's disease, polyarteritis nodosa, and systemic vasculitis. RPF is associated with the major histocompatibility complex HLA-B27.

RADIOLOGIC

◆ On intravenous urography there is hydronephrosis with medial deviation of the middle third of the ureters, which then taper near the L4–5 level. This is in contrast to most cases of lymphoma and other causes of lymphadenopathy, which are not associated with a desmoplastic response and thus cause lateral deviation of the ureters due to mass effect.

◆ On CT, a homogeneous mantle of soft-tissue envelopes, but does usually not displace, the aorta. It extends laterally to involve the IVC and ureters, but usually does not extend >1 cm lateral to the ureters. It may obstruct the gonadal vessels. The margins are usually sharply circumscribed and not nodular. However, it may be ill-defined, although the margin characteristics cannot be used to distinguish benign from malignant RPF reliably. Precontrast, it is isoattenuating with the psoas muscles. Postcontrast, the soft-tissue mass enhances uniformly, although enhancement diminishes with the chronicity of the disease.

◆ On ultrasound, a homogeneous hypoechoic perivascular mantle is characteristic.

◆ With MRI, the soft-tissue mass is relatively homogeneous on all imaging sequences. It is isointense to psoas muscle on T1-weighted images. The signal intensity on T2-weighted images and the enhancement on T1-weighted images post–gadolinium-chelate administration vary with the stage. Early in the disease, the cellular nature of the infiltrate results in high signal intensity on T2-weighted images and discernible contrast enhancement. Late in the disease, the signal intensity on T2-weighted images and contrast enhancement decreases, reflecting the fibrotic process. Heterogeneous high signal intensity on T2-weighted images suggests malignancy, while uniformly low signal suggests late-stage benign disease.

◆ SUGGESTED READING

Amis ES Jr. Retroperitoneal fibrosis. AJR Am J Roentgenol 1991; 157:321–329.

Arrive L, Hricak H, Tavares NJ, Miller TR. Malignant versus non-malignant retroperitoneal fibrosis: Differentiation with MR imaging. Radiology 1989;172:139–143.

Brooks AP, Reznek RH, Webb JA. Aortic displacement on computed tomography of idiopathic retroperitoneal fibrosis. Clin Radiol 1989;40:51–52.

Brun B, Laursen K, Sorensen IN, et al. CT in retroperitoneal fibrosis. AJR Am J Roentgenol 1981;137:535–538.

Degesys GE, Dunnick NR, Silverman PM, et al. Retroperitoneal fibrosis: Use of CT in distinguishing among possible causes. AJR Am J Roentgenol 1986;146:57–60.

Kottra JJ, Dunnick NR. Retroperitoneal fibrosis. Radiol Clin North Am 1996;34:1259–1275.

CASE 6

Jeremy A.L. Lawrance

HISTORY

A 67-year-old woman who was previously healthy presents with a 6-week history of epigastric pain.

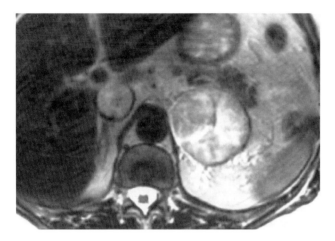

FIGURE 4-6A Axial T2-weighted MRI of the upper abdomen. There is a 5-cm left-upper quadrant mass. It is of relatively high signal intensity and heterogeneous in nature. In addition, a high-signal intensity mass is noted in the inferior vena cava.

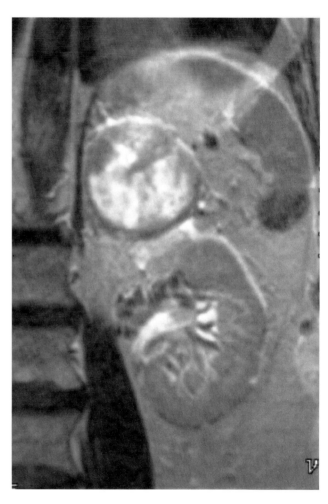

FIGURE 4-6B Coronal T2-weighted MRI of the upper abdomen. The mass is superior to and clearly separate from the left kidney.

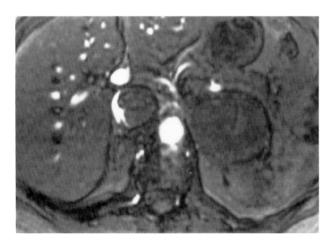

FIGURE 4-6C Axial T1-weighted gradient echo MRI of the upper abdomen shows a crescent of flow around the inferior vena cava filling defect.

◈ DIFFERENTIAL DIAGNOSIS

◆ **Renal carcinoma:** The mass is separate from the kidney; therefore this diagnosis is excluded.

◆ **Pheochromocytoma:** These tumors usually show very high signal on T2-weighted images. They are usually >3 cm and are frequently necrotic and hemorrhagic. Inferior vena cava (IVC) invasion, however, is not a feature of pheochromocytomas.

◆ **Adrenal metastasis:** Tumors >5 cm are more likely malignant. Furthermore, metastases are usually of higher signal intensity than adenomas. Apart from an adrenal metastasis in a patient with renal cell carcinoma, IVC invasion by an adrenal metastasis would be uncommon. The kidneys show no evidence of tumor in this case.

◆ **Adrenal adenoma:** This diagnosis is extremely unlikely unless IVC thrombosis is coincidental.

◆ **Adrenal carcinoma:** Although these tumors typically are larger at presentation, direct IVC invasion makes this the most likely diagnosis.

◈ DIAGNOSIS: Adrenal carcinoma with inferior vena cava invasion.

◈ KEY FACTS

CLINICAL

◆ Adrenal carcinomas are rare malignant tumors with an annual incidence of 0.5 to 2.0 cases per million per year.

◆ The average age in one large study was 47 years.

◆ There is a slight female preponderance.

◆ In a series of 156 cases, 53% had a functional endocrine syndrome. Cushing's syndrome is the most common, with virilization, hypertension, and feminization occurring less frequently.

◆ Up to 5% of cases are bilateral.

RADIOLOGIC

◆ Adrenal carcinomas tend to be large at presentation, usually >5 cm in diameter. Functional tumors tend to be smaller at presentation than nonfunctioning tumors. The range of sizes in one study was 3 to 30 cm, with a mean diameter of 12 cm.

◆ The problem with small adrenal carcinomas is that it is often impossible to differentiate benign from malignant tumors. Tumors >5 cm are more likely malignant, while evidence of local invasion into adjacent organs or distant metastases are features of malignant tumors.

◆ In recent studies, metastases from adrenal carcinoma were present in 22%, while older studies reported higher incidences of metastases. The most common sites are liver, lymph nodes, bone, and lungs.

◆ Areas of necrosis, hemorrhage, and calcification are common. The latter is best detected by CT and found in approximately 30% of cases.

◆ By MRI, adrenal carcinoma shows low signal intensity on T1-weighted images and signal intensity greater than liver on T2-weighted images. Pheochromocytomas tend to have very high signal intensity on T2-weighted images and can be difficult to distinguish from adrenal carcinomas with MRI. Detection and delineation of vascular invasion, as well as multiplanar capability, make MRI a useful diagnostic tool in cases of adrenal carcinoma.

◈ SUGGESTED READING

Dunnick NR. Adrenal carcinoma. Radiol Clin North Am 1994;32:99–108.

Icard P, Chapuis Y, Andreassian B, et al. Adrenocortical carcinoma in surgically treated patients: A retrospective study on 156 cases. French Assoc Endocrine Surg 1992;112:972–980.

Zografos GC, Driscoll DL, Karakousis CP, Humen RP. Adrenal adenocarcinoma: A review of 53 cases. Surg Oncol 1994;55:160–164.

CASE 7

Richard A. Leder

HISTORY

A 46-year-old man presents with urinary frequency.

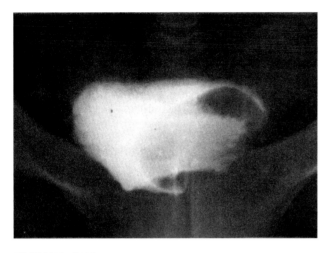

FIGURE 4-7A Anteroposterior supine 10-minute film of the bladder from an intravenous urogram demonstrates an oval to round filling defect along the left side of the bladder with no evidence of ureteral obstruction on that side.

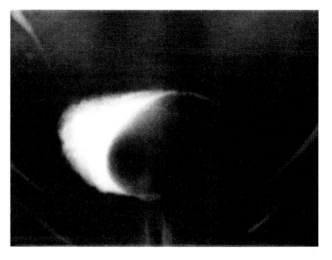

FIGURE 4-7B Anteroposterior postvoid film from the same intravenous urogram shows a smooth filling defect involving the left lateral wall of the bladder.

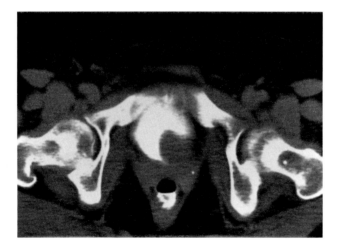

FIGURE 4-7C Contrast-enhanced CT through the urinary bladder shows a smooth, round filling defect in the left posterolateral wall of the bladder. The filling defect is of soft-tissue attenuation.

◆ DIFFERENTIAL DIAGNOSIS

◆ **Transitional cell carcinoma (TCC):** TCC must be included in the differential diagnosis of this lesion, but some features mitigate against this as the most likely diagnosis. Large intravesical transitional cell tumors are frequently of the papillary variety. They have a stippled surface and are unlikely to appear as smooth, as in this case. The location will dictate whether a large lesion of this size will obstruct the ureter. In this case, no ureteral obstruction was present.

◆ **Hematoma or fungus ball:** There are a multitude of nonfixed filling defects that can occur within the bladder. It is useful in cases where hematomas or fungus balls are being considered to image the patient using ultrasound to document that these are not fixed to the bladder wall. While ultrasound was not performed in this patient, it is essential to document whether filling defects within the bladder are likely to be mobile or fixed.

◆ **Bladder calculus:** All urinary calculi are hyperattenuating on CT (>+100 Hounsfield units [HU]). This filling defect measured soft-tissue attenuation.

◆ **Cystitis:** *Bullous cystitis* can appear as a bladder wall lesion. *Cystitis glandularis* is a proliferative lesion in which glandular elements of the bladder mucosa occur in the submucosa. Many patients have infections and associated *cystitis cystica*. These masses are typically villous. Submucosal fluid-filled cysts describe cystitis cystica, which can cause filling defects within the bladder. Chronic infection is postulated as the chief etiologic factor.

◆ **Bladder leiomyoma:** Smooth muscle tumors of the bladder wall may have this appearance and should be considered in the differential diagnosis of a smooth bladder wall filling defect.

◆ DIAGNOSIS: Leiomyoma of the bladder.

◆ KEY FACTS

CLINICAL

◆ Leiomyomas may occur in any site in the genitourinary tract. These lesions occur in all age groups and affect both sexes equally.

◆ Lesions may be endovesical (63%), intramural (7%), or extravesical (30%).

◆ The cause of these tumors is unknown.

◆ The tumor is usually asymptomatic and may be detected incidentally on physical examination or cystoscopy.

◆ The endovesical form may present with irritative urinary symptoms, gross hematuria, or obstructive symptoms.

◆ Small endovesical lesions can be managed with transurethral resection and fulguration. Larger endovesical, intramural, or extravesical tumors are best treated with segmental resection.

◆ The prognosis of this tumor is excellent. No malignant degeneration has been reported.

RADIOLOGIC

◆ Intravenous urography or cystography usually reveals a smooth filling defect within the bladder.

◆ CT is useful to determine consistency (attenuation), size, location, and possible adjacent organ involvement.

◆ The endovesical form can be sessile or pedunculated on cystoscopy and is usually covered with normal bladder mucosa.

◆ SUGGESTED READING

Illescas FF, Baker ME, Weinerth JL. Bladder leiomyoma: Advantages of sonography over computed tomography. Urol Radiol 1986;8:216–218.

Knoll LD, Segura JW, Scheithauer BW. Leiomyoma of the bladder. J Urol 1986;136:906–908.

CASE 8

John A. Stahl

HISTORY

A 40-year-old man with diabetes mellitus presents with fever, left flank pain, and pyuria.

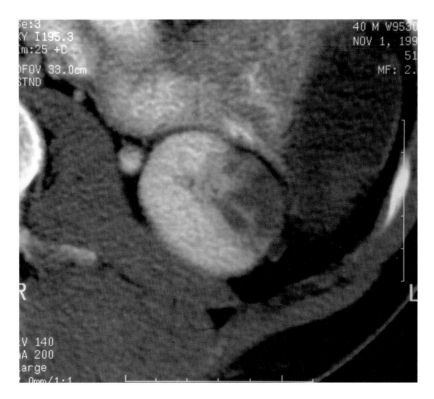

FIGURE 4-8 Contrast-enhanced CT focused on the left kidney. There is a focal, low-attenuation mass lesion in the left kidney that demonstrates both central and peripheral contrast enhancement.

◆ DIFFERENTIAL DIAGNOSIS

- **Renal abscess:** This diagnosis is unlikely since the central area of enhancement indicates viable tissue rather than liquefactive necrosis.
- **Renal cell carcinoma (RCC):** This is a possible diagnosis based on the CT appearance, but the clinical presentation mitigates against a malignant process.
- **Renal infarct:** This diagnosis is unlikely because infarcts are typically wedge-shaped and demonstrate a thin rim of cortical enhancement.
- **Focal xanthogranulomatous pyelonephritis (XGP):** The low-attenuation mass in XGP is typically associated with renal calculi (particularly staghorn) and a nonfunctional kidney, neither of which is present in this case.
- **Focal bacterial pyelonephritis (preabscess, lobar nephronia):** This is the most likely diagnosis based on the presence of an enhancing mass in the clinical setting of pyelonephritis.

◆ DIAGNOSIS: Focal bacterial pyelonephritis.

◆ KEY FACTS

CLINICAL

- Focal bacterial pyelonephritis (preabscess, lobar nephronia) represents progression from pyelonephritis to a more severe infection most commonly seen in patients who are immunocompromised (i.e., diabetes or patients on steroids/immunosuppressive therapy).
- *Escherichia coli* is the most common infecting organism.

- An elevated white blood cell count, pyuria, and bacteremia may occur.
- Failure to respond to appropriate antimicrobial therapy can cause pyelonephritis to progress to a renal abscess.

RADIOLOGIC

- Intravenous urography demonstrates a poorly functioning region of the affected kidney, with focal swelling and mass effect on adjacent calyces.
- On ultrasound, a hypoechoic mass with low-level internal echoes and attenuation of the ultrasound beam is present. The mass is poorly marginated, with disruption of the normal corticomedullary junction. Central anechoic areas may also be present.
- CT imaging displays a lobar inflammatory mass with mild contrast material enhancement (20 to 40 HU less than the surrounding enhanced parenchyma). The mass is typically irregular, rounded, and heterogenous in attenuation.

◆ SUGGESTED READING

Goldman S. Acute and chronic urinary infection: Present concepts and controversies. Urol Radiol 1988;10:17–24.

Pollack H. Clinical Urography. Philadelphia: Saunders, 1990;799–815.

Rabushka L, Fishman E, Goldman S. Pictorial review: Computed tomography of renal inflammatory disease. Urology 1994;44:473–480.

Zaontz M, et al. Acute focal bacterial nephritis: A systematic approach to diagnosis and treatment. J Urol 1985;133:752–756.

CASE 9

M. Gena Frederick

HISTORY

A 63-year-old woman has microscopic hematuria.

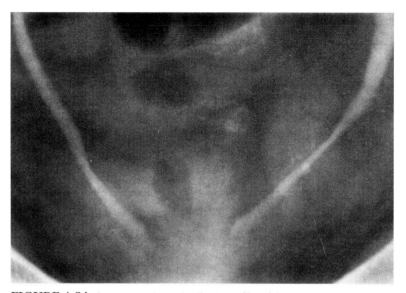

FIGURE 4-9A Anteroposterior supine 5-minute film of the urinary bladder from an intravenous urogram. There is bilateral columnation of both ureters to the level of the ureterovesical junction, with a rounded distal configuration.

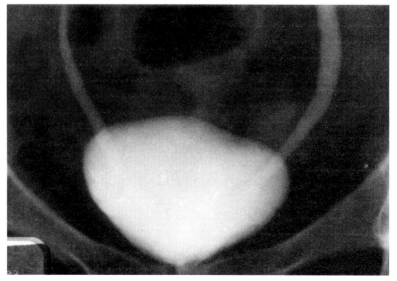

FIGURE 4-9B Anterosuperior supine 15-minute film of the urinary bladder from an intravenous urogram. Within the bladder, there is a "cobra head" appearance bilaterally. Note the lucent outline of the bulbous ureteral termination.

◆ DIFFERENTIAL DIAGNOSIS

- **Pseudoureterocele:** This appearance is caused by a transitional cell carcinoma (TCC) of the bladder or a stone obstructing the ureter. It is unlikely because of the lack of a filling defect or mass, as well as the bilaterality of the defects. Other less common causes of the "pseudoureterocele" appearance include cervical carcinoma invading the ureterovesical orifice, radiation cystitis, or edema of the ureterovesical junction from recent stone passage. However, these are unlikely in this case because the former are identified by asymmetry of the distal lumen and irregularity of the wall and generally do not have intravesicular protrusion. However, they are capable of distending the distal ureter and thus mimicking an orthotopic ureterocele.
- **Bilateral simple ureteroceles:** This is the most likely diagnosis given the lack of a bladder mass or irregularity, the intravesicular protrusion, the absence of upper tract dilatation, and the bilaterality.

◆ DIAGNOSIS: Bilateral simple ureteroceles.

◆ KEY FACTS

CLINICAL
- An orthotopic ureterocele forms in a ureter with a normal insertion into the trigone, as opposed to an ectopic ureterocele.
- Orthotopic ureteroceles usually occur in single systems, as opposed to ectopic ureteroceles, which occur in duplicated systems.
- Orthotopic ureteroceles are usually unilateral, asymptomatic, and incidental. However, a calculus may lodge or form in the ureterocele.
- A ureterocele is a congenital deformity.
- A ureterocele consists of a prolapse of the distal ureter into the bladder with associated dilation of the distal ureter.
- The wall of the ureterocele is composed of a thin layer of muscle between the outer surface of the bladder uroepithelium and the inner surface of the ureteral uroepithelium.

RADIOLOGIC
- The typical radiographic appearance is the so-called "cobra head" deformity, which is formed by the projection of the minimally dilated distal ureter into the lumen of the bladder, with opacified urine surrounding the ureterocele.
- The thin line of radiolucency represents the wall of the ureterocele.

◆ SUGGESTED READING
Davidson AJ, Hartman DS. Radiology of the Kidney and Urinary Tract (2nd ed). Philadelphia: Saunders, 1994;520–523.
Mitty HA, Schapira HE. Ureterocele and pseudoureterocele: Cobra versus cancer. J Urol 1977;117:557–561.

HISTORY

A 54-year-old man presents with abdominal pain.

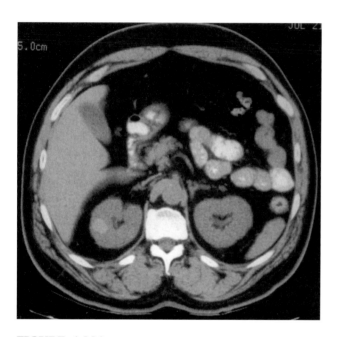

FIGURE 4-10A Noncontrast CT of the abdomen. An area of increased attenuation (+59 Hounsfield units [HU]) is seen in the lateral portion of the right kidney.

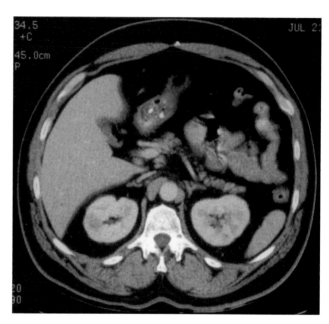

FIGURE 4-10B Contrast-enhanced CT of the abdomen. The same area appears low in attenuation (+60 HU) postcontrast.

◆ DIFFERENTIAL DIAGNOSIS

◆ **Hemorrhagic renal cell carcinoma (RCC):** This diagnosis is unlikely because the entire lesion is of uniform increased attenuation on the noncontrast study.

◆ **Angiomyolipoma that has bled:** This diagnosis is unlikely because no fat is demonstrated on the CT examination to raise the suspicion of an angiomyolipoma.

◆ **Hemorrhagic renal cyst:** This is the most likely diagnosis for a uniform, nonenhancing, high-attenuation renal mass.

◆ DIAGNOSIS: Hemorrhagic renal cyst.

◆ KEY FACTS

CLINICAL

◆ Renal cysts account for approximately 60% of all renal masses.

◆ Renal cysts increase in frequency with age (approximately 50% of cases occur past the age of 50).

◆ Most renal cysts are asymptomatic, whether hemorrhagic or not.

◆ Hemorrhagic cysts are frequently seen in patients with autosomal dominant polycystic kidney disease and acquired renal cystic disease.

RADIOLOGIC

◆ Noncontrast CT is absolutely necessary to evaluate the attenuation of the lesion before contrast material administration.

◆ Cysts that are "hyperdense" exhibit attenuation values between +50 and +90 HU. The high attenuation is due to a high content of protein, blood breakdown products, or iodine. To be considered a benign hyperdense cyst, the lesion must be sharply marginated, homogeneous, and nonenhancing (<10 HU increase postcontrast).

◆ Because of the thickness of the wall and the internal structure of the lesion, these cysts cannot be evaluated reliably with ultrasound, and only 50% of hyperattenuating lesions demonstrate typical sonographic cyst criteria. CT is necessary, particularly to evaluate for potential lesion enhancement.

◆ SUGGESTED READING

Bosniak MA. The small (≤3.0 cm) renal parenchymal tumor: Detection, diagnosis, and controversies. Radiology 1991;179:307–317.

Bosniak MA. Problems in the radiologic diagnosis of renal parenchymal tumors. Urol Clin North Am 1993;20:217–230.

Curry NS. Small renal masses (lesions smaller than 3 cm): Imaging evaluation and management. AJR Am J Roentgenol 1995;164:355–362.

HISTORY

A 33-year-old man has a history of urinary tract infections.

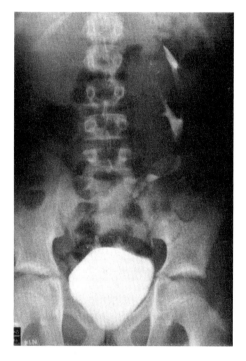

FIGURE 4-11A Anteroposterior film of the kidneys, ureters, and bladder from an intravenous urogram shows two collecting systems on the left side of the abdomen. On this film, only the distal left ureter is seen.

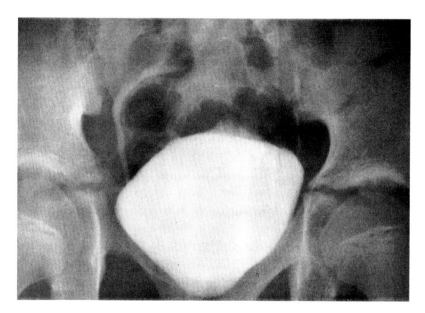

FIGURE 4-11B Anteroposterior coned view of the pelvis from the intravenous urogram shows both the distal left and distal right ureters entering the bladder in the expected location.

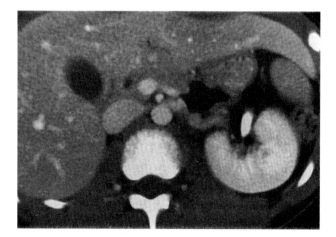

FIGURE 4-11C Contrast-enhanced CT of the mid abdomen shows enhancement of the left kidney, but no renal tissue is seen in the right renal fossa.

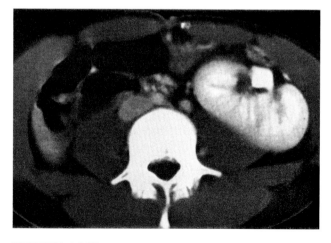

FIGURE 4-11D Contrast-enhanced CT of the lower abdomen. The right kidney is present in the left lower quadrant.

◆ DIFFERENTIAL DIAGNOSIS

◆ **Retroperitoneal mass with displacement of the kidney:** While a retroperitoneal mass can cause displacement of the kidney, the size of a mass required to displace the kidney into the opposite side of the abdomen would be quite large. One would expect such a mass to be obvious on physical examination.

◆ **Renal duplication with agenesis of the contralateral kidney:** Renal duplication would explain an enlarged kidney and would account for the presence of two ureters. However, noting that the ureter crosses into the opposite hemipelvis to enter in its normally expected location in the trigone excludes this diagnosis.

◆ **Crossed renal ectopia:** This is the most likely diagnosis given the position of the kidneys and the insertion of the ureters.

◆ DIAGNOSIS: Crossed renal ectopia.

◆ KEY FACTS

CLINICAL

◆ There are four types of crossed renal ectopia:
1. Crossed renal ectopia with fusion.
2. Crossed renal ectopia without fusion.
3. Solitary crossed renal ectopia: In this case, there is only one kidney, which lies in the abdomen opposite from the side of its ureteral insertion.
4. Bilateral crossed renal ectopia: In this case, both kidneys are crossed to the opposite side of the abdomen with their ureters inserting into the contralateral ureterovesicle junction.
5. The most common varieties are fused and unfused ectopia; crossed fused ectopia occurs in 85% to 90% of cases.

◆ Crossed renal ectopia is seen more commonly in males than females.

◆ The most common scenario is the left kidney crossing to the right side of the abdomen.

◆ There are associated urinary tract abnormalities, including obstruction, stones, infection, vesicoureteral reflux, primary mega-ureter, hypospadius, cryptorchidism, urethral valves, and multicystic dysplastic kidney.

◆ There are associated abnormalities of other organ systems, including skeletal anomalies, unilateral ovarian and fallopian tube agenesis, and cardiac and gastrointestinal anomalies.

◆ Theories of occurrence include faulty development of the ureteral bud with crossing of the midline to contact the contralateral metanephric blastema, obstruction of renal ascent by blood vessels, and local environmental factors involving surrounding tissues and organs.

RADIOLOGIC

◆ The most common scenario is crossed fused ectopia. Radiographically this can be diagnosed on either ultrasound, CT, or intravenous urography when renal tissue lies on the opposite side of the abdomen from its ureteral insertion, and renal tissue from the crossed kidney fuses with the kidney native to that side of the abdomen. Spiral CT, particularly using coronal reformation, or MRI may be useful in distinguishing fused from unfused ectopia.

◆ CT is also useful in establishing that a case of crossed ectopia is in fact a congenital abnormality and will help to exclude the presence of a retroperitoneal mass causing mass effect with renal displacement.

◆ Patients with this abnormality are usually asymptomatic, although they may present with a palpable abdominal mass or a history of urinary tract infection(s).

◆ SUGGESTED READING

Silva JM, Jafri SZH, Cacciarelli AA, et al. Abnormalities of the kidney: Embryogenesis and radiologic appearance. Appl Radiol 1995;24:19–24.

CASE *12*   *Richard A. Leder*

Richard A. Leder

HISTORY

A 60-year-old man presents with a palpable right-sided abdominal mass, flank pain, and hematuria.

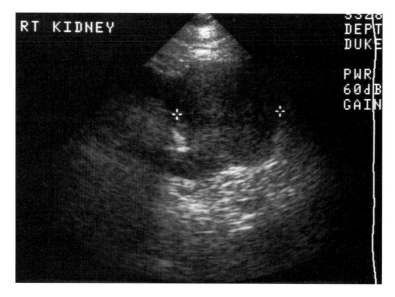

FIGURE 4-12A Transabdominal ultrasound of the right kidney in the longitudinal plane shows a solid, slightly hyperechoic mass projecting off the lower pole.

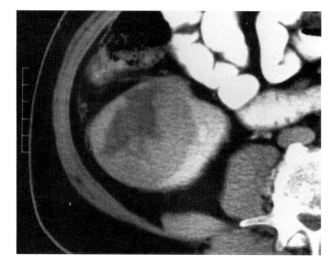

FIGURE 4-12B Contrast-enhanced CT shows a large, solid mass in the right kidney. Within the central and lateral portion of the mass, there is a broad area of decreased attenuation.

DIFFERENTIAL DIAGNOSIS

◆ **Renal cell carcinoma (RCC):** The imaging features in this case reveal the presence of a solid, enhancing right renal mass with features that are consistent with RCC. The broad area of low attenuation within the mass could represent internal hemorrhage or necrosis.

◆ **Oncocytoma:** There are no imaging features that confidently allow for the diagnosis of a benign oncocytoma. However, this diagnosis belongs in the differential diagnosis of a solitary renal mass in a patient who has no evidence of metastatic disease (no retroperitoneal lymphadenopathy and no osseous, hepatic, or pulmonary parenchymal metastases).

◆ **Renal metastasis:** If this patient had a history of a known primary malignancy, particularly in the lung, breast (this patient is a male), or colon, a renal metastasis would be a possibility. A percutaneous biopsy could be performed for further tissue diagnosis. No such history existed in this patient.

◆ **Angiomyolipoma:** The diagnosis of angiomyolipoma is made when fat is detected within a renal mass. It is possible that given sufficient hemorrhage within an angiomyolipoma no fat may be detected. Similarly, a small amount of fat may be present within an angiomyolipoma that cannot be detected unless thin sections are obtained. No fat was detected within this mass, and there was no evidence of subcapsular or perinephric hemorrhage.

◆ **Lymphoma:** This patient has no history of non-Hodgkin's lymphoma. Furthermore, no retroperitoneal lymphadenopathy is present, although lymphomatous masses may exist within the kidneys in the absence of lymphadenopathy.

DIAGNOSIS: Renal oncocytoma.

KEY FACTS

CLINICAL

◆ An "oncocyte" is a transformed epithelial cell with an enlarged, homogeneous, dense cytoplasm filled with acidophilic granules.

◆ Microscopically, a renal oncocytoma is characterized by eosinophilic epithelial cells with protuberant mitochondria within the cytoplasm.

◆ A renal oncocytoma has a distal tubular or collecting duct origin.

◆ On gross examination, lesions are well circumscribed, often encapsulated, without necrosis or hemorrhage. A central stellate scar may be present.

◆ The right kidney is affected as often as the left kidney. Cases of bilateral synchronous tumors have been reported.

◆ The tumor size ranges from 0.1 to 26.0 cm.

◆ The age at diagnosis ranges from 26 to 94 years.

◆ There is a 1.63 to 1.0 male-to-female ratio.

◆ Less than one-third of patients will present with the classic triad of a palpable mass, flank pain, and hematuria.

◆ Renal oncocytoma exhibits a limited, although real, potential for malignancy or metastasis.

RADIOLOGIC

◆ Ultrasound shows a homogeneous, iso- to hyperechoic, well-marginated mass. These are indistinguishable from RCC.

◆ Angiographic features include a "spoke-wheel" appearance to the internal vascular architecture. These lesions have a dense parenchymal blush and lack angiographic features of contrast media puddling, arteriovenous shunting, or renal vein invasion (all characteristics of RCC).

◆ On CT, these lesions have a distinct margin and smooth contour, with or without a central stellate scar. The lesions enhance homogeneously.

◆ A study performed to differentiate renal oncocytoma from RCC showed that among oncocytomas >3 cm, 67% exhibit criteria for oncocytoma (homogeneous attenuation throughout the tumor, a central, sharply marginated stellate area of low attenuation), while 33% met the criteria for adenocarcinoma. Among smaller oncocytomas, 82% met the criteria for oncocytoma, and 18% met the criteria for adenocarcinoma. CT, therefore, is a poor predictor of the diagnosis of oncocytoma.

◆ On MRI, oncocytomas are of homogenous, low signal intensity on T1-weighted images and high signal intensity on T2-weighted images. The presence of a capsule or a central stellate scar and the absence of either internal hemorrhage or necrosis also favor this diagnosis.

SUGGESTED READING

Cohan RH, Dunnick NR, Degesys GE, Korobkin M. Computed tomography of renal oncocytoma. J Comput Assist Tomogr 1984;8:284–287.

Davidson AJ, Hayes WS, Hartman DS, et al. Renal oncocytoma and carcinoma: Failure of differentiation with CT. Radiology 1993;186:693–696.

Harmon WJ, King BF, Lieber MM. Renal oncocytoma: Magnetic resonance imaging characteristics. J Urol 1996;155:863–867.

Honda H, Bonsib S, Barlon TJ, Masuda K. Unusual renal oncocytomas: Pathologic and CT correlations. Urol Radiol 1992;14:148–154.

Levine E, Huntrakoon M. Computed tomography of renal oncocytoma. AJR Am J Roentgenol 1983;141:741–746.

Morra MN, Das S. Renal oncocytoma: A review of histogenesis, histopathology, diagnosis and treatment. J Urol 1993;150:295–302.

Velasquez G, Glass TA, D'Souza VJ, Formanek AG. Multiple oncocytomas and renal carcinoma. AJR Am J Roentgenol 1984;142:123–124.

Wasserman NF, Ewing SL. Calcified renal oncocytoma. AJR Am J Roentgenol 1983;141:747–749.

CASE 13

Richard A. Leder

HISTORY

A 48-year-old man was referred for CT after seeing his ophthalmologist.

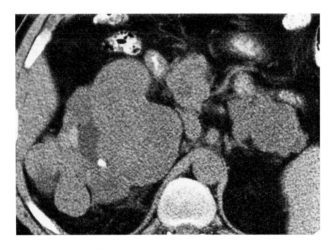

FIGURE 4-13A Noncontrast CT through the upper abdomen shows enlargement of both the head and tail of the pancreas, although it is difficult to determine whether there are solid or cystic lesions present. There is marked deformity of the right kidney, with a hydrocalyx containing a small calculus in the upper pole, exophytic renal masses, and a solid mass medially.

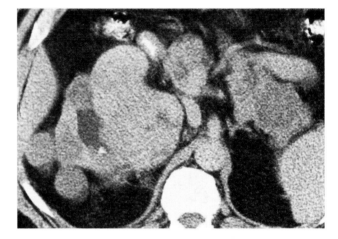

FIGURE 4-13B Contrast-enhanced CT at the same level as Figure 4-13A. Low-attenuation lesions are seen in the enlarged pancreatic head and tail. An enhancing solid mass is present in the medial aspect of the right kidney. Additional exophytic renal masses are also noted on the right.

◆ DIFFERENTIAL DIAGNOSIS

◆ **Multiple renal cell carcinomas (RCCs) in a patient with von Hippel-Lindau disease (VHL):** The constellation of bilateral renal enlargement with multiple solid and cystic lesions in combination with solid and cystic pancreatic lesions is virtually diagnostic of VHL. The patient was seeing the ophthalmologist because of a retinal angioma.

◆ DIAGNOSIS: von Hippel-Lindau disease with multiple renal cell carcinomas.

◆ KEY FACTS

CLINICAL

◆ VHL is characterized by retinal angiomas, central nervous system hemangioblastomas, cystic and solid tumors of the pancreas, pheochromocytomas, renal cysts, and RCCs.

◆ Inheritance follows an autosomal dominant pattern. Clinical situations leading to a suspicion of VHL include a family history of VHL, pheochromocytoma or RCC, an epididymal cystadenoma, bilateral multifocal RCC, bilateral multifocal renal cysts, bilateral pheochromocytomas, an RCC in a patient <30 years of age, pancreatic cysts, multiple hemangioblastomas of the central nervous system, and retinal angiomas.

◆ Early symptoms are usually caused by cerebellar and retinal tumors.

◆ Renal involvement is characterized by multiple bilateral cysts and RCCs. The mean age of presentation of RCC is approximately 39 years; this is 20 years younger than the mean age for the discovery of sporadic RCC. RCC in VHL has a slight male predominance.

RADIOLOGIC

◆ RCC has been reported to occur in 28% to 45% of patients with VHL. Renal cysts are present in 59% of patients, renal adenomas in 14%, and retinal angiomas in 7%.

◆ Renal involvement is characterized by multiple bilateral cysts and RCCs.

◆ Renal involvement in VHL is multicentric and bilateral in up to 75% of patients.

◆ Renal cysts in VHL may occur as simple cysts or complex papillary projections into cystic lumina. Small nodules of tumor may be found in the walls of cysts. Cysts may grow, typically at a rate of 0.5 cm/year; other cysts involute over time, leaving small scars on the renal surface. Extensive cystic disease in VHL can mimic autosomal dominant polycystic kidney disease.

◆ RCCs in patients with VHL grow at the rate of 0.2 to 2.2 cm/year, which is faster than patients observed with sporadic RCC.

◆ CT is more sensitive for small lesions (<2 cm). Thin section, contrast-enhanced CT is mandatory for the evaluation of renal lesions in patients with VHL.

◆ Yearly radiographic imaging is recommended to survey for renal lesions.

◆ An approach to renal lesion management is to wait until solid lesions obtain a size of 2 to 3 cm, and then perform nephron-sparing surgery. After surgery is performed, close follow-up is recommended. CT scanning every 6 months for 2 years, followed by lifetime annual screening, has been advocated.

◆ Approximately 7% to 18% of all patients with VHL have pheochromocytomas. Pheochromocytomas when associated with VHL are often multiple and ectopic; approximately 50% to 80% are bilateral.

◆ Pancreatic lesions also occur in the setting of VHL, including pancreatic cysts, serous microcystic adenomas, and adenocarcinomas. Cysts are present throughout the pancreas and have no predilection for a particular site. Lesions range from several millimeters in size to >10 cm.

◆ A serous cystadenoma is a grape-like cluster of multiple microscopic and macroscopic cysts separated by thickened walls of stroma. There may be a central nidus, which may be calcified or scar-like.

◆ Cysts and cystadenomas of the pancreas are benign in patients with VHL and need not be removed.

◆ Additional lesions present in a patient with VHL include papillary cystadenomas of the epididymis (10% to 26% of men with VHL). Epididymal cystadenomas can be unilateral or bilateral and are often found in the globus major. Lesions range in size from 1 to 5 cm but are typically 2 to 3 cm.

◆ SUGGESTED READING

Choyke PL, Glenn GM, Walther MM, et al. The natural history of renal lesions in von Hippel-Lindau disease: A serial CT study in 28 patients. AJR Am J Roentgenol 1992;159:1229–1234.

Choyke PL, Glenn GM, Walther MM, et al. von Hippel-Lindau disease: Genetic, clinical, and imaging features. Radiology 1995;194:629–642.

Fill WL, Lamiell JM, Polk NO. The radiographic manifestations of von Hippel-Lindau disease. Radiology 1979;133:289–295.

Levine E, Collins DL, Horton WA, Schimke RN. CT screening of the abdomen in von Hippel-Lindau disease. AJR Am J Roentgenol 1982;139:505–510.

CASE 14

Kelly S. Freed

HISTORY

A 41-year-old man involved in a motor vehicle accident presents with microscopic hematuria.

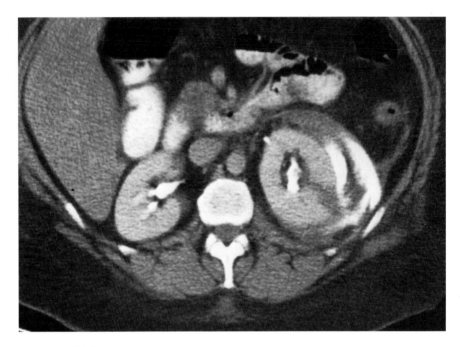

FIGURE 4-14 Contrast-enhanced CT at the level of the kidneys. A linear defect is noted in the lateral aspect of the lower pole of the left renal parenchyma. There is disruption of the renal capsule, with blood and extravasated contrast material in the left perirenal space.

◆ DIFFERENTIAL DIAGNOSIS

◆ **Renal contusion:** A renal contusion can be diagnosed as a hypoperfused area on postcontrast CT. There may be subtle changes in the perirenal fat and subcutaneous tissues to indicate a traumatic injury.

◆ **Renal laceration:** A renal laceration appears as a linear defect in the nephrogram on the CT evaluation. Lacerations may be either minor or major. A minor laceration does not extend to the level of the collecting system, whereas a major laceration involves the collecting system. A minor laceration will most often be accompanied by a perirenal hematoma; a major laceration is accompanied by both hematoma and urinoma.

◆ **Renal fracture:** A renal fracture is diagnosed when there is cleavage of the kidney into two separate portions. These injuries often occur along planes that spare renal vasculature; therefore, enhancement is seen in both portions of the fractured kidney.

◆ **Subcapsular hematoma:** A subcapsular hematoma is identified as a fluid collection contained within the renal capsule. This is easily diagnosed on noncontrast CT as a high-density fluid collection.

◆ **Renovascular injury:** Renovascular injuries are identified by nonenhancement of the kidney. Absence of the nephrogram is referred to as a *negative CT nephrogram*. Loss of the pyelogram postcontrast is called a *negative CT pyelogram*. Arterial renal vascular injuries may be secondary to thrombosis or laceration; thrombosis is more common. Given appropriate imaging, cut-off may be seen in the renal artery after a bolus of contrast material, the so-called "renal artery cut-off sign." Renal vein injuries tend to be lacerations as opposed to thrombotic in nature. In these cases, large retroperitoneal hematomas can occur without significant renal parenchymal injury.

◆ DIAGNOSIS: Renal laceration with perinephric hematoma/urinoma.

◆ KEY FACTS

CLINICAL

◆ Hematuria may be found in patients with injury to the genitourinary system, as well as in patients with intra-abdominal injury not related to the genitourinary system. The degree of hematuria does not reflect the severity of the injury. Furthermore, patients may have severe injury to the genitourinary system, including a renal pedicle injury, without the presence of hematuria.

◆ Traumatic injury to the kidney may cause a renal laceration or fracture, a contusion, a subcapsular hematoma,

or a renovascular injury. Although many renal injuries, such as contusions or minor lacerations, are managed conservatively, surgery is generally indicated in patients with a shattered kidney or a renovascular injury.

RADIOLOGIC

◆ A contrast-enhanced CT of the abdomen and pelvis is the single best imaging modality to evaluate the nature and extent of renal injury in the trauma setting. However, if renal vascular injury is suspected and the CT is negative or equivocal, angiography may be required.

◆ Renal contusion is manifest as a focal area of renal parenchyma that does not enhance to the degree of normal renal parenchyma, without evidence of laceration or fracture.

◆ A renal laceration is a focal parenchymal tear, demonstrated as an area of decreased attenuation within the renal parenchyma, as in this case. The tear often extends to involve the collecting system, resulting in extravasation of blood and urine into the perinephric space. In the early phase of contrast media excretion, the perinephric fluid may be of relatively low attenuation. Delayed images, however, are very helpful in confirming extravasation, because there will be progressive opacification of this fluid.

◆ A renal fracture implies cleavage or transection of the kidney into two poles, with extravasation of blood and urine.

◆ A shattered kidney denotes multiple fractures or fragments.

◆ On CT, a subcapsular hematoma is seen as a high-attenuation fluid collection in the perinephric region, often lenticular in shape, that may cause mass effect or flattening of the renal cortex.

◆ A renal vascular injury may be identified by extravasation of venous or arterial contrast material, or as focal or global areas of nonenhancement of renal parenchyma.

◆ SUGGESTED READING

Husmann DA, Gilling PJ, Perry MO, et al. Major renal lacerations with a devitalized fragment following blunt abdominal trauma: A comparison between nonoperative (expectant) versus surgical management. J Urol 1993;150:1774–1777.

Knudson MM, McAninch JW, Gomez R, et al. Hematuria as a predictor of abdominal injury after blunt trauma. Am J Surg 1992;164:482–485.

Moss AA, Bush WH. The Kidneys. In AA Moss, G Gamsu, HK Genant (eds), Computed Tomography of the Body. Philadelphia: Saunders, 1992;987–1003.

Udekwu PO, Gurkin B, Oller DW. The use of computed tomography in blunt abdominal injuries. Am Surg 1996;62:56–59.

HISTORY

A 52-year-old Asian woman presents with left flank pain.

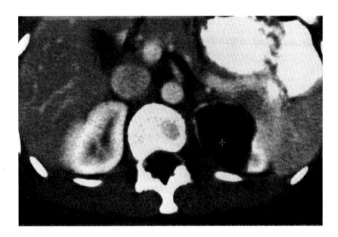

FIGURE 4-15A Contrast-enhanced CT of the upper portion of the kidneys shows a water attenuation mass (+10 Hounsfield units) in the left upper pole. The wall of this lesion is thick and enhances medially.

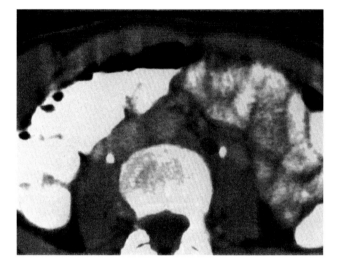

FIGURE 4-15B Contrast-enhanced CT through the proximal ureters shows contrast enhancement of each ureter, with a water attenuation tubular structure adjacent and medial to the proximal left ureter. This was seen in continuity with the cystic mass in the left upper pole.

◆ DIFFERENTIAL DIAGNOSIS

◆ **Complicated renal cyst of the left upper pole:** The water attenuation of the lesion fits for a simple cyst; however, the perceptible wall excludes the diagnosis of a simple cyst. A cyst that is infected or hemorrhagic could have this appearance.

◆ **Cystic renal cell carcinoma (RCC):** Some RCCs are cystic; others can measure in the range of water attenuation due to extensive necrosis or hemorrhage.

◆ **Renal abscess:** An infection within the kidney that has liquefied could have this appearance. It is helpful in these cases to correlate imaging findings with urinalysis, as well as possible clinical symptoms such as pyrexia, leukocytosis, and flank pain.

◆ **Ureteral duplication with obstruction of the upper pole moiety:** This diagnosis can be made due to the presence of the fluid attenuation tubular structure adjacent to the left ureter. This tubular structure may be confused with a thrombosed gonadal vein, and therefore its path must be followed. If this tubular structure enters the left renal vein, a thrombosed gonadal vein can be diagnosed. If this tubular structure is in continuity with the cystic upper pole mass, the diagnosis of an obstruction duplicated system can be made with confidence. This will subsequently be confirmed by cystoscopy, with the identification of two ureteral orifices on this side.

◆ DIAGNOSIS: Obstruction of the upper pole collecting system in complete ureteral duplication.

◆ KEY FACTS

CLINICAL

◆ Patient with obstruction of the upper pole moiety may present with nonspecific abdominal pain; this is the most common factor leading to clinical evaluation.

◆ Alternatively, patients may present with lower tract signs and symptoms related to the ectopic insertion of the duplicated ureter—e.g., incontinence.

◆ Other presentations may be related to obstruction of the upper pole moiety and the presence of calculus disease (hematuria) or stages of urine (infection).

RADIOLOGIC

◆ Duplication anomalies of the kidney are common. In patients with a completely duplicated system, both ureters may insert orthotopically; however, the ureter arising from the upper pole moiety frequently inserts ectopically either intravesically or extravesically. Patients most often present with symptoms related to upper pole obstruction or lower pole reflux.

◆ Imaging is useful for documenting the presence of complete duplication and whether the upper pole is obstructed. CT is useful for evaluating the amount of residual parenchyma in the upper pole. Cystography is frequently used to document reflux. Ultrasound can image the obstructed upper pole but usually cannot image the entire ureter.

◆ SUGGESTED READING

Cramer BC, Twomey BP, Katz D. CT findings in obstructed upper moieties of duplex kidneys. J Comput Assist Tomogr 1983; 7:251–253.

Cronan JJ, Amis ES, Zeman RK, Dorfman GS. Obstruction of the upper-pole moiety in renal duplication in adults: CT evaluation. Radiology 1986;161:17–21.

CASE *16*

Vincent G. McDermott

HISTORY

A 48-year-old woman is referred for renal ultrasound following a urinary tract infection.

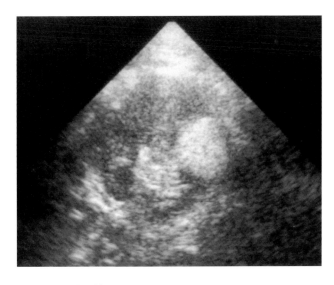

FIGURE 4-16A Ultrasound of the left kidney in the transverse plane. There is a 2.5-cm diameter, well-demarcated, uniformly echogenic mass in the posterior mid cortex.

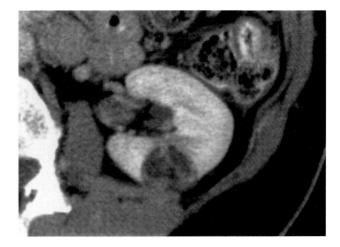

FIGURE 4-16B Contrast-enhanced CT of the left kidney. There is a corresponding mass that is of mixed soft tissue and fatty attenuation. A region-of-interest measurement obtained from a low-attenuation area of the mass reads –18 Hounsfield units (HU). This suggests the presence of fat.

◆ DIFFERENTIAL DIAGNOSIS

- **Renal cell carcinoma (RCC):** Approximately 30% of small RCCs are markedly hyperechoic. The presence of either small intratumoral cyst or an anechoic rim can suggest RCC. Thin-section CT must be performed for characterization of a hyperechoic mass. Fat-containing RCCs with osseous metaplasia have also been reported, although they are extremely rare. RCCs can also contain low attenuation of foci due to lipid-producing necrosis. These tumors contain lipid vacuoles and amalgamated cholesterol clefts. An RCC can also grow by extension and entrap perirenal fat. RCCs that behave in this fashion tend to be large, >5 cm in diameter, and have irregular margins.
- **Lipoma:** A lipoma is a rare benign tumor of the kidney composed of adipose tissue.
- **Liposarcoma**: A renal liposarcoma is usually located peripherally, beneath the renal capsule. The tumor is large and bulky and extends into the perirenal space.
- **Fat-containing renal oncocytoma:** Fat may be present within an oncocytoma that grows sufficiently large to entrap perirenal or sinus fat.
- **Adrenal myelolipoma:** A full examination of ultrasound and CT images should help distinguish a fat-containing adrenal mass from a fat-containing renal mass. MRI with sagittal and coronal imaging may improve the ability to distinguish a renal angiolipoma from an adrenal myelolipoma.
- **Renal angiomyolipoma (AML):** This is the most likely diagnosis for a fat-containing renal mass.

◆ DIAGNOSIS: Renal angiomyolipoma (AML).

◆ KEY FACTS

CLINICAL

- AMLs are benign hamartomas composed of fat, smooth muscle, and blood vessels.
- Eighty percent of AMLs are solitary; they occur sporadically, and they are most common in women 40 to 60 years of age.
- Twenty percent are multiple and bilateral, usually in association with tuberous sclerosis.
- These tumors are usually an incidental finding.
- Hemorrhage may occur when lesions are large, producing hematuria, flank pain, and in severe cases, shock.
- Treatment of AMLs includes embolization or resection, especially if the AML is >4 cm in diameter, to avoid the threat of spontaneous hemorrhage.

RADIOLOGIC

- Plain films may reveal subtle lucencies due to fat content; however, this finding is seen in <10% of cases. Calcifications are seldom seen, and when present, suggest an RCC.
- Intravenous urography reveals a nonspecific mass, which is frequently exophytic.
- Ultrasound demonstrates a well-demarcated, highly echogenic renal mass, although echo-poor areas may be seen due to internal necrosis or hemorrhage, particularly in larger tumors.
- On CT, either with or without contrast material, the presence of fat (< −10 HU) is virtually diagnostic. In some AMLs, however, the fat is microscopic, and because of partial volume averaging, no fatty attenuation will be appreciated.
- With angiography, 95% of the tumors are hypervascular, with dilated arteries. Angiography, however, is rarely performed unless embolization is anticipated.
- On MRI, there is variable high signal intensity on T1-weighted images and intermediate signal intensity on T2-weighted images depending on the fat content.

◆ SUGGESTED READING

Amis ES, Newhouse J. Essentials of Genitourinary Radiology. Boston: Little, Brown, 1991;124–125.

Barbaric ZL. Principles of Genitourinary Radiology. New York: Thieme, 1994;160–161.

Dunnick NR, McCallum RW, Sandler CM. Textbook of Uroradiology. Baltimore: Williams & Wilkins, 1991;125–127.

Resnick MI, Rifkin MD. Ultrasound of the Urinary Tract. Baltimore: Williams & Wilkins, 1991;187–189.

CASE 17

Richard A. Leder

HISTORY

A 60-year-old man has a palpable abdominal mass on the left.

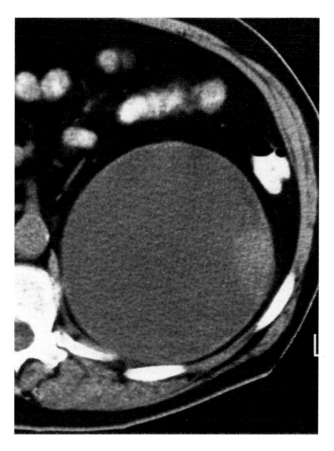

FIGURE 4-17A Noncontrast CT through the mid-abdomen shows a large cystic mass. This cystic mass arises from the left kidney. Of note is a mural soft-tissue nodule along the lateral wall of the cystic lesion.

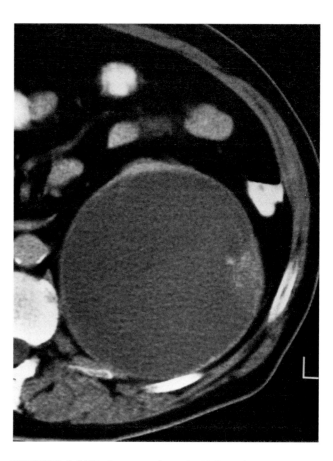

FIGURE 4-17B Contrast-enhanced CT through the left kidney again shows the large cystic renal mass. The soft tissue nodule in the lateral aspect of the cyst wall demonstrates enhancement. The wall is thickened and enhances as well.

◈ DIFFERENTIAL DIAGNOSIS

◆ **Renal abscess:** One would expect appropriate symptomatology in a patient with an abscess of this size. A thickened wall that enhances can be seen in a renal abscess. However, lack of inflammatory changes in the perinephric fat may suggest other diagnostic possibilities.

◆ **Hemorrhagic cyst:** Over time the attenuation within a hemorrhagic renal cyst may decrease, causing an old hemorrhagic cyst to have a more cystic appearance. The eccentric, lateral wall prominence that enhances, however, prevents one from calling this lesion a hemorrhagic cyst.

◆ **Cystic RCC:** This is the most likely diagnosis for a cystic renal mass with an enhancing mural nodule.

◈ DIAGNOSIS: Cystic renal cell carcinoma, Bosniak type 4 lesion.

◈ KEY FACTS

CLINICAL

◆ Patients with RCC may present with the classic triad of pain, mass, and hematuria.

◆ Other symptoms include fatigue, malaise, anorexia, weight loss, fever, and anemia.

◆ Men are most commonly afflicted, with a male-to-female ratio of 2 to 1.

◆ Patients are typically in the sixth to seventh decade.

RADIOLOGIC

◆ A Bosniak type 4 cyst is one that clearly has malignant features as well as large cystic components. Lesions in this category show irregular margins and solid enhanc-

ing elements. They are clearly malignant and should be treated surgically.

◆ Cysts are sometimes complicated by the presence of calcifications, septations, abnormal attenuation, wall thickening, or nodularity. A solid nodule within a cyst lumen that enhances is a feature that indicates the presence of a malignancy with high reliability. Vascularity within the nodule combined with nodular thickening of a cyst wall is also a clear indication of malignancy.

◆ This lesion should not be classified as a Bosniak type 3 lesion. Type 3 cysts exhibit some of the features of malignant lesions and radiographically cannot be distinguished from malignancy. Resection is necessary to distinguish a benign from a malignant lesion.

◆ A multilocular cystic nephroma is a benign Bosniak type 3 lesion, while a multicystic RCC is a malignant Bosniak type 3 lesion. These two tumors may be indistinguishable radiographically.

◈ SUGGESTED READING

Bosniak MA. The current radiological approach to renal cysts. Radiology 1986;158:1–10.

Dalla-Palma L, Pozzi-Mucelli F, Donna AD, Pozzi-Mucelli RS. Cystic renal tumors: US and CT findings. Urol Radiol 1990;12:67–73.

Parienty RA, Pradel J, Parienty I. Cystic renal cancers: CT characteristics. Radiology 1985;157:741–744.

Rofsky NM, Bosniak MA, Weinreb JC, Coppa GF. Giant renal cell carcinoma: CT and MR characteristics. J Comput Assist Tomogr 1989;13:1078–1080.

Waguespack RL, Kearse WS Jr. Renal cell carcinoma arising from the free wall of a renal cyst. Abdom Imag 1996;21:71–72.

Wilson TE, Doelle EA, Cohan RH, et al. Cystic renal masses: A reevaluation of the usefulness of the Bosniak classification system. Acad Radiol 1996;3:564–570.

HISTORY

A 62-year-old man has a history of chronic urinary tract infections.

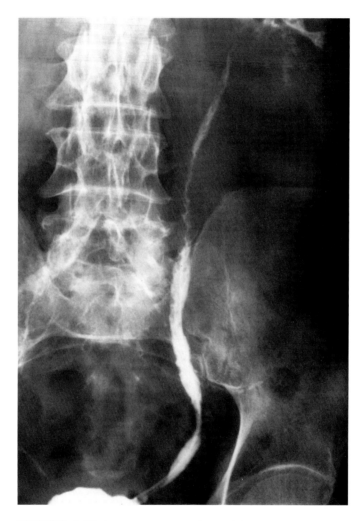

FIGURE 4-18 Anteroposterior view from a left retrograde pyelogram. Multiple small filling defects are present in the left ureter.

◆ DIFFERENTIAL DIAGNOSIS

- **Blood clots:** Blood clots can cause multiple ureteral filling defects. One would expect that the patient would have an accompanying history of hematuria. Additional history may be helpful and could include known bleeding disorders or trauma.
- **Multiple ureteral stones:** Stones can cause multiple filling defects, although typically, due to their calcium content, stones are most often radiopaque. This limits their detectability on contrasted examinations. The fixed nature of the filling defects, as seen in this patient, would make this an unlikely possibility.
- **Multiple ureteral transitional cell carcinomas (TCCs):** While TCC has a propensity to be multifocal, this would represent an extremely rare manifestation of urothelial carcinoma. Correlation should be made with findings of urine cytology to establish whether malignant cells are present.
- **Ureteritis cystica:** This is one of several causes of multiple ureteral filling defects. Ureteritis cystica is often seen in the setting of chronic urinary tract infections.

◆ DIAGNOSIS: Ureteritis cystica.

◆ KEY FACTS

CLINICAL

- Ureteritis cystica is associated with chronic mucosal irritation secondary to inflammation.
- These lesions are secondary to degeneration and cavitation of metaplastic surface urethelium or submucosal Brunn's cell nests.
- Patients may be asymptomatic or have hematuria and symptoms of a urinary tract infection.
- These lesions are not premalignant.
- The lesions may be unilateral or bilateral.
- Females are affected slightly more with ureteritis cystica than males.
- Patients are typically 50 to 60 years old.

RADIOLOGIC

- Lesions are typically 2 to 3 mm in size, although they can range from 1 mm to 2 cm in size.
- Lesions are multiple, smooth, well-rounded or oval filling defects with sharp borders.
- Lesions are said to predominate in the proximal ureter but may be seen throughout the ureter, in the renal pelvis (pyelitis cystica), or in the bladder (cystitis cystica).

◆ SUGGESTED READING

Frederick MG, Kakani L, Dyer RB. Ureteritis cystica and pseudodiverticulosis in ureteral stumps. Appl Radiol 1995;24:32–33.

Loitman BS, Chiat H. Ureteritis cystica and pyelitis cystica. Radiology 1957;68:345–351.

Richard A. Leder

HISTORY

A 76-year-old man has benign prostatic hypertrophy and bladder outlet obstruction.

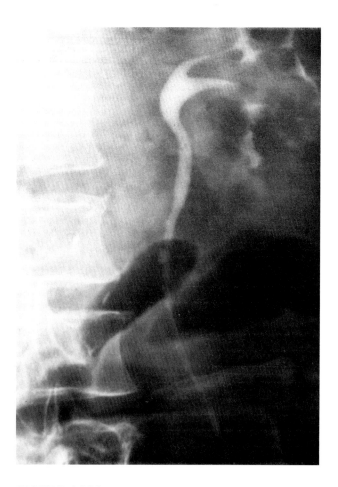

FIGURE 4-19A Anteroposterior compression view from an intravenous urogram shows multiple small left ureteral outpouchings.

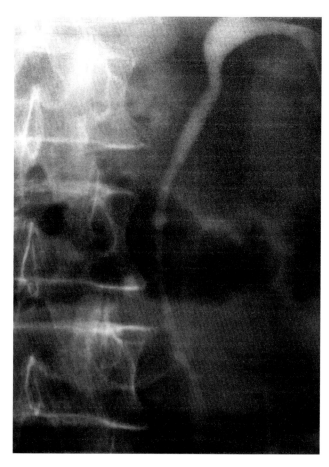

FIGURE 4-19B Oblique compression view from an intravenous urogram confirms the presence of multiple proximal left ureteral outpouchings.

◆ DIFFERENTIAL DIAGNOSIS

- **True ureteral diverticula:** True diverticula are typically large, saccular, round or oval, and usually solitary. True diverticula fill slowly with contrast material during an intravenous urogram. Depending on their location, they may be confused with a hydroureter, a bladder diverticulum, or a large ureterocele.
- **Ureteritis cystica:** It is important to recognize that in ureteritis cystica there are filling defects within the ureteral lumen. This case demonstrates ureteral outpouchings as opposed to mural filling defects.
- **Ureteral pseudodiverticulosis:** The small ureteral outpouchings present in this patient are virtually pathognomonic of ureteral pseudodiverticulosis.

◆ DIAGNOSIS: Ureteral pseudodiverticulosis.

◆ KEY FACTS

CLINICAL

- Ureteral pseudodiverticulosis is associated with urinary tract infections, obstruction, and stones.
- Patients may present with hematuria or symptoms of a urinary tract infection.
- Pathologically, these lesions are outpouchings of proliferated hyperplastic transitional epithelium extending into loose subepithelial connective tissue.

- The lesions do not extend through the muscularis propria; therefore, they are not true diverticula.
- Fifty percent of patients have atypica on urine cytology. A similar percentage have or will develop a TCC (most common site is the bladder).

RADIOLOGIC

- The outpouchings are small, typically measuring 2 to 4 mm in diameter.
- The outpouching are nearly always multiple, numbering three to eight lesions per ureter.
- The findings are bilateral in 70% of cases.
- The abnormalities predominate in the proximal and mid ureter (85% of cases).
- Retrograde or antegrade urography is better than intravenous urography, which is positive in only 60% of cases.

◆ SUGGESTED READING

Wasserman NF. Pseudodiverticulosis: Unusual appearance for metastases to the ureter. Abdom Imag 1994;19:376–378.

Wasserman NF, Pointe SL, Posalaky IP. Ureteral pseudodiverticulosis. Radiology 1985;155:561–566.

Wasserman NF, Zhang G, Posalaky IP, Reddy PK. Ureteral pseudodiverticula: Frequent association with uroepithelial malignancy. AJR Am J Roentgenol 1991;157:69–72.

HISTORY

A 22-year-old man presents with weight loss.

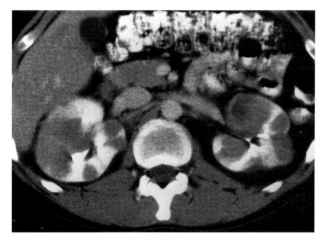

FIGURE 4-20A Contrast-enhanced CT of the mid abdomen. There are multiple hypoattenuating soft-tissue masses in the kidneys bilaterally. Both kidneys are also enlarged. Attenuation measurements show that the lesions are solid (+35 Hounsfield units [HU]).

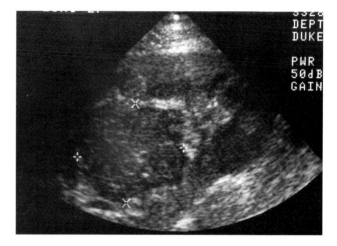

FIGURE 4-20B Transabdominal ultrasound of the right kidney in the longitudinal plane shows a large hypoechoic but solid mass in the upper pole. Other solid lesions were also seen on adjacent images of the right kidney.

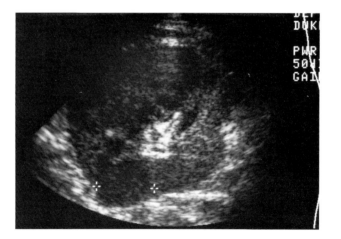

FIGURE 4-20C Transabdominal ultrasound of the lower pole of the left kidney in the transverse plane shows a hypoechoic but solid mass in the lower pole. Other images of the left kidney revealed additional mass lesions.

◆ DIFFERENTIAL DIAGNOSIS

◆ **Renal metastases:** Renal metastases typically arise from primary cancers of the lung, breast, colon, or melanoma. Renal metastases are usually discovered at autopsy rather than radiographically. To make a diagnosis of renal metastases, careful inspection should be made for potential additional sites of metastatic disease (lung, liver, adrenals, lymph nodes) as well as determination of appropriate clinical history.

◆ **Multifocal renal cell carcinoma (RCC):** While RCC can be multifocal, particularly in patients with von Hippel-Lindau disease (VHL), this would be an uncommon appearance and presentation for this renal malignancy.

◆ **Lymphoma:** The most common presentation of renal lymphoma is that of bilateral renal masses. This can occur with or without accompanying retroperitoneal lymphadenopathy.

◆ **Hemorrhagic renal cysts:** Patients with autosomal-dominant polycystic kidney disease often experience hemorrhage into renal cysts. Clinical history as well as noncontrast imaging should permit the radiologist to determine whether the lesions are solid and enhancing or hemorrhagic.

◆ DIAGNOSIS: Renal lymphoma.

◆ KEY FACTS

CLINICAL

◆ Genitourinary lymphoma is most commonly of the non-Hodgkin's variety.

◆ Lymphoma involves the genitourinary tract in 10% to 50% of cases.

◆ Of patients with non-Hodgkin's lymphoma, 10% to 20% either present with or eventually suffer from genitourinary-related symptoms.

◆ Sites of involvement in the genitourinary tract in descending order of frequency include the kidneys, testes, bladder, and prostate.

◆ Symptomatically, patients may have vague abdominal pain, weight loss, fever, night sweats, anemia, and hematuria. Additional manifestations may include lymphadenopathy, hepatosplenomegaly, and a palpable abdominal mass.

RADIOLOGIC

◆ The most common presentation of renal lymphoma on CT is bilateral soft-tissue masses (61%). This can often occur without accompanying retroperitoneal lymphadenopathy.

◆ The second most common presentation of renal lymphoma is that of invasion from retroperitoneal or perinephric masses.

◆ A third presentation is that of a single, bulky renal mass.

◆ The least common presentation is isolated lymphomatous disease in the perirenal space.

◆ Intravenous urography may show enlargement of one or both kidneys, a localized expanding mass, or masses with calyceal distortion.

◆ On ultrasound, lymphomatous masses are typically anechoic without posterior acoustical enhancement or hypoechoic.

◆ MRI may be used in patients in whom iodinated contrast material cannot be given. The multifocal nature of the disease process is usually readily apparent, particularly following the intravenous administration of a gadolinium-chelate.

◆ SUGGESTED READING

Cohan RH, Dunnick NR, Leder RA, Baker ME. Computed tomography of renal lymphoma. J Comput Assist Tomogr 1990; 14:933–938.

Dimopoulos MA, Moulopoulos LA, Costantinides C, et al. Primary renal lymphoma: A clinical and radiological study. J Urol 1996;155:1865–1867.

Heiken JP, Gold RP, Schnur MJ, et al. Computed tomography of renal lymphoma with ultrasound correlation. J Comput Assist Tomogr 1983;7:245–250.

Salem YH, Miller HC. Lymphoma of genitourinary tract. J Urol 1994;151:1162–1170.

HISTORY

A 15-year-old boy has a history of urinary tract infections.

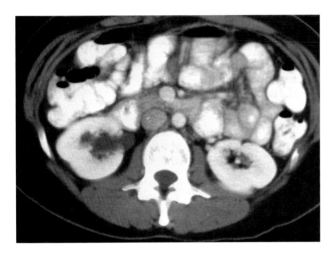

FIGURE 4-21A Contrast-enhanced CT of the kidneys. There is relatively equivalent enhancement of both kidneys, although there is apparent pelvocaliectasis on the right.

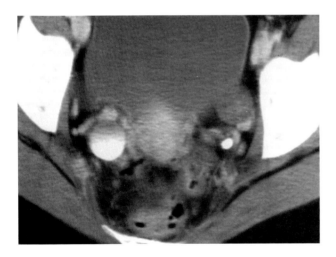

FIGURE 4-21B Contrast-enhanced CT through the pelvis. There is a contrast/urine level within the dilated distal right ureter. The distal left ureter is normal in caliber.

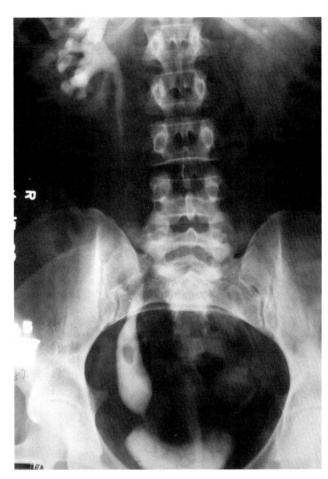

FIGURE 4-21C Anteroposterior supine postvoid film from an intravenous urogram shows a markedly dilated, sausage-shaped distal ureter with "rat tail" narrowing at the ureterovesicle junction. The ureter is also dilated proximally, and there is mild pelvicaliectasis.

◆ DIFFERENTIAL DIAGNOSIS

- **Right renal "obstruction" secondary to a distal right ureteral calculus:** While a stone with secondary edema could explain the narrowing of the distal ureter, the CT clearly shows that there was no delay in enhancement on the right side, and the "pelvicaliectasis" is more likely on the basis of congenital megacalyces. Clinically, the patient did not have renal colic, nor did he have hematuria.
- **Distal right ureteral stricture:** While a stricture could cause narrowing of the distal ureter, the appearance of the proximal ureter and kidney suggests that there is no obstruction of the distal ureter.
- **Primary megaureter:** The fusiform dilatation of the distal ureter above a narrowed segment is classic for primary megaureter. The associated megacalyces on the right also support this diagnosis.

◆ DIAGNOSIS: Primary megaureter.

◆ KEY FACTS

CLINICAL

- Primary megaureter has also been called *megaloureter*, *primary megaloureter*, *aperistaltic megaureter*, or *achalasia* of the ureter.
- In this condition, ureteral dilation occurs above a short, adynamic, extravesicle distal ureteral segment.
- The abnormal segment of distal ureter may have increased collagen between the muscle fibers at this level or a deficiency in longitudinal muscle.

- In adults, the lesion is 2.5 times more frequent on the left. In children, it is four times more frequent in boys, and bilateral involvement is almost exclusively a male disease. In all age groups, 20% of cases are bilateral.
- Surgery is considered in patients with infection, stones, persistent symptoms, or significant hydronephrosis. Mild cases may be followed radiographically.

RADIOLOGIC

- This abnormal distal ureteral segment is approximately 1.5 cm long and does not transmit a peristaltic wave when examined fluoroscopically.
- There is a high association with other abnormalities of the genitourinary system. Ureteropelvic junction obstruction may be found in 25% of cases. Contralateral reflux has been reported in 6% to 8% of cases, contralateral renal agenesis in 4% to 15%, contralateral ureteral duplication in 4% to 6%, a calyceal diverticulum in 4%, and contralateral ureterocele in 3%.
- Megacalyces, ipsilateral cryptorchidism, and ectopic ureteroceles have also occurred in association with this condition.

◆ SUGGESTED READING

MacKinnon KJ, Foote JW, Wiglesworth FW, Blennerhassett JB. The pathology of the adynamic distal ureteral segment. J Urol 1970;103:134–137.

McLaughlin AP, Pfister RC, Leadbetter WF, et al. The pathophysiology of primary megaloureter. J Urol 1973;109:805–811.

Mellins HZ. Cystic dilatations of the upper urinary tract: A radiologist's developmental model. Radiology 1984;153:291–301.

CASE 22

Douglas H. Sheafor

HISTORY

A 32-year-old diabetic woman presents with dysuria.

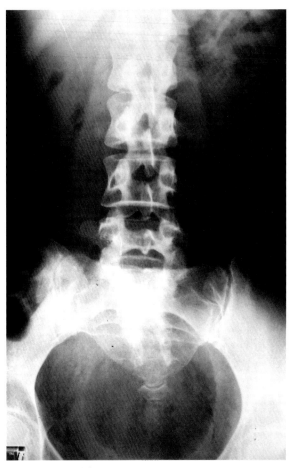

FIGURE 4-22A Anteroposterior supine radiograph of the pelvis. Curvilinear and small rounded lucencies outline the expected location of the urinary bladder wall.

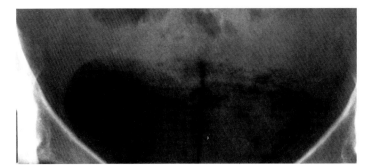

FIGURE 4-22B Anteroposterior coned down radiograph of the bladder dome. There are central lucencies within the bladder, with a suggestion of bladder wall thickening.

◆ DIFFERENTIAL DIAGNOSIS

- **Enterovesicle fistula:** This is most commonly caused by diverticulitis, inflammatory bowel disease, or colorectal carcinoma. While intraluminal gas is characteristic, submucosal gas collections are uncommon.
- **Penetrating trauma:** In a patient with a history of knife or gunshot injury, a small amount of pelvic gas is possible, but it should not create such a large collection.
- **Instrumentation:** Intraluminal gas may be seen following cystoscopy, cystography, or Foley catheter placement. Again, linear submucosal gas would not be expected.
- **Pneumatosis intestinalis:** Gas within the wall of small or large bowel can have a linear appearance; however, the size and location of this abnormality strongly suggest bladder pathology.
- **Emphysematous cystitis:** This diagnosis is most likely in a diabetic patient with gas in the expected position of the bladder lumen and wall.

◆ DIAGNOSIS: Emphysematous cystitis (cystitis emphysematosa).

◆ KEY FACTS

CLINICAL
- This is an uncommon inflammatory condition of the urinary bladder, usually with a transient and benign course.
- Gas localizes in the bladder submucosa, and often within the bladder lumen.
- *E. coli* is the most common causative organism, with glycosuria, stasis, neurogenic bladder, and chronic urinary tract infection as predisposing factors.
- The female-to-male ratio is 2 to 1.
- Symptoms include frequency, dysuria, and, occasionally, pneumaturia.
- Treatment consists of antibiotics, control of diabetes, and relief of obstruction, if present.

RADIOLOGIC
- The plain radiograph is often diagnostic.
- Gas within the submucosa may be linear or have a cobblestone appearance.
- CT is rarely indicated but elegantly demonstrates gas within the lumen and within a thickened bladder wall.
- Ultrasound also depicts a thickened bladder wall and irregular echogenic foci with acoustic shadowing.

◆ SUGGESTED READING

Bailey H. Cystitis emphysematosa. AJR Am J Roentgenol 1961;86: 850–862.

Katz DS, Aksoy E, Cunha BA. *Clostridium perfringens* emphysematous cystitis. Urology 1993;41:458–460.

Kauzlaric D, Barmer E. Sonography of emphysematous cystitis. J Ultrasound Med 1985;4:319–320.

Ney C, Kumar M, Billah K, Doerr J. CT demonstration of cystitis emphysematosa. J Comput Assist Tomogr 1987;11:552–553.

CASE 23

Richard A. Leder

HISTORY

A 72-year-old woman presents with hematuria.

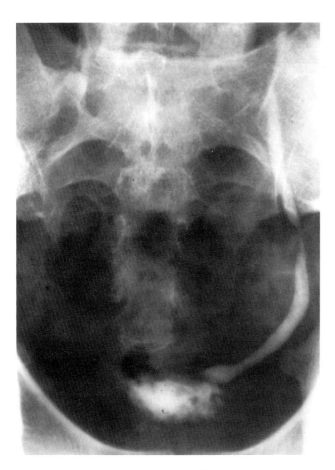

FIGURE 4-23A Anteroposterior postvoid film of the distal left ureter and bladder from an intravenous urogram shows a small "cobra head" deformity of the distal left ureter. There is also columnation on this side.

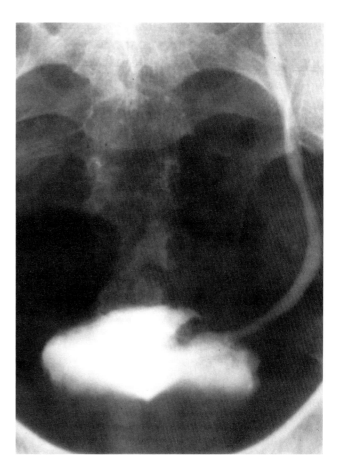

FIGURE 4-23B Anteroposterior film of the distal left ureter and bladder obtained before the postvoid film shows nodular thickening of the bladder wall just medial to the "cobra head" deformity in the distal left ureter.

◆ DIFFERENTIAL DIAGNOSIS

- **Pseudoureterocele:** The eccentric halo just medial to the distal left ureterocele indicates there is a left pseudoureterocele.
- **Ureterocele:** The postvoid film shows no evidence of a periureteral abnormality. The mucosa adjacent to the left ureterocele is not optimally imaged on the postvoid film and precludes the diagnosis of a pseudoureterocele. Given the patient's history of hematuria and what would otherwise appear to be a negative study, cystoscopy would follow, revealing bladder pathology adjacent to the distal left ureter.

◆ DIAGNOSIS: Left-sided pseudoureterocele secondary to a transitional cell carcinoma of the bladder.

◆ KEY FACTS

CLINICAL

- Ureteroceles are due to a defect in the muscular layer of the ureter, often with a defect in the bladder wall itself.
- There are two types of ureteroceles: intravesicle and ectopic.
- Intravesicle ureteroceles may be unilateral or bilateral, and they are more often seen in females than in males.

A "cobra head" defect is seen in the bladder, with a thin lucent line or halo around the lumen.

- Ectopic ureteroceles insert medially and caudally to the site of the normal ureteral orifice, often extending into the bladder neck or urethra.
- Pseudoureteroceles are secondary to edema from a ureteral stone, bullous edema of the bladder, or neoplastic disease. Neoplasms that can cause this appearance include transitional cell carcinoma (TCC) of the bladder or invasion of the bladder by squamous cell carcinoma of the cervix. Radiation cystitis can also lead to the appearance of a pseudoureterocele.

RADIOLOGIC

- The cobra head deformity with a thin lucent halo is the typical finding in a ureterocele. Deformity or thickening of the surrounding halo is a worrisome finding. Further work-up should include cystoscopy.
- Pseudoureteroceles are distinguished by asymmetry of the dilated ureteral lumen, moderate to severe obstruction of the upper tract, and evidence that this is an acquired abnormality.

◆ SUGGESTED READING

Thornbury JR, Silver TM, Vinson RK. Ureteroceles vs. pseudoureteroceles in adults. Radiology 1977;122:81–84.

CASE 24   *John A. Stahl*

HISTORY

A 60-year-old man presents with left flank pain.

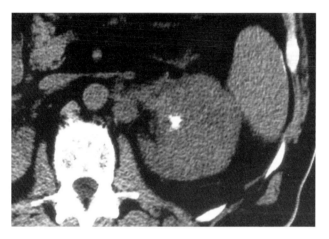

FIGURE 4-24A Noncontrast CT of the left kidney. There is a large, low-attenuation mass with calcifications located centrally within the left kidney.

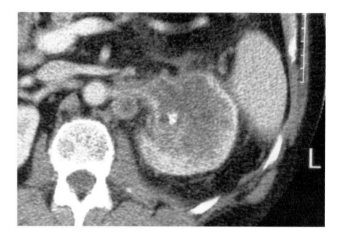

FIGURE 4-24B Contrast-enhanced CT of the left kidney. The mass is seen to infiltrate both the hilum and parenchyma on the left. Tumor is also noted to extend beyond the renal capsule anteriorly, although it remains within Gerota's fascia. The left renal vein is uninvolved.

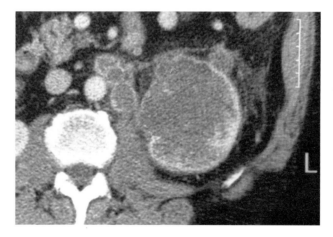

FIGURE 4-24C Contrast-enhanced CT of the left kidney at a more caudal level. Retroperitoneal lymphadenopathy, which has similar enhancement properties to the renal mass, is also seen in the left paraortic region.

◆ DIFFERENTIAL DIAGNOSIS

- **Renal cell carcinoma (RCC):** RCC can occasionally present as an infiltrative central renal mass. The presence of retroperitoneal lymphadenopathy is consistent with regional involvement in a patient with a left-sided RCC, although other causes of primary renal tumor must also be considered. Typically, RCCs are exophytic, contour-deforming lesions.
- **Transitional cell carcinoma (TCC):** TCC originates from the urothelium of the pelvicaliceal system. There are many manifestations of TCC, one of which is an infiltrative renal mass. Regional lymphadenopathy and vascular invasion are seen less commonly than in patients with RCC.
- **Lymphoma:** A solitary infiltrative renal mass is one of the presentations of renal lymphoma. More common presentations include multifocal renal masses and infiltration from bulky retroperitoneal lymphadenopathy.
- **Metastasis:** A renal metastasis can cause a mass with this appearance, and the presence of retroperitoneal lymphadenopathy does not exclude the possibility of a renal metastasis. It is useful to investigate for a history or the presence of common primary neoplasms in patients with this CT appearance, particularly of the lung, colon, and breast.

◆ DIAGNOSIS: Transitional cell carcinoma.

◆ KEY FACTS

CLINICAL

- Peak incidence of TCC is in the seventh decade.
- TCC occurs most often in men, with a male-to-female ratio of 2 to 1.
- Presenting symptoms include hematuria, flank pain, and either or both dysuria and an abdominal mass.
- The upper urinary tract is the site of 10% to 15% of TCCs.
- TCC comprises <10% of malignant renal tumors.
- Renal parenchymal invasion by TCC results in a poor prognosis.
- Risk factors for TCC of the upper tract:
  High-grade bladder TCC
  Analgesic abuse
  Cigarette smoking
  Cyclophosphamide therapy
  Radiation exposure
  Aniline dye workers
  Chronic inflammation (pyelitis cystica/glandularis)
- TCC may contain coarse punctate calcific deposits in <10% of cases.

RADIOLOGIC

- The radiologic manifestations of TCC are varied.
- On intravenous urography, TCC may appear as a discrete filling defect within the renal collecting system, a filling defect within a distended calyx, caliceal obliteration, caliceal amputation, hydronephrosis with renal enlargement, or reduced function without renal enlargement.
- The surface of a pelvicaliceal filling defect may be smooth, irregular, or stippled (the "stipple-sign"). An oncocalyx occurs when transitional cell tumor distends a calyx.
- A phantom calyx occurs when tumor obstructs a caliceal infundibulum.
- CT manifestations of TCC mimic their appearance on intravenous urography. Patterns of disease include caliceal or renal pelvis filling defect, pelvicaliceal irregularity, infundibular stenosis, caliceal cut-off, caliceal expansion, and focal or global nonvisualization.
- Differentiation of TCC from RCC is aided by the more modest enhancement of a transitional cell lesion as opposed to the typical hypervascular, nonnecrotic, and noncystic RCC.
- Transitional cell tumors are typically centrally located, with either or both centrifugal expansion and invasion of the kidney.
- There are unusual forms of TCC on CT, including the hydronephrotic form where an enhancing soft-tissue mass may be seen at the apex of a dilated renal pelvis indicative of tumor-causing ureteropelvic junction obstruction. Nodular thickening of the wall of the renal pelvis may also occur.

◆ SUGGESTED READING

Dinsmore BJ, Pollack HM, Banner MP. Calcified transitional cell carcinoma of the renal pelvis. Radiology 1988;167:401–404.

Gatewood OMB, Goldman SM, Marshall FF, Siegelman SS. Computerized tomography in the diagnosis of transitional cell carcinoma of the kidney. J Urol 1982;127:876–887.

Leder RA, Dunnick NR. Transitional cell carcinoma of the pelvicalices and ureter. AJR Am J Roentgenol 1990;155:713–722.

HISTORY

A middle-aged woman has a several-month history of chronic flank pain and a palpable flank mass.

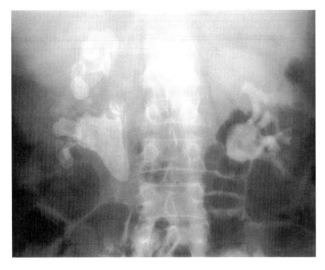

FIGURE 4-25A Anteroposterior postvoid film of the kidneys from an intravenous urogram. There is a large staghorn calculus in the right kidney. Enhancement of the right kidney is not demonstrated, nor is there excretion into the collecting system or ureter. The left kidney is normal.

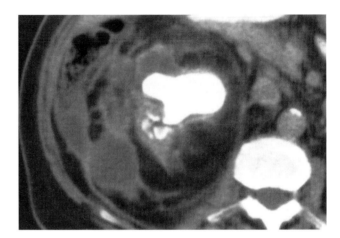

FIGURE 4-25B Noncontrast CT through the mid-right kidney. There is a dense staghorn calculus in the renal pelvis. There is a small amount of low-attenuation material surrounding this staghorn calculus, as well as low-attenuation fluid collections in the perirenal space.

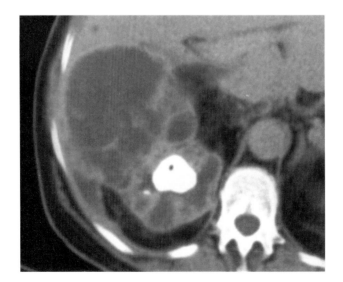

FIGURE 4-25C Contrast-enhanced CT through the upper pole of the right kidney. There is a staghorn calculus in the right upper pole calyx with fluid replacement of the kidney extending into Morrison's pouch. Rim enhancement is present secondary to inflammatory tissue.

◆ DIFFERENTIAL DIAGNOSIS

◆ **Pyonephrosis secondary to an obstructing calculus:** While this may have been a possibility at an earlier stage, one can no longer discern dilated calyces, and the kidney appears destroyed by a process more extensive than one would expect for pyonephrosis.

◆ **Xanthogranulomatous pyelonephritis (XGP):** A poorly or nonfunctioning kidney with an associated staghorn calculus makes this the most likely diagnosis, although this requires pathologic confirmation.

◆ **Chronic pyelonephritis secondary to calculus disease:** Since XGP is a pathologic diagnosis, the possibility exists that this is a nongranulomatous response of the kidney to chronic obstruction. The spread of disease into the perirenal space, however, makes XGP a more likely diagnosis.

◆ **Replacement lipomatosis of the kidney (RLK):** This can be differentiated from XGP by its fibrofatty proliferation. The attenuation of the tissue replacing the kidney in this case is near that of water and is not characteristic of fat, therefore this is not a case of RLK.

◆ DIAGNOSIS: Xanthogranulomatous pyelonephritis.

◆ KEY FACTS

CLINICAL

◆ XGP is a chronic granulomatous inflammation of the kidney. The parenchyma is replaced by xanthoma cells, which are lipid-laden macrophages.

◆ The etiology of XGP is unknown, though it may be caused by chronic urinary tract obstruction with superimposed recurrent infection. Diabetes mellitus and primary hyperparathyroidism may be associated with XGP in some cases.

◆ Fever, dysuria, and flank pain in a middle-aged woman is the classic presentation. Approximately 70% of patients are women. Tenderness in the renal area and a palpable abdominal or flank mass is found in approximately 50% of cases.

◆ Multiorganism urinary tract infections are characteristic. While *Proteus* is common, *E. coli, Klebsiella, Pseudomonas,* and *Enterobacter* may also be cultured. More than 80% of patients have pyuria and proteinuria. Laboratory studies show elevated erythrocyte sedimentation rate, anemia, and leukocytosis.

◆ Reversible hepatic dysfunction has been reported in association with XGP.

◆ A staghorn calculus is often found. An acalculous variety of XGP has been reported.

◆ Both diffuse and focal (tumefactive) varieties exist. The diffuse form is more common, occurring in 85% of cases.

◆ Involvement of the perirenal spaces, psoas muscles, small bowel, diaphragm, lung, or soft tissues of the flank may occur.

RADIOLOGIC

◆ The plain radiograph typically demonstrates enlargement of the infected kidney with evidence of a staghorn calculus. Extension into the perirenal space or pararenal space is suggested by indistinct outlines of the kidney or psoas muscle.

◆ The intravenous urogram shows nonfunction or faint opacification of the kidney.

◆ On ultrasound, the kidney is typically enlarged, with multiple fluid collections representing dilated calyces and areas of parenchymal destruction. Irregular masses, either anechoic or hypoechoic, with low-level internal echoes and varying degrees of through-transmission are frequently seen. Acoustical shadowing of the central staghorn calculus may be obscured by peripelvic fibrosis. Hypoechoic fluid in the perirenal space is secondary to extension of disease.

◆ On CT, the kidney is enlarged diffusely, and the renal parenchyma is replaced by low-attenuation masses. These masses measure between –20 and +10 HU depending on lipid content. True fat density is not seen in XGP. Rim enhancement of well-vascularized granulation tissue may occur. Central calcification is seen frequently, as well as calyceal calculi or small areas of calcification in the adjacent parenchyma. The renal pelvis is contracted. Gerota's fascia may be thickened. Low-attenuation masses may be present in the pararenal and perirenal spaces. Less common CT findings include acalculous XGP, a small contracted kidney with parenchymal destruction, and massive pelvic dilation mimicking obstructive hydronephrosis. Focal (tumefactive) XGP can mimic an RCC. Enhancement is demonstrated on postcontrast CT. Typically, a calculus is seen at the apex of the focal mass.

◆ Approximately 70% of patients have either staghorn calculi or multiple calyceal stones.

◆ XGP can extend to involve the perirenal and pararenal spaces or ipsilateral psoas muscle. Rarely XGP can involve the diaphragm, the paraspinal muscles, and the skin.

◆ SUGGESTED READING

D'Amelio F, Smathers R. CT of acalculous xanthogranulomatous pyelonephritis. Appl Radiol 1990;19:25–27.

Goldman SM, Hartman DS, Fishman EK, et al. CT of xanthogranulomatous pyelonephritis: Radiologic–pathologic correlation. AJR Am J Roentgenol 1984;141:963–969.

Hayes WS, Hartman DS, Sesterbenn IA. Xanthogranulomatous pyelonephritis. Radiographics 1991;11:485–498.

Kenney PJ. Imaging of chronic renal infections. AJR Am J Roentgenol 1990;155:485–494.

Subramanyam BR, Megibow AJ, Raghavendra BN, Bosniak MA. Diffuse xanthogranulomatous pyelonephritis: Analysis by computed tomography and sonography. Urol Radiol 1982;4:5–9.

CASE 26

Erik K. Paulson

HISTORY

A 39-year-old man presents with right flank pain.

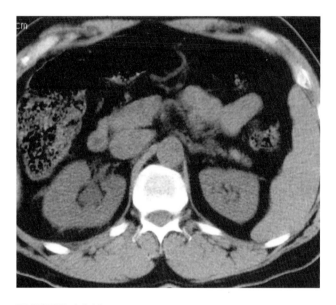

FIGURE 4-26A Noncontrast CT of the upper pole of the kidneys. There is right nephromegaly, stranding of the perinephric fat, and pelvicaliectasis. The left kidney is normal.

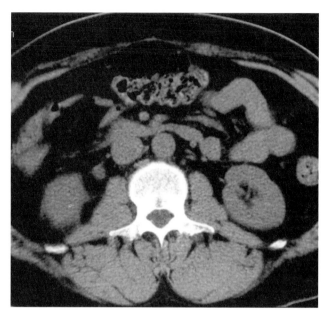

FIGURE 4-26B Noncontrast CT of the lower pole of the kidneys. There is dilation of the right proximal ureter. The left ureter is normal. There is stranding of the perinephric and peri-ureteric fat.

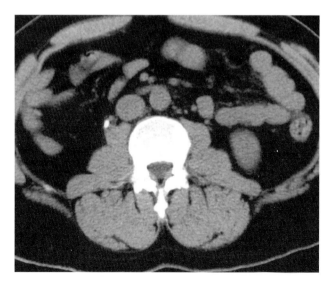

FIGURE 4-26C Noncontrast CT at the level of the ureters. A 3- to 4-mm calcification is identified in the right midureter.

◆ DIFFERENTIAL DIAGNOSIS

- **Pyelonephritis:** Patients with this common condition present with flank pain, fever, nausea, and vomiting. Imaging studies, including intravenous urography, ultrasound, and CT, are usually normal, although on contrast-enhanced CT, parenchymal striations may be seen. While acute pyelonephritis may cause nephromegaly and stranding of the perinephric fat, the ureteral dilation and ureteral calculus argue against this being the primary diagnostic choice.

- **Renal lymphoma:** Lymphoma involves the kidneys either by hematogeneous spread or by direct extension of hilar adenopathy. On CT, renal lymphoma may present as multiple masses, a solitary mass, or a renal hilar/retroperitoneal mass directly invading the kidney.

- **Ureteral obstruction due to a calculus:** The unilateral nephromegaly, perinephric fluid, pelvicaliureterectasis, and ureteral calcification all indicate an obstruction caused by a ureteral calculus.

◆ DIAGNOSIS: Acute ureteral obstruction caused by a calculus.

◆ KEY FACTS

CLINICAL

- The most common cause of ureteral obstruction is a calculus lodged in the ureter.
- Common sites of obstruction include the ureteropelvic junction, sites of blood vessels crossing the ureter, the pelvic brim, and the ureterovesical junction.
- Most small stones <5 mm in diameter will pass spontaneously.
- Calcium oxalate and calcium oxalate mixed with phosphate are the most common stones.
- Uric acid stones are associated with acidic urine, uricosuric drugs, and hyperuricemia. These stones are often radiolucent on plain radiographs but are always hyperattenuating on CT.

RADIOLOGIC

- Intravenous urography is the traditional method to confirm a suspected ureteral obstruction in a patient with renal colic. Classic findings include delayed parenchymal enhancement, delayed excretion, and collecting system dilation to the level of the calculus.
- CT has been shown to be accurate in the work-up of patients with renal colic. These studies are best performed using a spiral technique without intravenous or oral contrast material. Classic findings include nephromegaly, perinephric stranding, and collecting system dilation that extends to the level of the calculus.
- Advantages of spiral CT over intravenous urography include elimination of the need for intravenous contrast material, the occasional demonstration of nonurinary causes of flank pain, and a shorter examination time.
- Disadvantages of spiral CT include difficulty in differentiating vascular calcifications and phleboliths from ureteral stones, inaccurate demonstration of stone size, particularly along the cranial-caudal axis of stones, and lack of "functional" information in regard to the degree of obstruction.

◆ SUGGESTED READING

Dunnick NR, McCallum RW, Sandler CM. Nephrocalcinosis and Nephrolithiasis. In Textbook of Uroradiology. Baltimore: Williams & Wilkins, 1991;189–214.

Smith RC, Rosenfield AT, Choe KA, et al. Acute flank pain: Comparison of non-contrast-enhanced CT and intravenous urography. Radiology 1995;194:789–794.

Sommer FG, Jeffrey RB Jr, Rubin GD, et al. Detection of ureteral calculi in patients with suspected renal colic: Value of reformatted noncontrast helical CT. AJR Am J Roentgenol 1995;165: 509–513.

HISTORY

A 67-year-old asymptomatic man has a prostate-specific antigen (PSA) level of 12.0 ng/dL (normal < 4.0 ng/dL).

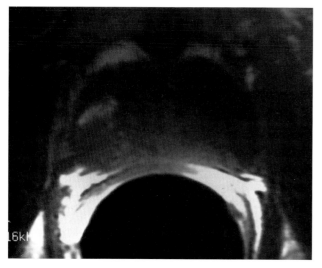

FIGURE 4-27A Axial T1-weighted MRI of the prostate. There is a focal area of high signal intensity on the right side of the prostate gland.

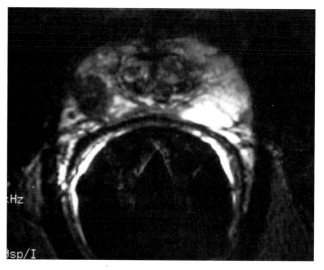

FIGURE 4-27B Axial T2-weighted MRI of the prostate. There is a well-demarcated, 1-cm focus of low signal intensity in the right peripheral zone of the gland. Note the right neurovascular bundle adjacent to this on the axial image.

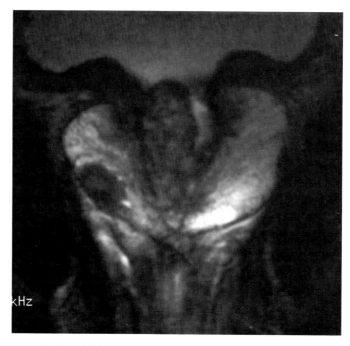

FIGURE 4-27C Coronal T2-weighted MRI of the prostate also demonstrate a focal area of low signal intensity in the right peripheral zone. The capsular surface appears relatively intact.

◆ DIFFERENTIAL DIAGNOSIS

◆ **Adenocarcinoma of the prostate, postbiopsy hemorrhage, and focal scar:** This appearance has a limited differential diagnosis. Well-defined, focal, low signal intensity in the peripheral zone of the prostate gland on T2-weighted images is usually due to adenocarcinoma, postbiopsy hemorrhage, or occasionally, a focal scar. Hemorrhage can be diagnosed when there are foci of high signal intensity on T1-weighted images. Diffuse low signal intensity in the peripheral zone on T2-weighted images may also be seen in cases of prostatitis or postradiotherapy.

◆ DIAGNOSIS: Adenocarcinoma of the prostate with postbiopsy hemorrhage.

◆ KEY FACTS

CLINICAL

◆ Adenocarcinoma of the prostate is the second leading cause of cancer death among American men.

◆ Prostate cancer is most commonly detected by routine screening, which includes a digital rectal examination and a serum PSA level.

◆ Any suspicious findings should lead to a transrectal ultrasound-guided biopsy which samples all quadrants of the gland (sextant biopsies).

◆ Staging of prostate carcinoma is by the Whitmore-Jewitt system, which is as follows: (A) nonpalpable, confined to prostate; (B) palpable, confined to prostate; (C) extracapsular extension; (D1) regional nodes; (D2) distant nodes.

◆ The 5-year survival for stage D1 is 50%.

◆ The treatment for stage A or B prostate carcinoma includes a radical prostatectomy or radiotherapy depending on the age of the patient. The treatment for stages C or D includes hormone therapy or radiotherapy.

RADIOLOGIC

◆ Plain films or intravenous urography may demonstrate osteoblastic metastases, particularly in the bony pelvis.

◆ With ultrasound, most prostate cancers are hypoechoic, but only about 20% of hypoechoic lesions noted are malignant. The larger the lesion, the more likely it is to be malignant.

◆ On CT, prostate carcinoma may be seen as a low-attenuation lesion in the peripheral zone; however, this is not the imaging modality of choice.

◆ On MRI, prostate carcinoma is of low signal intensity on both T1- and T2-weighted images. The presence of postbiopsy hemorrhage is seen as a focus of high signal intensity on the T1-weighted image. MRI is much more useful for staging prostate carcinoma than for screening.

◆ SUGGESTED READING

Choyke PL. Imaging of prostate carcinoma. Abdom Imag 1995;20:505–515.

Scheibler ML, Schnall MD, Pollack HM, et al. Current role of MR imaging in the staging of adenocarcinoma of the prostate. Radiology 1993;189:339–352.

CASE 28 *Kelly S. Freed*

HISTORY

A 75-year-old asymptomatic woman with a history of colon cancer.

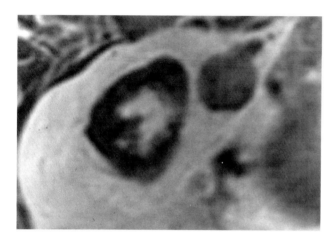

FIGURE 4-28A Axial T1-weighted MRI of the upper abdomen. There is a well-defined, 2-cm, right adrenal mass with a relative signal intensity of 168.

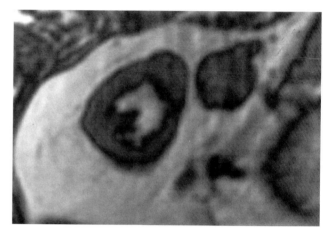

FIGURE 4-28B Axial opposed-phase (Dixon) T1-weighted MRI of the upper abdomen. The right adrenal mass darkens on the opposed-phase image with a relative signal intensity of 88.

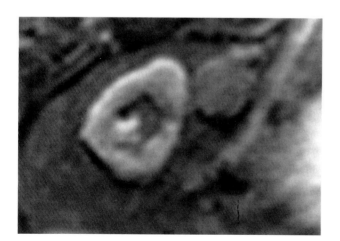

FIGURE 4-28C Axial T2-weighted MRI of the upper abdomen. The calculated T2 value of the right adrenal mass is 56 ms.

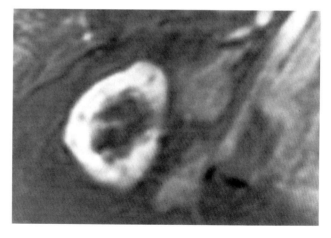

FIGURE 4-28D Axial contrast-enhanced, fat-suppressed T1-weighted MRI of the upper abdomen. The right adrenal mass demonstrates mild contrast enhancement.

◆ DIFFERENTIAL DIAGNOSIS

◆ **Metastasis:** This diagnosis is unlikely because the mass has a high lipid content, as evidenced by the loss of signal intensity on the opposed phase image. The T2 value would likely be >60 ms in metastases.

◆ **Pheochromocytoma:** A much higher signal intensity on the T2-weighted image and, therefore, a longer calculated T2 value would be expected in this diagnosis.

◆ **Nonhyperfunctioning adenoma:** This is the most likely diagnosis given the size and loss of signal intensity on the opposed-phase images, even though the patient has a known malignancy.

◆ DIAGNOSIS: Nonhyperfunctioning adenoma.

◆ KEY FACTS

CLINICAL

◆ Adrenocortical adenomas may be nonhyperfunctioning or hyperfunctioning. The incidence of nonhyperfunctioning adenomas in the general population is 1% to 3%.

◆ Hyperfunctioning adenomas may secrete:

　Cortisol: Cushing's syndrome (adenoma are usually >4 cm in diameter)

　Aldosterone: Conn's syndrome (adenomas are usually <2 cm in diameter)

　Androgens: virilization

RADIOLOGIC

◆ On CT, a precontrast attenuation value <0 Hounsfield units (HU) signifies a benign condition; a precontrast attenuation value +1–10 HU signifies that the adenoma is likely benign and may warrant follow-up based on the clinical setting.

◆ Opposed-phase MRI results in lower signal of the lesion compared with conventional in-phase MRI due to intracytoplasmic lipid. Calculated T2 values are generally <60 ms.

◆ Malignant imaging features include large size (>5 cm), heterogeneity, intense contrast enhancement, and an increase in size on follow-up imaging.

◆ Imaging studies cannot differentiate hyperfunctioning from nonhyperfunctioning adenomas.

◆ SUGGESTED READING

McLoughlin RF, Bilbey JH. Tumors of the adrenal gland: Findings on CT and MR imaging. AJR Am J Roentgenol 1994;163: 1413–1418.

Ros PR, Bidgood WD. Abdominal Magnetic Resonance Imaging. St. Louis: Mosby, 1993;348–362.

CASE 29

Bruce P. Hall

HISTORY

A 67-year-old woman presents with vaginal bleeding.

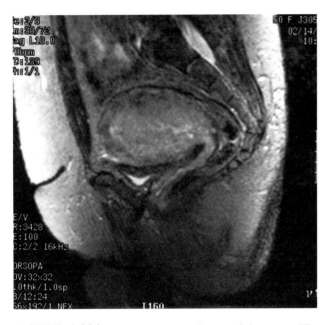

FIGURE 4-29A Sagittal T2-weighted MRI of the uterus. The low signal intensity junctional zone is not seen, and the myometrium is significantly thinned by an invasive mass.

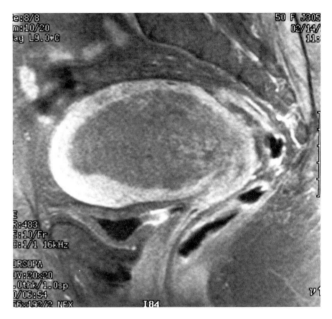

FIGURE 4-29B Sagittal T1-weighted MRI of the uterus following the intravenous administration of a gadolinium-chelate. The endometrial mass is hypointense relative to the myometrium, filling the endometrial cavity as well as the endocervical canal. There is thinning of both the cervical stroma and the myometrium.

◆ DIFFERENTIAL DIAGNOSIS

◆ **Endometrial carcinoma with extension to the uterine cervix:** This should be the primary consideration in this postmenopausal patient.

◆ **Endometrial polyp:** This is a possibility; however, polyps typically appear more focal and round. Only when it is surrounded by endometrial fluid can one make the definitive diagnosis of a polyp.

◆ **Endometrial hyperplasia:** This entity can be impossible to differentiate from endometrial carcinoma when the disease process is confined to the uterus. However, the disease process in this case clearly extends into the cervix, making endometrial hyperplasia very unlikely.

◆ **Retained placenta with hemorrhage or pus:** These processes tend to be more heterogeneous and, of course, would not be supported by the history.

◆ **Invasive molar pregnancy:** This would also be a consideration in a patient with the appropriate history and elevated human chorionic gonadotropin values.

◆ DIAGNOSIS: Endometrial carcinoma with invasion of the myometrium and cervix, FIGO stage II.

◆ KEY FACTS

CLINICAL

◆ Although 80% of cases of endometrial carcinoma occur in postmenopausal women, 90% of postmenopausal bleeding is caused by benign disease.

◆ Endometrial carcinoma is staged as follows according to the FIGO system:

Stage	Description
I	Confined to the uterine corpus
IA	Confined to the endometrium
IB	Invasion confined to the inner 50% of the myometrium
IC	Invasion extends into the outer 50% of the myometrium
II	Extension to the uterine cervix
III	Extrauterine spread limited to the true pelvis
IVA	Extension to the bladder or rectum
IVB	Distant metastases

◆ The incidence of pelvic lymph node involvement increases dramatically with stage IC and II lesions.

◆ Endometrial carcinoma can be either focal or diffuse. The current case is a good example of diffuse disease.

RADIOLOGIC

◆ Ultrasound is somewhat limited in its ability to distinguish between endometrial carcinoma and other causes of endometrial thickening.

◆ The accepted range of normal for endometrial thickness, as determined by adding the measurements of the anterior and posterior components of the endometrium, depends on the hormonal status of the patient, as follows:

Hormonal status	Normal range
Premenopausal	
Proliferative phase	4 to 8 mm
Secretory phase	7 to 14 mm
Postmenopausal	
Without estrogen replacement	4 to 8 mm
With estrogen replacement	<10 mm

◆ In two studies of patients with postmenopausal bleeding, no patient with an endometrial thickness of <5 mm had malignant pathology.

◆ On sagittal T2-weighted MR images, the junctional zone will clearly separate the endometrium from the myometrium in most patients. Disruption of the junctional zone is evidence for invasion into the myometrium. However, approximately 50% of postmenopausal women will not have a visible junctional zone on T2-weighted images. The use of gadolinium-enhanced dynamic imaging produces improved contrast between the enhancing endometrial carcinoma and the even more strongly enhancing myometrium. Because endometrial carcinoma enhances more than normal endometrium, superficial lesions are more easily recognized after enhancement. The junctional zone can also be delineated better using this technique.

◆ The accuracy of endovaginal ultrasound and MRI, using T2-weighted imaging, in the determination of the depth of myometrial invasion is approximately 76%. The recent use of contrast-enhanced dynamic MRI of the uterus has increased the accuracy to approximately 90% in the best hands.

◆ SUGGESTED READING

Chan FY, Chau MT, Pun TC. Limitations of transvaginal sonography and color Doppler imaging in the differentiation of endometrial carcinoma from benign lesions. J Ultrasound Med 1994; 13:623–628.

Goldstein SR, Nachtigall M, Snyder JR, Nachtigall L. Endometrial assessment by vaginal ultrasonography before endometrial sampling in patients with postmenopausal bleeding. Am J Obstet Gynecol 1990;163:119–123.

Lin MC, Gosink BB, Wolf SI. Endometrial thickness after menopause: Effect of hormonal replacement. Radiology 1991;180:427–432.

Mogavero G, Sheth S, Hamper UM. Endovaginal sonography of the nongravid uterus. Radiographics 1993;13:969–981.

Smith RC, McCarthy S. Magnetic resonance staging of neoplasms of the uterus. Radiol Clin North Am 1994;32:109–131.

Yamashita Y, Mizutani H, Torashima M. Assessment of myometrial invasion by endometrial carcinoma: Transvaginal sonography vs. contrast-enhanced MR imaging. AJR Am J Roentgenol 1993;161:595–599.

CHAPTER 5

MUSCULO-SKELETAL IMAGING

D. Lawrence Burk, *chapter editor*

D. Lawrence Burk, Andrew J. Collins,
Salutario J. Martinez, Joseph W. Melamed,
Charles E. Spritzer, and Robert M. Vandemark

CASE 1

Salutario J. Martinez

HISTORY

A 10-year-old boy with acute onset of right hip pain, fever, and a stiff ankle.

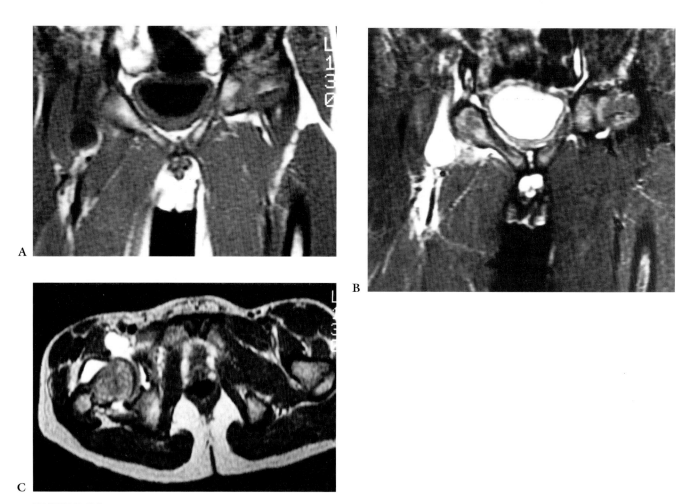

FIGURE 5-1 **(A)** Coronal unenhanced T1-weighted MRI of the pelvis. **(B)** Coronal short tau inversion recovery (STIR) MRI of the pelvis. **(C)** Axial T2-weighted MRI through the hips. All images demonstrate a focal, round, homogeneous mass anterior to the right hip joint. The mass is deep to the psoas muscle and lateral to the femoral neurovascular bundle. The mass is of low signal intensity on T1-weighted images and high signal intensity on STIR and T2-weighted images, consistent with fluid. There is also a hip joint effusion.

◆ DIFFERENTIAL DIAGNOSIS

◆ **Iliopsoas bursitis (IPB):** The location of the mass anterior to the hip joint, lateral to the femoral vessels, and deep to the psoas tendon, the teardrop or round configuration, and its fluid signal intensity characteristics are in favor of this diagnosis. The associated effusion indicates communication of the bursa with the hip joint. The cystic nature can be depicted further with T1-weighted gadolinium-enhanced MRI. The wall of the inflamed bursa would be expected to enhance uniformly without nodularity, while the fluid will not enhance. Other studies documented a seronegative arthropathy.

◆ **Neoplasm:** Most tumors have a heterogeneous signal intensity pattern. T1-weighted gadolinium-enhanced MRI helps differentiate tumors like intramuscular myxoma, synovial sarcoma, and hemangioma, which can imitate bursitis.

◆ **Femoral hernia:** Lack of gas and the signal characteristics indicating fluid in this mass exclude this condition.

◆ **Abscess:** Intramuscular abscess can be excluded because the collection of fluid is not intramuscular. However, in general, septic bursitis cannot be excluded unless noninfected fluid is obtained by percutaneous aspiration.

◆ **Femoral artery aneurysm:** Normal femoral vessels are seen in this patient. Furthermore, the location, fluid nature, age of the patient, and the communication with joint space are not consistent with this diagnosis.

◆ DIAGNOSIS: Iliopsoas bursitis associated with seronegative spondyloarthropathy.

◆ KEY FACTS

CLINICAL

◆ The iliopsoas bursa is the largest bursa in the body and is present in 98% of adults, interposed between the iliacus muscle/psoas tendon and the anterior capsule of the hip, lateral to the femoral artery, vein, and nerve. Communication exists between the iliopsoas bursa and the hip joint in 14% of adults.

◆ Inflammation and enlargement of the iliopsoas bursa may occur secondary to hip joint disease or, occasionally, as a primary bursal process.

◆ Diseases associated with IPB include seropositive and seronegative arthropathies, osteoarthritis, pigmented villonodular synovitis, synovial chondromatosis, infection, hip prosthesis, occupational trauma, and sports injuries.

◆ Clinical presentation in IPB includes pain, mass lesion, and compression syndromes of the inguinal compartment (pseudothrombophlebitis, femoral nerve neuropathy that may simulate L4 radiculopathy). Retroperitoneal extension of the iliopsoas bursa may present as a palpable abdominal or pelvic mass.

◆ IPB is frequently confused with a femoral hernia, lymphadenopathy, neoplasms, or a femoral artery aneurysm.

◆ Therapy for IPB is variable. Rest and nonsteroidal anti-inflammatory drugs are indicated for mild cases. Aspiration and corticosteroid injection may be required in more severe cases. Occasionally, surgical resection of the bursa is necessary.

RADIOLOGIC

◆ Early, accurate diagnosis of IPB is facilitated by appropriate radiologic studies.

◆ Conventional radiographs can help assess underlying hip joint disorders such as osteoarthritis or rheumatoid arthritis.

◆ Ultrasound may demonstrate the fluid-filled nature of palpable lesions and can guide needle aspiration.

◆ Contrast bursography outlines the extent of bursal enlargement.

◆ Hip arthrography is definitive in establishing the diagnosis when a communication exists.

◆ On CT, a water attenuation mass is typically seen in close apposition to the tendon muscle at the level of the hip joint and lateral to the femoral vessels. When a communication exists, an associated hip effusion may be seen. If the bursitis is secondary to a hip arthropathy, evidence of osteoarthritis or rheumatoid arthritis may be seen. Intravenous contrast material enhances the wall of the bursa but not the contents, as expected for a fluid collection in an inflamed bursa. In primary IPB, the hip joint may be normal. If there is no communication with the joint, there will be no evidence of a hip effusion.

◆ The soft-tissue contrast, noninvasiveness, and multiplanar capability of MRI make it superior for assessing IPB. Underlying arthropathic changes can be characterized in a case of secondary IPB. The signal intensity of uncomplicated bursitis is that of fluid. Debris, loose bodies, or blood yield different signal intensities. Contrast enhancement of the inflamed wall due to hypervascularity is typically seen. Signal intensity in synovial chondromatosis of the iliopsoas bursa varies depending on the degree of calcification of the cartilaginous nodules. However, in pigmented villonodular IPB, the hemosiderin will typically be of low signal intensity on all sequences.

◆ MRI will make the positive diagnosis of IPB in most clinical situations and exclude other conditions such as a hernia, tumor, lymph node, hematoma, aneurysm, and abscess. Ultrasound or CT-guided bursal aspiration can exclude septic bursitis, detect the presence of crystals, and provide a means of drainage of the bursa and injection of corticosteroids.

◆ SUGGESTED READING

Sartoris D, Danzig L, Gilula L, et al. Synovial cysts of the hip and iliopsoas bursitis: A spectrum of imaging modalities. Skeletal Radiol 1985;14:85–94.

Toohey AK, LaSalle TL, Martinez S, Polisson RP. Iliopsoas bursitis: Clinical features, radiographic findings, and disease associations. Semin Arthritis Rheum 1990;20:41–47.

Varma DGK, Richli WR, Charnsangavej C, et al. MR appearance of the distended iliopsoas bursa. AJR Am J Roentgenol 1991;156: 1025–1028.

CASE 2

Robert M. Vandemark

HISTORY

A 35-year-old woman who fell and twisted her ankle while running downstairs.

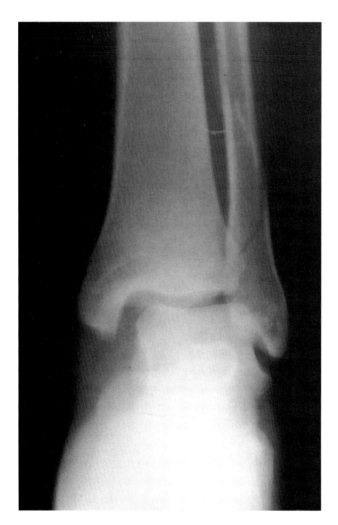

FIGURE 5-2A Anteroposterior radiograph of the ankle. This view gives the false impression of a nondisplaced spiral fracture of the distal fibula and widened medial joint space.

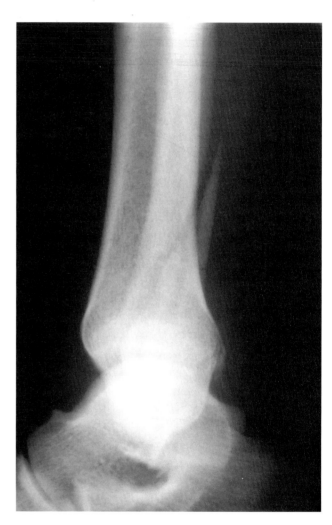

FIGURE 5-2B Lateral radiograph of the ankle. Fracture displacement is more readily apparent on the lateral view.

◆ DIFFERENTIAL DIAGNOSIS

- **Pronation-abduction injury:** This is an uncommon fracture pattern characterized by a low, oblique fibular fracture at the level of the ankle joint.
- **Supination-external rotation (SER) injury:** These injuries are characterized by a long oblique fracture of the distal fibula usually measuring 2 to 4 cm in length. Not uncommonly, the fracture is most apparent on the lateral view of the ankle.
- **Supination-adduction injury:** This injury causes a horizontally oriented fracture in the distal fibula, usually below the joint line.
- **Pronation-external rotation injury:** This injury produces a relatively horizontal fracture of the fibular diaphysis approximately 5 to 8 cm above the ankle joint.

◆ DIAGNOSIS: Supination-external rotation injury.

◆ KEY FACTS

CLINICAL

- SER is the most commonly observed ankle fracture pattern.
- The fracture is preceded by ankle inversion and rupture of the anterior tibiofibular ligament.
- Asymmetric widening of the ankle mortise denotes instability, an indication for open reduction with internal fixation.

RADIOLOGIC

- There is typically a long (2 to 4 cm), oblique-spiral fracture of the distal fibula.
- The fracture is often seen best on the lateral view.
- SER injury may be associated with either or both posterior and medial malleolus fractures or a tear of the deltoid ligament.
- The patterns of ankle fractures described in the differential diagnosis are derived from the Lauge-Hansen classification system. Although other classification schemes exist, it is the most widely used for communicating radiographic findings, determining appropriate orthopedic therapy, and predicting the prognosis.
- The importance of the classification system is the recognition that ankle fractures are not randomly oriented fractures through the medial, lateral, and posterior malleoli, but rather occur in a stereotypical and predictable manner based on the mechanism of injury, the position of the foot and ankle at the time of injury, and the relative strength and weakness of the bony and ligamentous structures about the ankle.
- The four types of fractures cause a relatively unique pattern of injury to the fibula, which is so characteristic it allows one to easily classify the four fracture types.

◆ SUGGESTED READING

Berquist TH. Imaging of Orthopedic Trauma. New York: Raven, 1992;512–517.

CASE 3

D. Lawrence Burk

HISTORY

A 33-year-old woman with diffuse bone pain and a chronic disease.

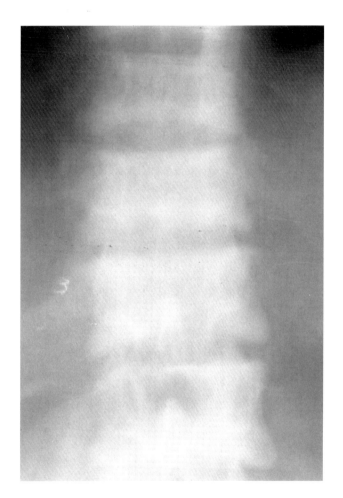

FIGURE 5-3A Anteroposterior radiograph of thoracic spine. The vertebral bodies are diffusely sclerotic.

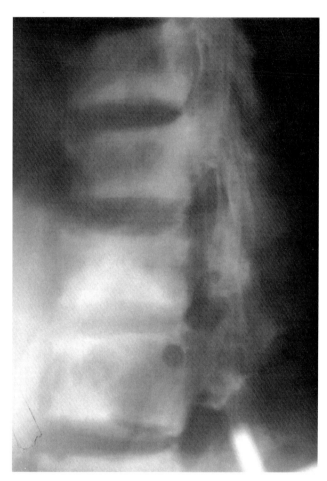

FIGURE 5-3B Lateral radiograph of thoracic spine. Band-like areas of sclerosis are noted to involve the superior and inferior endplates. Erosive changes are present in the anterior cortices of multiple vertebral bodies. A single small lytic lesion is seen in the posterior aspect of a lower vertebral body.

◆ DIFFERENTIAL DIAGNOSIS

- **Osteopetrosis:** Diffuse sclerosis results in a bone-within-bone appearance or a sandwich vertebra appearance. Anterior vascular notches may be seen in the vertebral bodies, but lytic lesions do not occur.
- **Systemic mastocytosis:** Osteosclerosis may be diffuse or patchy and multifocal. Multiple lytic lesions can also occur, which are usually surrounded by a halo of sclerosis.
- **Renal osteodystrophy and secondary hyperparathyroidism:** Osteosclerosis manifests as a rugger-jersey spine appearance. Subligamentous bone resorption simulating erosions and lytic brown tumors are additional features. This is the most likely diagnosis.
- **Myelofibrosis:** A diffuse increase in bone density is most commonly seen, but small areas of relative radiolucency or lytic lesions can also be present.

◆ DIAGNOSIS: Renal osteodystrophy and secondary hyperparathyroidism.

◆ KEY FACTS

CLINICAL

- Musculoskeletal manifestations of chronic renal insufficiency are increasingly common due to prolonged survival with hemodialysis.
- Symptomatic bone disease may consist of pain, tenderness, swelling, and deformity.
- The most common cause of chronic renal insufficiency is glomerulonephritis.
- Hyperphosphatemia results in hyperplasia of the parathyroid gland chief cells and increased levels of parathyroid hormone.

RADIOLOGIC

- Osteosclerosis most commonly involves the cancellous bone of the spine, but it may also involve the pelvis, ribs, clavicle, and the ends of long bones.
- Bone resorption occurs in subperiosteal, subchondral, subligamentous, and endosteal locations.
- Brown tumors or osteoclastomas are well-defined lytic lesions that may heal with sclerosis after treatment of the hyperparathyroidism.

◆ SUGGESTED READING

Murphey MD, Sartoris DJ, Quale JL, et al. Musculoskeletal manifestations of chronic renal insufficiency. Radiographics 1993;13:357–379.

Resnick D. Bone and Joint Imaging. Philadelphia: Saunders, 1989;630–646.

CASE 4

Andrew J. Collins

HISTORY

An 86-year-old woman with arthralgia of the knees, hips, and wrists with periodic exacerbations. She has recently complained of increasing right hip pain.

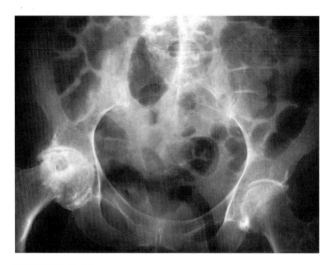

FIGURE 5-4A Anteroposterior radiograph of the pelvis. There is severe superomedial and moderately severe superior joint space narrowing of the right hip. There is associated subchondral sclerosis and osteophytosis on both sides of the joint. A large area of radiolucency appears at the superior aspect of the femoral head, with some surrounding sclerosis. There is articular collapse in this region, with flattening and undulation of the articular surface of the femoral head superolaterally. There are relatively mild osteophytic proliferative changes of the left hip. There is a linear density at the symphysis pubis consistent with chondrocalcinosis.

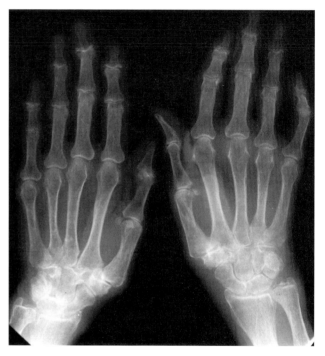

FIGURE 5-4B Posteroanterior radiograph of both hands and wrists. There are calcifications compatible with chondrocalcinosis in the region of the triangular fibrocartilages bilaterally and in the region of the hyaline cartilage of the right lunate, the right second and third metacarpophalangeal (MCP) joints, and the left second, third, and fourth MCP joints all along the radial aspect. Degenerative-appearing changes are noted at the first carpometacarpal joints and multiple distal interphalangeal joints.

◆ DIFFERENTIAL DIAGNOSIS

◆ **Calcium pyrophosphate deposition disease (CPPD):** This diagnosis is favored given the distribution of the process and the presence of chondrocalcinosis of fibro-cartilaginous and hyaline cartilaginous structures. Also supporting this diagnosis is the prominent subchondral cyst formation in the right femoral head.

◆ **Osteoarthritis:** Many of the features noted on these films are consistent with osteoarthritis, but the presence of chondrocalcinosis is in keeping with the diagnosis of CPPD. Some of the findings, such as the degenerative changes in the distal intraphalangeal joints, could represent osteoarthritis, but the arthritis of CPPD can have features identical to osteoarthritis or the degenerative process may be accelerated by CPPD.

◆ **Erosive (inflammatory) osteoarthritis:** Central depressions of the articular surfaces of the distal phalanges of the left second, fourth, and fifth digits and right fourth digit are seen in the case shown. This appearance, which gives a gull-wing appearance at the left fifth distant phalanx, can be seen with the central erosions of erosive osteoarthritis. Relatively mild deformities, as noted in this case, can be seen in osteoarthritis or with degenerative type changes associated with CPPD.

◆ **Osteonecrosis:** The area of lucency with adjacent sclerosis in the right femoral head with associated articular collapse makes osteonecrosis a consideration, but collapse can occur secondary to structural weakening associated with subchondral cyst formation. In addition, a fair amount of acetabular proliferative change is seen, and the joint space narrowing is most pronounced superomedially.

◆ DIAGNOSIS: Calcium pyrophosphate deposition disease.

◆ KEY FACTS

CLINICAL
◆ CPPD mainly affects middle-aged and elderly subjects.
◆ CPPD is clinically similar to osteoarthritis but has a greater tendency for acute exacerbations of the disease.
◆ Pseudogout occurs in approximately 10% to 20% of cases.
◆ Conditions that are strongly associated with CPPD include primary hyperparathyroidism, hemochromatosis, and, to a lesser extent, gout.

RADIOLOGIC
◆ The features of CPPD are similar to osteoarthritis, but CPPD has a greater tendency for subchondral cyst formation, destructive changes of the osteochondral articular surfaces, and joint effusion.
◆ Osteophyte formation is variable.
◆ Soft-tissue calcifications typically involve fibrocartilages (such as the menisci of the knee, triangular fibrocartilage, acetabular labrum, symphysis pubis, or annulus fibrosis) and the hyaline cartilage (particularly in the wrist, knees, elbows, and hips). Other periarticular soft tissues may also be involved.
◆ The distribution of CPPD includes areas less typical for osteoarthritis, such as the radiocarpal joints, elbows, or glenohumeral joints. There may be isolated or accelerated abnormalities at the metatarsophalangeal joints, patellofemoral joints, or talonavicular joints.

◆ SUGGESTED READING

Resnick D. Diagnosis of Bone and Joint Disorders (2nd ed). Philadelphia: Saunders, 1989;1672–1732.

Steinbach LS, Resnick D. Calcium pyrophosphate dihydrate crystal deposition disease revisited. Radiology 1996;200:1–9.

Uri DS, Martel W. Radiologic manifestations of the crystal-related arthropathies. Semin Roentgenol 1996;31:229–238.

HISTORY

A 34-year-old man with tenderness along the medial joint line of the right knee.

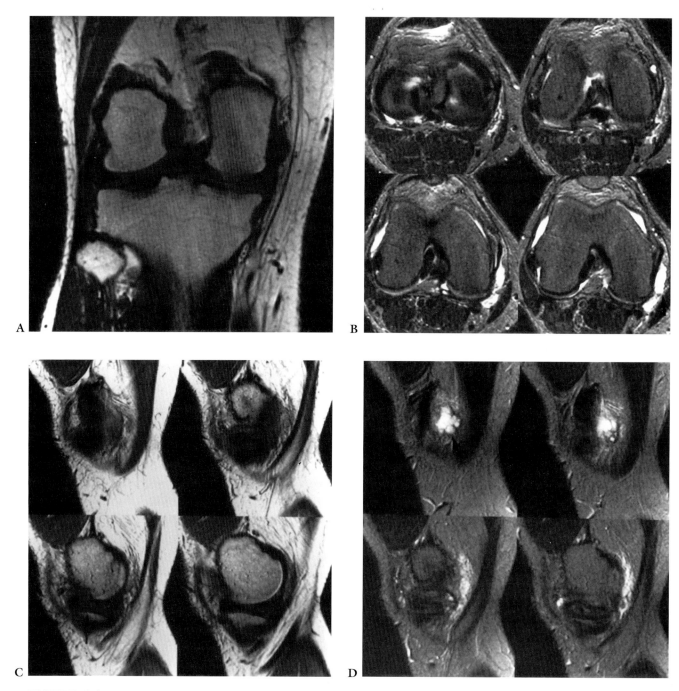

FIGURE 5-5 **(A)** Coronal spin echo T1-weighted MRI of the knee. **(B)** Axial T2-weighted MRIs of the knee. **(C)** Sagittal proton density-weighted MRIs of the knee. **(D)** Sagittal T2-weighted MRIs of the knee. A loculated fluid collection is seen adjacent to the medial femoral condyle just cephalad to the joint space (**B** and **D**). A tear of the medial meniscus is also appreciated (**A** and **C**), involving both the anterior and posterior horn and extending to the meniscocapsular junction. Intermediate signal intensity is seen in this area on the T1-weighted coronal image.

◆ DIFFERENTIAL DIAGNOSIS

- **Popliteal cyst:** These cysts tend to be located more posteriorly and not as medially as in this case. The neck of a popliteal cyst typically protrudes through the space between the medial head of the gastrocnemius and the semimembranosus muscles, not through the medial joint capsule as in this case.
- **Ganglion cyst:** The signal intensity of the loculated collection is consistent with a fluid-filled/jelly-like viscous substance. The presence of an associated meniscal tear makes this diagnosis less likely.
- **Meniscal cyst:** A horizontal meniscal tear with an associated cyst is characteristic of this diagnosis.
- **Pes anserinus bursitis:** Either or both fluid and edema are often seen in association with inflammation of the pes anserine, namely, the semitendinosis, sartorius, and gracilis muscles.

◆ DIAGNOSIS: Meniscal cyst.

◆ KEY FACTS

CLINICAL

- Meniscal cysts contain jelly-like mucinous or synovial fluid. The neck of the meniscal cyst is often traced to the joint line.
- Meniscal cysts are thought to occur more commonly on the lateral side of the knee rather than the medial side, although Burk et al. found more medial meniscal cysts in their series.
- For ganglion cysts, excision of the lesion is sufficient. However, if a meniscal cyst is excised in a similar fashion, it will typically recur. As such, the diagnosis of a meniscal cyst in this situation requires treatment of the underlying meniscal abnormality to prevent recurrence.
- It has been suggested that cysts located posteriorly to the medial collateral ligament are more apt to penetrate the capsule and to expand in an unrestricted fashion. These cysts may be misdiagnosed as ganglion cysts or popliteal cysts.

RADIOLOGIC

- On T2-weighted MRI, a loculated fluid collection extending from the joint line is seen.
- On proton density or T1-weighted MRI, the tear of the underlying meniscus is identified. These tears are typically horizontal, with the defect extending to the meniscocapsular junction rather than to the superior or inferior articular surface.

◆ SUGGESTED READING

Burk DL Jr, Dalinka MK, Kanal E, et al. Meniscal and ganglion cysts of the knee: MR evaluation. AJR Am J Roentgenol 1988; 150:331–336.

Stoller D, Dillworth W, Anderson LJ. The Knee. In D Stoller (ed), Magnetic Resonance Imaging in Orthopaedics and Sports Medicine. Philadelphia: Lippincott, 1995;139–372.

CASE 6

Robert M. Vandemark

HISTORY

Patient A: a 35-year-old man who fell from a ladder onto an outstretched hand and now complains of shoulder pain. Patient B: a 45-year-old woman who complains of severe shoulder pain following a grand mal seizure.

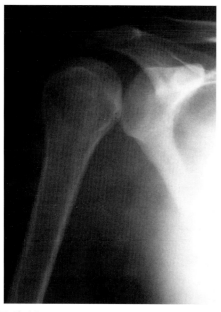

FIGURE 5-6A Anteroposterior internal rotation radiograph of the shoulder in patient A. There is widening of the joint space.

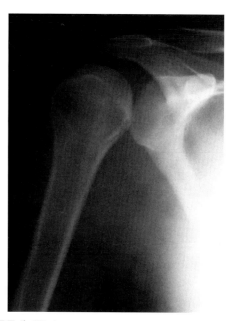

FIGURE 5-6B Anteroposterior external rotation radiograph of the shoulder in patient A. This view also shows identical joint space widening, which indicates lack of any motion at the glenohumeral joint.

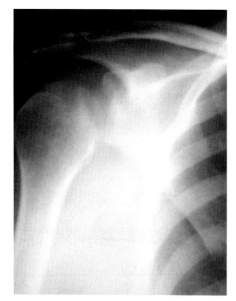

FIGURE 5-6C Anteroposterior radiograph of the shoulder in patient B. There is widening of the joint space and an oblique sclerotic band through the articular segment of the humerus.

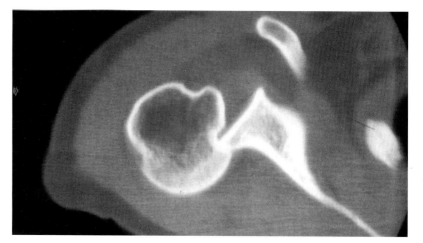

FIGURE 5-6D Axial CT of the glenohumeral joint in patient B. There is an impaction fracture produced by collision of the posterior glenoid rim on the humeral head.

◆ DIFFERENTIAL DIAGNOSIS

- **Anterior dislocation of the shoulder:** Anterior shoulder dislocations characteristically cause anteroinferior displacement of the humeral head relative to the glenoid. This position of the humeral head is never seen in patients with posterior dislocation. In addition, anterior dislocation leads to total obscuration of the normal glenohumeral joint space due to overlap of the humeral head and the glenoid.

- **Posterior dislocation of the shoulder:** Posterior dislocations are rare but are characteristic in patients with seizures, electrical injury, and, occasionally, blunt injury to the anterior aspect of the shoulder. In virtually all cases of posterior dislocation, the humeral head and glenoid remain in the same transverse plane, unlike anterior dislocation, where the humeral head displaces inferomedially. Some posterior dislocations give the appearance of a widened glenohumeral joint space, caused by "perching" of the humeral head on the posterior labrum. As a result, the distance between the humeral head and the anterior labrum is widened, which gives the false impression of a widened joint space. This feature is never seen in anterior dislocation.

- **Pseudodislocation of the shoulder:** This term applies to a clinical presentation in which physical findings suggest an abnormal position of the humeral head consistent with a shoulder dislocation. Subsequent radiographs fail to show a dislocation but do demonstrate inferior subluxation of the humeral head relative to the glenoid. Pseudodislocation can be seen in the setting of brachial plexus injury, chronic shoulder joint instability, hemarthrosis, and, occasionally, pyarthrosis.

◆ DIAGNOSIS: Posterior dislocation of the shoulder.

◆ KEY FACTS

CLINICAL

- Less than 3% of all shoulder dislocations are posterior.
- The characteristic setting for this injury is in a patient after a seizure.

RADIOLOGIC

- "Fixed" internal rotation should immediately raise the possibility of posterior dislocation of the shoulder.

- A "positive" rim sign is present when the distance between the anterior glenoid rim and the humerus is ≤6 mm.
- A post-traumatic "dent" in the anterior aspect of the articular segment is called the "trough sign."
- Posterior dislocation remains a challenging diagnosis when the axillary or "Y" views are unavailable. Such would be the case on portable chest radiographs obtained for patients with blunt trauma, electrical injury, or seizure disorders. Under these circumstances, it is important to recognize the clues of posterior dislocation on an anteroposterior view alone. The radiologist must recognize fixed internal rotation, widening of the joint space (rim sign), and loss of the overlap appearance (half moon) of the normal shoulder joint as characteristic findings of posterior dislocation on a frontal film.
- A post-traumatic dent in the humeral head (trough sign) is a helpful sign but is not always present. Posterior dislocations can also be seen in conjunction with comminuted fracture-dislocations of the proximal humerus. In any event, the reader should keep in mind that posterior dislocations when missed can easily escape clinical detection and become chronic dislocations. It is not unusual for patients with chronic posterior dislocation to remain undiagnosed for months at a time. The radiologist must always have a high index for a "missed" posterior dislocation when reviewing outpatient radiographs in patients with chronic shoulder pain.
- A clinical history of any or all of the following symptoms—a frozen shoulder, limited range of motion, and old trauma—should motivate the radiologist to obtain a dislocation view (axillary view preferred) to exclude the possibility of a chronic posterior dislocation.

◆ SUGGESTED READING

Berquist TH. Imaging of Orthopedic Trauma. New York: Raven, 1992;639–643.

Post M. The Shoulder: Surgical and Non-Surgical Management. Philadelphia: Lea & Febiger, 1988;550–566.

CASE 7

Andrew J. Collins

HISTORY

A 29-year-old man who presents with left heel pain as well as pain and swelling of multiple fingers. On physical examination, there is redness and scaling of the skin in the right groin.

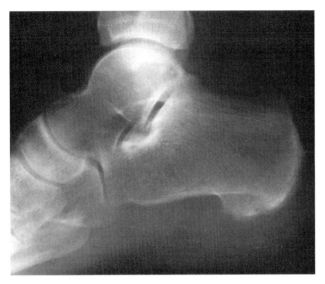

FIGURE 5-7A Lateral radiograph of the left heel. There is an erosion of the calcaneus at the plantar fascia insertion site with associated proliferative changes.

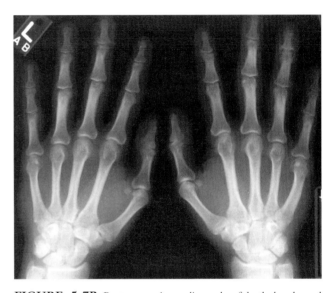

FIGURE 5-7B Posteroanterior radiograph of both hands and wrists. There is soft-tissue swelling in multiple digits, with fairly diffuse swelling noted in the right thumb, index finger, middle finger, and left index finger. There is erosion of the acral tuft of the right thumb. The right fourth distal interphalangeal joint reveals uniform space narrowing, marginal erosions with proliferative changes, central erosions, and soft-tissue swelling. Bone density appears preserved. There is erosion of the left first interphalangeal joint at the base of the distal phalanx.

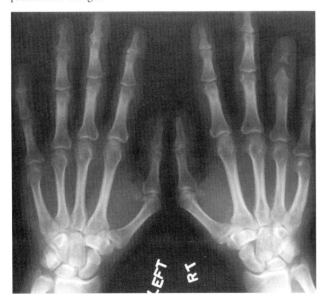

FIGURE 5-7C Posteroanterior radiograph of both hands and wrists 4 years later. There is progression of disease, with extensive destruction of bone in the periarticular and para-articular regions of the fourth distal interphalangeal joint with pencil-in-cup deformity, telescoping of the digit, and sausage digit soft-tissue swelling. Multiple other distal interphalangeal joints are now involved with less severe inflammatory arthritis.

◆ DIFFERENTIAL DIAGNOSIS

◆ **Reiter's syndrome:** Calcaneal erosions with proliferative changes at the plantar fascia insertion site in a male patient make Reiter's syndrome an important consideration. The arthritis of Reiter's syndrome, however, more typically involves the lower extremities. Skin abnormalities that may be encountered include keratoderma blennorrhagica (reddened palms and soles) and balanitis (penile rash).

◆ **Ankylosing spondylitis:** This diagnosis is unlikely given the extent of inflammatory arthritis of the peripheral appendicular skeleton and no history of sacroiliitis, spine disease, or hip or shoulder disease.

◆ **Rheumatoid arthritis:** The extensive and predominant distal interphalangeal (DIP) involvement, reactive proliferative changes, and preservation of bone density are all atypical for rheumatoid arthritis, making this diagnosis unlikely.

◆ **Psoriatic arthritis:** This is the favored diagnosis given the predominant involvement of DIP joints, presence of erosions with reactive proliferative bone formation, the preservation of bone mineral density, and findings of pencil-in-cup deformity and telescoping of the fourth digit. The skin changes are also consistent with psoriatic disease.

◆ **Septic arthritis:** This disorder is unlikely because it most commonly involves a single joint. Septic arthritis, however, can occur secondarily in a joint affected by a noninfectious inflammatory arthritis.

◆ DIAGNOSIS: Psoriatic arthritis.

◆ KEY FACTS

CLINICAL

◆ The arthritis usually is diagnosed *after* the skin condition develops. Typical skin findings include a scaly, micaceous rash involving extensor surfaces.

◆ Nail abnormalities such as pitting are common in patients with psoriatic arthritis.

◆ Of patients with psoriatic arthritis, 25% to 60% are HLA-B27 positive.

RADIOLOGIC

◆ The hands are the most common target site, with many cases showing predominant involvement of DIP joints.

◆ Erosions typically have proliferative change associated with them, which may give a "Mickey Mouse ears" appearance or a shaggy, frayed, irregular border to the erosions.

◆ Bone density is typically preserved.

◆ Acro-osteolysis may occur.

◆ Classic deformities include pencil-in-cup deformity and telescoping of digits. Subluxations, dislocations, swan neck deformities, or boutonniere deformities may also occur.

◆ Aggressive central erosions may result in joint space widening.

◆ The axial skeleton may be involved, with bilateral symmetrical or bilateral asymmetrical sacroiliitis and non-marginal asymmetric syndesmophyte formation at the discovertebral joints of the spine.

◆ SUGGESTED READING

Brower AC. Arthritis in Black and White. Philadelphia: Saunders, 1988;167–184.

Resnick D, Niwayama G. Diagnosis of Bone and Joint Disorders (2nd ed). Philadelphia: Saunders, 1988;1171–1198.

HISTORY

A 21-year-old man who was a restrained passenger in a head-on collision with another vehicle.

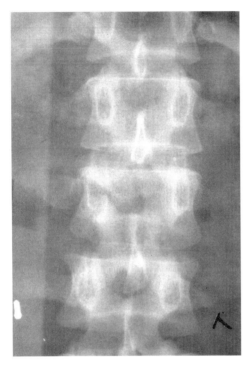

FIGURE 5-8A Anteroposterior radiograph of the lumbar spine. There is a subtle horizontal lucency through the right pedicle of L2.

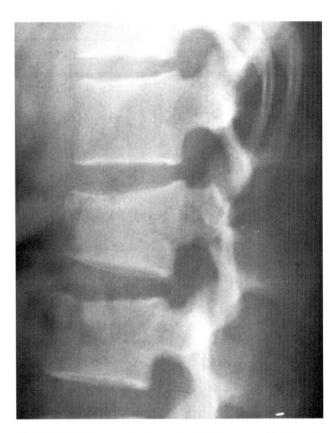

FIGURE 5-8B Lateral radiograph of the lumbar spine. There is only a minor compression fracture of the body of L2.

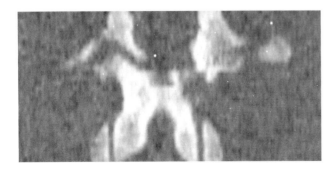

FIGURE 5-8C Axial CT scan of the lumbar spine reformatted in the coronal plane. There is a horizontally oriented fracture of the posterior elements.

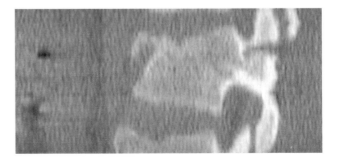

FIGURE 5-8D Axial CT scan of the lumbar spine reformatted in the sagittal plane shows both the anterior and posterior components of the fracture.

◆ DIFFERENTIAL DIAGNOSIS

◆ **Simple compression:** Minor compression fractures of the vertebral column are common but do not usually disrupt the middle or posterior columns of stability. Usually the degree of compression is <25% of the vertebral body height, and there is no evidence of retropulsion or extension of the fracture into the posterior elements.

◆ **Burst fracture:** Burst fractures are caused by an axial load on the vertebral column as would occur during a fall from a significant height. CT examination would demonstrate radial dispersion of the vertebral body fragments with retropulsion into the spinal canal.

◆ **Chance fracture:** The chance fracture is produced by a flexion-distraction mechanism. Fracture lines are typically seen extending into the posterior elements of the vertebrae on a lateral view. Characteristically, subtle bilateral pedicle fractures can be seen on the AP view and should be sought. Chance fractures sometimes produce only minimal anterior compression and can be confused with simple compression fractures when the pedicle and posterior element extension of the fracture are not appreciated.

◆ DIAGNOSIS: Chance fracture.

◆ KEY FACTS

CLINICAL

◆ Chance fractures are flexion-distraction injuries of the thoracolumbar region.

◆ They are associated with seatbelt/lapbelt restraint.

◆ There is a high association with intra-abdominal injuries.

RADIOLOGIC

◆ Chance fractures can be difficult to diagnose when undue emphasis is placed on the lateral view of the spine. The degree of vertebral compression may be slight, giving the false impression of a simple compression fracture. Regardless of the site of trauma, it is imperative to give equal time to the inspection of the AP view and lateral views in spine trauma. This is particularly true for chance fractures in which the posterior element component is often quite impressive on the AP view while unappreciated on the lateral view.

◆ Despite the substantial posterior element injury seen in chance fractures, neurologic deficits are less common than with other serious lumbar injuries such as burst fractures or fracture-dislocations of the spine.

◆ Simple compression fractures of the spine are common, and although they produce severe back pain, they do not cause neurologic injury. Simple compression fractures with <25% loss in vertical body height can be treated conservatively; additional imaging is not needed.

◆ Compression fractures >25% can be deceptive on radiographs, and CT can be helpful in excluding retropulsion of fragments, a finding that is commonly underestimated from plain film analysis.

◆ Burst fractures, regardless of their location in the spine, imply an axial load with radial dispersion of fracture fragments. An increase in the interpediculate distance on the frontal film is a key finding. This further emphasizes the importance of viewing the anteroposterior view in spinal trauma. CT and sometimes MRI are used in the evaluation of burst injuries due to the high propensity for spinal canal compromise.

◆ SUGGESTED READING

Berquist TH. Imaging of Orthopedic Trauma. New York: Raven, 1992;169–194.

Harris JH, Harris WH, Novelline RA. The Radiology of Emergency Medicine. Baltimore: Williams & Wilkins, 1993;247–280.

CASE 9

Andrew J. Collins

HISTORY

A 3-year-old boy with pain and a firm mass at the upper part of his left knee.

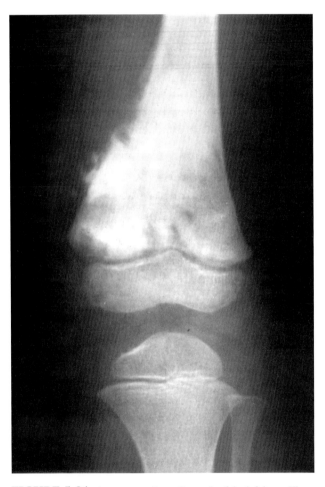

FIGURE 5-9A Anteroposterior radiograph of the left knee. There is an aggressive lesion in the distal femoral metaphysis with cumulus cloud–like mineralization and a permeative pattern of bone destruction with a wide transition zone. Medially, there is cortical destruction, a mineralized soft-tissue mass, and Codman's triangle–type periosteal reaction proximally.

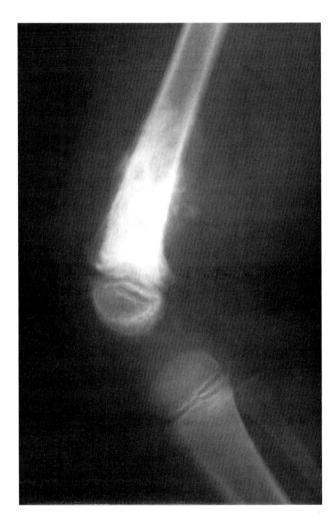

FIGURE 5-9B Lateral radiograph of the left knee. There is a soft-tissue mass at the posterior aspect of the distal femoral metaphysis with cumulus cloud–like mineralization. Fat planes are displaced posteriorly. There is multilayer periosteal reaction.

◆ DIFFERENTIAL DIAGNOSIS

◆ **Ewing's sarcoma:** In favor of this possibility is the presence of a soft-tissue mass, the multilayer or onion-skin periosteal reaction, and the fact that there is sclerosis, which is related to reactive bone formation. Ewing's sarcoma, however, more typically produces a longer diaphyseal lesion. It is excluded in this case by the presence of cumulus cloud–like malignant osteoid tumor bone mineralization in the soft tissues.

◆ **Central osteogenic sarcoma:** The location of this lesion, aggressive bone destruction, soft-tissue mass formation, and cumulus cloud–like mineralization both within the bone and in the soft-tissue mass overwhelmingly favor this diagnosis even though the patient is relatively young.

◆ **Osteomyelitis:** Osteomyelitis is typically metaphyscal and can cause bone destruction, reactive bone formation in the region of trabecular bone, and periosteal reaction that can be multilayered. However, this diagnosis is excluded because of the presence of a soft-tissue mass with malignant osteoid type mineralization and because infection would tend to make fascial planes indistinct rather than simply displace them.

◆ DIAGNOSIS: Central osteogenic sarcoma of the distal femur.

◆ KEY FACTS

CLINICAL

◆ This is the most common primary malignant tumor of bone in childhood.

◆ The patients are between 15 and 25 years of age in about 75% of cases.

◆ Approximately 70% of cases occur in long bones, and approximately 55% occur about the region of the knee.

RADIOLOGIC

◆ These tumors are typically eccentric in location and metaphyseal.

◆ Radiologic features include permeative bone destruction with cortical disruption and soft-tissue mass formation.

◆ Periosteal reaction is uncommonly present, having a "sunburst," "onion peel," "onion skin," or Codman's triangle appearance.

◆ Tumor bone formation has a cloud-like appearance, typically involving the tumor within the bone and within the soft tissue mass.

◆ MRI is the modality of choice for staging.

◆ SUGGESTED READING

Edeiken J. Roentgen Diagnosis of Diseases of the Bone (3rd ed) (Vol I). Baltimore: Williams & Wilkins, 1981;181–227.

Mirra JM, Piero P, Gold RH. Bone Tumors, Clinical, Radiologic-Pathologic Correlation. Philadelphia: Lea & Febiger, 1989;248–389.

Onikul E, Fletcher BD, Parham DM, Chen G. Accuracy of MR imaging for estimating intraosseous extent of osteosarcoma. AJR Am J Roentgenol 1996;167:1211–1215.

Sundaram M, McGuire MH, Herbold DR, et al. Magnetic resonance imaging in planning limb salvage surgery for primary malignant tumors of bone. J Bone Joint Surg Am 1986;68:809–819.

CASE 10

Salutario J. Martinez

HISTORY

A 58-year-old man with insulin-dependent diabetes mellitus presents with a several-week history of fever and an enlarging mass on the posterior aspect of his right arm.

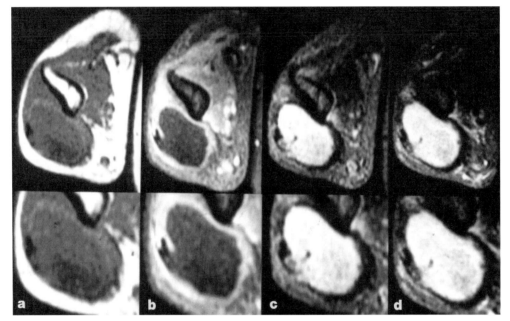

FIGURE 5-10 (a) Axial T1-weighted MRIs of the right arm. (b) Axial T1-weighted gadolinium-enhanced MRIs of the right arm with fat suppression. (c) Axial T2-weighted MRIs of the right arm. (d) Axial T2-weighted MRIs of the right arm at a slightly different level. A rim is depicted in all images that is of increased signal intensity on the T1-weighted images both pre- (a) and postcontrast (b), and of decreased signal intensity compared to muscle on the T2-weighted images (c, d). The cavity encircled by the rim is of low signal intensity on the T1-weighted images (a, b) and of high signal intensity on the T2-weighted images (c, d). These characteristics suggest the presence of fluid. The humeral marrow is normal, but edema and stranding are noted in the subcutaneous tissues on the T2-weighted images.

◆ DIFFERENTIAL DIAGNOSIS

◆ **Pyomyositis (PM):** In the case shown, the intramuscular cavitation that is hyperintense on T2-weighted image, has rim enhancement on T1-weighted postgadolinium images, and is associated with edema of adjacent tissues is consistent with the diagnosis of PM.

◆ **Neoplasm:** Tumors and PM both present clinically as a mass. Malignant tumors may have central necrosis that could be confused with PM. Sarcomas are limited to a compartment and are not associated with cellulitis unless they have been treated with radiation or a biopsy has been performed. PM is a diffuse process that extends beyond the compartments involving the subcutaneous fat and the skin. Soft-tissue lymphomatous masses may be diffuse and involve the subcutaneous fat, but they do not cavitate like PM.

◆ **Hematoma:** In most instances, there is a clear history of trauma, and blood components are seen (not present in this case). Central cavitation with rim enhancement is not a feature of traumatic lesions.

◆ **Myonecrosis:** This is a very rare complication of diabetes mellitus secondary to small vessel disease. Rim enhancement is not a feature of this condition.

◆ **Myositis:** There are numerous conditions associated with myositis, particularly the connective tissue diseases. These conditions produce multiple lesions that do not cavitate, making this an incorrect diagnosis.

◆ DIAGNOSIS: Pyomyositis.

◆ KEY FACTS

CLINICAL

◆ PM is a primary bacterial infection involving skeletal muscles. It is also known as *tropical PM* because it is endemic to warm climates. However, incidence of PM is increasing in temperate countries as well.

◆ PM tends to occur in the large muscles of the lower extremities.

◆ It is caused by *Staphylococcus aureus* in 90% of cases.

◆ Contributing factors include trauma, diabetes mellitus, human immunodeficiency virus (HIV) infection, chronic steroid use, connective tissue disorders, history of malignancy, and various hematologic disorders.

◆ PM has a predictable clinical course that consists of four stages. Stage 1 has a characteristic insidious onset with diffuse pain and swelling. In stage 2, there is progressive pain and enlargement of the extremity. Stage 3 denotes suppuration, and stage 4, resolution. Alternatively, progression to shock and death occurs in 2% of patients.

◆ Most PM cases are treated with surgical drainage and appropriate intravenous antibiotics.

RADIOLOGIC

◆ Plain radiographs are nondiagnostic in most instances. On occasion, they may show an associated osteomyelitis.

◆ On nuclear scintigraphy, the blood pool phase may demonstrate nonspecific muscular uptake. Late images demonstrate osseous uptake in cases with osteomyelitis.

◆ Ultrasound may detect and localize the process and demonstrate the presence of cavitation.

◆ Contrast-enhanced CT defines the abscess wall by the presence of rim enhancement. PM very often is associated with cellulitis, which on CT is seen as skin thickening, stranding of subcutaneous fat, blurring of intramuscular fat and fascial planes, and distention of subcutaneous veins.

◆ MRI is best for assessing the extent and location of the process and the presence or absence of osteomyelitis. Contrast-enhanced T1-weighted images often depict rim enhancement of the abscess. The rim of the abscess may be of subtle increased signal intensity in comparison with the rest of the muscle on T1-weighted images even before contrast material administration. The central collection of pus is hypointense to adjacent muscles on T1-weighted images. T2-weighted images are characterized by a diffuse increase in signal intensity in all involved muscles, very high signal intensity within the central fluid collection, a rim of low signal intensity, and increased signal intensity in the fascia, subcutaneous fat, and skin consistent with edema and cellulitis. The distal joint may also reveal an effusion.

◆ SUGGESTED READING

Gordon BA, Martinez S, Collins AJ. Pyomyositis: Characteristics at CT and MR imaging. Radiology 1995;197:279–286.

HISTORY

A 14-year-old boy with left hip pain. He has no history of trauma.

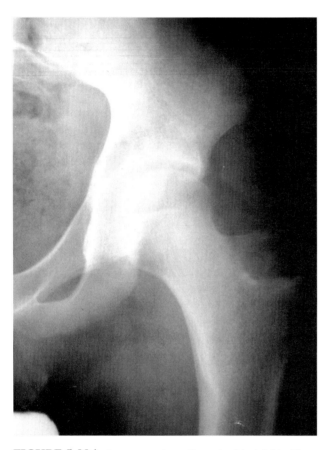

FIGURE 5-11A Anteroposterior radiograph of the left hip. There is a lucent expansile lesion of the apophysis of the left greater trochanter with a thin sclerotic margin. Thick periosteal reaction is present away from the lesion along the medial proximal metadiaphysis.

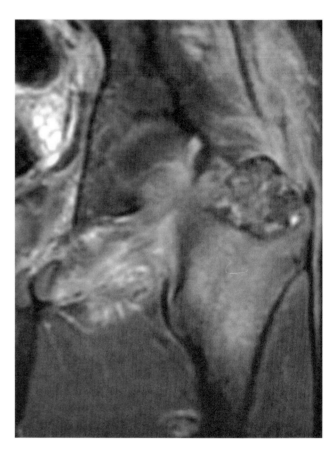

FIGURE 5-11B Coronal T2-weighted MRI of the left hip. There is a well-circumscribed lesion of the left greater trochanter of predominantly low signal intensity containing a few cystic foci of increased signal intensity. The adjacent marrow and muscles demonstrate diffuse increased signal intensity related to edema.

◆ DIFFERENTIAL DIAGNOSIS

- **Brodie's abscess:** This process is usually localized to the metaphysis. Extensive bone destruction and the presence of marrow and muscle edema are uncommon in this subacute infection.
- **Eosinophilic granuloma:** These lesions are most often metaphyseal and multifocal with less marrow and muscle edema.
- **Aneurysmal bone cyst (ABC):** The expansile radiographic appearance favors this diagnosis but would not account for the marrow and muscle edema.
- **Chondroblastoma:** This is essentially the only tumor to involve the greater trochanter, and may have an aneurysmatic component with edema of adjacent muscle and marrow. The radiographic and MRI features and the patient's age are most consistent with a chondroblastoma and a secondary ABC.
- **Clear cell chondrosarcoma:** These tumors mimic chondroblastomas and are usually found in older patients. They most often involve the femoral head and are not typically aneurysmal.

◆ DIAGNOSIS: Chondroblastoma of the greater trochanteric apophysis with secondary aneurysmal bone cyst.

◆ KEY FACTS

CLINICAL

- Chondroblastoma is a benign cartilaginous tumor comprising <1% of all primary bone tumors.
- Its incidence is intermediate among other benign cartilaginous tumors; it is more common than chondromyxoid fibroma but rarer than enchondroma or osteochondroma.
- The second decade of life is the most common age of presentation (70%). The male-to-female ratio is 3 to 1.
- Symptoms are nonspecific and include pain referred to the joint adjacent to the lesion.

- Curettage and bone grafting is the treatment of choice.
- Local recurrence can occur following surgery. However, malignant transformation is rare.

RADIOLOGIC

- Chondroblastoma is a geographic lucent lesion with thin sclerotic margins arising eccentrically in an epiphysis or apophysis, with or without extension into the metaphysis.
- The most common sites of involvement, in descending order, are the epiphyses of the distal femur, proximal tibia, proximal humerus, and apophysis of the greater trocanter. Occurrence in the greater trochanter is three times more common than in the femoral head.
- Detectable punctate calcified chondroid matrix is found in 60% of patients.
- Up to 60% of patients have benign-appearing periosteal reaction away from the lesion in the adjacent metadiaphysis.
- On MRI, chondroblastomas have a lobulated margin. The signal intensity characteristics are distinct from those of hyaline cartilage (i.e., enchondroma). Chondroblastomas appear homogeneously isointense to muscle on T1-weighted images and heterogeneously hypo- or isointense to fat on T2-weighted images. However, the 10% to 15% of chondroblastomas with an associated ABC are characterized by scattered foci of high signal intensity on T2-weighted images.

◆ SUGGESTED READING

Brower AC, Moser RP, Gilkey FW, Kransdorf MJ. Chondroblastoma. In RP Moser (ed), Cartilaginous Tumors of the Skeleton. AFIP Atlas of Radiologic-Pathologic Correlation. Fascicle II. Philadelphia: Hanley & Belfus, 1990;74–113.

Brower AC, Moser RP, Kransdorf MJ. The frequency and diagnostic significance of periostitis in chondroblastoma. AJR Am J Roentgenol 1990;154:309–314.

Weatherall PT, Maale GE, Mendelsohn DB, et al. Chondroblastoma: Classic and confusing appearance at MR imaging. Radiology 1994;190:467–474.

CASE 12

Charles E. Spritzer

HISTORY

A 19-year-old woman with an acute injury to the knee.

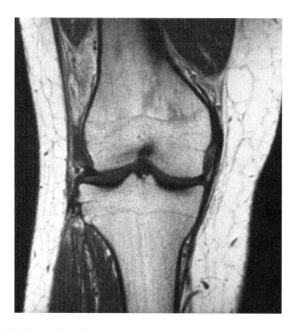

FIGURE 5-12A Coronal T1-weighted MRI of the knee. The body of the medial meniscus appears truncated. There also appear to be meniscal fragments within the intercondylar notch.

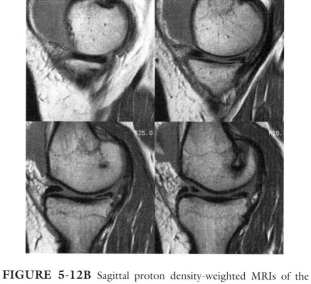

FIGURE 5-12B Sagittal proton density-weighted MRIs of the knee. The abnormal appearance of the medial meniscus suggests two anterior horns.

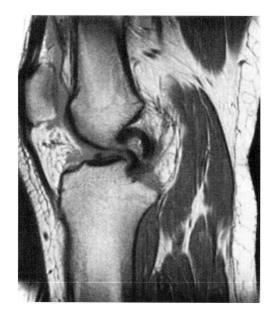

FIGURE 5-12C Sagittal proton density-weighted MRI through the intercondylar notch. There appear to be two posterior cruciate ligaments (PCL) within the intercondylar notch.

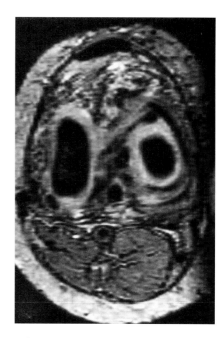

FIGURE 5-12D Axial reformatted three-dimensional gradient echo MRI of the knee. An attenuated body of the medial meniscus is seen, with meniscal material extending into the intercondylar notch.

◆ DIFFERENTIAL DIAGNOSIS

- **Prior arthroscopic meniscectomy:** Meniscal material in the intercondylar notch following an arthroscopy would not be expected. Furthermore, the patient has no history of arthroscopic surgery.
- **Bucket handle meniscal tear:** The body of the medial meniscus is truncated and in direct continuity with meniscal material in the intercondylar notch. On the axial view, the bucket and its handle can be visualized as it extends into the intercondylar notch.
- **Loose osteochondral fragments:** The linear appearance of the loose fragment is more in keeping with a meniscal fragment than osteochondral bodies, which are typically round or oval in shape. In addition, no donor site is seen on the available images.
- **Anterior cruciate ligament (ACL) injury:** The linear shape of the fragment does not exclude an ACL tear. However, meniscal tears of this type are _not_ typically associated with ACL injury.

◆ DIAGNOSIS: Bucket handle meniscal tear.

◆ KEY FACTS

CLINICAL

- This type of meniscal injury may be associated with rotation of either the femur or the tibia.
- There may be associated pain and effusion.
- Patients often present with a locked knee or inability to extend the knee fully.

RADIOLOGIC

- A thinned and somewhat truncated appearance to the body of the meniscus extending into the posterior horn is characteristic. There may be foreshortening of the posterior horn without a history of prior arthroscopy.
- Careful examination of the intercondylar notch typically reveals the sheared component of the meniscus. This is often seen beneath the ACL or posterior cruciate ligament (PCL) (as in this case, Figure 5-12C), producing the double PCL or double ACL sign.
- In the descriptive term "bucket handle tear," the posterior horn and body of the meniscus in anatomic position are analogous to a bucket, whereas the portion of the meniscus in the notch is analogous to a bucket handle.
- Tears may also be present within the handle.

◆ SUGGESTED READING

Stoller D, Dillworth W, Anderson LJ. The Knee. In D Stoller (ed), Magnetic Resonance Imaging in Orthopaedics and Sports Medicine. Philadelphia: Lippincott, 1995;139–372.

HISTORY

A 45-year-old man who was lifting a heavy object when he heard and felt a pop in his right shoulder.

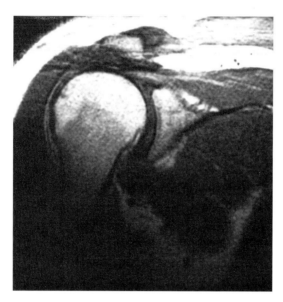

FIGURE 5-13A Oblique coronal T1-weighted MRI of the shoulder. The humeral head is slightly high riding.

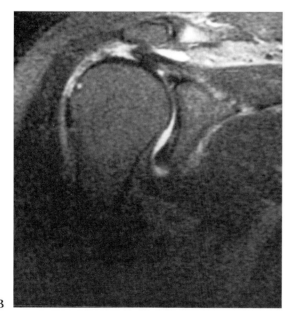

B

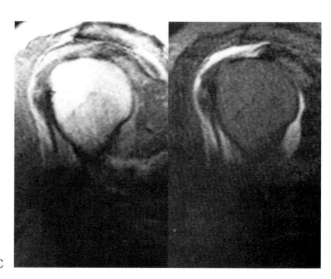

C

FIGURES 5-13B and 5-13C Oblique coronal T2-weighted MRI (**B**) and oblique sagittal proton density (left) and T2-weighted (right) MRIs (**C**) of the shoulder. Fluid is identified in the subacromial/subdeltoid bursa. There is high signal intensity equivalent to fluid in the expected position of the supraspinatus tendon. The normal low signal intensity of the tendon terminates abruptly 4 cm from its expected insertion on the humeral head.

◆ DIFFERENTIAL DIAGNOSIS

- **Complete tear of the rotator cuff tendon:** The constellation of findings is consistent with this diagnosis. There is abrupt termination of the low signal intensity in the supraspinatus tendon just beneath the acromion. This is associated with some muscle retraction. At the expected point of insertion of the supraspinatus tendon on the humeral head, there is high signal intensity approaching that of fluid. In addition, fluid is seen in the subacromial/subdeltoid bursa.
- **Partial tear of the rotator cuff tendon:** In the case shown, a full- rather than a partial-thickness tear is present, as evidenced by high signal intensity equal to the width of the supraspinatus tendon. The abrupt cut-off of the low signal intensity in the normal tendon implies a complete, not partial, tear.
- **Tendinopathy:** While tendinopathy may show slightly increased signal intensity on T2-weighted images, it should not be equal to the signal intensity of fluid and usually does not involve the entire tendon width.
- **Bursitis:** Bursitis could produce fluid in the subacromion-subdeltoid bursa, but the fluid would not be expected to extend into the glenohumeral space in the presence of an intact rotator cuff tendon.

◆ DIAGNOSIS: Complete tear of the rotator cuff tendon.

◆ KEY FACTS

CLINICAL

- Neer believed that impingement and rotator cuff tears represent a continuum from less severe to most severe injury. The latter is associated with increasing age and repetitive activity.
- Impingement is presumed to lead to edema and hemorrhage, which are reversible changes within the rotator cuff (stage I). Continued use of the shoulder causes more fibrosis and tendinitis (stage II), finally resulting in a complete or partial tear (stage III).
- Other investigators have suggested that since bursal site injuries are more common, rotator cuff tears may represent tensile strength failure from overuse. However, both theories suggest that it is a combination of mechanical factors, repetitive use, age, and associated degeneration of the cuff.

RADIOLOGIC

- The findings of rotator cuff tears include full-thickness tendon defect with fluid signal intensity on T2-weighted images, retraction, tendon atrophy, and fluid within the subacromial/subdeltoid bursa.
- According to Farley et al., a full-thickness tendon defect with fluid signal intensity on T2-weighted imaging, the accuracy of MR imaging in detecting full thickness tears is approximately 90%.
- Other associated findings include a hook (type 3) acromion, posterior-to-anterior downward sloping of the acromion, acromioclavicular joint degeneration, and a thickened coracoacromion ligament with or without associated spur formation.

◆ SUGGESTED READING

Farley TE, Neumann CH, Steinbach LS, et al. Full thickness tears of the rotator cuff of the shoulder: Diagnosis with MR imaging. AJR Am J Roentgenol 1992;158:347–351.

Neer CS. Anterior acromioplasty for the chronic impingement syndrome: A preliminary report. J Bone Joint Surg Am 1972;54:41.

Rafii M, Firooznia H, Sherman O, et al. Rotator cuff lesions: Signal patterns at MR imaging. Radiology 1990;177:817–823.

Stoller DW, Wolfe EM. The Shoulder. In DW Stoller (ed), Magnetic Resonance Imaging in Orthopaedics and Sports Medicine. Philadelphia: Lippincott, 1993;511–632.

CASE 14

Charles E. Spritzer

HISTORY

A 47-year-old man with a history of right hip pain.

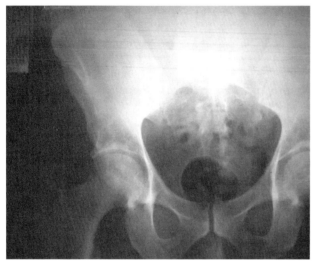

FIGURE 5-14A Anteroposterior supine radiograph of the pelvis. There are no abnormalities in either hip on this plain radiograph.

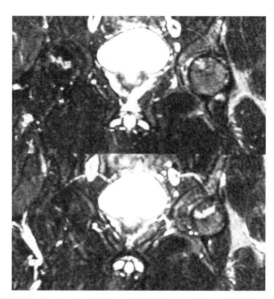

FIGURE 5-14B Coronal T2-weighted MRIs of the hips. High signal intensity lines are seen. These high signal intensity bands are adjacent to low signal intensity bands ("double line" sign) that are more conspicuous in Figures 5-14C and 5-14D. Small joint effusions are appreciated, although these are better seen on images not shown here.

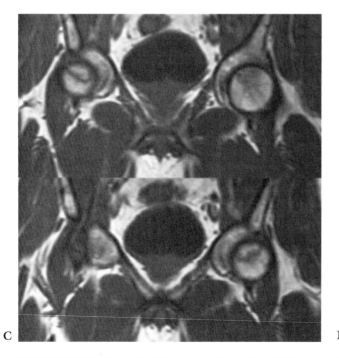

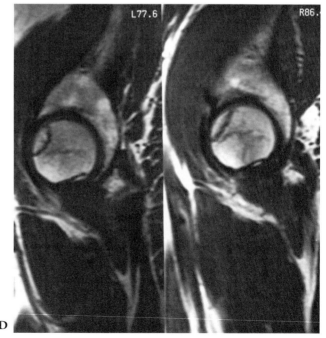

FIGURES 5-14C and 5-14D Coronal T1-weighted MRIs of both hips (**C**) and sagittal T1-weighted MRIs of the right hip (**D**). Serpiginous bands of decreased signal intensity are seen in both femoral heads.

◆ DIFFERENTIAL DIAGNOSIS

- **Osteoarthritis:** While subcortical cysts associated with osteoarthritis may have areas of high signal intensity on T2-weighted images, the absence of plain film findings and lack of changes on the acetabular side of the joint argue against this diagnosis.
- **Osteochondral injury:** The bilaterality of this process would be atypical for an osteochondral injury. The osseous abnormalities also appear farther away from the articular surface than would be expected. Osteochondral injuries would be expected to be associated with secondary degenerative changes, given the size of the abnormality in each femoral head.
- **Inflammatory arthritides:** This diagnosis is unlikely given preservation of the joint space on the plain film and the constellation of findings on MRI.
- **Avascular necrosis (AVN):** Preservation of the articular surface plus the underlying bony abnormalities are consistent with this diagnosis.

◆ DIAGNOSIS: Avascular necrosis of both femoral heads.

◆ KEY FACTS

CLINICAL

- AVN is a consequence of vascular injury resulting in bone death.
- The causes of AVN are numerous, including drugs such as corticosteroids and ethanol, marrow replacement processes such as sickle cell disease and Gaucher's disease, radiation- or lupus-induced vasculitis, and embolic etiologies including emboli secondary to trauma or Caisson disease. Other etiologies, in which the pathophysiology is less well understood, include idiopathic disease, Legg-Perthes disease, and pancreatitis.
- Early diagnosis (i.e., before plain radiographs demonstrate collapse and subcondylar lucency) is associated with less morbidity.

- Standard treatment consists of a decompression procedure. More recently, the placement of vascularized grafts has been used.

RADIOLOGIC

- MRI has been shown to be more sensitive than both radionuclide imaging and CT for the detection of early AVN. This is important since early intervention in these patients is associated with a better prognosis.
- Abnormalities typically occur in the weight-bearing region of the femoral head. The process is bilateral in 40% of cases.
- A well-demarcated serpiginous band of low signal intensity is seen on all pulse sequences and is visualized in approximately 90% of cases. In many cases, T2-weighted images reveal a band of increased signal intensity along the inner margin of this low signal intensity band. This is the so-called "double line" sign of AVN. It is unclear at present whether this represents a true reactive interface between viable and ischemic tissue or simply chemical shift artifact.
- Other associations with AVN include hip effusions (seen in 85% of cases) and early conversion of hematopoietic marrow to fatty marrow, especially in men.

◆ SUGGESTED READING

Coleman BG, Kressel HY, Dalinka MK, et al. Radiographically negative avascular necrosis: Detection with MR imaging. Radiology 1988;168:525–528.

Glickstein MF, Burk DL Jr, Schiebler ML, et al. Avascular necrosis versus other diseases of the hip: Sensitivity of MR imaging. Radiology 1988;169:213–215.

Mitchell DG, Kressel HY, Arger PH, et al. Avascular necrosis of the femoral head: Morphologic evaluation with MRI and CT correlation. Radiology 1986;161:739–742.

Mitchell DG, Kundel JL, Steinberg ME, et al. Avascular necrosis of the hip: Comparison of MR, CT and scintigraphy. AJR Am J Roentgenol 1986;147:67–71.

Mitchell DG, Rao VM, Dalinka M, et al. The distribution of hematopoietic and fatty marrow in the normal and ischemic hip: New observations with 1.5 Telsa MRI. Radiology 1986;161:191–202.

CASE 15

Charles E. Spritzer

HISTORY

A 28-year-old man who twisted and injured his knee.

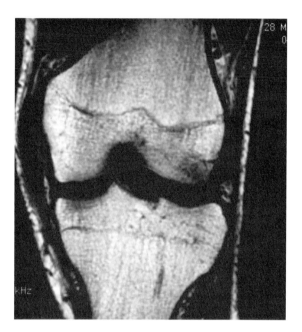

FIGURE 5-15A Coronal T1-weighted MRI of the knee. There is abnormal thickening of the medial collateral ligament consistent with a tear. A small bone bruise is noted as an area of decreased signal intensity in the lateral femoral condyle.

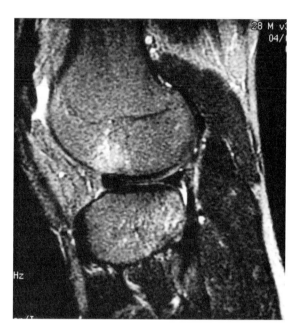

FIGURE 5-15B Sagittal T2-weighted MRI of the knee. High signal intensity consistent with bone bruises of the lateral femoral condyle and lateral tibial plateau is noted.

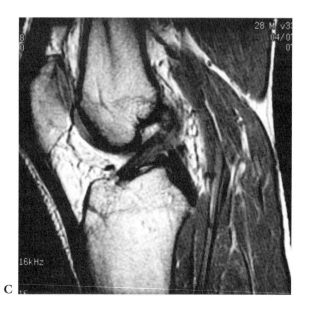

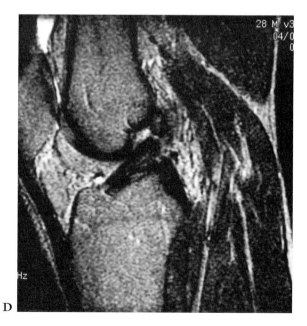

FIGURES 5-15C and 5-15D Sagittal proton density-weighted (**C**) and sagittal T2-weighted (**D**) MRIs of the knee. There is discontinuity and high signal intensity within the anterior cruciate ligament.

◆ DIFFERENTIAL DIAGNOSIS

- **Osteochondral injury of the lateral femoral condyle:** This diagnosis is unlikely as the overlying cartilage appears grossly intact. In addition, the pattern of edema is more in keeping with an acute injury rather than a more chronic insult. Finally, this diagnosis does not explain the other observed abnormalities.
- **Acute tear of the anterior cruciate ligament (ACL):** There is discontinuity of the ACL with associated edema. Other findings in keeping with an acute injury include the bone bruises that occur on both the femoral condyle and the tibial plateau laterally. In addition, the edema surrounding the medial collateral ligament (MCL) injury and the joint effusion suggest an acute injury.
- **Chronic tear of the ACL:** While the ACL is indeed torn, the high signal intensity within it and the high signal intensity within the lateral osseous structures on T2-weighted images suggest an acute injury.
- **Sprain of the ACL:** While there is certainly either or both edema and hemorrhage within the ACL, the discontinuity proves that this is more than just a simple sprain.

◆ DIAGNOSIS: Acute tear of the anterior cruciate ligament.

◆ KEY FACTS

CLINICAL

- The classic mechanism of ACL injury is external rotation of a minimally flexed femur on a fixed tibia.
- In addition to nonspecific pain and swelling, the patient often remembers a "popping" sensation during the traumatic insult.
- A positive drawer or Lochman's sign may be present. In patients with either or both acute pain and muscle spasms, these signs may be difficult to elicit.

RADIOLOGIC

- The normal ACL has low signal intensity on all pulse sequences. Discontinuity of the ACL confirms the diagnosis.
- Thickening of the ACL with high signal intensity within its fibers and around the ACL also indicate tendon injury. The high signal intensity may look like a mass adjacent to the femoral attachment of the ACL, aptly named the "bulge" sign. The overall accuracy of MRI in determining the presence of ACL injury is 95%.
- Osseous injuries are typically associated with acute tears of the ACL. In one study, 83% of patients with ACL injuries had "bone bruises" directly over the lateral femoral condyle terminal sulcus, and 96% had posterolateral joint injury involving the tibia.
- As with the ACL, discontinuity of the MCL is indicative of MCL injury. In 30% of MCL tears, there is a concomitant ACL injury.

◆ SUGGESTED READING

Berquist TH. MRI of the Musculoskeletal System (2nd ed). New York: Raven, 1990;195–252.

Feagin JA Jr. The Crucial Ligaments (2nd ed). New York: Churchill Livingstone, 1994;1–38.

Mink JH, Levy T, Crues JV III. Tears of the anterior cruciate ligament and menisci of the knee: MR imaging evaluation. Radiology 1988;167:769–774.

Speer KP, Spritzer CE, Bassett FH III, et al. Osseous injury associated with acute tears of the anterior cruciate ligament. Am J Sports Med 1992;20:382–389.

Stoller D, Dillworth W, Anderson LJ. The Knee. In D Stoller (ed), Magnetic Resonance Imaging in Orthopaedic and Sports Medicine. Philadelphia: Lippincott, 1995;139–372.

CASE 16

Charles E. Spritzer

HISTORY

A 16-year-old boy with knee pain and swelling. Plain films (not shown) are normal, with the exception of a joint effusion.

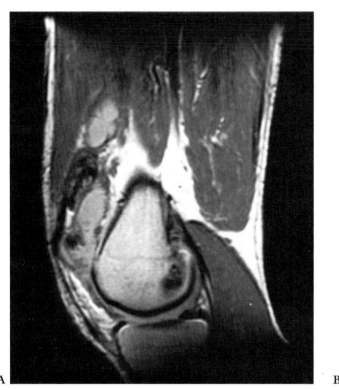 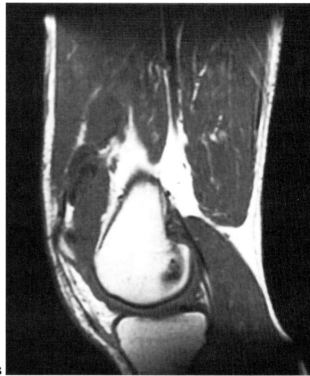

A   B

FIGURE 5-16 Sagittal T1-weighted (**A**) and sagittal T2-weighted (**B**) MRIs of the knee. A joint effusion is seen. On all pulse sequences, there are areas of decreased signal intensity within the synovium that protrude into the suprapatellar bursa. No osseous abnormalities are present. Plain films (not shown) did not show calcifications around the joint space.

◆ DIFFERENTIAL DIAGNOSIS

- **Synovial sarcoma:** These tumors are often para-articular and associated with calcifications in one-third of cases (none was present on the plain film in this case). The decreased signal intensity within the synovium is not typical of a sarcoma.
- **Synovial chondromatosis:** With this entity, calcifications are typically visualized on plain film. In addition, multiple nodules should be seen. In this case, the abnormality is synovial-based and not multinodular.
- **Rheumatoid arthritis:** This entity is a synovial process that may contain hemorrhage. However, it is not typically a mono-articular arthritis. This patient had no other symptoms.
- **Synovial hemangioma:** This entity may have a similar appearance to the case shown here, although the plain films often reveal phleboliths. They are commonly associated with adjacent hemangiomas, which are not identified in this case.
- **Pigmented villonodular synovitis (PVNS):** This typically produces a nodular pattern with areas of hemorrhage and hemosiderin deposition, as seen in this case.

◆ DIAGNOSIS: Pigmented villonodular synovitis.

◆ KEY FACTS

CLINICAL

- PVNS is an uncommon synovial abnormality of unknown etiology. It is not felt to represent a neoplastic condition, but whether it is an inflammatory or hyperplastic process due to an unknown stimulus or the consequence of repeated trauma and hemorrhage is controversial.
- PVNS is almost always a monoarticular process. The knee is the most frequently affected joint, involved in 66% to 80% of all cases.

- The typical presentation of PVNS is pain, swelling, and decreased range of motion.
- When fluid is aspirated from the joint, it is usually serosanguineous, although it may be yellow or chocolate brown in 30% of cases.

RADIOLOGIC

- On plain films, a joint effusion is typically seen. The effusion may be of increased density due to hemosiderin deposition.
- Bony erosions are visualized in 15% to 50% of patients, although these are less frequently seen in joints that are naturally capacious such as the knee.
- On noncontrast CT, those portions of the synovial membrane containing hemosiderin often are found to have high attenuation characteristics.
- On MRI, hemosiderin deposition results in low signal intensity on both T1- and T2-weighted spin echo images as well as on T1-weighted gradient-recalled echo acquisitions. The nodular appearance of the synovium projecting into a joint effusion is typically seen and reminiscent of the appearance seen by arthrography.

◆ SUGGESTED READING

Jelinek JS, Kransdorf MJ, Utz JA, et al. Imaging of pigmented villonodular synovitis with emphasis on MR imaging. AJR Am J Roentgenol 1989;152:337–342.

Myers BW, Masi AT. Pigmented villonodular synovitis and tenosynovitis: A clinical epidemiologic study of 166 cases and literature review. Medicine 1980;59:223–238.

Resnick DL. Diagnosis of Bone and Joint Disorders (3rd ed). Philadelphia: Saunders, 1995;3063–3065, 4565–4567.

Spritzer CE, Dalinka MK, Kressel HY. Magnetic resonance imaging of pigmented villonodular synovitis: A report of two cases. Skeletal Radiol 1987;16:316–319.

CASE *17*

D. Lawrence Burk

HISTORY

A 16-year-old girl with a mass behind her knee of several months' duration.

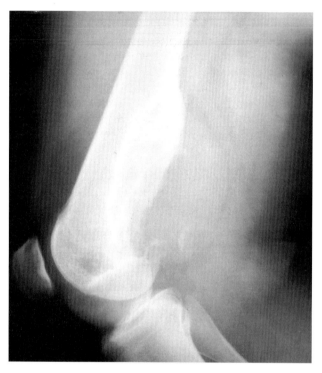

FIGURE 5-17A Lateral radiograph of the knee. There is a calcified soft-tissue mass along the posterior aspect of the knee, which is outlined by a popliteal fat plane posteriorly. The posterior cortex of the distal femoral metaphysis is remodeled, and periosteal elevation is seen at the superior aspect of the mass.

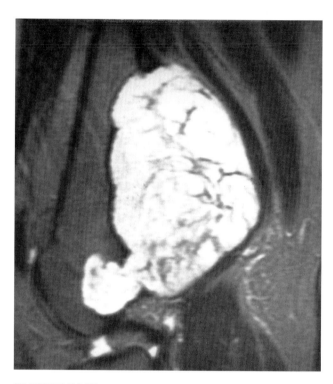

FIGURE 5-17B Sagittal T2-weighted MRI of the knee. The mass demonstrates high signal intensity except for central curvilinear fibrous tissue, which is of low signal intensity. Extension of the tumor into the epiphysis is seen, which was not evident on the radiograph.

◆ DIFFERENTIAL DIAGNOSIS

- **Parosteal sarcoma:** This form of osteosarcoma frequently occurs in this location but demonstrates central ossification rather than calcification. The tumor is usually connected to the underlying cortex by a narrow stalk.
- **Chondrosarcoma:** Central calcification, high signal intensity on T2-weighted MRI, and cauliflower morphology are consistent with a cartilaginous tumor. The large size and marrow invasion indicate a malignant process.
- **Periosteal chondroma:** The periosteal location and high signal intensity on T2-weighted MRI would be typical for this benign lesion. The lesions are usually much smaller in size, however, with infrequent calcification and no cortical invasion.
- **Periosteal Ewing's sarcoma:** Saucerization of cortex may yield a similar radiographic appearance to that seen in this case. Calcification within the soft-tissue component, however, would not be expected.

◆ DIAGNOSIS: Peripheral chondrosarcoma.

◆ KEY FACTS

CLINICAL

- Chondrosarcomas occur most often in the femur, pelvis, humerus, ribs, and scapula.
- These tumors are most commonly seen in elderly men.
- Secondary chondrosarcomas may arise from a pre-existing benign cartilaginous lesion.
- The incidence of malignancy is increased in hereditary multiple exostoses and in enchondromatosis (Ollier's disease).

RADIOLOGIC

- Chondrosarcomas are classified as central or peripheral depending on the location with respect to the medullary cavity.
- MRI frequently shows these tumors to have a lobulated morphology with a high water content due to the hyaline cartilage matrix.
- Differentiation between benign enchondroma or osteochondroma and chondrosarcoma cannot be made on the basis of the MR signal intensity characteristic alone. Secondary signs of malignancy such as cortical destruction and the presence of a soft-tissue mass may be helpful in making this distinction.

◆ SUGGESTED READING

Cohen EK, Kressel HY, Frank TS, et al. Hyaline cartilage-origin bone and soft-tissue neoplasms: MR appearance and histologic correlation. Radiology 1988;167:477–481.

Kenan S, Abdelwahab IF, Klein MJ, Herman G. Lesions of juxtacortical origin (surface lesions of bone). Skeletal Radiol 1993;22: 337–357.

Varma DGK, Ayala AG, Carrasco CH, et al. Chondrosarcoma: MR imaging with pathologic correlation. Radiographics 1992;12:687–704.

HISTORY

A 19-year-old man who lifts weights has persistent pain in his right shoulder.

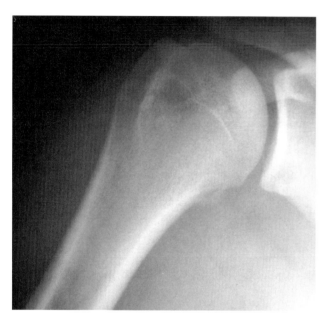

FIGURE 5-18A Anteroposterior radiograph of the right shoulder. A small cortical lesion is seen in the medial proximal humerus, with associated ill-defined periosteal reaction.

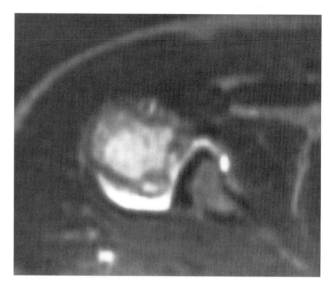

FIGURE 5-18B Axial T2-weighted MRI of the right shoulder. A focal, well-circumscribed, oval lesion is present in the posterior medial cortex of the humerus. The signal intensity in the adjacent bone marrow of the humerus is higher than in the glenoid, and there is a large joint effusion.

◆ DIFFERENTIAL DIAGNOSIS

- **Stress fracture:** Focal periosteal reaction without a visible fracture line suggests the possibility of a stress-related injury. Bone marrow edema may be much more extensive than the size of the cortical abnormality.
- **Osteomyelitis:** Bone marrow involvement and ill-defined metaphyseal periosteal reaction could represent evidence of infection. A joint effusion would also raise the possibility of septic arthritis.
- **Ewing's sarcoma:** Periosteal reaction could be an early sign of malignancy. A nidus can be overlooked in the presence of extensive bone marrow abnormality.
- **Osteoid osteoma:** In the case shown, a noncalcified nidus is seen surrounded by reactive bone marrow edema. The periarticular location is associated with a reactive joint effusion. This is the most likely diagnosis.

◆ DIAGNOSIS: Osteoid osteoma.

◆ KEY FACTS

CLINICAL
- The typical history is chronic pain that is worse at night.
- The pain is usually relieved by aspirin.
- Osteoid osteomas occur in children and young adults.
- Periarticular lesions may present with premature arthritis due to chronic reactive synovitis.

RADIOLOGIC
- The nidus, which may be calcified, can be identified more effectively with CT than MRI.
- Inflammatory changes can be present in adjacent bone marrow and soft tissue, which may mistakenly be taken as evidence of malignancy.
- Radiographs often show reactive bony sclerosis and periosteal reaction.

◆ SUGGESTED READING

Assoun J, Richardi G, Railhac J-J, et al. Osteoid osteoma: MR imaging versus CT. Radiology 1994;191:217–223.

Hayes CW, Conway WF, Sundaram M. Misleading aggressive MR imaging appearance of some benign musculoskeletal lesions. Radiographics 1992;12:1119–1134.

CASE 19

Robert M. Vandemark

HISTORY

A 49-year-old man who fell from a ladder onto his outstretched left hand.

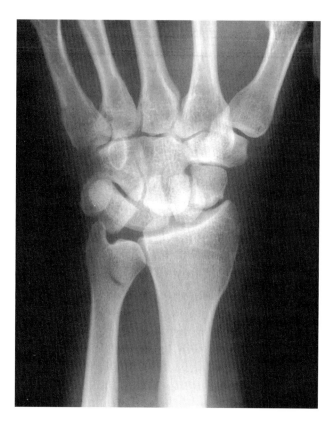

FIGURE 5-19A Posteroanterior radiograph of the left wrist. There is discontinuity of the normal carpal arcs and a displaced scaphoid waist fracture.

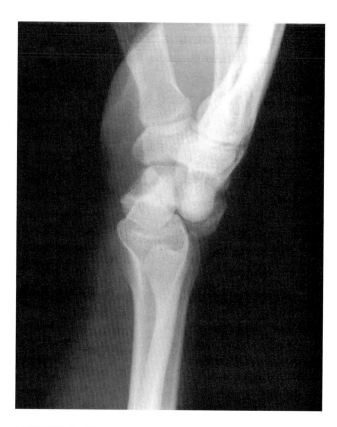

FIGURE 5-19B Lateral radiograph of the left wrist. The lunate and proximal scaphoid fragments remain aligned with the radius, while all other carpal bones are dislocated dorsally.

◆DIFFERENTIAL DIAGNOSIS

- **Isolated lunate dislocation:** This injury can be excluded by noting the position of the lunate, which is in contact with the distal radius. With isolated lunate dislocation, the capitate aligns with the radius, while the lunate is usually dislocated into the palmar aspect of the wrist.
- **Dorsal perilunate dislocation:** This diagnosis would be correct if no other carpal fractures were identified. In the illustrated case, the presence of a scaphoid fracture (or other carpal fracture) indicates a more severe fracture-dislocation.
- **Trans-scaphoid dorsal perilunate fracture-dislocation:** This injury is distinguished from dorsal perilunate dislocation by the presence of a displaced fracture through the scaphoid waist. Typically, the proximal scaphoid fragment remains in anatomic position, adjacent to the lunate, while the distal fragment travels dorsally with the remainder of the carpus.

◆DIAGNOSIS: Trans-scaphoid dorsal perilunate fracture-dislocation.

◆KEY FACTS

CLINICAL
- The typical mechanism of injury is a fall onto a hyperextended wrist.

- This type of injury usually requires open reduction, fracture fixation, and ligamentous repair.
- The synonym for this condition is *de Quervain's fracture-dislocation.*

RADIOLOGIC
- It is important to assess the scaphoid for a fracture when confronted with an apparent case of carpal dislocation.
- Fundamentally, the detection of carpal dislocations relies on recognizing the abnormal relationships of the carpal bones on properly positioned radiographs. When patients are badly injured, positioning can be difficult, with obliquity and various degrees of flexion and extension leading to distortion and misdiagnosis. If the distal radius and ulna are properly positioned on posteroanterior and lateral views, disorganization of the carpal landmarks usually will be apparent. Obscuration or overlap of the normal carpal arcs is the sine qua non of carpal fracture-dislocations.
- Long-term consequences of these injuries include chronic carpal instability, post-traumatic arthritis, and osteonecrosis when associated with a scaphoid fracture.

◆SUGGESTED READING
Berquist TH. Imaging of Orthopedic Trauma. New York: Raven, 1992;827–831.
Gilula LA, Yin Y. Imaging of the Wrist and Hand. Philadelphia: Saunders, 1996;303–309.

CASE 20

D. Lawrence Burk

HISTORY

A 17-year-old girl with a palpable mass in the distal thigh deep to the quadriceps muscle.

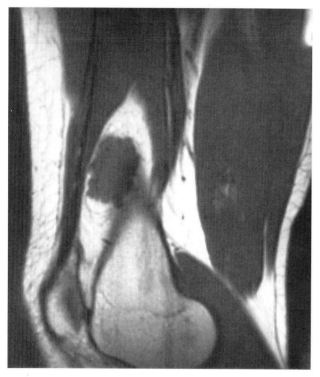

FIGURE 5-20A Sagittal T1-weighted MRI of the distal thigh. There is a lobulated, suprapatellar soft-tissue mass adjacent to the distal femur. The lesion is isointense with muscle and is completely surrounded by fat.

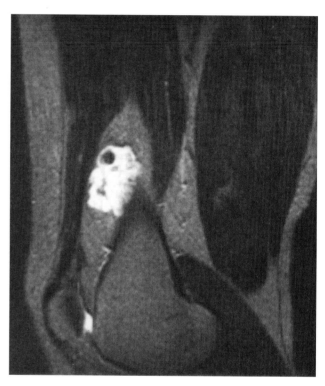

FIGURE 5-20B Sagittal T2-weighted MRI of the distal thigh. The mass demonstrates high signal intensity, with multiple well-defined internal areas of low signal intensity and a few fibrous strands or septations.

◆DIFFERENTIAL DIAGNOSIS

◆ **Neurofibroma:** These fusiform tumors typically infiltrate nerves in a diffuse fashion. On T2-weighted MRIs, peripheral high signal intensity myxoid material surrounds central low signal intensity fibrous tissue in a concentric fashion.

◆ **Schwannoma:** This tumor arises from the nerve sheath and is usually surrounded by fat within a fascial plane. Irregular, internal low signal intensity areas are commonly seen on T2-weighted MRIs.

◆ **Hemangioma:** These tumors have large, vascular channels that are high signal intensity on T2-weighted MRIs. The mass may have multiple lobulated compartments that are separated by fibrous septae. Focal thrombi or phleboliths may be seen internally without evidence of rapid flow or hemorrhage.

◆ **Ganglion cyst:** Although high signal intensity juxta-articular lesions may contain septations on T2-weighted MRIs, the internal architecture is otherwise homogeneous, without focal areas of decreased signal intensity. Therefore, this is an unlikely diagnosis.

◆DIAGNOSIS: Soft-tissue hemangioma.

◆KEY FACTS

CLINICAL

◆ These lesions may occur within muscle, fascial planes, or subcutaneous tissues.

◆ Hemangiomas may be difficult to diagnose in the absence of cutaneous manifestations.

◆ Intramuscular hemangiomas may be an occult cause of muscle pain. Hemangiomas are seen in Maffucci syndrome associated with multiple enchondromas.

RADIOLOGIC

◆ Hemangiomas are one of the benign lesions that can often be distinguished definitively from malignant soft-tissue masses.

◆ A histologic diagnosis can be made if calcified phleboliths are seen on plain radiographs.

◆ The diagnosis of hemangioma can be strongly suggested if small, high signal intensity compartments are seen on T2-weighted MRIs with internal low signal areas representing thrombi (see Figure 5-20B).

◆SUGGESTED READING

Burk DL Jr, Brunberg JA, Kanal E, et al. Spinal and paraspinal neurofibromatosis: Surface coil MR imaging at 1.5 T. Radiology 1987;162:797–801.

Cohen EK, Kressel HY, Perosio T, et al. MR imaging of soft-tissue hemangiomas: Correlation with pathologic findings. AJR Am J Roentgenol 1988;150:1079–1081.

Moulton JS, Blebea JS, Dunco DM, et al. MR imaging of soft-tissue masses: Diagnostic efficacy and value of distinguishing between benign and malignant lesions. AJR Am J Roentgenol 1995;164: 1191–1199.

CASE 21

Andrew J. Collins

HISTORY

A 43-year-old woman with morning stiffness, pain, and swelling in the joints of the wrists and fingers bilaterally.

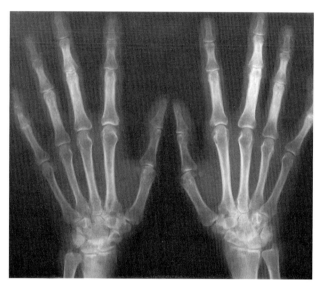

FIGURE 5-21A Posteroanterior radiograph of both hands and wrists. There is soft-tissue swelling about the wrists, metacarpophalangeal (MCP) joints (especially the first and second), and fusiform swelling at the second and third proximal interphalangeal (PIP) joints bilaterally. There is uniform joint space narrowing of the joints of the wrist, especially the intercarpal joints, where there are multiple erosions. Marginal erosions are noted at the radial aspects of the second MCP joints, radial aspects of the third PIP joints, and at the head of the right first metacarpal. There is juxta-articular osteoporosis.

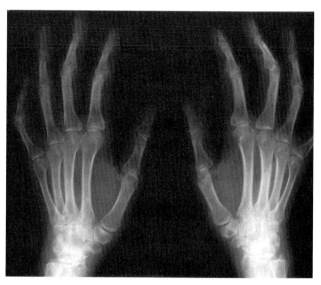

FIGURE 5-21B Oblique radiograph of both hands and wrists. Marginal erosions at the waist of the scaphoid bones are profiled bilaterally. The erosion of the right second metacarpal head, which interrupted the subchondral white line on the posteroanterior film, is profiled to better advantage on this oblique film.

◆ DIFFERENTIAL DIAGNOSIS

◆ **Gouty arthritis:** The erosions involving the left scaphoid have an appearance that could represent gout, with fairly defined margins and edges that appear to be overhanging. Gout is unlikely for multiple reasons, including the extensive joint space narrowing in the wrists, the juxta-articular osteoporosis, and the fact that this is a relatively young woman with no known disorder or enzymatic defect that would predispose to gout.

◆ **Rheumatoid arthritis:** This diagnosis is overwhelmingly favored in a female patient with bilateral symmetrical erosive disease involving the wrists, metacarpophalangeal (MCP) joints, and proximal interphalangeal (PIP) joints. The presence of juxta-articular osteoporosis and the absence of reactive bone formation also favor this diagnosis.

◆ **Psoriatic arthritis:** This is unlikely given the sparing of the distal interphalangeal (DIP) joints, the bilateral symmetrical distribution, and the lack of proliferative changes.

◆ DIAGNOSIS: Rheumatoid arthritis.

◆ KEY FACTS

CLINICAL
◆ Rheumatoid arthritis has a female prominence and tends to involve young to middle-aged individuals.

◆ The "morning gel" (i.e., morning stiffness) phenomenon is typical.
◆ The rheumatoid factor is positive (seropositive).
◆ Subcutaneous nodules are present in 25% of patients.

RADIOLOGIC
◆ The hands and wrists are the most common target sites. Distribution is typically bilateral and symmetrical.
◆ In the digits, MCP joints are typically involved earlier and more severely than PIP joints. On the other hand, PIP joints are typically involved earlier and more severely than DIP joints, which may be spared.
◆ Periarticular soft-tissue swelling, juxta-articular osteoporosis, marginal erosions, and uniform joint space narrowing are typical early findings.
◆ A striking lack of reactive proliferative bone formation is typical.
◆ The feet are commonly involved. Large joints of the appendicular skeleton may also be involved.
◆ Involvement of the axial skeleton most commonly affects the cervical spine, particularly the upper portion, often resulting in atlantoaxial subluxation.

◆ SUGGESTED READING
Brower AC. Arthritis in Black and White. Philadelphia: Saunders, 1988;137–165.
Resnick D, Niwayama G. Diagnosis of Bone and Joint Disorders (2nd ed). Philadelphia: Saunders, 1989;955–1067.

HISTORY

A 62-year-old, previously healthy woman presents with a 1-week history of chills, fever, and left hip pain of such severity that she is unable to walk. A pelvic radiograph and a left hip arthrogram/aspiration are negative. A bone scan revealed increased activity in the left sacroiliac joint.

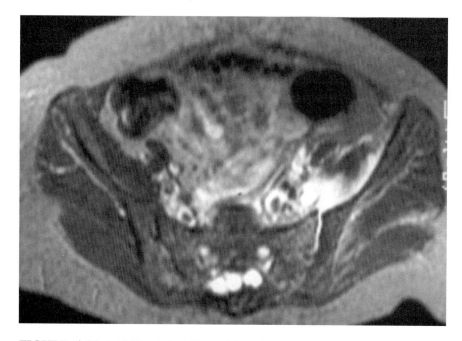

FIGURE 5-22 Axial T2-weighted MRI of the pelvis. Diffuse, increased signal intensity is noted in the marrow of the left wing of the sacrum. Fluid is seen in the adjacent sacroiliac joint. The left iliacus muscle is of high signal intensity, consistent with edema, and there is an adjacent fluid collection.

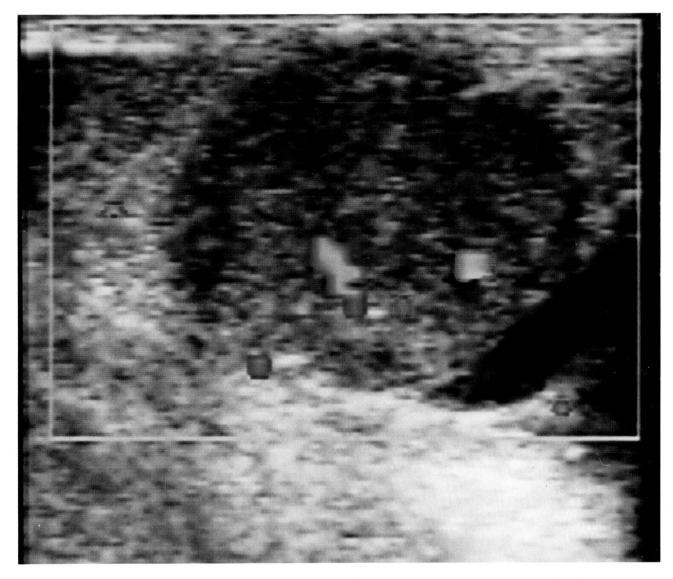

PLATE 1 Longitudinal testicular image with color Doppler ultrasound. The hypoechoic testicular mass has increased blood flow compared to the adjacent normal testis. [See Chapter 9, Case 14.]

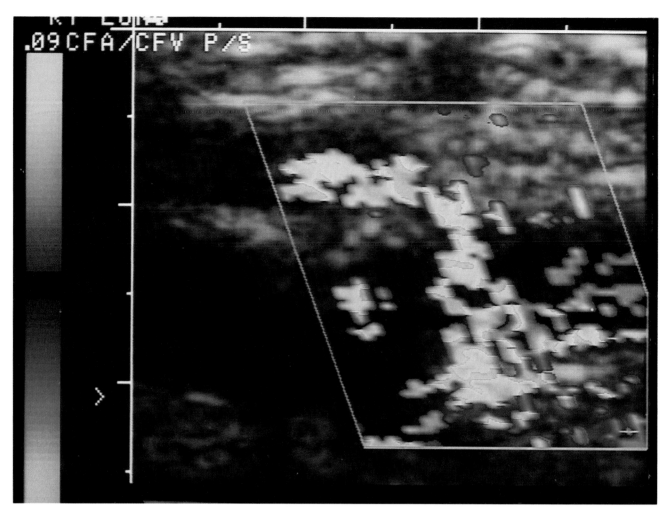

PLATE 2   A color Doppler ultrasound in the region of the puncture. A color Doppler "bruit" is manifested as scattered color Doppler pixels in the soft tissues surrounding the femoral artery and vein. [See Chapter 9, Case 15.]

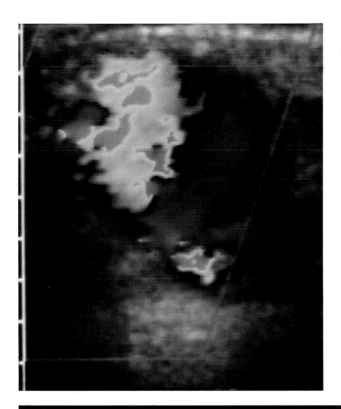

PLATE 3 A transverse color Doppler image of the right groin in the region of the visible catheterization puncture site demonstrates a "yin-yang" appearance of swirling bidirectional color flow within a hypoechoic mass. The short "neck" of flow can be seen between the mass and the common femoral artery. [See Chapter 9, Case 16.]

▼ **PLATE 4** Pulsed Doppler spectral waveform in the region of the "neck" shows a "to-and-fro" waveform. [See Chapter 9, Case 16.]

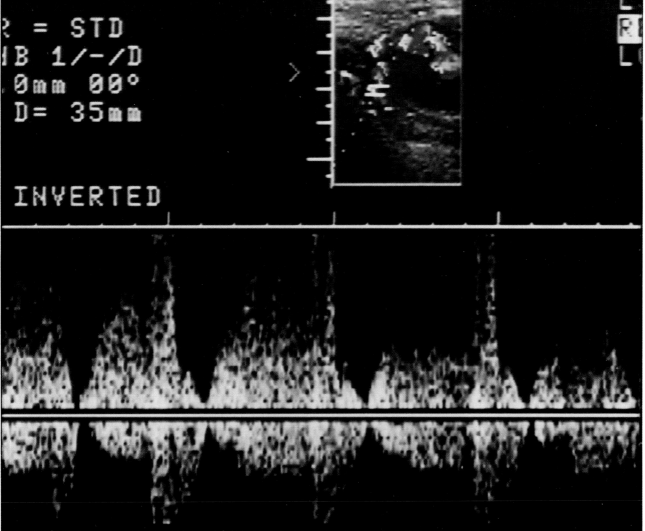

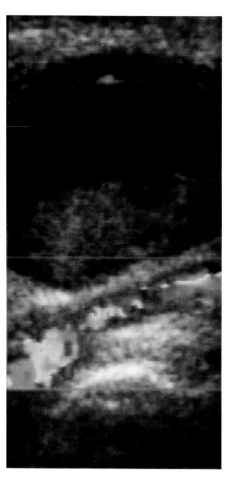

PLATE 5 A longitudinal color Doppler image of the right groin following ultra-sound-guided compression repair shows no flow within the mass, which now contains a layer of echogenic material. Flow is maintained in the underlying common femoral artery. [See Chapter 9, Case 16.]

▼ **PLATE 6** A color Doppler ultrasound of the right internal carotid artery demonstrates an extremely high-grade stenosis with flow disturbance and a relatively hypoechoic plaque. Tiny areas of slow reversed flow are seen within the hypoechoic plaque, a finding that can be suggestive of plaque ulceration. [See Chapter 9, Case 17.]

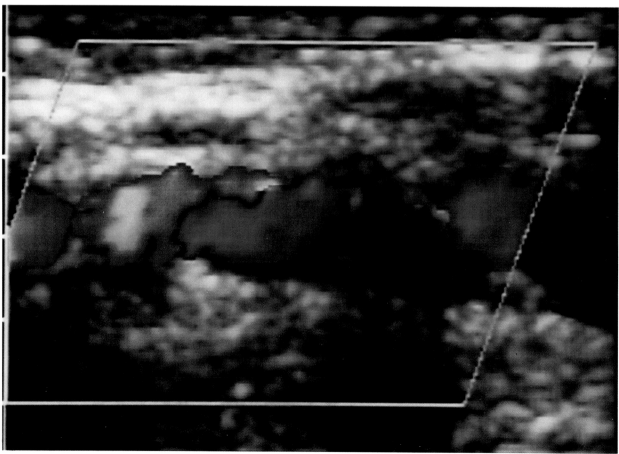

◆ DIFFERENTIAL DIAGNOSIS

- **Unilateral septic sacroiliitis:** The negative radiograph and positive bone scan indicate a sacroiliac joint process. The joint fluid, capsular distention, and irregular joint space on MRI reflect an articular process. The marked and diffuse marrow edema and iliacus muscle abscess are most consistent with an infectious sacroiliitis.
- **Unilateral seronegative sacroiliitis:** This entity has a more insidious onset than in the case presented. There may be a prior history of a seronegative arthropathy. There is much less subchondral edema than in the case shown. The myositis and abscess formation are more typical of septic sacroiliitis.
- **Ewing's sarcoma and lymphoma:** These neoplasms often present in young patients (i.e., at the same age as septic sacroiliitis). They target the marrow of the iliac bone adjacent to the sacroiliac joint. Unfortunately, this misdiagnosis is *not* uncommon. As a rule, the joint space is normal, and the epicenter of the tumor is in the iliac tuberosity and may extend to the posterior ligaments of the joint. Furthermore, it is often associated with a large soft tissue mass.

◆ DIAGNOSIS: Unilateral septic sacroiliitis.

◆ KEY FACTS

CLINICAL

- This entity accounts for only 1% to 2% of all cases of septic arthritis and osteomyelitis. For example, in 1988, only 166 cases were reported. Before antituberculous drugs, tuberculosis (TB) of the sacroiliac joints was 10 times more common.
- This disorder is often not suspected clinically because of the lack of localizing symptoms, unfamiliarity with the variability of presentation, and an incomplete physical examination.
- Septic sacroiliitis is very often misdiagnosed initially.
- Acute onset of fever and pain in the ipsilateral hip are present in 75% of patients.
- A delayed diagnosis is associated with increasesd morbidity and rate of complications, including abscess formation, osteomyelitis, and ankylosis.
- In 60% of patients, there is an associated preexisting condition, such as a focus of infection (skin: 8%; lung: 5%; ear, nose, and throat: 5%; gastrointestinal tract: 4%; gynecologic: 4%; and intravenous [IV] drug abuse: 13%) or trauma (6%).
- It is most often seen in young males (60%), with an average age of 22 years.
- The erythrocyte sedimentation rate is almost uniformly elevated.
- The most common infecting organism is *Staphylococcus aureus. Pseudomonas aeruginosa* is essentially only seen in IV drug abusers. Organisms may be obtained from blood cultures (23%), image-guided sacroiliac joint aspiration (50% to 88%), or by open biopsy. An organism is not identified in 25% of cases.
- Treatment includes high doses of oral and IV antibiotics. Surgery is occasionally needed for open biopsy or abscess drainage.

RADIOLOGIC

- Plain radiographs are usually insensitive and misleading in early stages because of obscured anatomy and lack of soft-tissue detail. Later, widening of the joint space and superficial erosions with some reactive sclerosis may be seen. After treatment, subchondral sclerosis increases, the joint becomes narrow, and 20% will ankylose. An abscess with calcification strongly suggests TB.
- Bone scintigraphy is more sensitive than plain radiography. It is the ideal modality for identifying a suspected infectious process because localizing signs are typically poor and, as a rule, unilateral. False-negative studies are possible, such as in bilateral sacroiliitis or in infants. Scintigraphy is also better than MRI for initial evaluation.
- CT is more sensitive than plain radiography and is particularly good for defining erosive changes. False-negative studies are uncommon. IV contrast material is essential for diagnosing an abscess. CT is usually reserved for guiding needle aspiration of the joint or percutaneous abscess drainage.
- On MRI, the infected and inflamed sacroiliac, synovial, and articular cartilages are typically accompanied by a joint effusion and distention of the capsule. In contrast to unilateral seronegative sacroiliitis, subchondral edema is prominent and diffuse on both sides of the joint. This results in decreased signal intensity on T1-weighted images and increased signal intensity on T2-weighted images, short tau inversion recovery (STIR), and post-gadolinium images. As with seronegative spondyloarthropathies, fluid in the joint with a distended anterior capsule is often noted on T2-weighted images. Unique to septic sacroiliitis is the fact that the adjacent muscles (iliacus, psoas, and gluteus) are inflamed. Focal, very intense signal intensity in the marrow on T2-weighted images and on T1-weighted post-gadolinium images suggests osteomyelitis.

◆ SUGGESTED READING

Ariza J, Pujol M, Valverde J, et al. Brucellar sacroiliitis: Findings in 63 episodes and current relevance. Clin Infect Dis 1993;16: 761–763.

Ballow M, Braun J, Hamm B, et al. Early sacroiliitis in patients with spondyloarthropathy: Evaluation with dynamic gadolinium-enhanced MR imaging. Radiology 1995;194:529–536.

Haliloglu M, Kleiman MB, Siddiqui AR, Cohen MD. Osteomyelitis and pyogenic infection of the sacroiliac joint: MRI findings and review. Pediatr Radiol 1994;24:333–335.

Nguyen T, Burk DL. Tuberculous sacroiliitis. AJR Am J Roentgenol 1995;165:205–206.

Vyskocil JJ, McIlroy MA, Brennan TA, Wilson FM. Pyogenic infection of the sacroiliac joint. Case report and review of the literature. Medicine 1991;70:188–197.

CASE 23

D. Lawrence Burk

HISTORY

A 12-year-old boy with a painless palpable mass along the lateral aspect of the left knee.

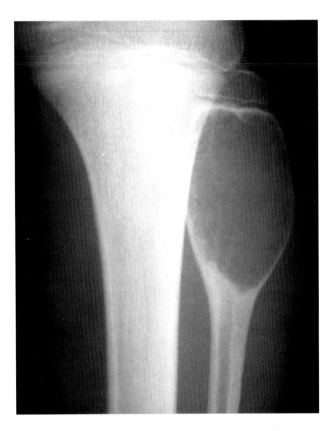

FIGURE 5-23A Anteroposterior radiograph of the left knee. A well-circumscribed, expansile lytic lesion is seen in the metaphysis of the left proximal fibula.

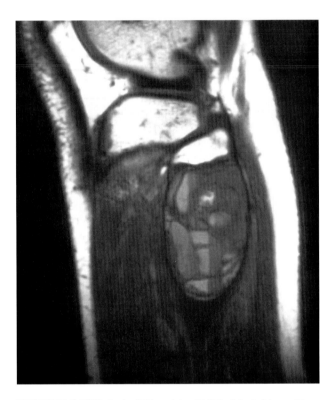

FIGURE 5-23B Sagittal T1-weighted MRI of the left knee. Many fluid-fluid levels are seen in multiple small compartments. A layer of high signal intensity fluid is noted along the ventral, nondependent aspect, and low signal intensity fluid is noted dorsally.

◆ DIFFERENTIAL DIAGNOSIS

◆ **Telangiectatic osteosarcoma:** This predominantly lytic lesion may demonstrate hemorrhage and fluid-fluid levels. However, these lesions usually have more destructive and aggressive features than the case shown here.

◆ **Simple bone cyst:** Fluid-fluid levels may be seen in bone cysts. These lesions, however, do not usually expand the cortex to a significant degree.

◆ **Aneurysmal bone cyst:** These expansile lesions are characterized by multiple compartments containing internal fluid-fluid levels on MRI. Extracellular methemoglobin (high signal intensity) in the supernatant contrasts with intracellular methemoglobin (low signal intensity) within intact, dependent red blood cells.

◆ **Fibrous dysplasia with cystic degeneration:** With these lesions, cyst formation may occur with expansion of the cortex and fluid-fluid levels. A ground-glass appearance is often noted in the noncystic portions of the lesion.

◆ DIAGNOSIS: Aneurysmal bone cyst.

◆ KEY FACTS

CLINICAL

◆ Aneurysmal bone cysts occur in pediatric patients and young adults.

◆ These lesions may present with a pathologic fracture.

◆ An enlarging palpable mass may be painless, as in this patient.

◆ The location is usually the metadiaphyseal region of long bones, but the pelvis and spine may also be involved.

RADIOLOGIC

◆ The typical appearance is an expansile lytic lesion surrounded by a thin shell of bone.

◆ Multiple small compartments are usually seen with a layered hematocrit effect due to previous hemorrhage.

◆ Fluid-fluid levels can also be seen with CT, but after positioning, a short waiting period before scanning is needed to allow layering to occur and the fluid-fluid level to be shown.

◆ SUGGESTED READING

Beltran J, Simon DC, Levy M, et al. Aneurysmal bone cysts: MR imaging at 1.5T. Radiology 1986;158:689–690.

Hudson TM. Fluid levels in aneurysmal bone cysts: A CT feature. AJR Am J Roentgenol 1984;141:1001–1004.

Tsai JC, Dalinka MK, Fallon MD, et al. Fluid-fluid level: A nonspecific finding in tumors of bone and soft tissue. Radiology 1990;175:779–782.

CASE 24

Andrew J. Collins

HISTORY

A 39-year-old woman with bilateral hip pain. She has a prior history of precocious puberty and a left scaphoid fracture.

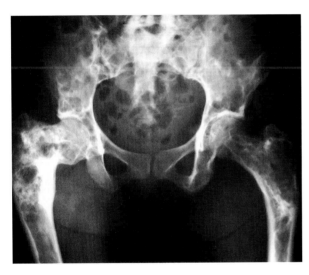

FIGURE 5-24A Anteroposterior radiograph of the pelvis. There are areas of lucency and sclerosis about the pelvis and proximal femur bilaterally. In some of these regions, there is a smudged or ground-glass appearance to the trabeculae. Several of the lesions have sclerotic margins. There is a shepherd's crook deformity of the right proximal femur and an incomplete fracture of the left proximal femur inferior to the greater trochanter laterally.

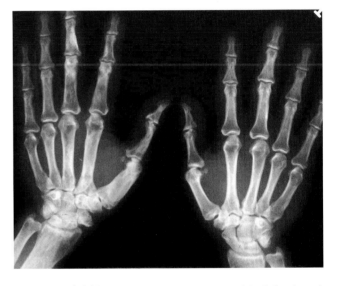

FIGURE 5-24B Posteroanterior radiograph of both hands and wrists. There is an old left scaphoid fracture with nonbony union. There are areas of increased density in the left first through third rays, with some thinning of the cortices and expansion of the bones. The left distal radius is also abnormal in appearance, with mixed lucency and sclerosis.

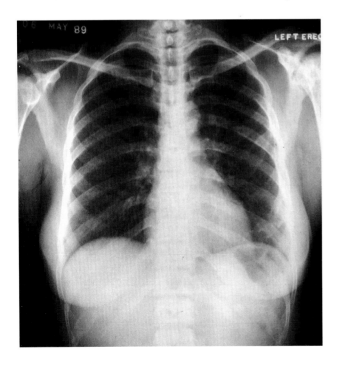

FIGURE 5-24C Posteroanterior radiograph of the chest. There is mixed lucency and sclerosis in the region of the left glenoid and proximal humerus. There are expansile lesions of multiple ribs with a ground-glass appearance, most notable in the left fourth and sixth ribs anteriorly and bilateral eleventh ribs posterolaterally. Some lucency is noted in the posterior elements of C7 on the left.

◆ DIFFERENTIAL DIAGNOSIS

◆ **Neurofibromatosis:** Although rare, precocious sexual development has been reported with neurofibromatosis. Neurofibromatosis can cause bone lesions with changes in bone density and shape, but the bone lesions in the case shown are atypical in distribution and appearance for neurofibromatosis.

◆ **Metastatic disease:** This diagnosis is unlikely because there is no history of a primary malignancy and there is relative sparing of the spine.

◆ **Fibrous dysplasia:** This is the most likely diagnosis given the expansile lesions of the ribs, the mixed lucent and sclerotic lesions of the pelvis and proximal femurs, the "shepherd's crook" deformity of the right femur, and the somewhat more pronounced overall involvement on the left side of the body. The history of precocious puberty and café-au-lait spots would fit with McCune-Albright syndrome.

◆ **Paget's disease:** This diagnosis is unlikely given the patient's age, relative sparing of the epiphyseal regions in the proximal femurs, and lack of classic pattern of enlargement of bone, trabecular coarsening, and cortical thickening.

◆ DIAGNOSIS: McCune-Albright syndrome with polyostotic fibrous dysplasia.

◆ KEY FACTS

CLINICAL

◆ The classic triad for McCune-Albright syndrome includes: (1) polyostotic fibrous dysplasia with a unilateral tendency, (2) café-au-lait spots, and (3) precocious puberty. This syndrome was originally described in female patients.

◆ McCune-Albright syndrome is not a familial condition.

◆ Proximal femoral deformities can result in limb shortening or a limp or be painful. Fractures are the most common complication.

RADIOLOGIC

◆ The lesions of fibrous dysplasia have variable density.

◆ A ground-glass appearance is typical. There is often a sclerotic rim or rind.

◆ Endosteal scalloping and bone expansion may occur.

◆ Common sites of involvement include the ribs, femur, tibia, pelvis, and skull. Vertebral involvement is rare. There is a unilateral predominance.

◆ A shepherd's crook deformity of the proximal femur is classic.

◆ In the skull, the outer table is involved earlier and more extensively than the inner table. There is also sclerosis at the base of the skull.

◆ SUGGESTED READING

Edeiken J. Roentgen Diagnosis of Diseases of the Bone (3rd ed) (vol II). Baltimore: Williams & Wilkins, 1981;994–1027.

Kransdorf MJ, Moser RP Jr, Gilkey FW. Fibrous dysplasia. Radiographics 1990;10:519–537.

Mirra JM, Gold RH. Fibrous Dysplasia. In JM Mirra, P Piero, RH Gold (eds), Bone Tumors. Philadelphia: Lea & Febiger, 1989;191–226.

Resnick D, Niwayama G. Diagnosis of Bone and Joint Disorders (2nd ed). Philadelphia: Saunders, 1988;4057–4072.

CASE 25

Andrew J. Collins

HISTORY

A 61-year-old man presents with right hip pain. His prostate is enlarged on physical examination.

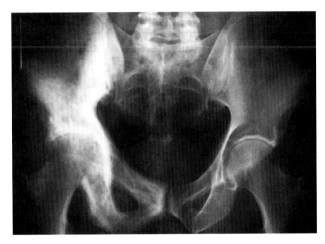

FIGURE 5-25A Anteroposterior radiograph of the pelvis. The right innominate bone is enlarged and exhibits mixed lucency and increased density, coarsening of trabeculae with an irregular pattern, and cortical thickening. The iliopectineal and ilioischial lines are thickened. There is mild superomedial right hip joint space narrowing.

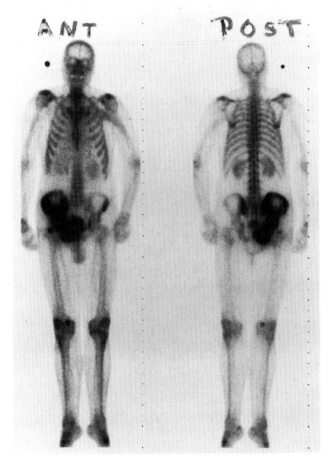

FIGURE 5-25B Whole body radionuclide bone scan in the anteroposterior and posteroanterior projections. There is intense increase in radiotracer uptake in the region of the right innominate bone. Incidentally noted is a second small focus of increased activity over the base of the right femoral neck anterolaterally. This corresponds to a focus of heterotopic bone that is vaguely evident on the anteroposterior radiograph as lucency and sclerosis over the base of the right femoral neck laterally.

◆ DIFFERENTIAL DIAGNOSIS

◆ **Skeletal metastasis from prostate carcinoma:** Metastasis is a consideration given the fact that there are multiple abnormal foci on the bone scan and a sclerotic lesion in the pelvis. However, the diagnosis is unlikely given the pattern of trabecular coarsening and cortical thickening and extensive involvement of one innominate bone without disease elsewhere in the axial skeleton.

◆ **Myelofibrosis:** This entity is unlikely given the asymmetric involvement.

◆ **Mixed phase of Paget's disease:** This is the best diagnosis because of its typical location in the innominate bone, bone enlargement, mixed lucency and sclerosis, trabecular coarsening, cortical thickening, and a positive bone scan.

◆ DIAGNOSIS: Mixed-phase Paget's disease of the right innominate bone.

◆ KEY FACTS

CLINICAL

◆ Paget's disease occurs in middle-aged to elderly subjects, and more commonly in men.

◆ The most common complication is a pathologic fracture. Bowing of bones may also occur.

◆ Other complications include spinal stenosis, cranial nerve compression, and degenerative joint disease.

◆ Secondary neoplasms may develop, such as sarcomatous transformation (<1%) and giant cell tumors (also uncommon).

RADIOLOGIC

◆ Three phases are recognized in Paget's disease: lytic, mixed, and sclerotic. Bone scintigraphy shows intensely increased activity in the lytic and mixed phases, and a variable pattern in the sclerotic phase.

◆ The disease tends to progress from one end of a long bone toward the other, sometimes with an advancing lytic edge having a flame-shaped or blade-of-grass–shaped margin.

◆ The lytic phase may show regional lucency in the skull and flat bones, which is known as _osteoporosis circumscripta._

◆ SUGGESTED READING

Lakhanpal S, O'Duffy JD. Paget's disease and osteoarthritis. Arthritis Rheum 1986;29:1414–1415.

Mirra JM, Brien EW, Tehranzadeh J. Paget's disease of bone: Review with emphasis on radiologic features. Parts I and II. Skeletal Radiol 1995;24:163–171 (part I), 173–184 (part II).

Moore T, King A, Kathol M, et al. Sarcoma in Paget disease of bone: Clinical, radiologic and pathologic features in 22 cases. AJR Am J Roentgenol 1991;156:1199–1203.

HISTORY

A 25-year-old hitchhiker who was struck in the back of the head by a trucker's side mirror.

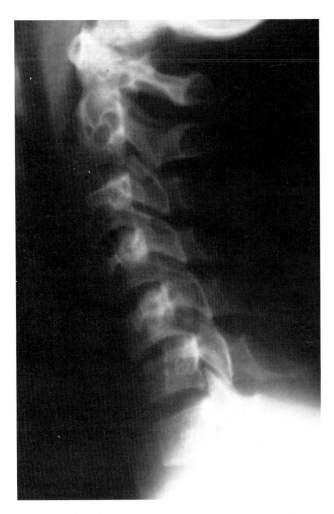

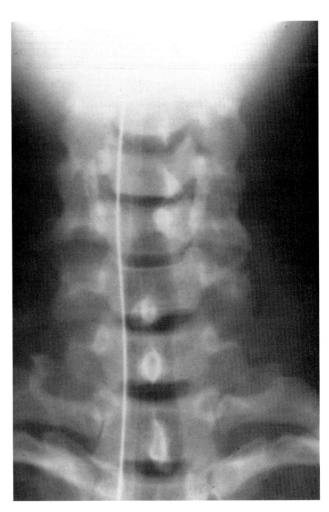

FIGURE 5-26A Lateral radiograph of the cervical spine. There is a 3-mm anterolisthesis of C5 on C6 with slight angular deformity.

FIGURE 5-26B Anteroposterior radiograph of the cervical spine. The C5 spinous process is deviated to the right side of the midline.

◆ DIFFERENTIAL DIAGNOSIS

- **Hyperflexion sprain:** Hyperflexion sprain is characterized by focal angulation of the spine and widening of the interspinous distance. On the anteroposterior (AP) view, the spinous process would not be deviated from the midline, which distinguishes it from unilateral interfacetal dislocation (UID).
- **Bilateral interfacetal dislocation (BID):** This severe cervical spine injury is distinguished from hyperflexion sprain by complete disruption of all ligamentous integrity at the injured level. BID is, therefore, a grossly unstable injury. It is distinguished from unilateral interfacetal dislocation by a lack of rotation of the spinous process on the AP view and by significant anterolisthesis (usually ≥50%) of one vertebral body on the subadjacent vertebra.
- **UID:** UID injuries are produced by flexion and rotation of the spine. The rotational component leads to a unilateral dislocation of the cervical apophyseal joint. The unilateral dislocation can be identified by displacement of the spinous process of the affected vertebra toward the side of the dislocation. Oblique views of the cervical spine also demonstrate the site of UID.

◆ DIAGNOSIS: Unilateral interfacetal dislocation on the right.

◆ KEY FACTS

CLINICAL

- The mechanism of injury is fundamentally flexion with rotation.
- This injury should be approached initially as unstable but may later prove to be mechanically stable if the ipsilateral fracture is minimal and the contralateral liga-

ments are intact. Based on review of the initial radiographs, such distinctions can be difficult and, for patient safety, it is best to consider these injuries as unstable until proven otherwise.
- Profound neurologic deficits are rare in patients with UID injuries, but radiculopathy is common.

RADIOLOGIC

- BID is characterized by a traumatic anterolisthesis of ≥50%. In UID injuries, the degree of anterolisthesis is constrained by the nondislocated side with anterolisthesis in the range of 25%. There may be slight angular deformity and fanning of the involved spinous processes on the lateral film. On the AP view, deviation of the spinous process of the involved vertebra toward the side of the dislocated facet is characteristic.
- In patients with a hyperflexion sprain injury, rotational abnormalities of the spine are not noted on either AP or lateral views. Typically, the degree of posterior ligamentous injury in patients with hyperflexion sprain is less than that in patients with UID. Nonetheless, some patients with a hyperflexion sprain injury have severe ligamentous damage that remains undetected for some time, and they can present with frank instability days to weeks after the initial trauma (delayed instability). It is for this reason that all hyperflexion sprain injuries should be considered as important soft-tissue injuries requiring both clinical and radiographic follow-up within 5 to 10 days of injury.

◆ SUGGESTED READING

Berquist TH. Imaging of Orthopedic Trauma. New York: Raven, 1992;123–169.

Harris JH, Harris WH, Novelline RA. The Radiology of Emergency Medicine. Baltimore: Williams & Wilkins, 1993;177–179.

HISTORY

Patient A: a 25-year-old woman involved in a head-on motor vehicle accident.
Patient B: a 30-year-old sign painter who fell 30 feet from a scaffold, landing on his right leg.

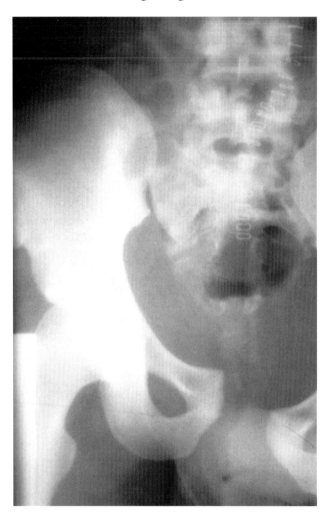

FIGURE 5-27A Anteroposterior radiograph of the right hemipelvis in patient A. There is cephalad displacement of the right hip and hemipelvis with symphyseal and sacroiliac joint diastasis.

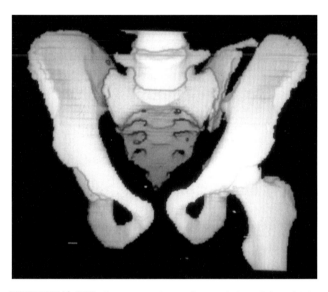

FIGURE 5-27B Anteroposterior surface rendering of the pelvis in patient B from a spiral CT data set. There is a vertical fracture through the left iliac wing, diastasis of the symphysis pubis, and slight elevation of the left hip.

◆ DIFFERENTIAL DIAGNOSIS

- **Lateral compression injury:** Lateral compression injuries are relatively uncommon but can be confused with vertical shear injuries. The two injuries are usually distinguished by the oblique orientation of the fractures in lateral compression injury and the cephalad displacement of the hemipelvis in vertical shear injury.
- **Anteroposterior compression injury:** This mechanism usually produces mirror image fractures of the pubic rami or traumatic diastasis of the symphysis pubis. In the posterior pelvis, one usually sees bilateral traumatic diastasis of the sacroiliac joints. The so-called "open book pelvis" is an example of an AP compression injury.
- **Vertical shear injury (formerly known as Malgaigne fracture dislocation):** This injury is produced by a forceful axial load on the hemipelvis that might occur from a fall onto one leg, as in patient B. A distinguishing feature of vertical shear injuries is the cephalad displacement of the hemipelvis, which is separated from the remainder of the pelvis by anterior and posterior ring disruptions.

◆ DIAGNOSIS: Vertical shear injury.

◆ KEY FACTS

CLINICAL

- This injury occurs when there is a vertical force directed along the axis of the femur.

- The physical examination can incorrectly suggest a hip dislocation.

RADIOLOGIC

- Vertical shear injury is caused by two disruptions of the pelvic ring, one anterior to the acetabulum and the other posterior to the acetabulum.
- The posterior disruption can occur through the sacral ala, sacroiliac joint, or posterior ilium. The anterior disruption can occur through the symphysis pubis, superior and inferior pubic rami, or acetabulum.
- The exact site of the anterior or posterior disruption is unimportant because any combination of pelvic disruptions from a vertical shear mechanism will produce an unstable, elevated hemipelvis.
- Lateral compression injuries can have a superficial resemblance to vertical shear injuries; however, cephalad displacement of the hemipelvis is not seen in lateral compression injuries.
- Distinction among anteroposterior compression, vertical shear, and lateral compression injuries is occasionally problematic. Furthermore, mixed injuries can occur.

◆ SUGGESTED READING

Berquist TH. Imaging of Orthopedic Trauma. New York: Raven, 1992;227–239.

Harris JH, Harris WH, Novelline RA. The Radiology of Emergency Medicine. Baltimore: Williams & Wilkins, 1993;693–764.

CASE 28

D. Lawrence Burk

HISTORY

A 66-year-old woman with chronic obstructive pulmonary disease (COPD) and back pain.

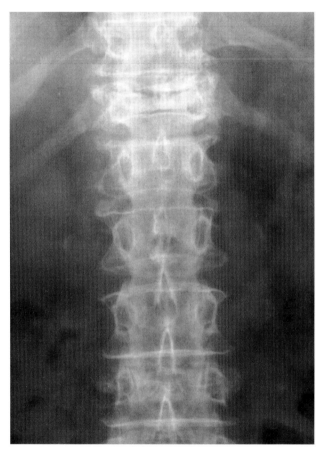

FIGURE 5-28A Anteroposterior radiograph of the lumbar spine. Multiple osteoporotic compression fractures are present, with a lower thoracic intravertebral vacuum phenomenon.

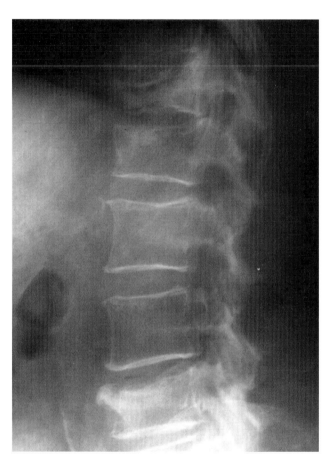

FIGURE 5-28B Lateral radiograph of the lumbar spine. Compression fractures and vacuum phenomenon are seen again. Deformed superior endplates demonstrate peripheral condensation of bone, resulting in increased subchondral density.

◆ DIFFERENTIAL DIAGNOSIS

◆ **Senile osteoporosis:** Intravertebral vacuum phenomenon may occur with this form of osteoporosis in a patient taking corticosteroids for COPD due to significant trauma or intraosseous prolapse of a vacuum disc. Concave endplates are often present.

◆ **Multiple myeloma:** The presence of a vacuum phenomenon in a collapsed vertebral body does not exclude malignancy as in multiple myeloma. Cortical destruction rather than subchondral endplate sclerosis would be expected.

◆ **Gaucher's disease:** Osteoporosis and multiple compression fractures are common with Gaucher's disease. Vertebra plana deformities may occur at multiple levels, but vacuum vertebral bodies are not typical.

◆ **Corticosteroid-induced osteoporosis:** This disorder is associated with peripheral condensation of bone at the site of endplate compression deformities. Vacuum vertebral bodies can be seen secondary to osteonecrosis. This is the most likely diagnosis for the case shown.

◆ DIAGNOSIS: Corticosteroid-induced osteoporosis and vertebral osteonecrosis.

◆ KEY FACTS

CLINICAL

◆ This condition may be caused by either Cushing's disease or exogenous corticosteroids.

◆ Endogenous Cushing's disease results from adrenal hyperplasia, adrenal adenoma or carcinoma, or ectopic adrenocorticotropic hormone–producing tumors.

◆ Increased bone resorption results in negative calcium balance and hypercalciuria.

◆ The bony manifestations may be accentuated in elderly women who have an underlying chronic disease.

RADIOLOGIC

◆ Subchondral endplate sclerosis is a result of inappropriate exuberant callus formation.

◆ The intravertebral vacuum phenomenon is most common at the thoracolumbar junction.

◆ The vacuum phenomenon is bordered frequently by sclerotic bone, suggesting the presence of a pseudoarthrosis.

◆ SUGGESTED READING

Kumar R, Guinto FC Jr, Madewell JE, et al. The vertebral body: Radiographic configurations in various congenital and acquired disorders. Radiographics 1988;8:455–485.

Kumpan W, Salomonowitz E, Seidl G, Wittich GR. The intravertebral vacuum phenomenon. Skeletal Radiol 1986;15:444–447.

Resnick D. Bone and Joint Imaging. Philadelphia: Saunders, 1989;650–651.

CASE 29

Joseph W. Melamed

HISTORY

A 50-year-old man with low back pain.

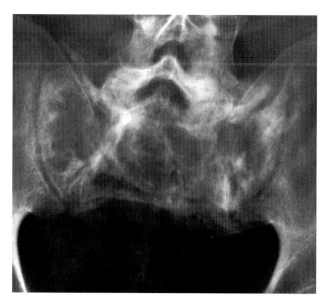

FIGURE 5-29A Anteroposterior view of the pelvis. A lytic, bubbly, expansile lesion is present in the sacrum.

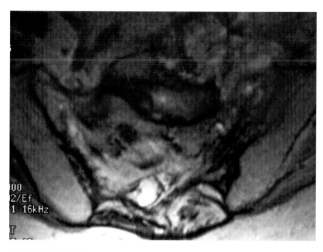

FIGURE 5-29B Fast spin echo T2-weighted axial MRI of the pelvis. A heterogeneous high signal mass corresponds to the plain radiographic abnormality.

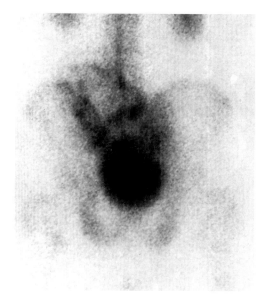

FIGURE 5-29C Tc^{99} MDP bone scan, posterior view, demonstrates a photopenic lesion in the region of the left sacral ala.

◆ DIFFERENTIAL DIAGNOSIS

◆ **Giant cell tumor:** The location of the lesion and radiographic appearance are compatible with this diagnosis. However, the patient's age makes this diagnosis unlikely, as giant cell tumor is usually seen in young adults.

◆ **Metastatic disease:** The age and radiographic appearance favor this diagnosis, especially for renal cell or thyroid carcinoma metastases. Renal cell carcinoma metastases, in particular, may be "cold" on a delayed-phase bone scan due to hypervascularity. The lack of other lesions, however, lowers the likelihood of this diagnosis.

◆ **Primary malignant bone tumor:** Chondrosarcoma and fibrosarcoma are possible considerations in this age group and may have a similar radiographic appearance. Chondrosarcoma, in particular, may occur in this location. However, chondrosarcoma would be expected to have a very bright signal on T2-weighted MRI (i.e., brighter than the abnormal signal seen in this case) due to the presence of chondroid matrix.

◆ **Brown tumor:** The radiographic appearance is compatible with this diagnosis, but there is no concomitant evidence or history of hyperparathyroidism.

◆ **Solitary myeloma:** The patient's age and the radiographic appearance of the lesion are compatible with this diagnosis.

◆ **Fibrous dysplasia:** Fibrous dysplasia typically demonstrates some increased uptake of tracer on a bone scan. Although the radiographic appearance of this lesion is compatible with this diagnosis, these lesions are usually healed by age 50.

◆ DIAGNOSIS: Solitary myeloma (plasmacytoma).

◆ KEY FACTS

CLINICAL

◆ This rare entity represents <5% of all plasma cell dysplasias. It tends to affect a younger population (mean age of 50 years) than multiple myeloma.

◆ Criteria for diagnosis are:
   Histologic proof
   Complete skeletal survey excluding other lesions
   Negative bone marrow biopsy
   Absence of dysproteinemia and Bence-Jones proteinuria (or if M-spike is present, disappearance after resection of the solitary lesion)

◆ The treatment is en bloc excision and radiation therapy.

◆ The clinical prognosis is much better than in multiple myeloma, even in those patients who eventually develop multiple lesions.

◆ The existence of this entity is controversial, and very few true cases are reported. At least 70% of patients presenting with solitary myeloma eventually progress to multiple myeloma.

RADIOLOGIC

◆ Plasmacytomas are variable in appearance. The lesions may be purely lytic without expansion, or bubbly and expansile with thickened trabeculae. Sclerotic plasmacytoma has also been reported. Calcifications may be present in plasmacytoma and can mimic chondrosarcoma.

◆ The most common sites of involvement are the vertebral bodies, pelvic bones, and shoulder girdle.

◆ When plasmacytoma occurs in the spine, it is often associated with a gibbous deformity and can cross the disk spaces.

◆ SUGGESTED READING

Bataille R, Sany J. Solitary myeloma: Clinical and prognostic features of a review of 114 cases. Cancer 1981;48:845–851.

Dichel J, Kirketerp P. Notes on myeloma. Acta Radiol 1938;19: 487–503.

Gootnick L. Solitary myeloma: Review of 61 cases. Radiology 1945;45:385–391.

Meyer J, Shulz M. Solitary "myeloma" of bone. A review of 12 cases. Cancer 1974;34:438–440.

Valderrama J, Bullough P. Solitary myeloma of the spine. J Bone Joint Surg 1968;50:82–90.

CHAPTER 6

NEURO-RADIOLOGY

James M. Provenzale, *chapter editor*

Joseph B. Cornett, Charles B. Donovan,
David S. Enterline, E. Ralph Heinz,
James M. Provenzale, Robert D. Tien,
and Fernando M. Zalduondo

HISTORY

A 14-year-old girl with morning headaches and papilledema.

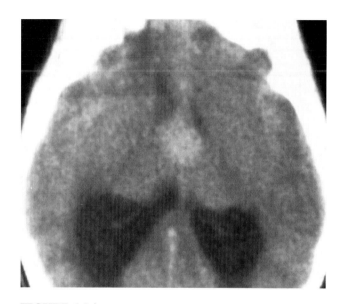

FIGURE 6-1A Noncontrast axial CT image shows a slightly hyperdense, homogeneous, round lesion between the two foramina of Monro. The lesion is located in the anterosuperior portion of the third ventricle. Hydrocephalus is present. The lesion did not enhance after contrast administration (not shown).

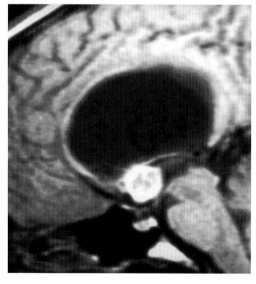

B

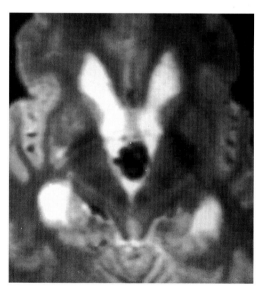

C

FIGURES 6-1B and 6-1C MRI in another patient with the same diagnosis and headaches that worsened when he leaned forward. **(B)** Noncontrast T1-weighted sagittal image shows a homogeneous, hyperintense mass in the anterior portion of the third ventricle. Marked hydrocephalus is present. The lesion did not enhance after contrast administration (not shown). **(C)** Axial T2-weighted image shows the lesion is markedly hypointense relative to brain tissue.

◆ DIFFERENTIAL DIAGNOSIS

- **Craniopharyngioma:** This diagnosis might be considered because the lesion is located in the midline near the suprasellar region. However, craniopharyngiomas are typically located in the suprasellar cistern or, on occasion, within the sella. They rarely originate in the third ventricle, although they can compress the third ventricle from below.
- **Arachnoid cyst:** This diagnosis might be considered because the lesions shown above are round, raising the possibility that they are cysts. However, arachnoid cysts are isodense with cerebrospinal fluid (CSF) on CT and are isointense on MRI, unlike the lesions shown above, making this an incorrect diagnosis.
- **Meningioma:** This entity can occasionally occur within the third ventricle. The hyperintense appearance on T1-weighted images would be very unusual, although it is conceivable that a densely calcified meningioma would be T1-bright and T2-dark. Furthermore, contrast enhancement would be expected in the case of meningioma but was not present in the lesions shown above.
- **Dermoid cyst:** This diagnosis might be considered because the lesions shown above are located in the midline, a feature that is typical of dermoid tumors. However, dermoid cysts are typically hypodense on CT relative to CSF due to their fat content, and are typically inhomogeneous on MR images.
- **Colloid cyst:** This lesion is commonly slightly hyperdense on noncontrast CT, hyperintense on noncontrast T1-weighted MR images, and hypointense on T2-weighted images. This is the correct diagnosis.

◆ DIAGNOSIS: Colloid cyst.

◆ KEY FACTS

CLINICAL

- Colloid cysts are benign neoplasms that account for <1% of intracranial neoplasms.
- These lesions are usually discovered in adolescence or young adulthood. The typical presentation is that of episodic symptoms or signs of increased intracranial pressure due to obstructive hydrocephalus. The headache is often positional (e.g., worsened by leaning forward).
- Colloid cysts are almost always located in the anterosuperior portion of the third ventricle and produce symptoms by intermittent ventricular obstruction at the level of the foramen of Monro.
- These lesions are thin-walled, well-circumscribed, round structures with various degrees of attachment to the roof of the third ventricle.

- Colloid cysts are thought to be a form of neuroepithelial cyst, produced by abnormal folding of the neuroepithelium in the anterior portion of the third ventricle during embryogenesis. More specifically, they are thought to be derived from the paraphysis, a stalked protuberance of extraventricular choroid plexus that is derived from the neuroepithelial lining of the roof of the diencephalon.
- Contents of colloid cysts include mucinous substances (including secretory products, such as fat and cholesterol crystals), hemorrhagic products, and variable degrees of ions, such as calcium, magnesium, and sodium.
- Various treatments are available, including treatment of hydrocephalus alone (via biventricular shunt placement), cyst aspiration via stereotactic guidance, and surgical excision.

RADIOLOGIC

- On CT, colloid cysts are typically hyperdense relative to CSF due to their mucinous contents. They are typically homogeneous.
- Variable degrees of obstructive hydrocephalus can be seen. Because the lesion is located in the anterior portion of the third ventricle, only the lateral ventricles would be expected to be enlarged.
- Calcification is rare and considered a finding that makes the diagnosis of colloid cyst less likely.
- Mild contrast enhancement can be seen occasionally, but dense enhancement is not a feature of these lesions.
- MRI can be used for localizing the lesion to the anterior third ventricle rather than adjacent sites such as the hypothalamus, optic tract, or suprasellar cistern.
- On MRI, the cyst will be seen to differ in signal intensity from CSF on one or more pulse sequences. The cysts are often hyperintense relative to CSF on T1-weighted sequences due to the mucinous contents and, possibly, presence of cholesterol crystals. Less commonly, they are hypointense to CSF on T2-weighted images, possibly due to paramagnetic properties of ions contained within the cyst fluid.

◆ SUGGESTED READING

Maeder PP, Holtas SL, Basibuyuk LN, et al. Colloid cysts of the third ventricle: Correlation of MR and CT findings with histology and chemical analysis. AJNR 1990;11:575–581.

Scotti G, Scialfa G, Colombo N, et al. MR in the diagnosis of colloid cysts of the third ventricle. AJNR 1987;8:370–372.

Waggenspack GA, Guinto FC. MR and CT of masses of the anterosuperior third ventricle. AJNR 1989;10:105–110.

CASE 2

Fernando M. Zalduondo

HISTORY

A 26-year-old woman with acquired immunodeficiency syndrome (AIDS) and deteriorating mental status.

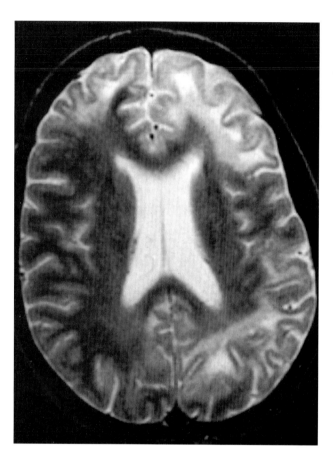

FIGURE 6-2A Axial T2-weighted MRI shows multiple, bilateral, subcortical, hyperintense white matter lesions, more numerous in the left hemisphere. The lesions extend up to the gray-white junction. No mass effect is seen. Instead, mild diffuse volume loss for age is seen.

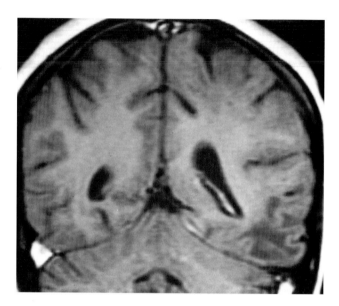

FIGURE 6-2B Coronal T1-weighted contrast-enhanced image shows a nonenhancing, hypointense lesion in the left temporal lobe. Again, no mass effect is present.

◆DIFFERENTIAL DIAGNOSIS

◆ **Toxoplasmosis:** This diagnosis might be considered because it is common in AIDS patients. Although lesions can occur anywhere in the brain, a more central location (in the periventricular regions) is typical. Furthermore, lesions generally contrast-enhance and have edema and mass effect, making this an unlikely diagnosis.

◆ **Lymphoma:** Primary B cell central nervous system (CNS) lymphoma is also relatively common in AIDS patients. However, in the immunocompromised patient, ring enhancement is typically and frequently accompanied by edema and mass effect. These features make lymphoma an unlikely diagnosis.

◆ **Cryptococcosis:** Cryptococcal infection is common in AIDS patients and can have a number of radiologic appearances: meningeal enhancement (due to meningitis), nonenhancing (or rim-enhancing) masses typically occurring in the basal ganglia (so-called gelatinous pseudocysts), ring-enhancing parenchymal masses (cryptococcomas), and intraventricular masses. Nonenhancing lesions lacking mass effect would be distinctly unusual.

◆ **Infarction:** Infarctions can occur in the periphery of the brain, usually in a setting of embolic infarction. However, the distribution of these lesions—i.e., abrupt termination at the gray-white junction with sparing of the cortex—would be very unusual for infarction. Instead, both gray and white matter would be expected to be involved. This is an unlikely diagnosis.

◆ **Progressive multifocal leukoencephalopathy (PML):** The typical appearance of PML is that of one or more nonenhancing white matter lesions lacking mass effect in an immunocompromised host. This is the correct diagnosis.

◆DIAGNOSIS: Progressive multifocal leukoencephalopathy.

◆KEY FACTS

CLINICAL

◆ PML is due to an oligodendroglial infection by the human papovavirus (also known as the JC virus, the initials of the patient in whom it was first described). The JC virus remains latent until reactivated by an immunodeficient state.

◆ This infection occurs primarily in immunocompromised patients. It occurs in 1% to 4% of adult AIDS patients but is extremely rare in children. Organ transplant recipients are another non-AIDS group at increased risk of acquiring the infection.

◆ Symptoms include visual deficits and cranial nerve palsy, focal neurologic deficits such as motor weakness and sensory loss, and nonfocal neurologic symptoms—e.g., encephalopathy or headache.

◆ The diagnosis should be considered in advanced cases of AIDS. The prognosis is very poor. There is no proven effective therapy, and death typically occurs within months of the onset of symptoms.

RADIOLOGIC

◆ On CT, lesions can be seen as nonenhancing, hypodense white matter lesions lacking mass effect. MRI is superior to CT in displaying the number and size of lesions.

◆ Lesions are frequently bilateral but distributed in an asymmetric manner between the hemispheres. The posterior centrum semiovale is the most common location. The subcortical white matter is affected initially. With the development of deep white matter lesions, large confluent lesions can result. External capsule and posterior fossa involvement is less common and can occur in the absence of centrum semiovale lesions.

◆ The absence of mass effect or contrast enhancement is a characteristic feature. Faint peripheral enhancement can be seen rarely. Nonetheless, the lack of contrast enhancement or mass effect is a useful finding in distinguishing PML from other AIDS-related lesions.

◆ Involvement of the basal ganglia and other gray matter structures is explained by contiguous involvement of white matter lesions and/or infiltration of myelinated white matter fibers that course through the basal ganglia.

◆ Cavitary changes can be seen as a late manifestation of PML.

◆SUGGESTED READING

Osborn AG. Diagnostic Neuroradiology. St. Louis: Mosby, 1994;700–701.

Post MJD, Seminer DS, Quencer RM. CT diagnosis of spinal epidural hematoma. AJNR 1982;3:109–192.

Wheeler AL, Truwit CL, Kleinschmidt-DeMasters BK, et al. Progressive multifocal leukoencephalopathy: Contrast enhancement on CT scans and MR images. AJR Am J Roentgenol 1993;161:1049–1051.

CASE 3

James M. Provenzale

HISTORY

A 16-year-old boy with lethargy, confusion, and increasing thirst and urination.

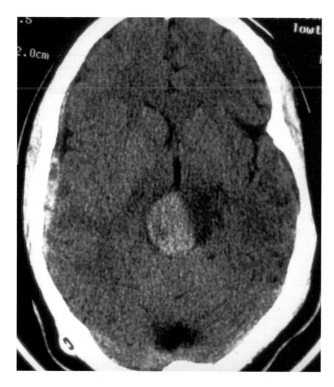

FIGURE 6-3A Noncontrast CT shows a hyperdense mass in the pineal region. The mass is relatively homogeneous except for a small hypodense region in the right half of the lesion. A hypodense crescentic region is seen to the left of the mass due to edema. A small, hyperdense, right subdural hematoma is present secondary to placement of a ventricular shunt for treatment of hydrocephalus.

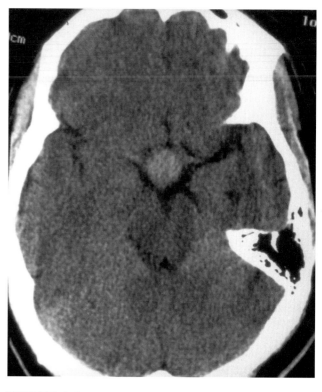

FIGURE 6-3B Image at a more caudal level from the same noncontrast CT shows a hyperdense mass in the suprasellar cistern.

◆ DIFFERENTIAL DIAGNOSIS

◆ **Primary CNS lymphoma:** This diagnosis would be considered because of the presence of multiple hyperdense masses. However, this would be an unlikely diagnosis in a child because most affected patients are in late adulthood (with the exception of immunocompromised patients, who can be affected at any age).

◆ **Pineoblastoma:** This tumor is a consideration when a pineal region tumor is seen in a child. Although these tumors are often large (>4 cm), they have an irregular contour, and are inhomogeneous, unlike the lesion shown in this case. This diagnosis would not account for the suprasellar mass, although it is conceivable that it could represent a metastasis from pineoblastoma.

◆ **Germinoma:** These tumors appear slightly hyperdense on CT, are smoothly contoured, and 95% are in the pineal or suprasellar region. Furthermore, this is the only tumor that might be expected to be found in both the pineal and suprasellar regions simultaneously.

◆ **Metastases:** Intracranial metastases are rare in childhood. The overwhelming majority of intracranial tumors are primary in origin. Furthermore, the vast majority of metastases would be hypodense, or occasionally isodense, on noncontrast CT and usually parenchymal, unlike the lesions shown in the case illustrated, making metastases an unlikely diagnosis.

◆ DIAGNOSIS: Germinoma.

◆ KEY FACTS

CLINICAL

◆ Germ cell tumors (GCTs) are an important category of pediatric brain tumors. However, it should be remembered that the vast majority of GCTs occur in an extracranial site and do not involve the central nervous system.

◆ Intracranial GCTs typically present in the second (70%) or third decades, possibly due to increased gonadotropin secretion during puberty. Symptoms depend on tumor location: Suprasellar GCTs typically present with neuroendocrine dysfunction, visual symptoms, or headache; pineal region GCTs present with features of elevated intracranial pressure or Parinaud's syndrome (failure of upward gaze and retractory nystagmus). The increased thirst and urination of the patient shown above was due to diabetes insipidus related to the suprasellar lesion.

◆ Two major forms of GCTs are recognized: germinomas and nongerminomatous GCTs. Germinomas are the least malignant type of GCTs. The spectrum of nongerminomatous GCTs includes embryonal carcinoma, endodermal sinus tumor, benign or malignant teratomas, and choriocarcinoma, all of which are more malignant than germinomas.

◆ GCTs account for 1% to 3% of pediatric brain tumors in the Western hemisphere, but they are reported to be more common in Japan, where they comprise 5% to 15%.

◆ Ninety-five percent of intracranial GCTs are located in the midline, along an axis from the suprasellar cistern to the pineal gland. About 55% solely involve the pineal region, 35% involve the suprasellar region, and about 5% involve both locations.

◆ About 70% of GCTs in the suprasellar region are germinomas. Conversely, 65% of GCTs in the pineal region are of the nongerminomatous type.

◆ Pineal region GCTs do not arise from the pineal gland itself but from rests of embryonic germ cells.

◆ Suprasellar GCTs are equally frequent in males and females, but the ratio of males to females with pineal GCTs is about 10 to 1.

◆ Germinomas are very radiosensitive tumors, usually rapidly shrinking within a few months of beginning radiation therapy. Nongerminomatous GCTs respond poorly to radiotherapy but are sometimes sensitive to chemotherapy.

◆ Overall prognosis for GCTs depends on patient age, tumor type, and tumor location. Patients <15 years at the time of diagnosis have a better 10-year survival rate (90%) than older patients (50%). The prognosis for suprasellar germinomas (90% survival at 10 years) is much better than for pineal germinomas. Prognosis for nongerminomatous GCTs, on the other hand, is generally poor, with about a 50% 1-year survival rate.

RADIOLOGIC

◆ Ideally, it would be helpful to distinguish, based on imaging studies, tumors arising from the pineal gland (e.g., pineoblastomas and pineocytomas) from those arising from nonpineal tissue (e.g., GCTs) by identification of the pineal gland as a separate structure. Unfortunately, the pineal gland is almost never seen as a separate structure from any pineal region tumor.

◆ The typical appearance of intracranial germinomas on noncontrast CT is that of a relatively homogeneous, mildly or moderately hyperdense mass that densely enhances after contrast administration.

◆ On noncontrast MRI, germinomas are generally isointense to gray matter on T1-weighted images, densely contrast-enhance, and (like most tumors) hyperintense on T2-weighted images.

◆ The finding of synchronous tumors both having a hyperdense appearance on noncontrast CT (as shown in the case above) is highly suggestive of the diagnosis of germinoma. Although only 5% of germinomas are found in both regions, no other tumor would be expected to be located at both sites and have this CT appearance.

◆ Brain imaging studies of patients with GCTs must be assessed for tumor extension into adjacent intracranial structures as well as dissemination throughout intracranial CSF spaces. Spinal imaging is usually indicated to exclude spinal metastases, seen in about 10% of cases.

◆ Determination of hormonal tumor markers in CSF is sometimes useful in attempting to establish the diagnosis of nongerminomatous GCTs. Alpha-fetoprotein is secreted by endodermal sinus tumors, human chorionic gonadotropin (HCG) by choriocarcinomas, and both markers by embryonal carcinomas. However, elevated CSF HCG levels can also be seen occasionally with germinomas.

◆ SUGGESTED READING

Chang T, Teng MM, Guo WY, Sheng WC. CT of pineal tumors and intracranial germ-cell tumors. AJNR 1989;10:1039–1044.

Deutsch M. Intracranial Germ Cell Tumors. In M Deutsch (ed), Management of Childhood Brain Tumors. Boston: Kluwer, 1990;383–399.

Jennings MT, Gelman R, Hochberg F. Intracranial germ cell tumors: Natural history and pathogenesis. J Neurosurg 1985;63:155–167.

CASE 4

E. Ralph Heinz

HISTORY

Two patients with the same diagnosis are presented. The patient in Figure 6-4A was noted to have seven cutaneous café-au-lait spots. The patient in Figure 6-4B has radicular pain along the course of the left second rib.

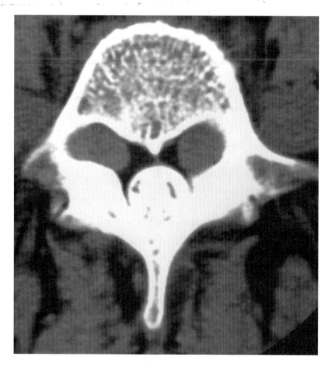

FIGURE 6-4A CT of the lumbar spine following myelography. Bilateral, symmetrical, oval soft-tissue masses fill the neural foramina. Note that the masses prevent passage of contrast material along the nerve root sheath. The neural foramina are smoothly dilated.

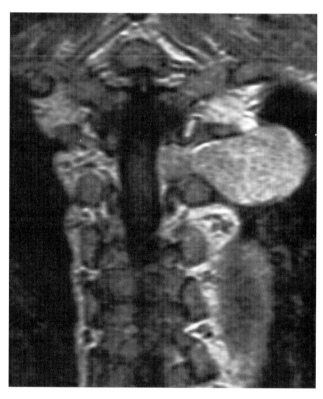

FIGURE 6-4B Contrast-enhanced coronal T1-weighted image at the level of the upper thoracic spine. A smoothly marginated, "dumbbell-shaped" mass exits between the T2 and T3 vertebrae, following the course of the intercostal nerve. The neural foramen is dilated by the mass. The mass homogeneously contrast-enhances.

◆ DIFFERENTIAL DIAGNOSIS

◆ **Spinal dural ectasia in the setting of neurofibromatosis:** This could be a consideration in Figure 6-4A as the cause of dilation of the thecal sac and nerve root sleeves. However, the dilated nerve root sleeves would be expected to be filled by contrast material or CSF, rather than by soft-tissue masses, making this an incorrect diagnosis.

◆ **Meningioma:** This is a possible consideration in Figure 6-4A because, on occasion, meningiomas can extend through the neural foramen. However, a nerve sheath tumor is more common and more likely to cause the "dumbbell" configuration seen in this case.

◆ **Drop metastases:** Solitary CSF metastases along the proximal nerve root can be seen occasionally but are rare. In the absence of any other likely cause, this consideration could be essentially excluded by imaging the remainder of the CNS.

◆ **Plexiform neurofibromas:** These tumors appear as multiple, tortuous, worm-like masses arising along the axis of a major nerve, unlike the solitary, smoothly marginated masses seen in these cases, making this an unlikely diagnosis.

◆ **Nerve sheath tumor:** These lesions are typically smoothly contoured masses that can assume a dumbbell configuration (like the appearance in Figure 6-4B). They densely enhance after contrast administration. These features make this diagnosis the most likely.

◆ DIAGNOSIS: Nerve sheath tumor.

◆ KEY FACTS

CLINICAL

◆ Schwannoma, neurinoma, and neurilemmoma are synonymous terms used to refer to Schwann cell tumors.

◆ Schwannomas and neurofibromas are collectively referred to as nerve sheath tumors but are different pathologic entities.

◆ Nerve root schwannomas do not encase the adjacent nerve root, usually involve the dorsal (sensory) root, are usually solitary, and are not associated with neurofibromatosis. In contrast, neurofibromas encase the dorsal nerve root, are usually multiple, and are frequently associated with neurofibromatosis, even when solitary.

◆ Nerve sheath tumors are often associated with radicular pain or motor dysfunction related to a specific nerve root.

◆ Nerve sheath tumors are found most frequently in the cervical region and usually located in the extra-medullary intradural compartment (about 60% of cases), but they are extradural in 25% of cases, and both extra- and intradural (in which case they often assume a dumbbell configuration) in 15% of cases. Rarely, these tumors can be intramedullary.

◆ Nerve sheath tumors can undergo malignant degeneration (seen in 5% to 10% of cases), usually after a latency period of 10 to 20 years. Thus, malignant degeneration would typically be seen in the third or fourth decade of life.

RADIOLOGIC

◆ From an imaging standpoint, schwannomas and neurofibromas resemble one another very closely. Furthermore, distinction of the two entities on imaging studies is not an important issue. For these reasons, they are generally reported on imaging studies simply as nerve sheath tumors.

◆ One feature that can occasionally be used to distinguish schwannomas from neurofibromas is the asymmetric location of schwannomas. Because schwannomas arise from one side of the nerve root, they displace and efface the normal nerve. They appear lobulated and eccentric, whereas neurofibromas typically have a fusiform shape.

◆ Nerve sheath tumors generally cause widening of the neural foramina. They can be associated with posterior scalloping of the vertebral bodies in neurofibromatosis due to dural ectasia.

◆ Nerve sheath tumors can have increased signal on T1-weighted images (probably related to mucopolysaccharide content) and dense contrast enhancement. Usually markedly increased signal is seen on T2-weighted images (due to high water content). Many neurofibromas have central areas of low signal on T2-weighted images.

◆ Differential diagnosis of benign versus malignant: On CT and MRI, malignant nerve sheath tumors usually have irregular, infiltrative margins, whereas benign nerve sheath tumors usually have smooth margins. In addition, malignant nerve sheath tumors are typically larger than benign lesions.

◆ SUGGESTED READING

Aoki S, Barkovich AJ, Nishimura K, et al. Neurofibromatosis types I and II: Cranial MR findings. Radiology 1989;172:527–534.

Atlas SW (ed). Magnetic Resonance Imaging of the Brain and Spinal Cord. New York: Raven, 1991;946–950.

Suh J-S, Abenoza P, Galloway HR. Peripheral (extra-cranial) nerve tumors: Correlation of MR imaging and histologic findings. Radiology 1992;183:341–346.

CASE 5

David S. Enterline

HISTORY

A 21-year-old woman with occipital headaches. She has previously undergone sub-occipital decompression surgery and C1 laminectomy.

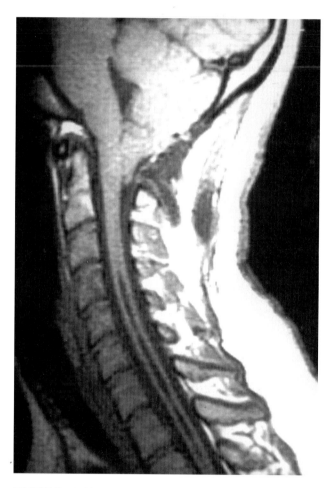

FIGURE 6-5A Sagittal T1-weighted MRI shows herniation of peg-like cerebellar tonsils to the mid C2 level. A hypointense linear abnormality is seen centrally in the spinal cord, extending from the C4 level to the thoracic level.

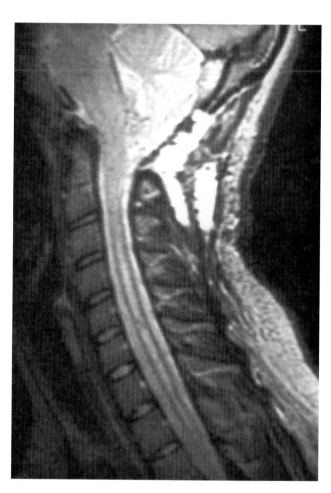

FIGURE 6-5B Sagittal T2-weighted MRI shows the linear abnormality has hyperintense signal on this pulse sequence. Postoperative changes are seen along the dorsal aspect of the spinal column.

◆ DIFFERENTIAL DIAGNOSIS

◆ **Chiari I malformation:** In this congenital malformation, herniation of the cerebellar tonsils occurs through the foramen magnum. The abnormality within the spinal cord is isointense to spinal fluid on all pulse sequences and is due to syringohydromyelia, which is commonly seen in patients with Chiari I malformation. These findings make Chiari I malformation the most likely diagnosis.

◆ **Chiari II:** This entity might be considered because of the herniation of cerebellar tissue. However, other manifestations of Chiari II—e.g., medullary kinking, tectal beaking, a towering cerebellum, hydrocephalus, and myelomeningocele—are not present.

◆ **Chiari III malformation:** In this malformation, herniation of the hindbrain into a low occipital or high cervical encephalocele is seen, often in association with aplasia of the posterior elements of the three highest cervical vertebral bodies. The absence of any of these features excludes this diagnosis in the case shown.

◆ **Other causes of cerebellar tonsillar herniation:** A posterior fossa mass can cause downward herniation of the cerebellar tonsils. Developmental disorders involving the craniovertebral junction (e.g., basilar impression or cranial settling) due to a variety of conditions (e.g., Paget's disease and rheumatoid arthritis) can cause an abnormal relationship of the cerebellar tonsils to the foramen magnum. None of these conditions is present in the case shown.

◆ DIAGNOSIS: Chiari I malformation.

◆ KEY FACTS

CLINICAL

◆ Congenital hindbrain dysgenesis characterized by downward herniation of the cerebellar tonsils was described in 1891 by Hans Chiari. In Chiari I malformation, there is downward herniation of the cerebellar tonsils into the spinal canal, with the fourth ventricle and vermis remaining in a relatively normal position, except in severe cases.

◆ This malformation is thought to result from a dysplasia of bone at the craniocervical junction.

◆ Patients with Chiari I malformation typically are first diagnosed in young adulthood. Almost all symptomatic patients have at least 5 mm of cerebellar herniation.

◆ Symptoms and signs can be on the basis of either compression of the cervicomedullary junction or syringohydromyelia.

◆ The most common clinical features are hypesthesia (decreased sensation) and weakness in the extremities (about 50%), headaches, cranial neuropathy, and long tract findings (e.g., gait disturbance, spasticity, and bowel and bladder dysfunction).

◆ Treatment is usually directed at decompression of the cervicomedullary junction and consists of suboccipital decompression of the foramen magnum with cervical laminectomy to the level of the tonsillar herniation. Some surgeons will place a shunt tube through the foramen of Magendie into the fourth ventricle. In addition, treatment of syringohydromyelia can be performed by decompression and, on occasion, shunting.

RADIOLOGIC

◆ The diagnosis is made by measuring the displacement of the tonsils below a line from the basion (anterior lip of foramen magnum) to the opisthion (posterior lip of the foramen magnum). The normal position of the tonsils varies with age. Tonsillar herniation is present when the tonsils are ≥6 mm (≤10 years), 5 mm (age 11 to 30), or 4 mm (age 31 to 80) below this line. Most patients present in late childhood or early adulthood—hence, the usual criterion of 5 mm. The tonsils are considered low lying rather than herniated when 3 to 5 mm of inferior displacement is present.

◆ The peg-like configuration of the tonsils narrows the posterior CSF space at the level of the foramen magnum, altering the CSF flow dynamics. This may be shown by cine MR flow techniques.

◆ Hydrocephalus is seen in 20% to 25% of Chiari I malformation patients.

◆ Compression of the brain stem and upper cervical cord may be an important cause of symptoms. Arachnoid adhesions may develop due to repeated trauma of the cerebellum, further compromising CSF flow.

◆ Syringohydromyelia occurs in 60% to 70% of patients, usually in symptomatic patients. This condition is more appropriately termed *hydromyelia* because the CSF-filled cavity develops in the ependyma-lined central canal. The most accepted theory of causation of syringohydromyelia is transmission of exaggerated CSF pulsations (due to restricted flow at the level of the fourth ventricle outlet foramina) into the central cavity of the spinal cord.

◆ Basilar invagination—i.e., extension of the tip of the odontoid process >5 mm above Chamberlain's line (a line drawn from the posterior margin of the hard palate to the posterior aspect of the foramen magnum)—is seen in about 25% of Chiari I malformation patients.

◆ Skeletal anomalies are common in Chiari I malformation and include assimilation of C1 to the occiput (10%), partial nonsegmentation of C2 and C3 (15%), and Klippel-Feil deformity (5%).

◆ SUGGESTED READING

Byrd SE, Osborn RE, Radkowski MA, et al. Disorders of midline structures: Holoprosencephaly, absence of corpus callosum, and Chiari malformations. Semin US CT MR 1988;9:201–215.

Elster AD, Chen MYM. Chiari I malformations: Clinical and radiologic reappraisal. Radiology 1992;183:347–353.

Mikulis DJ, Diaz O, Egglin TK, Sanchez R. Variance of the position of the cerebellar tonsils with age: Preliminary report. Radiology 1992;183:725–728.

Pillay PK, Awad IA, Little JR, Hahn JF. Symptomatic Chiari malformation in adults: A new classification based on magnetic resonance imaging with clinical and prognostic significance. Neurosurgery 1991;28:639–645.

CASE 6

Fernando M. Zalduondo

HISTORY

A 16-year-old boy with left proptosis, chemosis, decreased visual acuity, and a bruit heard over the left orbit.

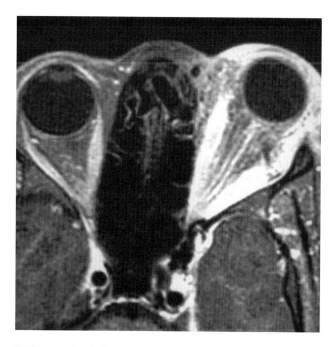

FIGURE 6-6A Contrast-enhanced T1-weighted axial MRI of the orbit. Left proptosis, dense enhancement, and thickening of the left extraocular muscles relative to those on the right, and dilation of the left cavernous sinus (which contains numerous flow voids) are seen.

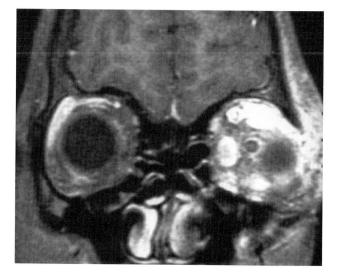

FIGURE 6-6B Contrast-enhanced T1-weighted coronal MRI of the orbit. Abnormal contrast enhancement and thickening of the left periorbital soft tissues and extraocular muscles are present. The left superior ophthalmic vein, seen at the 11 o'clock position, is dilated.

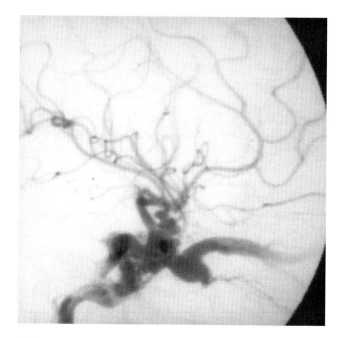

FIGURE 6-6C Early arterial phase of catheter angiogram of the left internal carotid artery, lateral view. Abnormal early opacification of a dilated left cavernous sinus and superior ophthalmic vein is seen.

◆ DIFFERENTIAL DIAGNOSIS

◆ **Orbital pseudotumor:** This diagnosis would not account for a number of features in the case shown—e.g., orbital bruit, dilatation of the superior ophthalmic vein (SOV), and abnormal communication between the internal carotid artery (ICA) and SOV. This diagnosis, therefore, is unlikely.

◆ **Thyroid orbitopathy (Graves' disease):** This diagnosis might be considered because of the proptosis and extraocular muscle enlargement. However, involvement of both orbits is typical, and patients are usually much older than in the case presented. Furthermore, Graves' disease would not account for some of the MRI findings (e.g., dilatation of the left cavernous sinus and SOV) or the angiographic findings.

◆ **Optic nerve plexiform neurofibroma:** Enlargement of the orbital or retro-orbital segments of the optic nerve would be expected but are not present in the case shown. Again, an orbital bruit, dilatation of the SOV, and the angiographic findings would not be expected.

◆ **Carotid-cavernous fistula (CCF):** Patients with this diagnosis typically present with orbital pain, proptosis, and a bruit. Imaging findings can include dilation of the SOV and widening of the cavernous sinus. This is the correct diagnosis.

◆ DIAGNOSIS: Carotid-cavernous fistula.

◆ KEY FACTS

CLINICAL

◆ Clinical features of CCF depend on the predominant route of venous drainage. When the majority of the venous drainage is into the superior and inferior ophthalmic veins, ocular chemosis, proptosis (secondary to venous congestion), glaucoma, and occasionally, unilateral visual loss are found. When the bulk of the venous drainage is into the superior, inferior, and petrosal sinuses, or when the cavernous sinus becomes greatly distended, a cavernous sinus syndrome consisting of ophthalmoplegia and facial pain occurs.

◆ In traumatic CCFs, a delay in symptom onset of days or weeks after the injury is common.

◆ CCFs are best classified by the nature of the arteriovenous connection, which is either direct or indirect.

◆ Direct CCFs are due to a direct connection between the internal carotid artery (ICA) and the veins of the cavernous sinus. Etiologies include (1) trauma, (2) rupture of an intracavernous ICA aneurysm, and (3) a fistulous communication due to an underlying vasculopathy (e.g., Ehlers-Danlos syndrome).

◆ Traumatic CCFs frequently follow skull base fracture or penetrating injuries but can be iatrogenic (e.g., after surgery at sites near the cavernous sinus, such as sphe-noidotomy or trigeminal rhizotomy). These lesions are often high-flow conduits between the arterial and venous circulation.

◆ Indirect CCFs are typically spontaneous and caused by development of multiple fistulous communications between dural branches of the carotid circulation and the cavernous sinus. The volume of blood shunted in indirect CCFs is usually much smaller than in direct CCFs.

◆ CCFs sometimes involve both cavernous sinuses (and hence both orbits) because communication between the cavernous sinuses is allowed by the circular sinus, the collective term for the anterior and posterior intercavernous sinuses that variably connect both cavernous sinuses.

◆ Conservative treatment of patients with indirect CCFs and mild symptoms is often attempted by frequent, self-administered external compression of the carotid artery and jugular vein for many minutes at a time. However, most patients need invasive treatment.

◆ Complications requiring emergency treatment are: (1) rapid progression of proptosis or visual loss, and (2) development of increased intracranial pressure (due to cortical venous hypertension, caused by diversion of blood flow into cortical veins) and intraparenchymal or subarachnoid hemorrhage (following rupture of a large cavernous sinus varix or congested cortical vein).

RADIOLOGIC

◆ Major findings on CT and MRI include extraocular muscle enlargement, proptosis, and dilation of the ipsilateral cavernous sinus and SOV.

◆ Reversal of flow through the SOV can be shown on phase-contrast MR angiography.

◆ The site of the fistula and exact arterial supply can only be shown by catheter angiography. This information is important for planning endovascular therapy. Findings include early opacification of the cavernous sinus, poor opacification of the ICA distal to the fistula, and retrograde filling of dilated venous tributaries.

◆ Endovascular therapy with preservation of distal ICA flow is the standard first-line therapy. Detachable balloons or, on occasion, coils are used for large-hole fistulas (e.g., direct CCFs). Embolic agents such as isobutyl-2-cyanoacrylate or polyvinyl-alcohol particles are used for indirect CCFs. Surgery is reserved for cases that fail endovascular therapy.

◆ SUGGESTED READING

Debrun GM. Treatment of traumatic carotid-cavernous fistula using detachable balloon catheters. AJNR 1983;4:355–356.

Mafee MF, Schatz CJ. The Orbit. In PM Som, RT Bergeron (eds), Head and Neck Imaging (2nd ed). St. Louis: Mosby, 1991;693–813.

Panasci DJ, Nelson PK. MR imaging and MR angiography in the diagnosis of dural arteriovenous fistulas. Magn Res Clin North Am 1995;3:493–508.

HISTORY

A 65-year-old woman with mild proptosis.

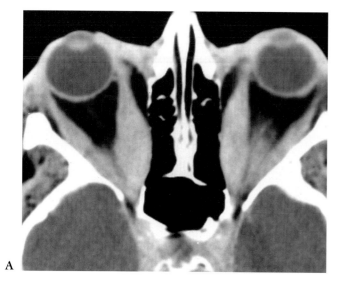

A

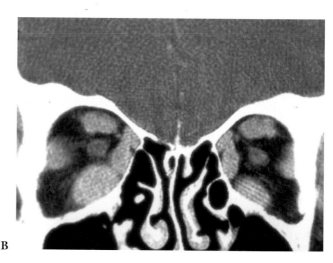

B

FIGURES 6-7A and 6-7B Contrast-enhanced axial CT of the orbits. **(A)** shows marked enlargement of the bellies of the medial rectus muscles and less prominent enlargement of the lateral rectus muscles. A portion of the inferior rectus muscle, which is also enlarged, is seen in the left orbit. Contrast-enhanced coronal CT **(B)** shows smooth enlargement of the extraocular muscles. The intraorbital fat is normal in appearance. These images show relatively symmetric enlargement of most of the extraocular muscles, with predominant involvement of the inferior rectus, medial rectus, and superior rectus muscles, and relative sparing of the lateral rectus muscles. The superior ophthalmic vein is normal in diameter. The bellies of the muscles are enlarged, with sparing of the muscle tendons.

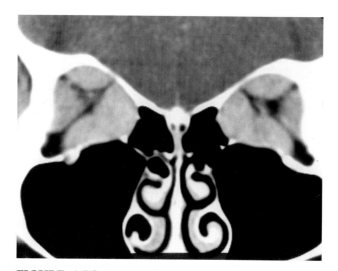

FIGURE 6-7C Contrast-enhanced coronal CT near the orbital apex in another patient with the same diagnosis shows enlargement of all the visualized extraocular muscles. The fat-containing spaces around the optic nerves are narrowed, especially on the patient's right side. The orbital veins are normal in size.

◆ DIFFERENTIAL DIAGNOSIS

◆ **Orbital pseudotumor (idiopathic orbital myositis):** Myositis is one of many manifestations of orbital pseudotumor. This is an unlikely diagnosis for the case shown above because diffuse enlargement of the entire extraocular muscle is usually seen in orbital pseudotumor, whereas the tendinous portions of the muscles are not enlarged in Figure 6-7A.

◆ **Neoplasm arising from muscle:** Tumors such as rhabdomyosarcoma, lymphoma, leukemia, and metastases can involve the extraocular muscles. However, bilateral, symmetric involvement makes this diagnosis unlikely.

◆ **Vascular congestion causing extraocular muscle enlargement:** Muscle enlargement can result from vascular congestion associated with high blood-flow states such as carotid cavernous fistula (see Case 6). This condition is often manifested clinically by chemosis and an orbital bruit (neither of which was present in this patient) and radiologic findings of dilatation and tortuosity of the superior ophthalmic vein (which is of normal size in this patient). This diagnosis is, therefore, unlikely.

◆ **Graves' ophthalmopathy:** This is the best diagnosis given the bilateral muscle enlargement, predominant involvement of the inferior, medial, and superior rectus muscles, and sparing of muscle tendons.

◆ DIAGNOSIS: Graves' disease (thyroid ophthalmopathy).

◆ KEY FACTS

CLINICAL

◆ Thyroid ophthalmopathy is a common cause of unilateral or bilateral proptosis in adults.

◆ Extraocular muscle enlargement occurs due to lymphocytic and plasmacytic infiltration of connective tissue (presumed to be autoimmune in origin) accompanied by mucopolysaccharide deposition, edema, and fibrosis.

◆ Enlargement of the extraocular muscles can produce proptosis, decreased range of globe motion and diplopia, and periorbital and conjunctival edema due to elevated orbital pressure.

◆ Visual loss is threatened in 10% of patients due to compressive optic neuropathy (caused by compression of the optic nerve at the orbital apex due to muscle enlargement) or corneal ulceration (due to corneal exposure secondary to lid retraction and exophthalmos).

◆ Thyroid ophthalmopathy usually occurs in patients with hyperthyroidism, but 10% of patients have no clinical or laboratory evidence of thyroid disease.

◆ Treatment is typically with corticosteroids. Occasionally, radiation therapy or surgical decompression of the optic nerve is performed is cases in which vision is threatened.

RADIOLOGIC

◆ Thyroid ophthalmopathy typically produces enlargement of the bellies of the extraocular muscles, with sparing of the tendinous insertions, which can be helpful in distinguishing it from other causes of extraocular muscle enlargement.

◆ The inferior rectus muscles and medial rectus are affected earliest and most severely. The lateral rectus muscle is usually the least involved. In 6% of cases, only one muscle is enlarged.

◆ Approximately 85% of cases have bilateral disease on CT or MRI.

◆ Imaging in the coronal or sagittal plane is better suited for determination of enlargement of the extraocular muscles, particularly the inferior rectus and superior rectus muscles (which are cut tangentially on axial images).

◆ Findings other than extraocular muscle enlargement that may be seen include an increase in the volume of orbital fat and enlargement or anterior displacement of the lacrimal gland.

◆ SUGGESTED READING

Carter JA, Utiger RD. The ophthalmopathy of Graves' disease. Annu Rev Med 1992;43:487–495.

Enzmann D, Donaldson SS, Kriss JP. Appearance of Graves' disease on orbital computed tomography. J Comput Assist Tomogr 1979;3:815–819.

Nugent RA, Belkin RI, Neigel JM, et al. Graves' orbitopathy: Correlation of CT and clinical findings. Radiology 1990;177:675–682.

Trokel SL, Jakobiec FA. Correlation of CT scanning and pathologic features of ophthalmic Graves' disease. Ophthalmology 1981;81:553–564.

CASE 8

Charles B. Donovan

HISTORY

A 6-year-old girl with short stature and diabetes insipidus.

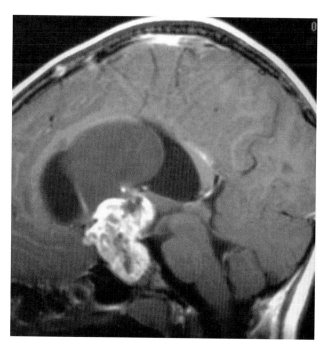

FIGURE 6-8A Contrast-enhanced T1-weighted sagittal MRI. A large, heterogeneously enhancing sellar and suprasellar mass is seen. The mass has both cystic and solid components. The contents of each cyst have signal characteristics that differ from one another and from cerebrospinal fluid.

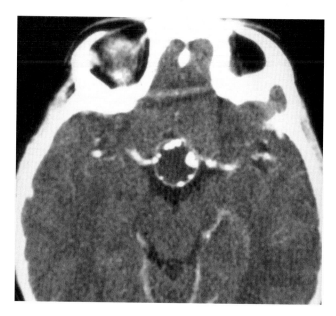

FIGURE 6-8B Contrast-enhanced axial CT image in another patient, a 5-year-old boy, with the same diagnosis. A round, partially calcified cystic mass is present in the suprasellar cistern.

◆ DIFFERENTIAL DIAGNOSIS

- ◆ **Chiasmatic/hypothalamic glioma:** These lesions usually spare the sella and are usually not cystic or calcified.
- ◆ **Craniopharyngioma:** These lesions account for 50% of suprasellar tumors in children. A typical MR appearance is that of a heterogeneously enhancing, calcified sellar and suprasellar mass with multilobulated cystic components, as in this case. This is the best diagnosis for the lesions shown.
- ◆ **Germ cell tumor (GCT):** The age of these patients and lesion location make this category of tumor (which includes a wide number of lesions; see Case 3) a possible consideration. However, germinomas typically have homogeneous signal intensity. Cystic components are occasionally seen but are not usually large. Teratomas have heterogeneous signal like the lesion shown here, but they usually have fat and calcium and are not typically cystic. These factors make GCT an unlikely diagnosis for the cases shown above.
- ◆ **Pituitary adenoma:** These lesions are very uncommon in children and, unlike the lesions shown here, do not usually have large cystic components and are not calcified.
- ◆ **Rathke's cleft cyst:** These lesions often contain mucoid material that is hyperintense on all pulse sequences. However, they are typically intrasellar (unlike the lesion shown above, which is predominantly suprasellar), usually much smaller than the lesion shown here, are not calcified, and do not contrast-enhance.

◆ DIAGNOSIS: Craniopharyngioma.

◆ KEY FACTS

CLINICAL

- ◆ Craniopharyngiomas are derived from squamous epithelial remnants of Rathke's cleft. Most involve both the sellar and suprasellar regions, but less commonly, they can be located solely within the sella or the third ventricle.
- ◆ These tumors represent 3% to 5% of all intracranial tumors, show no gender predilection, and have a bimodal age distribution. More than half occur in childhood (peak: ages 5 to10 years) and adolescence, but a second peak is seen in middle age.
- ◆ About 90% of craniopharyngiomas are partially cystic. Rarely, the lesion is purely cystic. The cyst contents consist of straw-colored or oily brownish fluid with variable amounts of cholesterol crystals.
- ◆ Clinical symptoms are typically due to mass effect on adjacent structures—e.g., visual field defects due to compression of the optic pathways and neuroendocrine dysfunction due to compression of the hypothalamus and pituitary gland.
- ◆ Two distinct clinicopathologic variants are recognized. The adamantinomatous type is the more common of the two variants. It can be seen in both adults and children but is more common in the latter. The papil-

lary form almost always occurs in adults, accounting for about one-third of adult craniopharyngiomas. It is more often solid, less frequently calcified, and has been reported to have a better surgical outcome than adamantinomatous tumors in the adult.

- ◆ Presenting symptoms and signs are usually those associated with increased intracranial pressure (headache, nausea, vomiting, papilledema) or visual disturbance. Craniopharyngiomas are hormonally inactive and can compress the pituitary gland and hypothalamus, causing neuroendocrine dysfunction.
- ◆ There is considerable debate regarding the best management of craniopharyngiomas—i.e., whether to use surgical resection or cyst aspiration followed by radiation therapy. Surgical excision is complicated by the fact that complete resection of the tumor away from the hypothalamus and pituitary stalk is often impossible.

RADIOLOGIC

- ◆ Calcifications are frequently present. CT is more sensitive than MRI in detection of these calcifications.
- ◆ The noncontrast CT appearance is that of an inhomogeneous mass that frequently has cystic components and punctate or clumpy calcifications. Occasionally, the cyst is hyperdense, thought to be due to very high protein concentration. Variable degrees of a soft-tissue component can be seen, which enhance after contrast administration. On CT and MRI studies, when cyst contents are identical in appearance to cerebrospinal fluid, the presence of calcifications and soft-tissue components helps to distinguish craniopharyngioma from arachnoid cyst, a lesion that also commonly occurs in the suprasellar region.
- ◆ The cystic components of craniopharyngiomas are variable on T1-weighted MRIs, varying from isointensity with CSF to hyperintensity. The hyperintense signal has been attributed to very high protein concentrations, although the presence of cholesterol crystals and triglycerides has also been suggested. Solid portions are frequently relatively isointense to brain on all pulse sequences.
- ◆ MRI is helpful in preoperative definition of the relationship of the tumor to the optic nerves and chiasm, internal carotid arteries and their branches, pituitary stalk, hypothalamus, and third ventricle.
- ◆ The papillary type has a more uniform CT and MR appearance with less frequent calcification and cyst formation.

◆ SUGGESTED READING

Ahmadi J, Destian S, Apuzzo ML, et al. Cystic fluid in craniopharyngiomas: MR imaging and quantitative analysis. Radiology 1992;182:783–785.

Dietman JL, Cromero C, Tajahmady T, et al. CT and MRI of suprasellar lesions. J Neuroradiol 1992;19:1–22.

Hald JK, Eldevik OP. Craniopharyngioma identification by CT and MR imaging at 1.5 T. Acta Radiol 1995;36:142–147.

Pusey E, Kortman KE, Flannigan BD, et al. MR of craniopharyngiomas: Tumor delineation and characterization. AJNR 1987;8:439–444.

CASE 9

James M. Provenzale

HISTORY

A 38-year-old man with spastic paraparesis. He experienced an episode of right facial paralysis of 2 weeks' duration 3 years earlier.

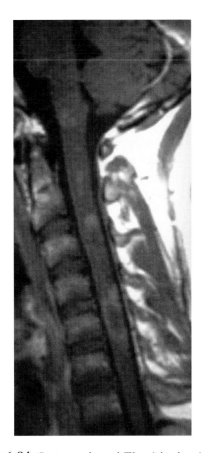

FIGURE 6-9A Contrast-enhanced T1-weighted sagittal MRI of the spine shows multiple enhancing lesions within the spinal cord.

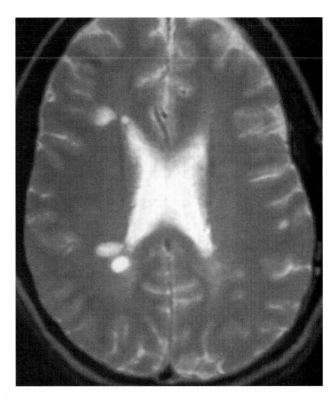

FIGURE 6-9B T2-weighted axial MRI of the brain shows multiple foci of hyperintense signal within the periventricular regions, aligned at right angles to the ventricular surface.

◆ DIFFERENTIAL DIAGNOSIS

◆ **Diffuse axonal injury:** This entity is seen as one or more hyperintense foci on T2-weighted images, but it is found following trauma, which was not present in this patient. Furthermore, a more random distribution of the cranial lesions, rather than an alignment at right angles to the ventricles, would be expected.

◆ **White matter lesions associated with aging:** Hyperintense foci can be seen as (usually incidental) findings in middle-aged and elderly patients. Although occasional foci can be seen in young patients, they are usually small, few in number, and confined to the brain, making this an incorrect diagnosis.

◆ **Vasculitis:** Scattered white matter hyperintense lesions are often seen in patients with vasculitis due to small infarcts. Central nervous system vasculitis is usually characterized by a relatively acute or subacute onset over the course of weeks or months. The history of repeated neurologic events occurring over the course of a few years makes this diagnosis unlikely.

◆ **Multiple sclerosis (MS):** MS typically produces multiple white matter lesions that are hyperintense on T2-weighted images. Characteristically, the lesions are aligned at right angles to the ventricular surface, as in the case shown above. Contrast enhancement is relatively commonly seen.

◆ **Neurosarcoidosis:** This disease generally affects leptomeninges but can produce lesions within the white matter and, on occasion, the spinal cord. It can have the same appearance on MRI as MS. The presence of systemic sarcoidosis (e.g., bilateral hilar lymphadenopathy, elevated angiotensin-converting enzyme levels), not mentioned as present in this patient, would be considered evidence that the central nervous system lesions are due to neurosarcodiosis.

◆ DIAGNOSIS: Multiple sclerosis.

◆ KEY FACTS

CLINICAL

◆ MS is a demyelinating disease typified by a remitting/relapsing course, with multiple exacerbations and remissions involving different parts of the central nervous system. Thus, lesions are characterized by being "multiple in space and time."

◆ The most common sites of involvement are the white matter tracts of the centrum semiovale, corona radiata, and brain stem.

◆ Spinal cord involvement is seen in about 10% of cases.

◆ Onset of symptoms is usually in the third to fifth decades.

◆ Optic neuritis is common. Furthermore, a significant proportion of patients with isolated optic neuritis later are diagnosed as having MS.

◆ The prevalence of MS is higher at northern and temperate climates compared to regions near the equator.

◆ Laboratory abnormalities include the presence of oligoclonal bands in cerebrospinal and abnormal electrophysiologic studies (i.e., visual, auditory, or somatosensory evoked potentials).

◆ The exact etiology is unknown, but MS is generally considered an autoimmune phenomenon.

RADIOLOGIC

◆ MS lesions are typically periventricular in location. Although many diseases can produce such lesions, MS plaques are often oval and have a perpendicular orientation to the lateral ventricles.

◆ MS plaques are generally much more obvious on MRI than CT.

◆ Lesions are characteristically hyperintense on T2-weighted images. Long TR/short TE ("proton density" weighted) images are most sensitive for detecting small lesions adjacent to ventricular surface because they are hyperintense relative to cerebrospinal fluid on this pulse sequence.

◆ MS plaques are generally either isointense (most commonly) or hypointense compared to white matter on T1-weighted images.

◆ Lesions in the corpus callosum, middle cerebellar peduncle, or spinal cord increase the likelihood of the diagnosis of MS.

◆ Optic nerve plaques can be seen using contrast-enhanced T1-weighted or T2-weighted images using fat saturation technique to diminish background signal from orbital fat.

◆ Contrast-enhancing lesions are relatively frequently seen and are generally considered to represent plaques in the acute ("active") stage of demyelination.

◆ SUGGESTED READING

Gean-Marton AD, Vezina LG, Marton KI, et al. Abnormal corpus callosum: A sensitive and specific indicator of multiple sclerosis. Radiology 1991;180:215–221.

Horowitz AL, Kaplan RD, Grewe G, et al. The ovoid lesion: A new MR observation in patients with multiple sclerosis. AJNR 1989;10:303–305.

Yetkin FZ, Haughton VM, Papke RA, et al. Multiple sclerosis: Specificity of MR for diagnosis. Radiology 1991;178:447–451.

CASE 10

E. Ralph Heinz

HISTORY

A 20-year-old man with a primary brain tumor.

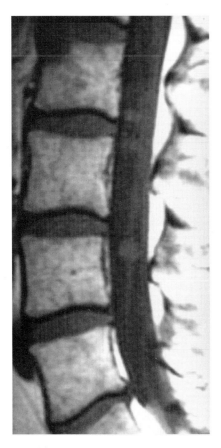

FIGURE 6-10A Noncontrast T1-weighted sagittal image of the spine. A number of nodules are seen within the thecal sac.

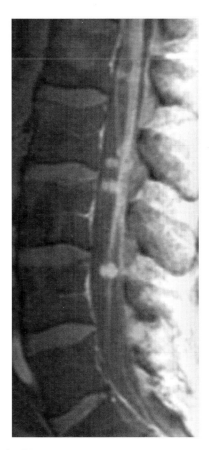

FIGURE 6-10B Contrast-enhanced T1-weighted sagittal image of the spine using fat saturation technique. The nodules densely contrast-enhance in a homogeneous manner.

◆ DIFFERENTIAL DIAGNOSIS

◆ **Leptomeningeal ("drop") metastases:** This term refers to leptomeningeal spread of tumor arising from a primary central nervous system (CNS) neoplasm. Small metastases disseminate through the cerebrospinal spaces and subsequently enlarge. The diffuse pattern of enhancing nodules along the entire length of the cauda equina in a patient with a known primary brain tumor makes this diagnosis the most likely consideration.

◆ **Neurofibroma of the spinal roots:** This diagnosis is considered because neurofibromas usually contrast-enhance. However, they are usually larger and oriented along the axis of the nerve root.

◆ **Granulomatous disease:** Granulomatous diseases—e.g., sarcoidosis—can coat the spinal cord and spinal nerve roots. The appearance is usually that of contrast-enhancing nodules accompanied by adjacent enhancement of the pia and arachnoid (not present in the case shown above). Granulomatous involvement at other cranial sites (e.g., the basilar meninges) or extra-CNS sites (e.g., the lungs) might be expected, which is not reported in this patient.

◆ **Contrast enhancement of spinal cord vessels:** Contrast enhancement of veins posterior to the spinal cord is often seen on MRI, even in normal subjects. On a single axial image, contrast enhancement within veins can be mistaken for enhancing metastases. The distinction between the two entities can be made by looking at serial axial images. Because veins are generally oriented along the craniocaudad axis, venous enhancement should be seen in the same site on serial axial images; metastases will be seen on only one or two of a series of axial images. The lesions shown above are not oriented along the spinal cord and do not represent enhancing vessels.

◆ DIAGNOSIS: Drop metastases.

◆ KEY FACTS

CLINICAL

◆ Between 5% and 30% of children with CNS tumors will have cerebrospinal fluid (CSF) metastasis at the time of diagnosis or at some point in the clinical course—i.e., at initial diagnosis or at time of recurrence.

◆ Clinical status is not a good predictor of the presence of drop metastases. Unless CSF metastases are quite large, patients with drop metastases are generally asymptomatic and appear well.

◆ Detection of drop metastases is vital, because survival is poor if early treatment of tumor dissemination is not performed.

◆ Imaging studies are frequently positive for drop metastases in patients in which cytologic examination of the CSF is negative. However, CSF cytologic findings are positive in 30% of cases in which imaging studies are negative. Therefore, CSF examination and imaging studies are complementary—either examination can be positive when the other examination is negative.

◆ Medulloblastoma is the most common source of drop metastasis (about 50% of all cases), followed by glioblastoma (about 15%).

◆ Two age peaks of drop metastases are seen in patients with childhood brain tumors. The first peak occurs at about age 6 years, at the time of initial diagnosis. The second occurs at about age 15 years and occurs in two conditions: (1) patients with an incompletely treated brain tumor who have had previous prophylactic spinal radiation but subsequently develop drop metastases, and (2) patients with previous remission of brain tumor who develop recurrence of the brain tumor with coexistent drop metastases.

◆ CSF cytology is still the most sensitive means for determining leptomeningeal tumor spread, being positive on initial lumbar puncture in about half of patients with proven CSF metastases.

RADIOLOGIC

◆ Drop metastases tend to be more frequent in the lower spinal canal—i.e., the lumbosacral area (73%), probably due to the effects of gravity.

◆ Metastases within the spinal canal are usually dorsal in location, reflecting CSF flow from the head; ventral CSF flow tends to be toward the head.

◆ The sensitivity of contrast-enhanced MRI is greater than CT myelography or myelography alone. Rapid screening of the entire spinal axis can be performed by MRI in a noninvasive manner. CT myelography is an invasive study in which the myelogram is typically used to direct CT imaging of only a portion of the spinal canal.

◆ SUGGESTED READING

Heinz ER, Weiner D, Friedman H, Tien RD. Detection of cerebral spinal fluid metastasis: CT myelography or MR. AJNR 1995;16:1147–1151.

Kramer ED, Rafto S, Packer RJ, Zimmerman RA. Comparison of myelography with CT follow-up vs. gadolinium MRI for subarachnoid metastatic disease in children. Neurology 1991;41:46–50.

Yousem DM, Patrone PM, Grossman RI. Leptomeningeal metastasis: MR evaluation. J Comput Assist Tomogr 1990;14:255–261.

HISTORY

A 50-year-old woman with sudden onset of low back pain and progressive paraparesis over 6 hours. Symptoms began suddenly after the patient sneezed.

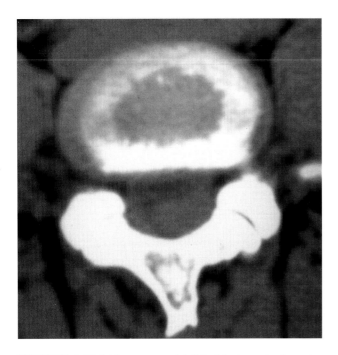

FIGURE 6-11A Noncontrast axial CT of the lower lumbar spine shows a round hyperdense mass in the posterior half of the spinal canal. The thecal sac is displaced anteriorly.

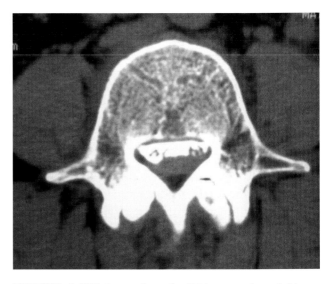

FIGURE 6-11B Postmyelography CT image performed 6 hours after the noncontrast CT shown in Figure 6-11A. The contrast-filled thecal sac is displaced anteriorly by the mass, which is border-forming with the posterior epidural fat.

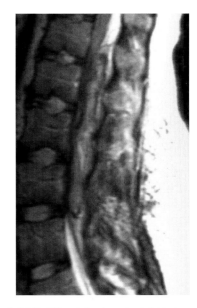

FIGURE 6-11C T2-weighted sagittal MR image in another patient with the same diagnosis. An inhomogeneous mass that is hypointense relative to epidural fat is seen displacing the thecal sac anteriorly. A sharp interface is seen with epidural fat along the superior aspect of the mass. This fact, and the displacement of the thecal sac, indicates that the mass is epidural in location.

◆ DIFFERENTIAL DIAGNOSIS

◆ **Epidural metastases:** These usually arise from vertebral body metastases and extend into the spinal canal, making this an unlikely diagnosis. Nonetheless, in rare instances, some metastases (e.g., lymphoma and leukemia) can infiltrate solely the soft tissues and dura. However, these diagnoses would be unlikely in light of the acute onset of symptoms and the hypointense signal of the lesion in the second patient shown above.

◆ **Spinal epidural abscess:** Risk factors include insulin-dependent diabetes mellitus, chronic renal failure, intravenous drug abuse, or recent spinal surgery (none of which was present in this patient). Usually osteomyelitis or discitis is present. However, in the patients shown above, only the posterior epidural space is involved.

◆ **Spinal epidural hematoma (SEH):** The rapid onset of neurologic deficit is consistent with this diagnosis. The absence of trauma in the first patient discussed above does not exclude SEH, because SEH sometimes occurs after Valsalva maneuvers that accompany exertion (e.g., weightlifting) or vigorous coughing or sneezing (as in this patient). The inhomogeneous, predominantly hypointense signal on T2-weighted images is compatible with acute hemorrhage and would be unexpected with other entities.

◆ **Spinal cord infarction:** This entity is a consideration based on the acute onset of neurologic findings in both patients. However, infarction would be expected to produce an intramedullary lesion, not an epidural lesion, and motor and sensory dysfunction rather than pain.

◆ DIAGNOSIS: Spinal epidural hematoma.

◆ KEY FACTS

CLINICAL

◆ SEH can occur spontaneously or after various degrees of spinal trauma, including minimal trauma, stretching or twisting of the vertebral column without vertebral fracture, Valsalva maneuvers (the first patient shown above), or spinal procedures (e.g., following lumbar puncture, which was the precipitating event in the second patient discussed above).

◆ The typical clinical presentation is acute onset of back pain and rapid development of myelopathy inferior to the level of the hematoma. Early diagnosis of SEH is critical because the likelihood of reversal of neurologic deficit is related to duration of symptoms.

◆ SEH can be seen at any age. About half of cases occur in patients >50 years. It is slightly more common in men. The two most common sites are the low cervical level and the thoracolumbar junction.

◆ Emergency laminectomy to evacuate the hematoma is usually performed. Preoperative radiologic demonstration of the extent of the hematoma is important for surgical planning.

◆ In most patients, the etiology of SEH is not known, even after surgery. Possible etiologies include a weakened spinal epidural vein (e.g., ruptured during Valsalva maneuver), spinal arterial hemorrhage, and rupture of a small arteriovenous malformation.

RADIOLOGIC

◆ SEHs are typically fusiform in shape, with their longest dimension along the craniocaudad axis. They are best seen on sagittal MRI.

◆ These lesions are usually located in the posterior epidural space and are typically three to four vertebral bodies in length.

◆ MRI is the most sensitive and specific means of making the diagnosis, but the diagnosis can also be made by CT alone, myelography alone, and CT myelography.

◆ The MR signal intensity of SEH depends on the age of the hemorrhage. In the acute stage (i.e., that of intracellular deoxyhemoglobin), the SEH is hypointense on T2-weighted images. After a few days, SEH becomes hyperintense on T1-weighted images.

◆ If MRI is unavailable or contraindicated, CT myelography is an acceptable means of making the diagnosis. On axial images, the lesion is seen as a (usually posterior) epidural mass that is isodense or hyperdense to spinal cord and displaces the thecal sac or spinal cord.

◆ Myelographic findings are nonspecific and consist of narrowing or block of the intrathecal contrast column. The lesion can often be seen to be smoothly tapered at each end.

◆ The diagnosis can be difficult to make by plain CT when the epidural mass is isodense to the spinal cord.

◆ SEH can be difficult to distinguish from spinal subdural hematoma, a very uncommon entity. The distinction is usually not important, because surgical evacuation is usually performed in both cases. On axial CT and MRI, subdural hematoma is frequently crescentic and sometimes separated from the lamina by epidural fat. On MRI, subdural hematoma can sometimes be seen to be separated from the epidural fat by the linear hypointense signal of the dura.

◆ SUGGESTED READING

Groen RJM, Ponssen H. The spontaneous epidural hematoma. A study of the etiology. J Neurol Sci 1990;98:121–138.

Holtas S, Heiling M, Lonntoft M. Spontaneous spinal epidural hematoma: Findings at MR imaging and clinical correlation. Radiology 1996;199:409–413.

Post MJD, Seminer DS, Quencer RM. CT diagnosis of spinal epidural hematoma. AJNR 1982;3:190–192.

CASE 12

Robert D. Tien and
James M. Provenzale

HISTORY

A 30-year-old woman with progressively worsening headaches.

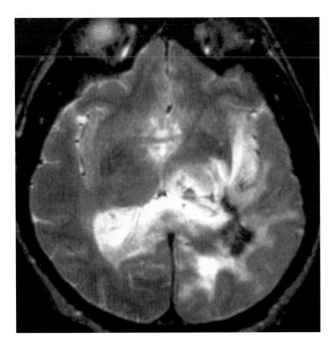

FIGURE 6-12A T2-weighted axial MRI shows an inhomogeneous mass involving much of the left temporal lobe, basal ganglia, and splenium of the corpus callosum. Regions of marked hypointensity are seen within the lesion, raising the possibility of internal hemorrhage or calcification.

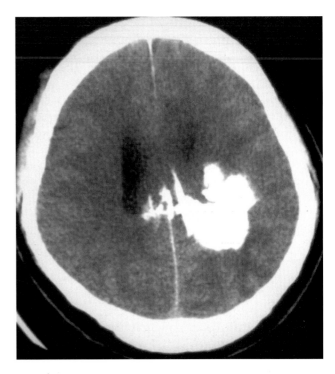

FIGURE 6-12B Noncontrast axial CT image shows that the mass is almost entirely calcified, which explains the hypointense signal seen on the MRI.

◆ DIFFERENTIAL DIAGNOSIS

◆ **Meningioma:** This tumor might be a consideration because meningiomas are commonly calcified, like the lesion shown. However, meningiomas are extra-axial lesions, whereas the lesion shown is intra-axial.

◆ **Tumor with previous radiation therapy:** It is common for tumors that have undergone radiation therapy to become calcified. However, a history of radiation therapy is not present in the case shown above.

◆ **Oligodendroglioma:** This diagnosis should be considered because the lesion shown above is heavily calcified. In particular, it is unusual for any tumor other than oligodendroglioma to develop calcification of this degree in the absence of prior radiation therapy.

◆ DIAGNOSIS: Oligodendroglioma.

◆ KEY FACTS

CLINICAL

◆ Oligodendrogliomas are tumors that arise from oligodendrocytes, the cells from which central nervous system myelin forms.

◆ These tumors account for 5% to 10% of intracranial gliomas.

◆ A 2 to 1 male predominance is seen. The peak age is in the fourth and fifth decades.

◆ Slightly more than half of oligodendrogliomas occur in the frontal lobes, and another 15% each in the temporal lobes and parietal lobes.

◆ Oligodendrogliomas most frequently occur in the periphery of the brain and involve brain cortex (accounting for the high prevalence of seizures). However, as in the cases shown above, it is not uncommon for lesions to occur centrally.

◆ Seizures are the most common presenting feature.

◆ These tumors are characteristically slow growing and can on occasion erode overlying skull. Peritumoral edema is mild or absent. Nodular calcification is the hallmark, seen in 70% to 90% of cases.

◆ About 50% of oligodendrogliomas have a mixed histology consisting of astrocytoma and anaplastic oligodendroglioma. These tumors have a poorer prognosis than the remainder of oligodendrogliomas.

RADIOLOGIC

◆ Between 80% and 90% of oligodendrogliomas are calcified. About two-thirds of oligodendrogliomas have a focus of calcification >1 cm.

◆ The CT scan appearance is that of an inhomogeneous hypodense mass that typically has dense nodular calcification. The tumor frequently extends to involve cortex and can erode the adjacent calvarium.

◆ Intratumoral cysts are common. Intratumoral hemorrhage can occasionally be seen.

◆ Overall, about one-third of oligodendrogliomas contrast-enhance, although it is usually mild. However, two-thirds of oligodendrogliomas with a histologic grade of III or IV contrast-enhance, often in a ring fashion.

◆ MRI is less sensitive than CT in detecting tumor calcification but is superior in defining tumor extent.

◆ MR scans show mixed hypo- and isointense areas on T1-weighted images and hyperintense foci on T2-weighted images. Regions of calcification can be seen as hyperintense foci on T1-weighted images and hypointense foci on T2-weighted images. As on CT, contrast enhancement is typically very mild. Dense contrast enhancement suggests an anaplastic component.

◆ SUGGESTED READING

Lee YY, Van Tassel P. Intracranial oligodendrogliomas: Imaging findings in 35 untreated cases. AJR Am J Roentgenol 1989; 152:361–369.

Rees JH, Smirniotopoulos JG, Jones RV, Mena H. Oligodendroglioma: Clinical and imaging features in 87 patients. Presentation at the 34th Meeting of the American Society of Neuroradiology, 1996.

Vanofakos D, Marcu H, Hacker H. Oligodendrogliomas: CT patterns with emphasis on features indicating malignancy. J Comput Assist Tomogr 1979;3:783–788.

CASE *13*

David S. Enterline

HISTORY

A 17-year-old girl with slow onset of mild spastic paraparesis and urinary incontinence.

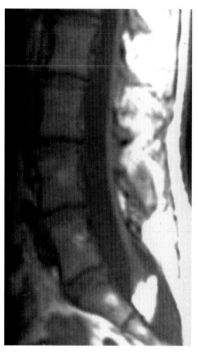

FIGURE 6-13A Noncontrast sagittal T1-weighted image shows that the spinal cord extends to the level of the S1 vertebral body, where it is in contact with a smoothly contoured, homogeneous, hyperintense mass. The posterior elements of the spinal column are absent at the level of the lumbosacral junction, and the caudal portion of the spinal canal is widened.

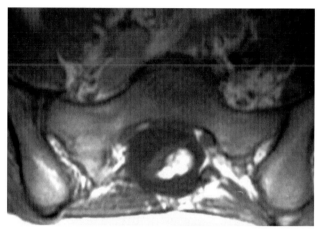

FIGURE 6-13B Noncontrast axial T1-weighted image at the level of the S1 vertebral body shows the thecal sac is widened and projects outside the expected confines of the spinal canal. Instead of a normal cauda equina, the neural elements are arranged as a flat structure (neural placode) abutting the surface of the hyperintense mass.

◆DIFFERENTIAL DIAGNOSIS

◆ **Tightened filum terminale syndrome:** In this syndrome, the conus medullaris is normal or near-normal in position, but clinical features of spastic paraparesis are present. These findings are solely due to the presence of a filum terminale that is thickened (≥3 mm), stretched, and under tension. As a result, the filum terminale often has a curved course, projecting along the posterior aspect of the spinal cord ("bowstring appearance"). However, in the case shown above, other abnormalities are present: the conus medullaris is markedly lower in position than normal, and the

neural elements have an abnormal appearance (the flat neural structure indicative of a neural placode).

◆ **Leptomeningeal ("drop") metastasis:** This entity might be considered because of the clinical features and the presence of a mass within the thecal sac. However, this entity occurs in the presence of a primary brain tumor, which has almost always been diagnosed prior to onset of spinal symptoms. Furthermore, the mass in the caudal end of the thecal sac is hyperintense on noncontrast T1-weighted images and most compatible with fat rather than a neoplasm.

◆ **Lipomyelomeningocele:** In this disorder, dysraphism of the lower lumbar and sacral posterior elements in association with a sac containing neural and fatty structures and projecting beyond the confines of the spinal canal is seen. These findings are present in the case shown above. The hyperintense mass is a lipoma, which has caused tethering of the spinal cord due to adherence of neural elements to the lipoma. The flat structure adherent to the lipoma is the neural placode often seen in this condition.

◆ **DIAGNOSIS: Tethered spinal cord due to a lipomyelomeningocele.**

◆ **KEY FACTS**

CLINICAL

- There are three main congenital causes of spinal cord tethering: (1) intradural lumbosacral lipoma, (2) tight filum terminale, and (3) diastematomyelia (splitting of the spinal cord with fixation due to a fibrocartilaginous or osseous septum within the spinal canal).
- Intraspinal lipomas causing spinal cord tethering can be seen in the setting of: (1) a thickened filum terminale that progressively widens into a lipoma, (2) a normally formed conus medullaris adherent to an adjacent lipoma, and (3) an incompletely closed conus medullaris (myeloschisis) attached to a lipoma.
- Presenting features of tethered cord can include (1) pain in the back, legs, buttocks, or perineum; (2) spastic paraparesis (i.e., abnormal gait, leg weakness and muscular atrophy, hyperreflexia, and urinary or fecal retention or incontinence); (3) sensory changes in the distribution of the lumbosacral roots; (4) tightened Achilles' tendon; (5) scoliosis; and (6) pes cavus deformity of the foot.
- Clinical features related to a tethered spinal cord typically begin in late childhood, adolescence, or early adulthood but can be seen in early childhood or middle age.
- Tethered cords can be seen in association with a variety of spinal lesions, most commonly a lipoma or lipomyelomeningocele.
- Intraspinal lipomas are not invariably associated with neurologic findings; only about half of subjects with these lesions develop symptoms. In particular, small lipomas within the thecal sac or within the filum terminale (sometimes termed a *fibrolipoma*) can be incidental findings seen at autopsy (about 20% of individuals) or on cross-sectional imaging studies.
- Tethered cord syndrome can also occur solely in the presence of a tight, slightly thickened filum terminale ("tightened filum" syndrome). When neurologic features suggestive of tethered cord syndrome are seen in the absence of other structural abnormalities on MRI, it is important to pay particular attention to the thickness and course of the filum terminale to exclude findings indicative of a tightened filum terminale (see the section on Differential Diagnosis).

- Symptoms related to a tethered spinal cord can be precipitated (or worsened) by many factors, including increased tension on the spinal cord (e.g., during pregnancy or following acute anterior flexion of the trunk), increased crowding of intraspinal contents (e.g., disc herniation), and minor trauma.
- Standard treatment for a tethered spinal cord is surgical untethering by release of the spinal cord, spinal nerve roots, or filum terminale from the lesion causing tethering (e.g., from a spinal lipoma), or sectioning of the filum terminale (in the case of a tightened filum). Intraoperatively, only slight cephalad movement of the spinal cord would be expected to be seen after untethering. Therefore, little change in the position of the conus medullaris would be expected on follow-up imaging studies.

RADIOLOGIC

- Findings on plain radiographs associated with a spinal dysraphic state are nonspecific but can include spina bifida occulta (e.g., bifid laminae and absence of the neural arches), widening of the spinal canal, and fusion of the vertebral bodies.
- The position of the conus below the inferior endplate of L2 is considered abnormal.
- MRI is the preferred method of diagnosis because it is (1) noninvasive, (2) the most sensitive method for determination of the level of the conus medullaris and detection of a tethering lesion, and (3) shows the dorsal placement of a tightened filum terminale well. T1-weighted images are the most sensitive pulse sequence for detection of a spinal lipoma.
- Myelography followed by CT is a less acceptable method of diagnosis than MRI but is performed when MRI is unavailable or contraindicated.
- During myelography in patients with a suspected tethered spinal cord, care must be taken to avoid puncture of the spinal cord or filum terminale, which is often close to the posterior wall of the thecal sac. This can be avoided by needle puncture from an oblique angle. Myelographic evaluation can be difficult, because the lumbosacral thecal sac is frequently enlarged due to dural ectasia, which promotes pooling of the contrast material.

◆ **SUGGESTED READING**

Hall WA, Albright AL, Brunberg JA. Diagnosis of tethered cords by magnetic resonance imaging. Surg Neurol 1988;30:60–64.

Levy LM, DiChiro G, McCullough DC, et al. Fixed spinal cord: Diagnosis with MR imaging. Radiology 1988;169:773–778.

McLendon RE, Oakes WJ, Heinz ER, et al. Adipose tissue in the filum terminale: A computed tomographic finding that may indicate tethering of the spinal cord. Neurosurgery 1988;22: 873–876.

E. Ralph Heinz

HISTORY

A 37-year-old man with mild right hemiparesis and headache.

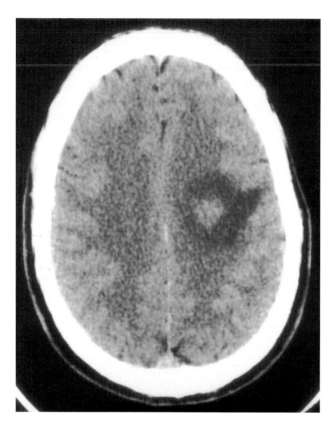

FIGURE 6-14A Noncontrast CT shows a mass that is mildly hyperdense compared to normal white matter with a surrounding rim of hypodense vasogenic edema.

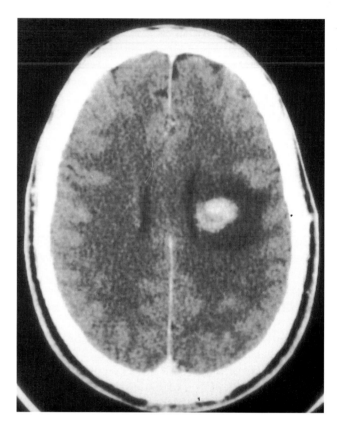

FIGURE 6-14B Postcontrast CT shows homogeneous enhancement of the mass.

◆ DIFFERENTIAL DIAGNOSIS

- **Primary brain tumors:** Primary brain tumors usually have inhomogeneous contrast enhancement and a more variegated appearance. However, lymphoma can appear hyperdense relative to white matter on non-contrast CT, thought to be due to a high nuclear to cytoplasmic ratio. Central nervous system (CNS) lymphoma is frequently solitary (as in the case shown above), but multiple homogeneously enhancing lesions (frequently abutting an ependymal surface) are also a common appearance.

◆ DIAGNOSIS: Primary lymphoma of the central nervous system.

◆ KEY FACTS

CLINICAL

- Primary CNS lymphoma accounts for about 1% of all primary brain tumors but is increasing in frequency as a complication of acquired immunodeficiency disorder (AIDS).
- The CNS does not have intrinsic lymphoid tissue, and the cell of origin of primary CNS lymphoma is unknown.
- Essentially all primary CNS lymphoma is composed of the non-Hodgkin's type.
- Unlike primary CNS lymphoma, CNS spread from systemic lymphoma is usually leptomeningeal, or dural-based, in location rather than parenchymal.
- Patients with non–AIDS-related primary CNS lymphoma usually present in later life (usually in the sixth decade) and are therefore older than the typical patient with AIDS-related lymphoma.
- In addition to AIDS patients, other immunocompromised patients (e.g., organ transplant recipients and patients with congenital immunodeficiency diseases) are at risk for primary CNS lymphoma.

RADIOLOGIC

- Lesions due to primary CNS lymphoma are often located in the white matter, corpus callosum, and basal ganglia. In about half of cases, multiple lesions are present.
- Ependymal extension of periventricular lesions is a common finding and, when seen, should raise the diagnosis of primary CNS lymphoma.

- Calcification and hemorrhage are rarely seen. In non–AIDS-related primary CNS lymphoma, peritumoral edema is usually absent or only mild. However, in the setting of AIDS, edema can sometimes be quite marked, causing lesions to simulate those of toxoplasmosis.
- Lymphoma not related to AIDS is often a homogeneous mass that is hyperdense relative to white matter on noncontrast CT. It thus differs in appearance from AIDS-related lymphoma, in which lesions are often inhomogeneous with hypodense components. Primary CNS lymphoma in the two populations also differs from the standpoint of contrast enhancement: non-AIDS lymphoma frequently contrast-enhances in a homogeneous manner, but AIDS-related lymphoma often has inhomogeneous enhancement in a ring-fashion, another feature causing it to simulate toxoplasmosis.
- Lymphoma, when located deep within the brain, is usually isointense to gray matter on spin echo MR sequences, a finding that is also seen in other hypercellular small cell-type tumors. However, on occasion, the lesions can be very hyperintense on T2-weighted images.
- Parenchymal brain metastases from systemic lymphoma can be indistinguishable from primary CNS lymphoma, but parenchymal metastases are rare in the absence of leptomeningeal lesions.
- AIDS-related primary CNS lymphoma can closely simulate toxoplasmosis. However, toxoplasmosis lesions frequently have a peripheral hyperintense rim on T1-weighted MR images, which is hypointense on proton density and T2-weighted images, a finding not generally seen in lymphoma. Thallium SPECT scans have shown usefulness in distinguishing the two entities, because scans are negative in toxoplasmosis and positive in lymphoma.
- If hemorrhage is present, this argues against lymphoma, and it is frequently seen in toxoplasmosis.

◆ SUGGESTED READING

Roman-Goldstein SM, Goldman DL, Howieson J, et al. MR of primary CNS lymphoma in immunologically normal patients. AJNR 1992;13:1207–1213.

Ruiz A, Ganz WI, Post MJD, et al. Use of thallium-201 brain SPECT to differentiate cerebral lymphoma from toxoplasma encephalitis in AIDS patients. AJNR 1994;15:1885–1894.

Russell DS, Rubinstein LJ. Pathology of Tumor of the Nervous System (5th ed). Baltimore: Williams & Wilkins, 1989.

HISTORY

A 21-year-old woman with seizures.

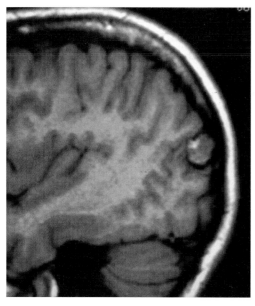

FIGURE 6-15A Noncontrast T1-weighted sagittal image shows an inhomogeneous lesion that is located in brain cortex and has a small focus of hyperintense signal along the superior surface. The hyperintense signal is consistent with hemorrhage.

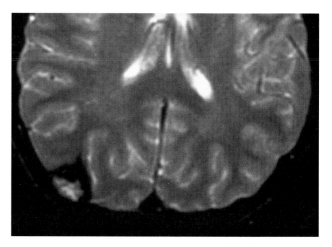

FIGURE 6-15B T2-weighted axial image shows two regions of signal abnormality. An inhomogeneous hyperintense focus is seen within brain cortex, which has a reticulated appearance. A surrounding region of markedly hypointense signal is also seen, consistent with hemosiderin deposition. No edema is seen surrounding the lesion.

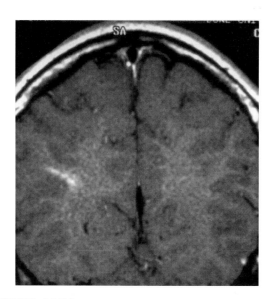

FIGURE 6-15C Contrast-enhanced coronal T1-weighted image shows a thin linear region of contrast enhancement. This abnormality was separate from, and located a few centimeters anterior to, the lesion shown in Figures 6-15A and 6-15B.

◆ DIFFERENTIAL DIAGNOSIS

◆ **Hemorrhagic contusion:** This diagnosis might be considered because of the superficial location of the lesion and the MR signal characteristics indicating hemorrhage. However, there is no history of trauma.

◆ **Hemorrhagic neoplasm:** Most or all of the lesion has signal characteristics compatible with hemorrhage. It is unusual for intratumoral hemorrhage to occupy the entire volume of the tumor.

◆ **Arteriovenous malformation (AVM):** This lesion might be considered because of the evidence of hemorrhage. However, AVMs typically appear on MRI as a conglomeration of flow-voids, rather than solely a focus of hemorrhage.

◆ **Embolic infarction:** This entity might be considered because embolic infarcts occur in the periphery of the brain and are frequently hemorrhagic. However, the reticulated appearance shown above would be unusual for a hemorrhagic infarction because they usually have homogeneous signal.

◆ **Cavernous angioma:** These lesions are associated with seizures and typically appear as rounded, reticulated regions of abnormal signal with internal foci of hemorrhage surrounded by dark signal on T2-weighted images due to hemosiderin deposition. This is the correct diagnosis. The entity shown in Figure 6-15C has features typical of a venous angioma, with which cavernous angiomas are associated.

◆ DIAGNOSIS: Cavernous angioma with an associated venous angioma.

◆ KEY FACTS

CLINICAL

◆ Cavernous angiomas consist of a cluster of enlarged vascular channels lacking intervening brain parenchyma. Unlike cavernous angiomas, AVMs have a nidus of abnormal vessels with well-defined feeding arteries and draining veins.

◆ Cavernous angiomas can be either sporadic or familial in nature.

◆ Multiple angiomas are found in 10% to 15% of patients with the sporadic variety and about 75% of those with the familial form.

◆ Symptom onset is typically in young adulthood. The most common clinical features are seizures (40% to 70% of patients), headache, and, on occasion, sudden onset of neurologic deficit.

◆ Cavernous angiomas, especially those located in the posterior fossa, are often found in association with venous angiomas, which are benign venous developmental abnormalities.

◆ Histologic examination of these lesions shows a cluster of thin-walled (often thrombosed and calcified) vascular channels that are not separated from one another by brain tissue.

◆ The rate of hemorrhage of cavernous angiomas has been determined to be between 0.25% and 0.70% per person year of exposure.

◆ Symptomatic cavernous angiomas that are superficial are often resected if they are not located in eloquent brain tissue. Brain stem lesions that are not amenable to excision can be treated by stereotactic radiosurgery.

RADIOLOGIC

◆ Cavernous angiomas are usually <2 cm in size but occasionally can be larger, particularly when substantial hemorrhage has occurred.

◆ These lesions are frequently found incidentally on MRI or CT studies performed for unrelated symptoms.

◆ These lesions are almost always occult on angiography, although rarely a small vascular blush (without arterial feeders or early draining veins) can be seen.

◆ On CT, these lesions can be seen as well circumscribed, frequently hyperdense lesions that often have one or more small foci of calcification due to previous hemorrhage. Often, however, lesions are isodense with brain, especially if they are small or have not undergone hemorrhage.

◆ These lesions typically do not contrast-enhance to a large degree on CT or MRI.

◆ Edema is typically not seen surrounding cavernous angiomas unless they have recently undergone a substantial amount of hemorrhage.

◆ Generally, cavernous angiomas are occult on catheter angiography but can occasionally be seen as a region of capillary blush or pooling of contrast material in the venous phase.

◆ MRI is very helpful in confirming the diagnosis when it is suspected on CT because it can show multiple lesions (making the diagnosis more likely) and reveal the typical hemosiderin halo around lesions.

◆ T2-weighted MRIs and gradient-echo images are sensitive to the magnetic susceptibility effect of chronic blood products.

◆ On occasion, cavernous angiomas can be difficult to distinguish from primary or secondary brain tumors. The presence of multiple lesions is helpful in excluding a primary tumor. The presence of calcification on CT or a characteristic hemosiderin rim on MRI (both features not expected with metastases) is helpful in making the distinction.

◆ SUGGESTED READING

Abe T, Singer RJ, Marks MP, et al. Coexistence of cavernous and developmental venous anomalies in the central nervous system: MR evaluation. Presentation at the 34th Meeting of the American Society of Neuroradiology, 1996.

Rigamonti D, Hadley MN, Drayer BP, et al. Cerebral cavernous malformations. N Engl J Med 1988;319:343–347.

Robinson JR, Awad IA, Little JR. Natural history of the cavernous angioma. J Neurosurg 1991;75:709–714.

HISTORY

A 38-year-old woman with visual loss over the period of a few weeks and mild diabetes insipidus over the course of a year.

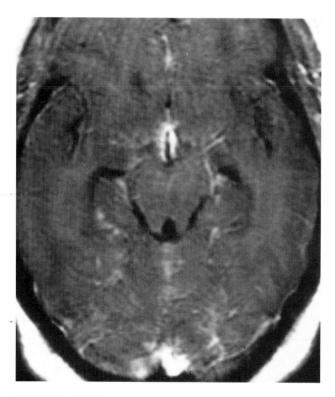

FIGURE 6-16A Contrast-enhanced T1-weighted axial MRI shows prominent enhancement of the hypothalamus and walls of the third ventricle. A lesser degree of contrast enhancement of the leptomeninges is seen throughout the supratentorial compartment.

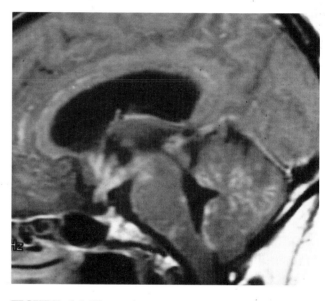

FIGURE 6-16B Contrast-enhanced T1-weighted sagittal MRI shows dense enhancement of the optic chiasm and anterior aspect of the third ventricle and leptomeningeal enhancement over the surface of the brain stem and cerebellum. Scattered foci of leptomeningeal enhancement are again seen throughout the supratentorial compartment, but to a lesser degree than at the base of the brain.

◆ DIFFERENTIAL DIAGNOSIS

◆ **Leptomeningeal carcinomatosis:** This diagnosis is unlikely in the absence of a prior history of a non-CNS neoplasm. Furthermore, preferential involvement of the cisternal spaces at the base of the brain would not be expected.

◆ **Viral meningitis:** Leptomeningeal enhancement due to viral meningitis is typically thin, unlike the relatively thick contrast enhancement seen at the level of the optic chiasm and third ventricle seen in the case shown above. Bacterial meningitis, another consideration in the case shown above, can be seen to produce thick leptomeningeal enhancement. However, neither bacterial nor viral meningitis would be expected to produce the preferential leptomeningeal involvement at the base of the brain seen in the case shown above.

◆ **Tuberculous meningitis:** This diagnosis should be strongly considered because tuberculous meningitis frequently produces thick exudates involving the leptomeninges on the undersurface of the brain. This diagnosis cannot be excluded on the basis of imaging features in the case shown above. Instead, clinical and laboratory data (including cerebrospinal fluid [CSF] analysis) would need to be evaluated. Patients with central nervous system (CNS) tuberculosis (TB) usually have active pulmonary disease, which was not present in the patient shown above. In the case shown above, the CSF did not stain positive for acid-fast bacilli.

◆ **Neurosarcoidosis:** This disease entity has a predilection for involvement of the leptomeninges on the undersurface of the brain and also often produces chronic symptoms, as in the case shown above. The diagnosis can be inferred on the basis of known extra-CNS sarcoidosis or directly obtained by biopsy of the leptomeninges or brain, which was performed in the case shown above and showed noncaseating granulomas.

DIAGNOSIS: Neurosarcoidosis.

KEY FACTS

CLINICAL

- Sarcoidosis is an idiopathic systemic disease characterized by formation of noncaseating granulomas in multiple organ systems. The disease usually affects young adults in the third or fourth decade of life, who usually present clinically with insidious onset of malaise, weight loss, and fatigue.

- Only about 5% of patients have CNS symptoms, but 25% of patients have findings of CNS involvement at autopsy. CNS symptoms usually begin within the first few years after onset of systemic disease. The predilection of the disease to involve the midline structures at the base of the brain is reflected by the symptom distribution outlined below.

- Cranial neuropathy (especially seventh nerve paresis) is the most common neurologic manifestation, seen in more than half of patients with CNS disease.

- Aseptic meningitis due to granulomatous infiltration of the leptomeninges is seen in about 20% of patients with neurologic disease.

- Neuroendocrinologic dysfunction due to infiltration of the hypothalamus or pituitary gland and stalk is seen in about 20% of patients with CNS involvement.

- Spinal disease manifestations are uncommon (about 5% of patients with neurologic disease) and can have a wide variety of presentations, including spinal cord findings (e.g., myelopathy due to spinal cord compression or infiltration) and involvement of single or multiple nerve roots.

- The clinical diagnosis of neurosarcoidosis is based on typical neurologic features, histopathologic evidence of systemic disease (e.g., from skin, bronchial washings, or lymph nodes), and CSF analysis (typically showing decreased glucose content, elevated protein, and elevated white blood cell count).

RADIOLOGIC

- Leptomeningeal contrast enhancement is the most common finding in neurosarcoidosis. In particular, the basilar meninges are affected, a finding that can simulate tuberculous meningitis. Contrast enhancement within the Virchow-Robin spaces due to disease extension along the subarachnoid space surrounding small penetrating vessels is a relatively common finding.

- White matter lesions that are hyperintense on T2-weighted MR images and often contrast enhancing are the most common form of brain parenchymal involvement. These lesions are frequently periventricular or subcortical in location.

- Gray matter lesions within brain cortex and in the deep gray matter structures that are difficult to detect with CT but that contrast-enhance on T1-weighted MRIs and are hyperintense on T2-weighted images are not uncommon.

- Involvement of the midline basilar structures—e.g., optic chiasm, hypothalamus, and pituitary stalk—is a common feature.

- On occasion, focal epidural masses can be seen. These lesions are usually isointense with brain on noncontrast T1-weighted images and can have variable signal intensity on T2-weighted images. These lesions can simulate a wide variety of epidural masses, particularly meningiomas.

- Contrast enhancement of the ventricular lining, representing ependymal involvement, and enhancing intraventricular lesions can sometimes be seen in association with hydrocephalus.

- Spinal disease is less common than brain involvement in neurosarcoidosis. The most common disease patterns include intramedullary lesions and intrathecal nodular masses over the surface of the spinal cord and nerve roots.

- Patients often have little or no pulmonary disease at the time of CNS symptoms. Therefore, a negative chest radiograph cannot be used as evidence against the diagnosis of neurosarcoidosis.

SUGGESTED READING

Nesbit GM, Miller GM, Baker HL, et al. Spinal cord sarcoidosis: A new finding at MR imaging with Gd-DTPA enhancement. Radiology 1989;173:839–843.

Seltzer S, Mark AS, Atlas SW. CNS sarcoidosis: Evaluation with contrast-enhanced MR imaging. AJNR 1991;12:1227–1233.

Sherman JL, Stern BJ. Sarcoidosis of the CNS: Comparison of unenhanced and enhanced MR images. AJNR 1990;11:915–923.

CASE 17

Fernando M. Zalduondo

HISTORY

A 57-year-old woman with fever, confusion, and a nonfocal neurologic examination.

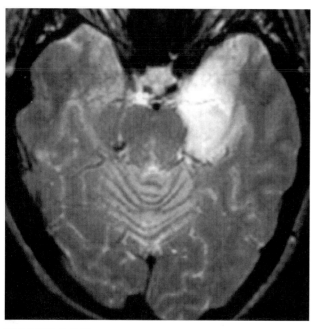

FIGURE 6-17A T2-weighted axial MRI shows abnormal hyperintense signal in the medial third of the left temporal lobe. On more superior images (not shown), the basal ganglia were not involved.

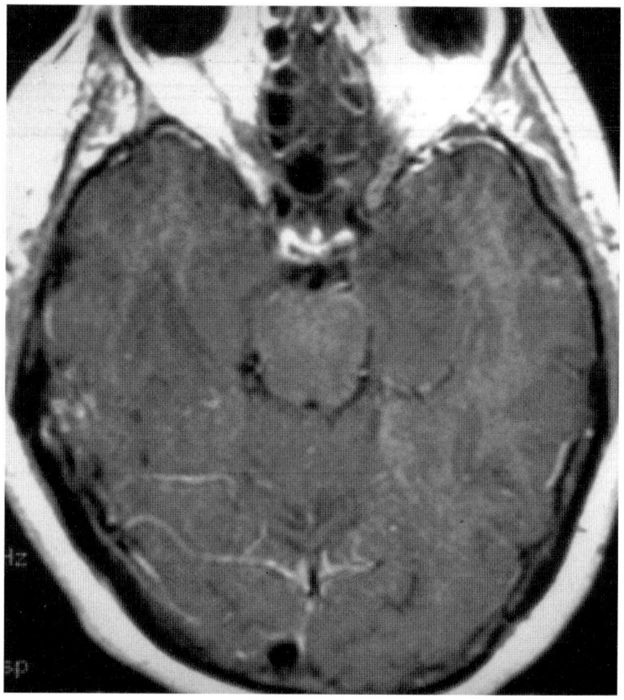

FIGURE 6-17B Contrast-enhanced T1-weighted axial MRI shows abnormal hypointense signal and loss of gray-white matter differentiation along the medial third of the left temporal lobe. No abnormal enhancement is seen.

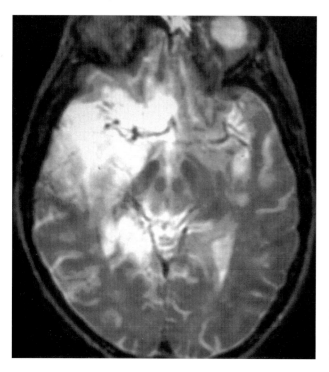

FIGURE 6-17C T2-weighted axial image in another patient with a 3-day history of confusion. Hyperintense signal is present throughout much of the right temporal lobe, as well as into the right subfrontal region and left insular cortex.

◆ DIFFERENTIAL DIAGNOSIS

◆ **Nonhemorrhagic contusion:** This diagnosis might be considered because the anterior portion of the temporal lobe is a region that is affected frequently in closed head injury. The absence of a history of trauma excludes this diagnosis. Furthermore, abnormal signal is seen in regions that would be atypical sites for contusion—e.g., the insula.

◆ **Infarction:** Infarction confined to the anterior portion of the temporal lobe is unusual. Instead, infarction usually involves either the lateral two-thirds of the temporal lobe (middle cerebral artery territory) or the medial third of the temporal lobe and the occipital lobe (posterior cerebral artery territory).

◆ **Tumor:** Low-grade infiltrating gliomas and neoplasms such as gliomatosis cerebri can produce abnormal MR signal with little or no contrast enhancement. However, the bilateral abnormality confined to the temporal lobes and insula in Figure 6-17C would not be expected with tumor.

◆ **Herpes simplex type 1 (HSV 1) encephalitis:** This is the correct diagnosis given the clinical history, primary involvement of both temporal lobes and the insula, and relative paucity of contrast enhancement.

◆ DIAGNOSIS: Herpes simplex virus type 1 encephalitis.

◆ KEY FACTS

CLINICAL

◆ The term *encephalitis* refers to a diffuse parenchymal inflammatory process that may be caused by a wide variety of etiologies, but most commonly has a viral etiology.

◆ The most common cause of nonepidemic acute viral encephalitis in immunocompetent patients in the United States and Europe is HSV type 1 (oral strand) infection. However, HSV 1 accounts for only about 10% of viral encephalitides.

◆ Nearly all adults have been exposed to this virus, which is responsible for "cold sores."

◆ HSV 1 encephalitis is thought to usually result from reactivation of latent viral infection of the trigeminal ganglion. The infection extends in a retrograde fashion along the meningeal innervation of the middle cranial fossa and inferior portion of the anterior cranial fossa.

◆ Clinical features include seizures, encephalopathy, headache, and low-grade fever.

◆ Because untreated HSV 1 encephalitis has a high mortality rate, prompt treatment with acyclovir is essential. Brain biopsy is the most specific means of diagnosis but is often deferred when the diagnosis is highly likely based on clinical, laboratory, and radiologic findings. In such cases, acyclovir therapy is started without a definitive diagnosis.

RADIOLOGIC

◆ The earliest CT findings, seen during the first few days after onset of overt symptoms, consist of hypodensity in one or both temporal lobes, typically in the medial portions. Over the course of the next few days, similar changes can be seen in the insula and inferior frontal lobes. Contrast enhancement is often absent or only mild. When present, contrast enhancement is often confined to small areas and sometimes follows a gyriform pattern.

◆ MRI is more sensitive than CT in establishing the early diagnosis. MR findings include temporal lobe swelling and hyperintense lesions on T2-weighted images in the same regions as described for CT. In comparison to CT, MRI shows the lesions earlier and shows more widespread involvement. As on CT, little or no contrast enhancement is typically seen.

◆ The bilateral involvement often seen in HSV 1 encephalitis is a useful feature in distinguishing this entity from a neoplasm.

◆ Sparing of the basal ganglia has been described as a useful feature in helping to distinguish HSV 1 encephalitis from infarction.

◆ Follow-up imaging after institution of intravenous acyclovir often shows a decrease in the signal abnormalities.

◆ SUGGESTED READING

Lester JW Jr, Carter MP, Reynolds TL. Herpes encephalitis: MR monitoring of response to acyclovir therapy. J Comput Assist Tomogr 1988;12:941–943.

Zimmerman RD, Russell EJ, Leeds NE, Kaufman D. CT in the early diagnosis of herpes simplex encephalitis. AJR Am J Roentgenol 1980;134:61–66.

CASE 18

E. Ralph Heinz

HISTORY

A 13-year-old girl with weakness in both legs and incontinence.

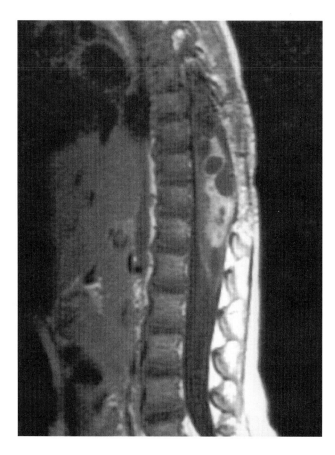

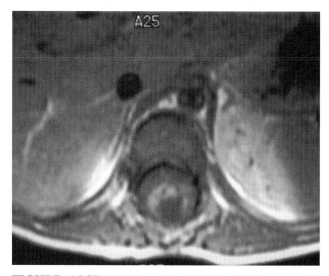

FIGURE 6-18B Axial T1-weighted MRI at T11 shows marked expansion of the spinal cord with a region of contrast enhancement of the rim of a cyst.

FIGURE 6-18A Contrast-enhanced sagittal T1-weighted MRI shows diffuse enlargement of the spinal cord with the maximum enlargement at T10–11. Inhomogeneous contrast enhancement of the spinal cord is seen. Hypointense cystic areas are seen throughout the spinal cord.

◆ DIFFERENTIAL DIAGNOSIS

- **Transverse myelitis secondary to multiple sclerosis (MS):** Spinal cord demyelinating lesions due to MS usually show spinal cord swelling over one or two spinal segments. In the acute stage, these lesions can contrast-enhance. However, the spinal cord swelling seen in MS is usually smoothly contoured and fusiform, unlike the exophytic expansion of the spinal cord seen in the case shown above. Furthermore, cystic regions would not be expected.
- **Metastasis:** Intramedullary spinal cord metastases are relatively rare. They can be seen as focal regions of abnormal signal and, often, contrast enhancement. This diagnosis would be unlikely because of the infiltrative appearance of the lesion shown above and the presence of multiple cysts.

- **Meningioma:** These tumors are extramedullary masses, whereas the mass shown above is intramedullary, making this an incorrect diagnosis.
- **Cavernous hemangioma:** These lesions are variable in appearance, often seen as inhomogeneous regions of abnormal signal. They are frequently hyperintense on T1-weighted images and have hypointense regions on T2-weighted images. However, these lesions are typically small and focal, rather than diffuse and infiltrative, as in the case shown above.
- **Spinal cord neoplasm:** This diagnosis should be considered given the expansion of the spinal cord, inhomogeneous contrast enhancement, and ill-defined borders of the mass. Given these features and the thoracic location of the mass, the most likely diagnosis is glioma.

◆**DIAGNOSIS: Spinal cord glioma.**

◆**KEY FACTS**

CLINICAL

◆ There are three major types of intramedullary spinal cord tumors: gliomas, ependymomas, and hemangioblastomas. The first two are malignant and the third is histologically benign.

◆ Gliomas account for about half of adult spinal cord tumors, but they account for a higher percentage in children. The peak incidence is in the third and fourth decade. They are most common in the thoracic region, are not usually encapsulated, and usually have ill-defined borders. They are most common in the thoracic region. These tumors tend to extend over the length of a few vertebral bodies but can be much longer.

◆ Ependymomas arise from ependymal cells in the central spinal canal. Thus, they tend to be central in location and expand the cord outward. They are soft tumors that usually have a delicate capsule that forms a plane of cleavage that allows surgical excision without damage to spinal cord tissue. They frequently form cysts. Ependymomas arising in the filum terminale are typically of the myxopapillary type, which are mucinous and may bleed, causing subarachnoid hemorrhage. They may be associated with extremely high levels of protein in the CSF. Ependymoma is the most common primary tumor of the lower spinal cord and the filum terminale. Two-thirds of intramedullary tumors at the conus medullaris are ependymomas. Following total removal of the tumor, there is only a small chance of recurrence (about 10%). If the absence of a well-defined capsule prevents total excision, tumor progression, often accompanied by metastases to the CSF or even to distant metastases, is common.

◆ Hemangioblastoma is a much less common primary spinal cord tumor (about 3%) than glioma and ependymoma. About 30% of patients with spinal cord hemangioblastoma have von Hippel-Lindau syndrome (VHL). However, <5% of VHL patients are reported to have spinal hemangioblastomas, although the common use of MRI to screen these patients may show that the incidence is, in fact, much higher.

◆ Most spinal hemangioblastomas are intramedullary. About half are associated with cysts. They are usually associated with dilated veins on the surface of the cord. Development of a long syrinx cavity is very common.

RADIOLOGIC

◆ The typical appearance of a spinal cord glioma on MRI is an infiltrative mass that is hypointense on T1-weighted images and hyperintense on T2-weighted images. The tumors essentially always contrast-enhance in an inhomogeneous manner and have poorly defined borders. Associated cysts are frequently seen at the cranial and caudal ends of the tumor. These cysts are typically benign and do not contrast-enhance. Malignant cystic portions of the tumor, on the other hand, typically rim-enhance.

◆ Ependymoma tends to arise in the center of the spinal cord and displaces the normal tissue toward the perimeter. The typical appearance is a mass in the center of the spinal cord extending both cephalad and caudad over a number of segments. The lesions generally homogeneously contrast-enhance and have well-defined margins. Focal sites of hemorrhage can occasionally be seen as hypointense areas on T2-weighted images.

◆ If the conus is involved as well as the filum terminale, the diagnosis is very likely to be ependymoma. The probability is further increased if the filum terminale is involved in isolation, in which case the myxopapillary type of ependymoma is highly likely.

◆ Hemangioblastomas appear as a focal, markedly enhancing nidus, often with an adjacent cyst and marked edema. A syrinx cavity is quite common. There are frequently very small associated vascular foci elsewhere in the spinal cord, particularly if the patient has VHL. Multiple associated vessels are often seen, particularly on the dorsal aspect of the spinal cord. They can sometimes be seen on myelography as focal enlargement of the spinal cord with serpiginous filling defects due to the presence of vessels on the dorsal surface of the spinal cord. These vessels can be mistaken for evidence of a dural arteriovenous fistula or a spinal cord arteriovenous malformation.

◆**SUGGESTED READING**

Dillon WP, Norman D, Newton TH, et al. Intradural spinal cord lesions: GD-DTPA: enhanced MR imaging. Radiology 1989;170:229–237.

Sze G. MR imaging of the spinal cord: Current status and future advances. AJR Am J Roentgenol 1992;159:149–159.

Sze G, Twohig M. Neoplastic Disease of the Spine and Spinal Cord. In SW Atlas (ed), Magnetic Resonance Imaging of the Brain and Spine. New York: Raven, 1991;921–962.

HISTORY

A 37-year-old woman with multiple renal cysts and bilateral renal cell carcinomas (RCCs).

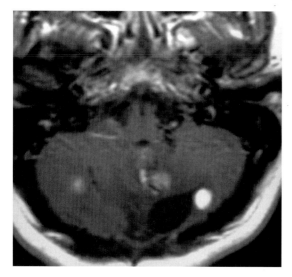

FIGURE 6-19A Contrast-enhanced T1-weighted axial MRI shows multiple, round, enhancing masses in the cerebellum. One of the lesions has an adjacent cyst.

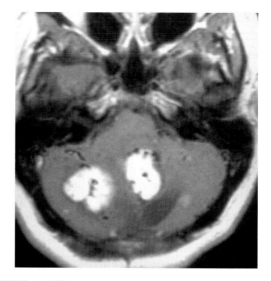

FIGURE 6-19B Contrast-enhanced T1-weighted axial MRI at a slightly more cephalad level shows solid masses with numerous flow voids representing vessels within the lesions and in the adjacent brain tissue.

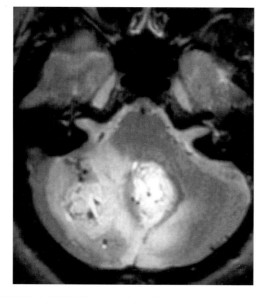

FIGURE 6-19C T2-weighted axial MRI shows the masses are hyperintense and having surrounding edema. Numerous associated flow voids are again seen.

◆ DIFFERENTIAL DIAGNOSIS

- **Metastasis:** This diagnosis might be considered because multiple lesions are present in a patient with RCC. However, the appearance is atypical for metastasis. The cystic lesions shown above consist of a cyst and a peripheral mural nodule, whereas cystic regions within metastasis (due to necrosis) are usually central. Although RCC metastases can be vascular, the actual presence of flow voids within the masses would be a very unusual finding.

- **Juvenile pilocytic astrocytoma:** This diagnosis might be considered because of the presence of a cyst with a contrast-enhancing mural nodule in the case shown above. This tumor is usually seen in children and young adults, but the age of the patient shown above does not exclude the diagnosis. However, these tumors are typically solitary and would not be expected to have the internal flow voids shown above.

- **Hemangioblastoma:** This is the correct diagnosis based on the presence of multiple posterior fossa cystic lesions having densely enhancing mural nodules in a young adult. Internal flow voids due to hypervascularity, as shown in the case above, are occasionally seen in this tumor, further supporting the diagnosis.

◆ DIAGNOSIS: Hemangioblastoma.

◆ KEY FACTS

CLINICAL

- Hemangioblastoma is a benign tumor of the CNS accounting for 1.0% to 2.5% of all intracranial neoplasms. The tumor is most commonly found in the cerebellum and, less commonly, in the spinal cord. Supratentorial hemangioblastomas are rare.

- The most common age at the time of discovery is the third through fifth decades. There is not a strong predilection for either gender.

- The tumor is histologically benign. Neurologic features occur on the basis of location—e.g., mass effect of posterior fossa lesions and involvement of spinal motor or sensory tracts by spinal lesions.

- Many patients with hemangioblastomas have an inherited genetic disorder termed von Hippel Lindau (VHL). Diagnostic criteria include at least one CNS hemangioblastoma in association with one of the following features: multiple cysts or neoplasms of the visceral organs or a family history of VHL.

- Sites of visceral organ system involvement in VHL include kidneys (RCC, cysts), pancreas (multiple cysts, microcystic adenoma or adenocarcinoma), adrenal gland (pheochromocytoma, which can also occur at other sites), epididymis (cysts), and liver (adenomas, cysts).

- Polycythemia is seen in some cases due to secretion of erythropoietin by the tumor.

RADIOLOGIC

- One-third of hemangioblastomas have a purely solid structure, one-third have a characteristic cyst with peripheral mural nodule (Figure 6-19A), and the remainder are cystic but with a more complex solid component than a simple mural nodule.

- Complete evaluation of patients with VHL should include MRI of both the brain and spine.

- On noncontrast CT and MRI, the cyst contents can often be seen to differ slightly from CSF due to a high protein content.

- Solid components of hemangioblastomas densely contrast-enhance on CT and MRI due to their high vascularity associated with breakdown of the blood-brain barrier.

- On MRI, flow voids can sometimes be seen within solid portions of hemangioblastomas (Figures 6-19B and 6-19C) due to (1) either feeding or draining vessels, or (2) large sinusoids within the tumor.

- At catheter angiography, the solid components are seen to have enlarged feeding arteries and densely stain with contrast material. Cystic portions of the tumor are seen as avascular regions next to the nodule.

◆ SUGGESTED READING

Sato Y, Waziri M, Smith W, et al. von Hippel-Lindau disease: MR imaging. Radiology 1988;166:241–246.

Smirniotopoulos JG. Congenital Syndromes with Neoplasms: The Phakomatoses. In BP Drayer, DR Enzmann, JG Smirniotopolous, RR Lukin (eds), Core Curriculum in Neuroradiology, Part II: Neoplasms and Infectious Diseases. American Society of Neuroradiology, 1996;61–69.

CASE 20

David S. Enterline

HISTORY

A 4-month-old boy with facial nevus.

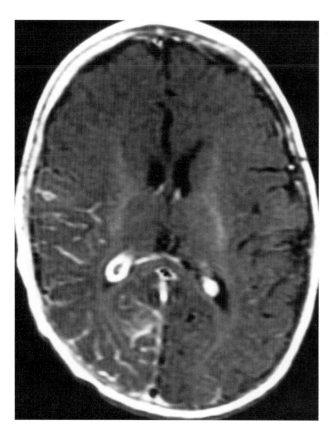

FIGURE 6-20A Contrast-enhanced axial T1-weighted MRI shows leptomeningeal enhancement in the right occipital, parietal, and posterior frontal lobes. Enlargement of the ipsilateral choroid plexus is present. The right hemisphere is slightly smaller than the left hemisphere.

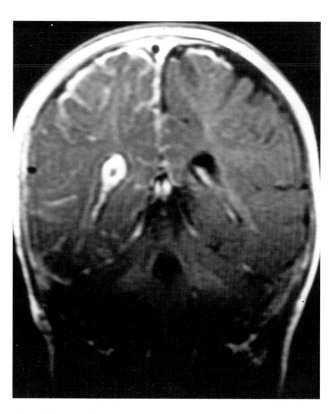

FIGURE 6-20B Contrast-enhanced coronal T1-weighted MRI shows marked enlargement of the right choroid plexus and right parietal-occipital leptomeningeal enhancement.

◆ DIFFERENTIAL DIAGNOSIS

◆ **Meningitis:** Prominent involvement of only a portion of one hemisphere with sparing of the remainder of the brain would be an atypical leptomeningeal enhancement pattern to be caused by meningitis. In addition, this diagnosis would not explain the facial nevus, the asymmetric size of the hemispheres, or the enlargement of the choroid plexus.

◆ **Leptomeningeal carcinomatosis:** This diagnosis would be unlikely because of many of the reasons cited against the diagnosis of meningitis. In addition, however, leptomeningeal infiltration by tumor would be distinctly unusual in a child of the age in the case shown above.

◆ **Subacute infarction:** Leptomeningeal enhancement can be seen in the first few days after cerebral infarction. Stroke in a child of the age in the case shown above is, however, quite uncommon. Furthermore, this diagnosis would not explain the other findings, which suggest a congenital cause.

◆ **Sturge-Weber syndrome:** The findings of leptomeningeal enhancement, underlying cortical atrophy and enlargement of the choroid plexus, as seen in the case shown above, are typical for this disorder.

◆ DIAGNOSIS: Sturge-Weber syndrome.

◆ KEY FACTS

CLINICAL

◆ The Sturge-Weber syndrome, also known as *encephalotrigeminal angiomatosis,* is a congenital neurocutaneous syndrome in which the main features are a facial cutaneous vascular nevus (port-wine stain), a leptomeningeal venous angiomatosis associated with cerebral cortical calcifications, and angiomatosis of the choroid of the eye.

◆ Congenital glaucoma, seizures, hemiparesis, hemianopsia, and mental retardation (two-thirds of cases) are the major clinical manifestations.

◆ The facial nevus is in the distribution of the trigeminal nerve, usually the first division, and typically ipsilateral to the intracranial lesions. However, only 10% of patients with such facial nevi have Sturge-Weber syndrome. In the remaining 90%, the facial nevus is a solitary dermatologic abnormality without associated findings.

◆ The intracranial lesion is a leptomeningeal vascular malformation, which is usually unilateral in the parietal-occipital region and ipsilateral to the facial nevus. A plethora of small, thin-walled structures, which resemble telangiectatic capillaries or venules, are seen to lie along the surface of the brain between the pia and the arachnoid membranes. The underlying cerebral cortex becomes dysfunctional and atrophic, and often calcifies. Abnormal venous drainage of the cortex develops, with increased collateral flow through the choroid plexus.

◆ Seizures are often the initial neurologic feature, frequently beginning in the first year of life and thereafter relentlessly progressing with advancing age. Progressive hemianopsia and hemiparesis contralateral to the leptomeningeal vascular abnormality are often seen.

◆ The choroid of the eye is involved by an angioma in 30% of cases, often causing buphthalmos (enlargement of the eye, or "cow eye"), a form of congenital glaucoma.

◆ Angiomas can be seen in other organs, including the kidneys, spleen, ovaries, intestines, adrenals, thyroid, pancreas, heart, thymus, and lungs.

◆ Laser therapy of the facial nevus yields cosmetic improvement. Intractable seizures in Sturge-Weber patients can be surgically treated by lobectomy or hemispherectomy and corpus callosum resection, if the patient is of a sufficiently young age (i.e., <2 years of age) that the remaining hemisphere can assume motor and sensory function for both sides of the body.

RADIOLOGIC

◆ A gyriform pattern of calcification is often seen at the site of the leptomeningeal vascular malformation. This finding is due to foci of calcification within the cerebral cortex rather than vascular calcifications. It is best seen on CT but can also be seen on plain radiographs and MRI, on which it is best delineated on gradient echo images.

◆ Other CT findings include cortical atrophy and enlargement of the choroid plexus. The extent of involvement as judged by cortical atrophy is often more extensive than the sites of parenchymal calcification. Cortical enhancement can be seen on contrast-enhanced CT, thought to be reflect impaired superficial cortical venous outflow associated with the leptomeningeal venous angioma.

◆ Findings on T2-weighted MRIs include hyperintense signal abnormality in areas of gliosis, ischemia, and demyelinization and hypointense gyriform signal due to cortical calcifications. As a reaction to the brain atrophy, the adjacent calvarium can thicken and the paranasal sinuses hypertrophy, changes that have been termed the *Dyke-Davidoff-Masson syndrome.*

◆ On contrast-enhanced T1-weighted MRIs, marked enhancement of the leptomeninges overlying the involved hemisphere, the enlarged choroid plexus ("choroidal angiomatosis"), enlarged deep medullary veins, and a retinal angioma can often be seen.

◆ At catheter angiography, abnormalities of the superficial cerebral venous drainage just deep to the area of leptomeningeal angiomatosis can be seen.

◆ SUGGESTED READING

Braffman B, Naidich TP. The phakomatoses: Part II. von Hippel-Lindau disease, Sturge-Weber syndrome, and less common conditions. Neuroimaging Clin North Am 1994;4:325–348.

Hiraldo E. Sturge-Weber syndrome: Study of 40 patients. Pediatr Neurol 1993;9:283–288.

Pascual-Castroviejo I, Diaz-Gonzalez C, Garcia-Melian RM, et al. The phakomatoses. AJNR 1992;3:725–746.

CASE 21

James M. Provenzale

HISTORY

A 38-year-old woman with unremitting left-sided headache and oculosympathetic paresis of 2 weeks' duration.

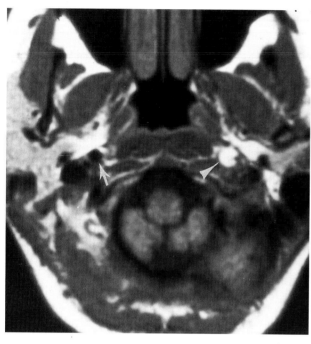

FIGURE 6-21A Noncontrast T1-weighted axial MRI near the level of the foramen magnum shows a focus of hyperintense signal (arrowhead) in the left internal carotid artery, with only a small residual flow void along the lateral surface of the artery. The external diameter of the left internal carotid artery is increased relative to that of the right internal carotid artery (arrow).

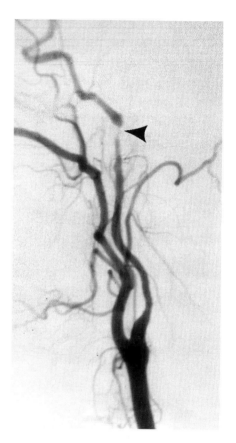

FIGURE 6-21B Lateral view from a catheter angiogram performed 1 day after the MRI study shows narrowing of the left internal carotid artery beginning about a centimeter above the carotid bifurcation and extending along the whole length of the remainder of the visualized portion of the artery. The contrast column is narrowest at the junction of the cervical and petrous segments of the artery, at about the level of the region shown in Figure 6-21A.

◆ DIFFERENTIAL DIAGNOSIS

- **Atherosclerotic narrowing:** This diagnosis would be unlikely in a young patient and would not be expected to cause the symptoms mentioned above. Furthermore, the site of arterial narrowing is above the level of the carotid bifurcation and extends into the level of the skull base. Atherosclerotic narrowing, on the other hand, typically occurs at the carotid bifurcation and does not extend the length of the internal carotid artery (ICA).
- **Vasospasm:** Arterial spasm in the extracranial portion of the ICA could be seen after trauma due to catheter placement or external trauma but does not usually affect a long segment of the artery and would not explain the MRI findings.
- **Arterial dissection:** This entity typically shows abnormal periarterial signal on MRI and increase in the external diameter of the artery (as in Figure 6-21A) due to intramural hemorrhage. Luminal narrowing over a variable length of the artery is commonly seen beginning a few centimeters above the carotid bifurcation (as in Figure 6-21B). This is the correct diagnosis.

◆ DIAGNOSIS: Arterial dissection.

◆ KEY FACTS

CLINICAL

- Dissections cause approximately 1% to 2% of all strokes in the general population but between 5% and 20% of strokes among patients <40 years old.
- Dissection can occur after trauma, on a spontaneous basis, or after movements of the head or neck that are generally considered benign ("trivial trauma").
- Headache or neckache is present in about 75% of patients. Oculosympathetic paresis (Horner's syndrome) is commonly seen in ICA dissection.
- Transient ischemic attacks and completed strokes occur in a minority of patients.
- Subarachnoid hemorrhage can accompany intracranial dissections.
- The most common sites are the cervical portion of the ICA (within a few centimeters of the carotid bifurca-

tion) and the vertebral artery at the level of the C1–2 vertebral bodies.
- Anticoagulation for a period of a few months is usually performed when subarachnoid hemorrhage is not present.

RADIOLOGIC

- The most common finding at catheter angiography is a site of smooth or irregular narrowing extending over a few centimeters in length. Other catheter angiography findings can include pseudoaneurysm formation, arterial occlusion, and, less commonly, an intimal flap. A double-lumen appearance is rare.
- The typical MRI finding is a narrowed arterial lumen (flow void) with an adjacent crescentic area of abnormal signal (usually hyperintense on T1- and T2-weighted images).
- At MR angiography, a narrowed arterial signal column, frequently with an adjacent region of hyperintense signal aligned parallel to the artery, can often be seen.
- Diagnostic features at ultrasonography include an echogenic intimal flap (the most specific sign, but present in only a minority of cases) and echogenic thrombus.
- CT is not usually performed to establish the diagnosis, but contrast-enhanced CT can demonstrate a narrowed arterial lumen with an eccentric region of mural thickening.
- Resolution or significant improvement at the time of a repeat imaging study performed a few weeks later is seen in about 80% of treated cases.

◆ SUGGESTED READING

Houser OW, Mokri B, Sundt TM, et al. Spontaneous cervical cephalic arterial dissection and its residuum: Angiographic spectrum. AJNR 1984;5:27–34.

Levy C, Laissy JP, Raveau V, et al. Carotid and vertebral artery dissections: Three-dimensional time-of-flight MR angiography and MR imaging versus conventional angiography. Radiology 1994;190:97–103.

Provenzale JM. Dissection of the internal carotid and vertebral arteries: Imaging findings. AJR Am J Roentgenol 1995;165:1099–1104.

HISTORY

A 51-year-old woman with visual field defect and headache.

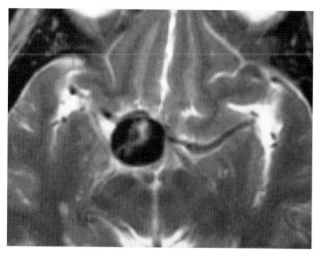

FIGURE 6-22A T2-weighted axial MRI shows a round mass just anterior to the midbrain. The mass is predominantly hypointense but has an ill-defined central region of higher signal.

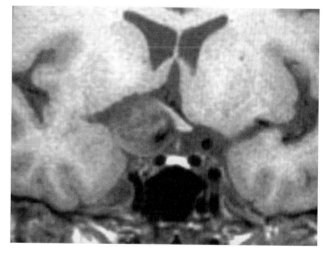

FIGURE 6-22B Noncontrast T1-weighted coronal image shows the mass is slightly hypointense to gray matter and extra-axial. The lesion surrounds a portion of the cavernous segment of the right internal carotid artery and elevates the right half of the optic chiasm.

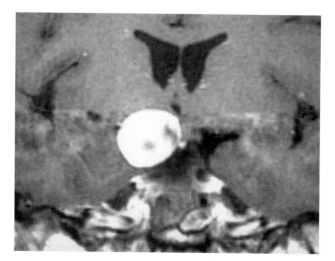

FIGURE 6-22C Contrast-enhanced T1-weighted coronal image shows that the mass densely enhances and has sharp margins. Abnormal signal is seen throughout the medial temporal lobes bilaterally.

◆ DIFFERENTIAL DIAGNOSIS

- **Meningioma:** This might be considered because the lesion is extra-axial and densely contrast-enhances. However, this diagnosis would not account for the abnormal signal in both temporal lobes.
- **Craniopharyngioma:** This diagnosis might be considered because a portion of the mass extends into the suprasellar cistern. However, craniopharyngiomas are typically cystic, often calcified, and do not generally diffusely contrast-enhance.
- **Epidermoid cyst:** This diagnosis might be considered because of the extra-axial suprasellar location of the lesion. However, epidermoids usually appear moderately hyperintense on T2-weighted images and do not contrast-enhance.
- **Pituitary adenoma:** On Figure 6-22B, the posterior lobe of the pituitary gland is seen between the two internal carotid arteries (ICAs). The lesion is clearly separate from the pituitary gland.
- **Aneurysm:** This diagnosis should be considered when a mass lesion is seen in the region of the circle of Willis. A wide range of signal intensities can be seen due to slow blood flow within an aneurysm or partial or complete thrombosis. Therefore, the fact that a normal flow void is not present in the lesion by no means excludes this diagnosis. The abnormal signal seen in the temporal lobes is a clue to the correct diagnosis. This signal is due to pulsation artifact in the phase-encoding direction produced by flow within the mass, which is an aneurysm.

◆ DIAGNOSIS: Giant aneurysm.

◆ KEY FACTS

CLINICAL

- Giant aneurysms are >25 mm in diameter and account for approximately 5% of all intracranial aneurysms.
- Presentation usually is in the fourth through sixth decades. Giant aneurysms typically become symptomatic due to mass effect on adjacent intracranial structures (which may raise clinical suspicion of a neoplasm) rather than aneurysmal rupture.
- Giant intracranial aneurysms are associated with substantial neurologic morbidity or death within 5 years of diagnosis if untreated.
- The optimal treatment options include (1) clipping of the neck of the aneurysm with preservation of the parent vessel, or (2) endovascular occlusion of the aneurysm by balloons or embolic coils. Less optimally, carotid artery ligation or wrapping of the aneurysm is performed in the uncommon instance in which the aneurysm cannot be treated definitively.

RADIOLOGIC

- About half of giant aneurysms involve the ICA and its distal branches. The most common sites in the carotid circulation are near the origin of the ophthalmic artery, ICA bifurcation, and cavernous segment of the ICA. The most frequent sites in the vertebrobasilar system are at the tip of the basilar artery, junction of the basilar and superior cerebellar arteries, and vertebrobasilar junction.
- At catheter angiography, partially thrombosed giant aneurysms often appear smaller than their actual size, which can be more accurately defined by CT and MRI.
- The CT and MRI appearance of a giant aneurysm can be mistaken for a tumor. In particular, giant aneurysms in the parasellar region and at other sites near the skull base can be mistaken for a meningioma. It is important to consider this entity in the differential diagnosis of masses in these regions if inadvertent biopsy or improper surgery is to be avoided.
- On noncontrast CT, aneurysms appear as rounded or oval masses that are relatively isodense or, frequently, hyperdense relative to adjacent brain tissue. Partially thrombosed aneurysms often have a hyperintense crescentic rim. Occasionally, the rim of an aneurysm can be seen to be calcified. Following contrast administration, nonthrombosed aneurysms densely and homogeneously contrast-enhance, while generally only the patent lumen of partially thrombosed aneurysms densely contrast-enhances.
- On MRI, a nonthrombosed aneurysm is seen as an oval or spherical extra-axial region of absent signal (flow void), continuous with a vessel. Partially thrombed aneurysms typically have a laminated appearance, due to layers of hemorrhage of different age. Occasionally, a thin circumferential region of abnormal perianeurysmal signal due to chronic hemorrhagic products can be seen.
- An important clue that a mass lesion seen on MRI is an aneurysm is a band of pulsation artifact extending from the aneurysm into adjacent tissues along the phase-encoding axis. This artifact is often increased after administration of contrast material (Figure 6-22C).

◆ SUGGESTED READING

Atlas SW, Grossman RI, Goldberg HI, et al. Partially thrombosed giant intracranial aneurysms: Correlation of MR and pathologic findings. Radiology 1987;162:111–114.

Kwan ESK, Wolpert SM, Scorr RM, Runge V. MR evaluation of neurovascular lesions after endovascular occlusion with detachable balloons. AJNR 1988;9:523–531.

Olsen WL, Brant-Zawadzki M, Hodes J, et al. Giant intracranial aneurysms: MR imaging. Radiology 1987;163:431–435.

CASE 23

Fernando M. Zalduondo

HISTORY

A 76-year-old woman with progressive visual deficits and headache.

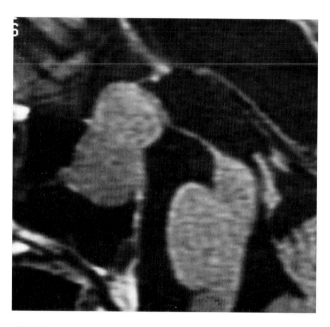

FIGURE 6-23A T1-weighted sagittal noncontrast MRI shows a homogeneous intermediate signal mass that fills and enlarges the sella turcica and extends into the suprasellar cistern, displacing the optic chiasm.

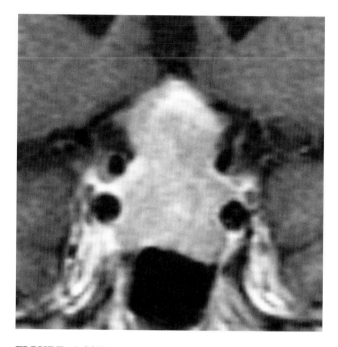

FIGURE 6-23B Contrast-enhanced T1-weighted coronal MRI shows relatively homogeneous enhancement of the mass. The optic chiasm is draped over the mass, which bulges into the cavernous sinuses without compressing the internal carotid arteries. A focal constriction is seen in the mid portion of the mass, producing a bilobed appearance.

◆ DIFFERENTIAL DIAGNOSIS

◆ **Rathke's cleft cyst:** This lesion typically has hyperintense signal on noncontrast T1-weighted images due to proteinaceous composition. Contrast enhancement is not seen. Therefore, this is the incorrect diagnosis for the case shown above.

◆ **Craniopharyngioma:** This lesion nearly always is centered in the suprasellar cistern, although an intrasellar component is often present. The vast majority are calcified and cystic, features not seen in the case shown above. Because craniopharyngioma can have a uniformly contrast-enhancing appearance suggesting a solid mass, the diagnosis cannot be absolutely excluded based on the imaging findings shown above but is considered unlikely.

◆ **Aneurysm:** This diagnosis might be considered because the lesion shown above is oval and close to the ICA. The absence of a flow void within the lesion is not evidence against the diagnosis of aneurysm, because aneurysms are frequently partially thrombosed. However, pulsation artifact in the phase-encoding direction, indicative of flow, would be expected in a nonthrombosed or partially thrombosed aneurysm. Such artifact is not present. In addition, sellar enlargement and the symmetric constriction seen in the middle of the lesion shown above would be atypical for an aneurysm.

◆ **Meningioma:** Meningioma is a consideration because of the homogeneous enhancement pattern. However, meningiomas are typically juxtasellar and rarely intrasellar. Furthermore, in the case of meningioma, the mass should be separable from the pituitary gland. The mass illustrated here is inseparable from the pituitary gland.

◆ **Pituitary microadenoma:** By definition, microadenomas are <1 cm in size. They do not extend to the suprasellar cistern and should appear as hypointense regions within an otherwise normally enhancing pituitary gland.

◆ **Pituitary macroadenoma:** This term refers to adenomas >10 mm in size. This is the correct diagnosis given the large size, intrasellar location, and diffuse enhancement pattern. This mass has grown superiorly, expanding the infundibular orifice of the diaphragma sella, producing a bilobed appearance.

◆ DIAGNOSIS: Pituitary macroadenoma.

◆ KEY FACTS

CLINICAL

◆ Adenomas are the most common neoplasm of the pituitary gland and arise in the adenohypophysis (anterior lobe of the pituitary gland). They comprise 10% to 15% of all intracranial tumors.

◆ Many hormonally active pituitary adenomas become clinically apparent while small. Three-fourths of all adenomas present with signs and symptoms related to hormonal overproduction.

◆ Many nonfunctioning tumors grow to large size before producing symptoms. One-fourth of all adenomas present with symptoms due to mass effect—e.g., headache, visual field defects, cranial nerve palsies, and cerebrospinal fluid (CSF) rhinorrhea due to sellar erosion.

◆ Hormonally active adenomas may secrete prolactin, thyroid-stimulating hormone, growth hormone, adrenocorticotropic hormone, follicle-stimulating hormone, and luteinizing hormone, alone or in various combinations. Hormonally inactive adenomas have been termed "null cell" adenomas or oncocytomas.

RADIOLOGIC

◆ Unless contraindicated, MRI is generally considered the first-line imaging study for detection of pituitary adenomas.

◆ During the evaluation of the lesion of the sellar/juxtasellar region, the radiologist's role is to establish the center of the lesion and its relationship to adjacent structures. Relevant features include the relation to the optic structures, course and caliber of the cavernous segment of the ICAs, and whether the cavernous sinuses are invaded.

◆ Pituitary adenomas can be diagnosed on any MRI pulse sequence, but contrast-enhanced T1-weighted images in the coronal plane are probably the technique that is most widely accepted. Nonetheless, they can be detected on noncontrast T1-weighted images as a hypointense region and in 30% to 50% of cases as a hyperintense lesion on T2-weighted images. The latter finding is more common in macroadenomas.

◆ MRI is optimally performed within a few minutes of contrast infusion. Microadenomas contrast-enhance less rapidly than the normal pituitary tissue in that time period and appear relatively hypointense to the normal gland. Further delay in imaging can lead to false-negative studies, because over many minutes, the lesion contrast-enhances to the same degree as normal pituitary tissue.

◆ Macroadenomas are typically isointense to gray matter on all pulse sequences and intensely contrast-enhance, often in an inhomogeneous manner.

◆ Complicated adenomas can have calcification, hemorrhage, cyst formation, and necrosis and will display corresponding focal signal changes. These features are more common following medical treatment.

◆ If MRI is unavailable or contraindicated, adenomas can be detected on contrast-enhanced CT imaging using thin-section axial and coronal images.

◆ Incidental macroadenomas of moderate size can easily be missed on routine axial CT images of the brain (i.e., CT studies not specifically performed to assess the pituitary gland). Enlargement of the sella turcica on the lateral scout topogram can be the only indication that a macroadenoma is present in a routine brain CT study.

◆ SUGGESTED READING

Elster, AD. Modern imaging of the pituitary gland. Radiology 1993;187:1–14.

Lundin R, Nyman R, Burman P, et al. MRI of pituitary macroadenomas with reference to hormonal activity. Neuroradiology 1992;34:43–51.

Newton DR, Dillon WP, Norman D, et al. GD-DTPA-enhanced MR imaging of pituitary adenomas. AJNR 1989;10:949–954.

HISTORY

A 12-year-old girl with seizures and headache.

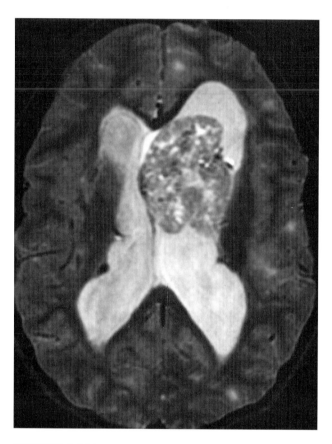

FIGURE 6-24A Axial T2-weighted MRI shows a large, inhomogeneous mass within the left lateral ventricle in the region of the foramen of Monro. Multiple small areas of abnormal hyperintense signal are seen in the cortical and subcortical regions of the left hemisphere. In addition, a small oval region of hypointense signal is seen on the ependymal surface of the right lateral ventricle projecting into the right atrium.

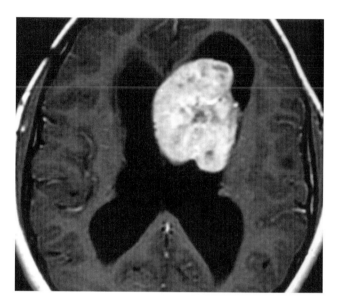

FIGURE 6-24B Contrast-enhanced axial T1-weighted image shows dense enhancement of the mass in the left lateral ventricle. An unenhancing small region of hypointense signal is seen in the left frontal lobe at the gray-white junction, lateral to the posterior surface of the mass. This lesion is at the same location as one of the hyperintense foci seen in Figure 6-24A.

◆ DIFFERENTIAL DIAGNOSIS

The differential diagnosis of mass lesions within the lateral ventricle includes:

◆ **Choroid plexus papilloma:** This lesion might be considered, because it is an intraventricular mass that is seen more frequently in children than adults. However, because it arises from choroid plexus, it is typically found in the atrium of the lateral ventricle and not near the foramen of Monro, as in the case shown above.

◆ **Neurocytoma:** This lesion typically arises in the lateral ventricle and is attached to the septum pellucidum. On the images shown above, it is difficult to determine whether the mass is attached to the septum pellucidum or merely abuts it. However, this diagnosis would not account for the presence of the multiple regions of hyperintense signal within brain parenchyma and the hypointense lesion in the right ventricle on the T2-weighted images.

◆ **Meningioma:** Meningiomas can arise within the ventricular system, but when they are located in the lateral ventricle, they are almost always attached to the choroid plexus, unlike the lesion shown above. Furthermore, as in the case of choroid plexus papilloma and neurocytoma, the diagnosis of meningioma would not adequately account for the parenchymal signal changes and the hypointense nodule seen on the ependymal surface of the right lateral ventricle.

◆ **Subependymal giant cell tumor (SGCT):** These tumors arise at the foramen of Monro, as in the case shown above. In the vast majority of cases, these tumors are seen in association with clinical and radiologic findings of tuberous sclerosis (TS). This diagnosis would account for the cortical and subcortical hyperintense signal (representing hamartomas) and the lesion on the surface of the right lateral ventricle (a calcified subependymal nodule).

◆ **DIAGNOSIS: Subependymal giant cell tumor in a patient with tuberous sclerosis.**

◆ **KEY FACTS**

CLINICAL

◆ TS is a phakomatosis with an autosomal dominant inheritance pattern associated with deletion on chromosome 9 and, in some cases, chromosome 11. However, about half of cases are spontaneous mutations.

◆ Initially, the disease was diagnosed by a clinical triad of adenoma sebaceum, seizures, and mental retardation, as described by Vogt. Although these three features are commonly seen, this has been replaced by a more inclusive set of diagnostic criteria (see below).

◆ The disease is characterized by the presence of hamartomas in multiple organs. In addition to brain, the skin (adenoma sebaceum in 95% of patients), eye (retinal hamartomas, 50%), kidneys (angiomyolipomas in 50% to 80%, renal cysts, and renal artery aneurysms), heart (rhabdomyomas, 30%), skeleton (multiple sclerotic bone islands), and, less commonly, the lungs (smooth muscle proliferation within the interstitial tissues, more common in women) are affected.

◆ Adenoma sebaceum is a form of facial angiofibroma. Subungual fibromas are another cutaneous manifestation of the disease.

◆ The retinal hamartomas are small rounded masses that overlie the optic nerve head, are histologically similar to subependymal tubers, and commonly calcify.

◆ Hamartomas are seen in two major locations in the brain: within the parenchyma (cortical and subcortical regions) and at subependymal sites. Histologically, these lesions consist of disorganized conglomerations of poorly differentiated neurons and are thought to result from disordered migration and differentiation of glial tissue.

◆ Subependymal hamartomas are typically arranged along the caudothalamic groove. In 15% of TS patients, they undergo malignant degeneration into a SGCT.

RADIOLOGIC

◆ Subependymal nodules are frequently calcified, allowing confident CT diagnosis of TS. When calcified, they are hypointense on T2-weighted sequences (Figure 6-24A). Noncalcified subependymal lesions are frequently hyperintense on T2-weighted MRIs.

◆ In addition to TS, calcifications arranged along the ventricular surface can be seen in various congenital infections, cysticercosis, and some treated neoplasms having subependymal disease (e.g., lymphoma).

◆ MRI is more sensitive than CT in the detection of cortical hamartomas, which appear as regions of gyral broadening. Cortical and subcortical hamartomas are typically hypointense on T1-weighted images and hyperintense on T2-weighted images.

◆ On occasion, a linear band of hyperintense signal on T2-weighted images can be seen traversing the white matter from a subependymal nodule to a cortical hamartoma, possibly an indication of a neuronal migration abnormality.

◆ SGCTs are grade I astrocytomas seen only in the setting of TS. They are thought to arise from subependymal nodules, are located at the foramen of Monro, and are usually detected in late childhood and adolescence.

◆ SGCTs can grow to large size and cause obstructive hydrocephalus. They do not invade brain parenchyma or metastasize through CSF pathways.

◆ Until relatively recently, it was assumed that contrast enhancement of a subependymal nodule was an indication of early malignant degeneration to an SGCT. However, it is now generally accepted that benign subependymal nodules can contrast-enhance on MRI.

◆ It is recommended that TS patients initially be screened with MRI for development of SGCT at 1- to 2-year intervals and then annually in the 8- to 18-year-old age range.

◆ **SUGGESTED READING**

Bell DG, King BF, Hattery RR, et al. Imaging characteristics of tuberous sclerosis. AJR Am J Roentgenol 1991;156:1081–1086.

Braffman BH, Bilaniuk LT, Naidich TP, et al. MR imaging of tuberous sclerosis: Pathogenesis of this phakomatosis, use of gadopentetate dimeglumine, and literature review. Radiology 1992;183: 227–238.

Braffman B, Naidich TP. The phakomatoses: Part I. Neurofibromatosis and tuberous sclerosis. Neuroimaging Clin North Am 1994; 4:299–324.

CASE 25

James M. Provenzale

HISTORY

An 11-year-old boy with mental retardation.

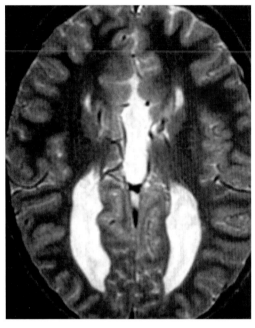

FIGURE 6-25A T2-weighted axial MRI shows a midline structure that is isointense with cerebrospinal fluid located just cephalad to the third ventricle. The corpus callosum is not seen. The lateral ventricles are aligned in a straight line from anterior to posterior and enlargement of the atria is seen.

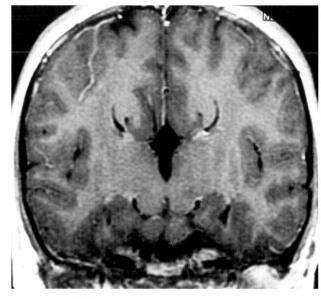

FIGURE 6-25B Contrast-enhanced T1-weighted coronal image shows cephalad extension of the third ventricle. The lateral ventricles are concave along their medial surface ("crescent-shaped"). White matter structures are aligned along the medial surface of both lateral ventricles. Vertically oriented gray matter structures (everted cingulate gyri) are seen medial to the aforementioned white matter structures. The hippocampi are malformed bilaterally and incompletely rotated.

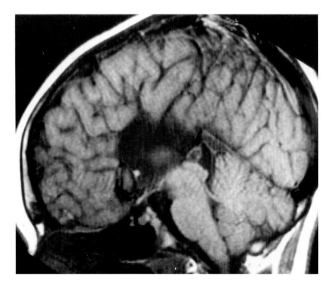

FIGURE 6-25C T1-weighted sagittal image shows cephalad extension of the third ventricle and absence of the cingulate gyrus and corpus callosum. The mesial hemispheric sulci extend all the way down to the third ventricle rather than ending at the cingulate sulcus.

◆ DIFFERENTIAL DIAGNOSIS

◆ **Interhemispheric cyst:** A congenital or acquired cyst located in the interhemispheric region could produce a space filled with cerebrospinal fluid (CSF) between the hemispheres but would not alone account for the abnormal shape of the ventricles and cingulate gyrus or the abnormal white matter tracts along the medial aspects of the ventricular surfaces.

◆ **Agenesis of the corpus callosum (ACC):** This is the correct diagnosis based on the abnormal CSF-filled space cephalad from the third ventricle ("high-riding third ventricle"), abnormal configuration of the ventricles and cingulate gyrus, and abnormal white matter tracts along the medial aspects of the ventricular surfaces (which are due to conglomeration of white matter fibers that run parallel to the medial walls of the lateral ventricles—the so-called bundles of Probst).

◆ DIAGNOSIS: Agenesis of the corpus callosum.

◆ KEY FACTS

CLINICAL

◆ The corpus callosum is formed between the eighth and twentieth weeks of gestation. The parts of the corpus callosum form in a specific order: genu, body, splenium, and rostrum.

◆ Three forms of callosal dysgenesis are recognized: ACC, hypogenesis (i.e., incomplete formation), and hypoplasia (resulting from an insult to cortex or white matter after the corpus callosum has been formed).

◆ A wide spectrum of potential mechanisms (e.g., infectious, toxic, metabolic, and mechanical) by which ACC can occur have been reported, but in the vast majority of instances, the exact etiology is not known.

◆ ACC usually occurs as an isolated finding but can be seen with other structural abnormalities of the brain—e.g., Dandy-Walker malformation, neuronal migration abnormalities, septo-optic dysplasia (hypoplasia of the optic discs, absence of the septum pellucidum, and hypopituitarism), Aicardi's syndrome (seizures, ocular abnormalities, and mental retardation), and malformations of the face (e.g., cleft lip or palate, hypertelorism, and hypoplastic mandible).

◆ ACC is often, but by no means always, associated with mental retardation (which is usually due to associated abnormalities). The incidence of callosal dysgenesis is 5 to 10 times higher in individuals with developmental delay than in individuals with normal cognitive development.

RADIOLOGIC

◆ CT findings include (1) absence of all or part of the corpus callosum, (2) a CSF-filled space extending cephalad from the third ventricle, (3) a parallel appearance of the lateral ventricles, and (4) dilatation of the occipital horns and posterior portions of the temporal horns ("colpocephaly") (Figure 6-25A).

◆ The term *high-riding third ventricle* is often used to refer to the abnormal cephalad extension of this ventricle. The cephalad portion of the ventricle is often dilated and can simulate an interhemispheric cyst.

◆ Colpocephaly associated with ACC is thought to be due to the combination of absence of the splenium of the corpus callosum and underdevelopment of the forceps major.

◆ MRI is more sensitive than CT in displaying the structural abnormalities in ACC. On sagittal MR images, the medial hemispheric sulci can be seen to extend down to the third ventricle (Figure 6-25C). These gyri normally terminate at the cingulate sulcus. In the normal brain, inversion of the cingulate gyri occurs in association with the crossing of white matter fibers in the corpus callosum. For this reason, in patients with ACC, the cingulate gyri remain everted (and formation of the normal cingulate sulcus and gyrus does not occur).

◆ On coronal MRIs, the lateral ventricles can be seen to have a crescentic shape (with a medial wall that is straight or concave) due to impression on their medial surface by heterotopic bundles of axonal fibers that have failed to cross the midline (longitudinal bundles of Probst). These bundles lie between the cingulate gyri and the ventricular surface (Figure 6-25B).

◆ SUGGESTED READING

Barkovich AJ, Norman D. Anomalies of the corpus callosum. AJNR 1988;9:493–501.

Jinkins JR, Whittemore AR, Bradley WG. MR imaging of callosal and corticocallosal dysgenesis. AJNR 1989;10:339–344.

Serur D, Jeret JS, Wisniewski K. Agenesis of the corpus callosum: Clinical, neuroradiological and cytogenetic studies. Neuropediatrics 1988;19:87–91.

CASE 26 *Joseph B. Cornett*

HISTORY

An 18-month-old girl with vomiting.

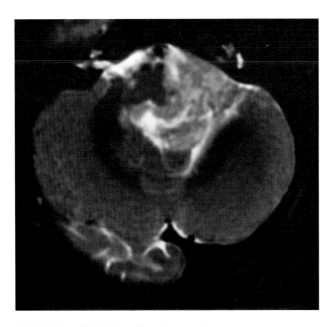

FIGURE 6-26A Axial T2-weighted MRI shows a solid, heterogeneous, hyperintense mass within the fourth ventricle. A thin crescentic rim of cerebrospinal fluid is seen posterior to the mass, representing the compressed fourth ventricle. The mass extends anterolaterally through an enlarged left foramen of Luschka, into the left cerebellopontine angle and up to the basilar artery.

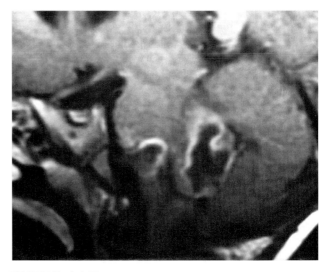

FIGURE 6-26B Contrast-enhanced sagittal T1-weighted image just to the left of midline shows that the mass contrast enhances in an inhomogeneous manner. The lesion fills and obstructs the fourth ventricle, and a portion of the mass is seen wrapping next to the anterior aspect of the lower pons. A small portion of the fourth ventricle can be seen posterior to the upper half of the mass.

◆ DIFFERENTIAL DIAGNOSIS

◆ **Medulloblastoma:** This tumor might be considered because it is a common posterior fossa neoplasm of childhood. This tumor usually arises from the cerebellar vermis and bulges forward from the roof of the fourth ventricle. The fourth ventricle would be expected to be displaced anteriorly (see Case 27). However, in this case, the fourth ventricle is displaced posteriorly. Furthermore, extension into the cerebellopontine angle by medulloblastoma is uncommon.

◆ **Choroid plexus papilloma:** In childhood, choroid plexus papillomas usually occur in the lateral ventricle, unlike the case shown above. Occurrence in the fourth ventricle is usually seen in adults. Furthermore, unlike the lesion shown above, choroid plexus papilloma generally contrast-enhances diffusely and has internal signal voids due to a high degree of vascularity.

◆ **Ependymoma:** Fourth ventricular ependymomas typically arise in the floor of the fourth ventricle, thereby displacing the ventricle posteriorly (as in the case shown above). They often extend through the foramen of Luschka and up to (and sometimes around) the anterior surface of the lower brain stem.

◆ DIAGNOSIS: Ependymoma.

◆ KEY FACTS

CLINICAL

◆ Intracranial ependymoma is largely a tumor of children and adolescents but does occur in adults. Most cases present prior to 5 years of age.

◆ Approximately 60% of brain ependymomas are infratentorial. The remaining 40% are supratentorial and typically occur in either a parenchymal or periventricular location.

◆ Infratentorial ependymoma arises from the ependymal lining of the fourth ventricle and is predominantly intraventricular. It is not uncommon for the tumor to invade the brain stem. Growth along adjacent brain cisterns is characteristic. The term *plastic ependymoma* is given to an ependymoma that has grown around the anterior surface of the brain stem or spinal cord.

◆ Fourth ventricular ependymoma often presents with signs and symptoms of obstructive hydrocephalus (headache, vomiting). Less often, gait or limb ataxia,

nystagmus, or cranial nerve dysfunction is a presenting feature.

◆ CSF dissemination is uncommon (about 10% of cases) at the time of presentation but is more common at a time of relapse.

◆ Treatment is generally surgical resection and radiation therapy. Prognosis is relatively poor, especially in young children with subtotal resection (adult 5-year survival: approximately 70%; pediatric 5-year survival: approximately 15%).

◆ Ependymoma can arise in the spinal cord as an intramedullary mass (see Case 18). The myxopapillary type characteristically arises from conus medullaris or filum terminale.

RADIOLOGIC

◆ The correct preoperative diagnosis of infratentorial ependymoma can be made based on location and morphology of the mass. This is a solid fourth ventricular mass, often with "plastic" extension into the cerebellopontine angle via the foramen of Luschka or into the foramen magnum via the foramen of Magendie.

◆ On noncontrast CT, posterior fossa ependymomas appear relatively isodense to gray matter but are inhomogeneous, with 50% having calcification and about 20% having cystic components. Inhomogeneous contrast enhancement is typical.

◆ On MRI, ependymoma often has inhomogeneous signal intensity due to hemorrhage, necrosis, cyst formation, calcification, and hemosiderin deposition. Like most tumors, the solid component is iso- or hypointense relative to brain parenchyma on T1-weighted images and hyperintense on T2-weighted images. Contrast enhancement is usually inhomogeneous.

◆ Cyst formation is much more common in supratentorial ependymomas (40% to 85% of cases) than infratentorial lesions.

◆ SUGGESTED READING

Furie DM, Provenzale JM. Supratentorial ependymomas and subependymomas: CT and MR appearance. J Comput Assist Tomogr 1995;19:518–526.

Lyons MK, Kelly PJ. Posterior fossa ependymomas: Report of 30 cases and review of the literature. Neurosurgery 1991;28: 659–664.

Spoto GP, Press GA, Hesselink JR, Solomon M. Intracranial ependymoma and subependymoma: MR manifestations. AJNR 1990;11:83–91.

HISTORY

A 6-year-old boy with headache and ataxia.

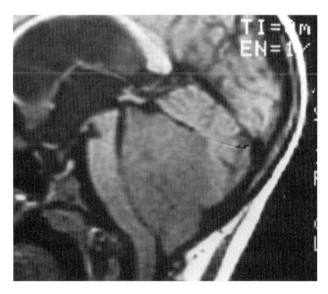

FIGURE 6-27A Noncontrast T1-weighted sagittal MRI shows a large homogeneous mass occupying the fourth ventricle, causing obstructive hydrocephalus and inferior displacement of the cerebellar tonsils. The brain stem is displaced forward, and the fourth ventricle can be seen as a thin rim of cerebrospinal fluid along the superior aspect of the ventral surface of the mass.

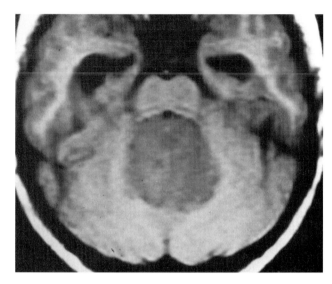

FIGURE 6-27B Noncontrast T1-weighted axial MRI shows the fourth ventricle as a slit-like, cerebrospinal fluid-filled structure ventral to the mass.

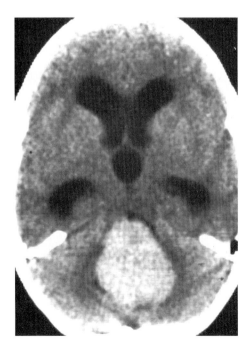

FIGURE 6-27C Noncontrast axial CT image shows the mass is intrinsically hyperdense relative to gray and white matter.

◆ DIFFERENTIAL DIAGNOSIS

◆ **Ependymoma:** This tumor might be considered because it is one of the common posterior fossa tumors in the pediatric population and is usually located within the fourth ventricle. However, ependymomas are frequently inhomogeneous, and about 50% are calcified. Furthermore, they typically arise in the floor of the fourth ventricle. In the case shown above, the fourth ventricle is displaced ventrally, indicating that the mass originated in the roof of the fourth ventricle.

◆ **Astrocytoma (juvenile pilocytic astrocytoma):** This tumor is also one of the common posterior fossa tumors of the pediatric population. Unlike the case shown above, however, these lesions are typically cystic and located in the cerebellar hemisphere.

◆ **Medulloblastoma:** This tumor typically arises from the roof of the fourth ventricle and is homogeneous and often hyperdense on noncontrast CT, all features of the lesion shown above.

◆ DIAGNOSIS: Medulloblastoma.

◆ KEY FACTS

CLINICAL

◆ Medulloblastoma is a highly malignant tumor that is usually seen between the ages of 3 and 10 years.

◆ Medulloblastoma is considered one type of primitive neuroectodermal tumor, along with ependymoblastoma, pinealoblastoma, and cerebral neuroblastoma.

◆ In childhood, the tumor typically arises in the midline, originating in the cerebellar vermis and extending into the fourth ventricle. When seen in young adults, it often occurs off the midline, in the cerebellar hemispheres. A 2 to 1 male predominance has been reported.

◆ Metastasis through the subarachnoid space of the brain and spine is common, being seen in 25% to 50% of patients at the time of diagnosis or early in the postoperative period.

◆ Because ventriculoperitoneal shunts are often placed in these patients for hydrocephalus, peritoneal metastasis can sometimes be seen.

◆ Medulloblastoma is one of the few CNS tumors that metastasizes with any notable frequency outside the central nervous system. Bone metastases are seen in about 5% of cases.

◆ The 5-year survival rate is estimated at 40% to 80%.

RADIOLOGIC

◆ On noncontrast CT, the tumor appears as a well-marginated, homogeneous, hyperdense mass (Figure 6-27C) that arises from the vermis and fills the fourth ventricle. The hyperdense appearance, although not invariably present, is a helpful feature in identifying the mass as medulloblastoma. Small cysts are sometimes seen. Calcification is seen in about 10% of cases, but it is not a prominent feature when present.

◆ Medulloblastoma must be distinguished from two other common pediatric posterior fossa tumors: cerebellar juvenile pilocytic astrocytoma (JPA) and ependymoma. JPA is usually hypodense on CT due to a large cystic component, and ependymoma is usually isodense or slightly hyperdense and calcified more commonly (50%) than medulloblastoma (and thus has an intrinsically inhomogeneous appearance).

◆ Following contrast administration, medulloblastoma typically densely enhances in a homogeneous pattern except for the usually small areas of necrosis. In comparison, only the solid portions of JPAs contrast-enhance, resulting in an inhomogeneous appearance. Ependymoma also often enhances in an inhomogeneous pattern, further allowing distinction from medulloblastoma in most cases.

◆ Atypical appearances of medulloblastoma at the time of presentation can occasionally be seen, including a mass that is wholly cystic, a mass arising in the cerebellopontine angle, and multifocal tumor.

◆ On MRI, the tumor is hypointense on T1-weighted images and iso- or hyperintense on T2-weighted images. The pattern of MR contrast enhancement is similar to that seen on CT.

◆ Sagittal MRIs are often helpful in distinguishing medulloblastoma from ependymoma. Because medulloblastoma typically originates in the roof of the fourth ventricle, a cleavage plane can often be seen between the mass and the brain stem (Figures 6-27A and 6-27B). Ependymomas are often adherent to the floor of the fourth ventricle and can grow into the brain stem. A cleavage plane, therefore, is often seen between the posterior aspect of the tumor and the vermis.

◆ Imaging of the entire neuroaxis is indicated early in the clinical course to assess for drop metastases. It is important to recognize that if spinal imaging is first performed after craniotomy, postoperative extradural spinal hemorrhage can simulate drop metastases.

◆ SUGGESTED READING

Ramsey RD. Posterior Fossa Tumor. In Neuroradiology (3rd ed). Philadelphia: Saunders, 1994;495–564.

Tomlinson FH, Scheithauer BW, Meyer FB, et al. Medulloblastoma I: Clinical, diagnostic and therapeutic overview. J Child Neurol 1992;7:142–155.

Truwit CL. Posterior Fossa Tumors. In BP Drayer, DR Enzmann, JG Smirniotopolous, RR Lukin (eds), Core Curriculum in Neuroradiology, Part II: Neoplasms and Infectious Diseases. American Society of Neuroradiology, 1996;97–102.

HISTORY

A 67-year-old woman with headache.

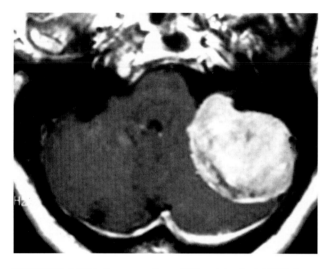

FIGURE 6-28A Contrast-enhanced T1-weighted axial MRI shows a slightly inhomogeneously contrast-enhancing mass in the posterior aspect of the left cerebellopontine angle cistern. The cisternal space along the left side of the pons is widened, consistent with the presence of an extra-axial mass.

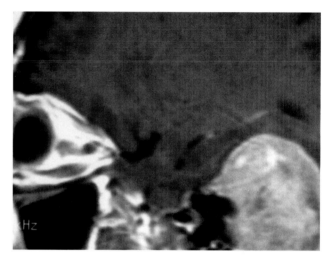

FIGURE 6-28B Contrast-enhanced T1-weighted sagittal MRI shows the mass elevating the posterior aspect of the temporal lobe. A small lip of contrast-enhancing tissue is seen extending forward along the dura from the anterior aspect of the mass.

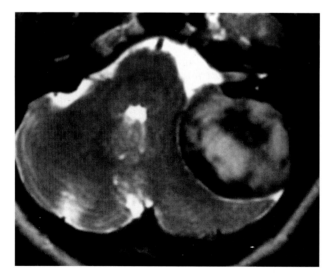

FIGURE 6-28C T2-weighted axial MRI shows the mass is generally slightly hyperintense to gray matter on this pulse sequence but has hypointense regions. A sharp interface between the mass and normal brain is seen, consistent with an extra-axial mass. The mass extends up to the level of the internal auditory canal but does not extend into it.

◆ DIFFERENTIAL DIAGNOSIS

- **Acoustic schwannoma:** This is the most common cerebellopontine angle (CPA) cistern mass lesion. However, this diagnosis is unlikely in the patient shown above because the mass does not extend into the internal auditory canal.
- **Arachnoid or epidermoid cyst:** Both of these lesions are extra-axial and can occur in the CPA cistern. Arachnoid cysts are isointense with cerebrospinal fluid (CSF), unlike the lesion shown above. Epidermoid cysts do not contrast-enhance or only minimally contrast-enhance, unlike the lesion shown above.
- **Meningioma:** This is the best diagnosis because of the extra-axial location of the mass, hypointense appearance on T2-weighted images, dense contrast enhancement, and the presence of a small portion of the lesion extending along the dura (so-called dural tail).

◆ DIAGNOSIS: Meningioma.

◆ KEY FACTS

CLINICAL

- Meningioma is the most common nonglial intracranial neoplasm.
- The peak incidence is the fifth through seventh decades. The female-to-male ratio is 2 to 1.
- Meningiomas are rare in the pediatric population. Approximately 25% of children with a meningioma will have neurofibromatosis.
- Meningiomas arise from meningothelial cells (arachnoid "cap" cells) of the arachnoid villi and occur most often where these cells are most numerous.
- Sites of occurrence, in order of decreasing frequency, are parasagittal convexity, sphenoid wing, planum spenoidale, supra- or parasellar region, falx, posterior fossa, and spine. Less common sites include the cavernous sinus, ventricle (especially trigone of the lateral ventricle), and orbit. These lesions may rarely occur in the diploic space and extracranial sites (nasal cavity, paranasal sinuses, nasopharynx, infratemporal fossa).

- Four classic histologic subtypes are described: meningothelial (syncytial), fibroblastic, transitional, and angioblastic. Malignant meningiomas are rare.

RADIOLOGIC

- Most meningiomas are well-defined, extra-axial masses. They may be broad-based, pedunculated, or flat ("en plaque").
- On CT, these lesions can be (1) isodense with brain, (2) intrinsically homogeneously hyperdense, or (3) calcified to varying degrees. They typically strongly contrast-enhance. Calcification is seen in 15% to 20% of cases. Atypical findings (necrosis, cyst formation, hemorrhage) occur in 15% of cases.
- On MRI, meningiomas are typically isointense (60%) or hypointense (30%) relative to gray matter on non-contrast T1-weighted images and usually densely contrast-enhance. They are isointense (50%) or hyperintense (40%) relative to gray matter on T2-weighted images. However, densely calcified or fibrous tumors can be very hypointense on T2-weighted images (Figure 6-28C). Peritumoral hyperintense signal on T2-weighted images due to edema is seen in 75% of tumors.
- A "dural tail" is seen in approximately 60% of tumors on MRI. This finding can represent either tumor or non-neoplastic dural reaction. Although this finding is highly suggestive of meningioma, it is not specific for meningioma because it can be seen in other entities.

◆ SUGGESTED READING

Black P McL. Meningiomas. Neurosurgery 1993;32:643–657.

Buetow MP, Burton PC, Smirniotopoulos JG. Typical, atypical, and misleading features in meningioma. Radiographics 1991;11: 1087–1100.

Elster AD, Challa VR, Gilders TH, et al. Meningiomas: MR and histopathologic features. Radiology 1989;170:857–862.

Sheporaitis LA, Osborn AG, Smirniotopoulos JG, et al. Radiologic-pathologic correlation. Intracranial meningioma. AJNR 1992;13:29–37.

HISTORY

A 73-year-old woman with right seventh nerve dysfunction.

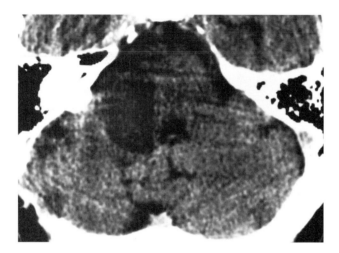

FIGURE 6-29A Noncontrast axial CT shows a hypointense right cerebellopontine angle mass that compresses the right side of the pons and the right cerebellar hemisphere. The mass is slightly hyperdense relative to cerebrospinal fluid.

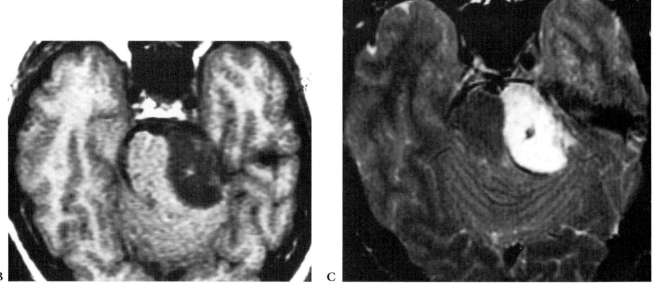

FIGURES 6-29B and 6-29C MRI study in a 43-year-old man with the same diagnosis. **(B)** Noncontrast T1-weighted axial image shows an extra-axial mass deforming the left side of the pons. The mass is inhomogeneous and slightly hyperintense relative to cerebrospinal fluid on this pulse sequence. **(C)** T2-weighted axial image shows that much of the mass is isointense to cerebrospinal fluid on this pulse sequence but that the lateral portion of the mass is hypointense.

◆ DIFFERENTIAL DIAGNOSIS

- **Arachnoid cyst:** This lesion might be considered because the lesions shown above are nearly isointense with CSF. However, arachnoid cysts are truly isodense to cerebrospinal fluid (CSF) on CT and isointense on all MR pulse sequences, unlike the lesions shown above.
- **Cysticercosis:** Extra-axial lesions can be seen due to cysticercosis infection in the "racemose" form of the disease, in which cystic lesions are found within the subarachnoid spaces and brain cisterns. The lesions can grow to large size and compress adjacent brain. However, they are typically isointense with CSF, unlike the lesion shown above.
- **Epidermoid cyst:** These lesions are frequently located in the cerebellopontine angle (CPA) and deform adjacent brain. They are isodense or slightly hyperdense to CSF on CT (Figure 6-29A). They are isointense to CSF on one or more MR pulse sequences but, in the majority of cases, differ in signal intensity from CSF on at least one MR pulse sequence (Figures 6-29B and 6-29C).

◆ DIAGNOSIS: Epidermoid cyst.

◆ KEY FACTS

CLINICAL

- Epidermoid cysts are thought to arise from inclusion of epithelial elements within the neural groove during its closure.
- Although epidermoid cysts grow with age, they are not considered neoplasms. Enlargement occurs due to progressive accumulation of breakdown products of desquamated epithelial cells, including keratin and solid cholesterol.
- Eighty percent of intracranial epidermoid cysts are intradural in location, often appearing in the infratentorial compartment. The CPA is one of the more common sites. Supratentorial epidermoid cysts are usually found in the parasellar region and medial aspect of the middle cranial fossa.
- Epidermoid cysts are slow-growing lesions that conform to the surface of the brain as they enlarge, infiltrate through the subarachnoid space, and surround vessels and cranial nerves. Symptoms have often been present for many months or a few years by the time of discovery.
- Because the surfaces of intracranial epidermoid cysts have a shiny, white surface appearance, they are sometimes referred to as "pearly tumors."
- Epidermoid cysts are similar to dermoid cysts in that both lesions have a stratified squamous epithelial lining

with a fibrous connective tissue capsule, but epidermoid cysts lack sebaceous and sweat gland secretory units.
- Arachnoid cyst is the principal diagnostic consideration from which epidermoid cyst must be distinguished. This is true because arachnoid cysts are frequently not treated because they are asymptomatic, stable congenital lesions. Epidermoid cysts, however, are often symptomatic and continue to grow with advancing age, necessitating resection.
- Total surgical resection of an epidermoid cyst is often impossible because portions of the lesion are buried in spaces that cannot be reached without causing undue traction on important neurologic or vascular structures and because the tumor is often tightly adherent to brain and blood vessels. In those instances, partial debulking is performed, which may need to be repeated as the lesion regrows.

RADIOLOGIC

- On noncontrast head CT, epidermoid cysts are hypodense extra-axial masses whose margins are often slightly lobulated or scalloped. Many lesions are slightly hyperdense relative to CSF and mildly inhomogeneous. However, they frequently are isodense to CSF, making distinction from arachnoid cyst difficult. Occasionally, a very small amount of calcification can be seen.
- Epidermoid cysts have a soft, pliable consistency, but they often exert a moderate degree of mass effect on adjacent brain structures.
- Lack of enhancement after contrast administration is the general rule, although sometimes very mild contrast enhancement can be seen around the rim of the lesion.
- MRI is frequently useful in distinguishing epidermoid cysts from arachnoid cysts because the lesion often appears inhomogeneous and has a signal intensity that differs from CSF on at least one pulse. MRI is also important in surgical planning because it is the best method for defining the limits of the mass and the spatial relationship to cranial nerves and blood vessels.
- When a suspected epidermoid cyst is isointense with CSF on all pulse sequences, the distinction from arachnoid cyst can be made by pulse sequences that are sensitive to water motion—e.g., diffusion-weighted images and steady-state free precession images.

◆ SUGGESTED READING

Latack JT, Kartush JM, Kemink JL, et al. Epidermoidomas of the cerebellopontine angle and temporal bone: CT and MRI aspects. Radiology 1985;157:361–366.

Tampieri D, Melanson D, Ethier R. MR imaging of epidermoid cysts. AJNR 1989;10:351–356.

Tsuruda JS, Chew WM, Moseley ME, Norman D. Diffusion-weighted MR imaging of the brain: Value of differentiating between extra-axial cysts and epidermoid tumors. AJNR 1990;11:925-931.

CHAPTER 7

VASCULAR RADIOLOGY

Tony P. Smith, *chapter editor*

James T.T. Chen, Michael J. Kelley,
Glenn E. Newman, Cynthia S. Payne,
Tony P. Smith, Daniel J. Stackhouse,
and Paul V. Suhocki

CASE 1

Glenn E. Newman

HISTORY

A 45-year-old woman with diabetes mellitus and exercise claudication. Both femoral pulses are markedly diminished, and the popliteal and pedal pulses are detectable only by Doppler recording. The ankle/arm index (AAI) at rest was 0.48 on the right and 0.47 on the left.

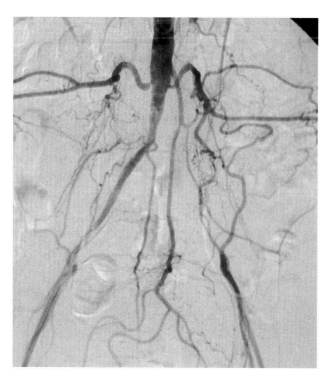

FIGURE 7-1A Anteroposterior view of a catheter angiogram of the distal aorta. The left common iliac artery is occluded and is reconstituted by collateral arteries at the bifurcation of the left common iliac artery. Stenoses of both proximal and distal segments of the right common iliac artery are seen.

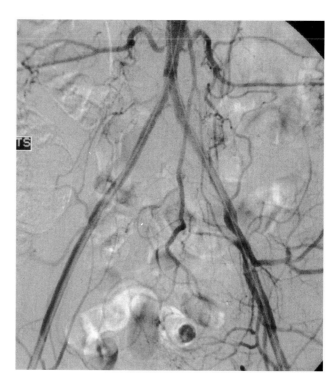

FIGURE 7-1B Catheter angiogram after percutaneous transluminal angioplasty and stenting of the distal aorta, entire left common iliac artery, and the proximal and distal segments of the right common iliac artery. The previously stenosed or occluded segments are now patent.

◆ DIFFERENTIAL DIAGNOSIS

◆ **Peripheral vascular disease (PVD) with claudication.**
◆ **Leriche's syndrome:** Symptoms include fatigue, symmetric muscle atrophy, pallor of the lower extremities, and impotence in males. Angiographically, these patients frequently have an occlusion of the infrarenal abdominal aorta.

◆ DIAGNOSIS: Bilateral aortoiliac atherosclerotic disease.

◆ KEY FACTS

CLINICAL

◆ In general, the diagnosis of claudication is a clinical one based on history, physical examination, and noninvasive testing. Physical examination findings include diminished or absent peripheral arterial pulses pattern and trophic changes in the affected extremities such as hair loss and muscle atrophy. Nonvascular diagnoses such as radiculopathy should be excluded before an invasive procedure such as angiography.

◆ Obstructive atherosclerotic disease of the infrarenal segment of the abdominal aorta and pelvic arteries supplying the legs is relatively common, with a prevalence of approximately 40/10,000 patients.

◆ Obstructive PVD is 5 to 10 times more common in men than women. It generally occurs after 50 years of age unless a concomitant disease such as diabetes mellitus or a family history of atheromatous disease is present.

◆ The choice of therapies is determined by the anatomic location and extent of arterial disease and comorbid features (e.g., cardiopulmonary status). Approximately 90% of patients have a clinical history of occlusive atheromatous disease in other locations—e.g., coronary or carotid circulation.

◆ Integration of the history, physical examination, and results of noninvasive tests allows preangiographic prediction of the disease site and severity, including the presence of inflow (i.e., suprainguinal) and ouflow (i.e., infrainguinal) disease.

◆ The AAI in the resting state, which decreases as disease severity increases, is used to quantitate disease severity. Note that arterial disease of the upper extremities could give a false-negative value. The following scale correlates disease severity with AAI: normal: ≥0.9; mild insufficiency: 0.7 to 0.9; moderate insufficiency: 0.5 to 0.7; severe insufficiency (i.e., a threatened limb): <0.5.

◆ Percutaneous transluminal angioplasty (PTA), alone or in combination with intravascular stenting, is the major nonsurgical means of treating atheromatous aortoiliac disease. PTA is not possible when occlusive lesions cannot be negotiated with a catheter-guidewire combination. PTA is contraindicated when lesions are immediately adjacent to arterial aneurysms.

◆ Aortobifemoral graft placement is generally reserved for patients who have extensive atheromatous disease and low surgical risk.

RADIOLOGIC

◆ Aortoiliac atheromatous disease frequently begins above the aortic bifurcation and sometimes extends as far as the distal iliac arteries. Alternatively, isolated stenoses of each common iliac origin can occur. The major aim of radiologic assessment is to determine preoperatively the extent of disease (i.e., detect the presence of either or both inflow and outflow disease), which will guide therapy.

◆ Although PTA alone is frequently successful, intravascular stenting is sometimes also necessary. Indications for stenting include (1) a high residual aortoiliac systolic blood pressure gradient (>15 mm Hg) or residual or recurrent stenosis (>30%) after PTA, and (2) arterial dissection at the angioplasty site that compromises blood flow.

◆ Factors that predict long-term patency after PTA can be divided into two categories: (1) clinical predictors, based on degree of ischemia as assessed by history and physical examination; and (2) anatomic predictors, based on lesion location (proximal versus distal) and lesion appearance (stenosis versus occlusion; short, concentric stenosis versus long, eccentric stenosis).

◆ Clinical predictors are based on the symptoms before PTA. In general, patients who present with claudication fare much better overall than those who present for limb salvage (nonhealing ulcers, skin changes, hair loss, etc.). This is not unexpected since the latter is a reflection of much more extensive vascular disease.

◆ Anatomic predictors are based on the location and angiographic appearance of the lesion. Proximal lesions (so-called inflow disease) have a much better prognosis than more distal lesions. Angiographic lesion appearance refers to the degree of vessel narrowing, the degree of irregularity of the lesion, and its length. In general, patients with stenoses have a better result from PTA than those with occlusions, and patients with short (i.e., <5 cm), concentric (smooth) lesions fare better than those with long (i.e., >5 cm), eccentric (irregular) lesions. Therefore, based on clinical and anatomic predictors, the patient who complains only of claudication and who has a short, smooth, proximal stenosis has the best chance of long-term patency after PTA.

◆ The 5-year patency rate of iliac PTA alone is approximately 70% to 75%, but that of PTA with intravascular stenting is 90% to 95%.

◆ SUGGESTED READING

Rholl KS, van Breda A. Percutaneous Intervention for Aortoiliac Disease. In DE Strandness Jr, A van Breda (eds), Vascular Diseases: Surgical and Interventional Therapy. New York: Churchill Livingstone, 1994;433–466.

CASE 2

James T.T. Chen

HISTORY

A 12-year-old girl with a 6-year history of exertional dyspnea and palpitations.

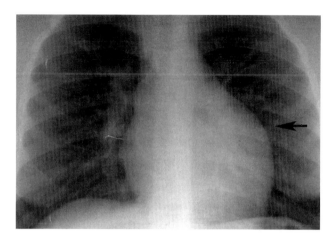

FIGURE 7-2A Frontal chest radiograph. A peculiar cardiac contour is seen with a straight-ending left upper border and a bulge in the left mid border (arrow). The normal "triad" of densities (ascending aorta, aortic knob, and pulmonary trunk) is absent.

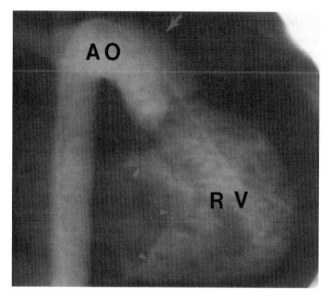

FIGURE 7-2B Right ventriculogram. The morphologic (trabeculated) right ventricle (RV) is reached by an aortic catheter. The right ventricle gives rise to the aorta (AO). The ascending segment of the aorta forms a leftward convexity (arrow). The right ventricle receives blood from the left atrium via the tricuspid valve (arrowheads).

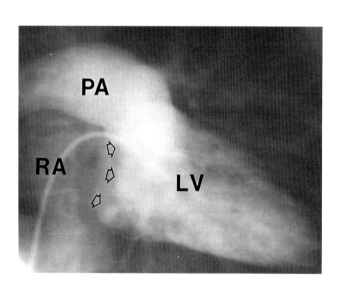

FIGURE 7-2C Left ventriculogram. The morphologic (nontrabeculated) left ventricle (LV) is reached by a venous catheter from the right atrium (RA) via the mitral valve (open arrows). The left ventricle gives rise to the pulmonary arteries (PA).

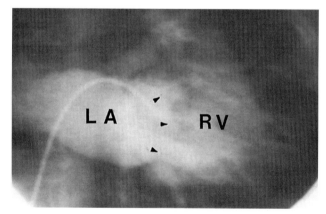

FIGURE 7-2D Levophase following left ventricular contrast injection. The levophase of the left ventriculogram shows sequential opacification of the pulmonary veins, the left atrium (LA), the tricuspid valve (arrowheads), and the right ventricle (RV).

◆ DIFFERENTIAL DIAGNOSIS

◆ **Left ventricular aneurysm:** This entity might be considered, because it can produce a left-sided contour irregularity on chest radiographs. However, it is rare at this age and is usually seen in the setting of left ventricular infarction from coronary artery disease in older adults. Furthermore, angiographic findings of an aneurysm are not present.

◆ **Idiopathic hypertrophic subaortic stenosis (IHSS):** IHSS is a consideration based on the history. However, the chest radiograph in IHSS is often either normal or shows diffuse cardiomegaly. The angiographic findings are not consistent with this entity, because in IHSS the ventriculoarterial relationships are normal and the ejection fraction is increased.

◆ **Loculated pericardial effusion:** The contour irregularity at the left heart margin makes this a diagnostic consideration. However, the symptoms of palpitation and chronic chest pain, as in the case shown above, would be unusual. Furthermore, the angiogram would be expected to be normal, unlike the findings in the case presented.

◆ **Partial absence of pericardium on the left:** The history is usual for this entity, because patients typically present with acute, occasionally intermittent, chest pain due to ischemia resulting from entrapment of the herniated portion of the left atrium. However, there is no irregularity of the left atrium on the angiogram shown above.

◆ **L-loop transposition of the great arteries:** This diagnosis is the most likely based on the history and radiographic and angiographic findings.

◆ DIAGNOSIS: L-loop transposition of the great arteries (congenitally corrected transposition of the great arteries).

◆ KEY FACTS

CLINICAL

◆ The patient shown above represents the 10% of patients with L-loop transposition of great arteries who do not have evidence of associated cardiac defects.

◆ Over 90% of patients with L-loop transposition of the great arteries will have or develop one or more of the following lesions: (1) left-sided atrioventricular (AV) (tricuspid) valve insufficiency, (2) heart block, (3) ventricular septal defect (VSD), or (4) pulmonary stenosis.

◆ Because of the risk for later development of either or both tricuspid insufficiency and heart block, patients need close clinical monitoring.

RADIOLOGIC

◆ Absence of the normal triad of densities on the frontal chest radiograph is explained on the following anatomic abnormalities: (1) the ascending aorta is left-sided, (2) the pulmonary trunk is more medial and posterior, (3) the aortic knob is formed at a more acute angle and is more medial on the posteroanterior projection.

◆ Periodic radiographic evaluations are a helpful adjunct to the clinical examination in the detection of associated lesions. Interim development of left atrial and right ventricular enlargement with either or both cephalization of the pulmonary vasculature and pulmonary edema are diagnostic signs of left-sided AV valve insufficiency.

◆ Enlarging heart size in these patients can be seen in the setting of heart block or AV valve insufficiency.

◆ Cardiomegaly and increased pulmonary vascularity suggested an associated VSD.

◆ Decreased pulmonary vascularity is suggestive of pulmonary stenosis only if a VSD is present.

◆ SUGGESTED READING

Chen JTT. Essentials of Cardiac Roentgenology. Boston: Little, Brown, 1987.

Kelley MJ, Jaffe CC, Kleinman CS. Cardiac Imaging in Infants and Children. Philadelphia: Saunders, 1982.

Nugent EW, Plauth WH, Edwards JE, Williams WH. The Pathology, Pathophysiology, Recognition, and Treatment of Congenital Heart Disease. In RC Schlant, RW Alexander (eds), The Heart (8th ed). New York: McGraw-Hill, 1994;1761–1828.

90% Cardiac defects

CASE 3

Tony P. Smith

HISTORY

A 40-year-old woman with nephrotic syndrome and sudden onset of right-sided pleuritic chest pain.

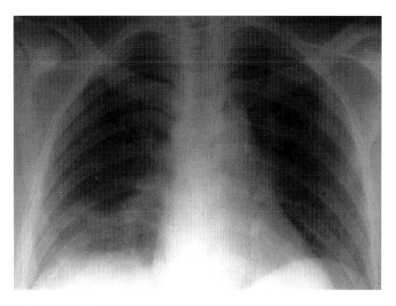

FIGURE 7-3A Posteroanterior chest radiograph. A homogeneous opacity is seen in the right lower lobe that was not present on a prior study.

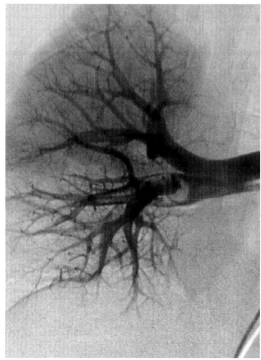

FIGURE 7-3B Right pulmonary artery angiogram. A filling defect is seen in the interlobar artery extending into the right middle and lower lobe branches.

◆ DIFFERENTIAL DIAGNOSIS

◆ The differential diagnosis on the chest radiograph is that for any focal lung opacity and therefore includes a wide spectrum of entities. However, given the unilateral and focal nature of the pulmonary opacity, pneumonia and lung infarct are the best considerations.

◆ The findings on the pulmonary angiogram are diagnostic for acute pulmonary embolism (PE).

◆ DIAGNOSIS: Acute pulmonary embolus.

◆ KEY FACTS

CLINICAL

◆ PE is a common, life-threatening entity with an estimated 600,000 cases per year in the United States alone. Approximately 10% of the patients with PE do not survive the initial event.

◆ The clinical signs of PE are nonspecific and typically can include dyspnea, tachypnea, pleuritic pain, and hemoptysis.

◆ Treatment usually consists of anticoagulation with heparin followed by warfarin. If there is a contraindication to anticoagulation, an inferior vena cava filter can be placed at the time of angiography.

◆ Acute treatment of PE with thrombolytic agents has not yet definitively demonstrated advantages over long-term anticoagulation and is usually reserved for very acutely ill patients to decrease their clot burden.

◆ Recurrent PE occurs in only a minority of patients treated with anticoagulant therapy.

RADIOLOGIC

◆ Most patients with PE do have abnormal chest radiographs, but the findings are nonspecific—e.g., either or both atelectasis and pulmonary parenchymal opacities. In the appropriate circumstances, however, it is actually a normal radiograph that is most helpful in assessment for PE. A normal chest radiograph in a patient with dyspnea and hypoxia (PaO_2 ≤70 mm Hg) should strongly raise the possibility of PE, because it effectively excludes other entities that clinically mimic PE. The other main function of the chest radiograph is to aid in interpretation of the ventilation-perfusion imaging in a patient with suspected PE (see Chapter 10, Case 17).

◆ Pulmonary angiography is usually performed using a pigtail-type catheter placed from the common femoral vein. Other access sites include the jugular and brachial veins. Selective angiography is usually performed with the catheter placed into the right or left pulmonary artery. More subselective angiography can be performed if there is concern regarding a specific region of a lung.

◆ The contrast infusion for pulmonary angiography is usually 15 to 25 ml/sec for a total of 30 to 50 ml in each pulmonary artery, depending on arterial flow. Filming is usually at three or four films per second.

◆ The presence of intra-arterial filling defects on pulmonary angiography is indicative of PE. Complete arterial occlusion (vessel cutoff) is also highly suggestive of the diagnosis.

◆ Secondary signs of PE on pulmonary angiography include parenchymal staining, decreased perfusion to an area, crowding of vessels, delayed venous return from the affected area, and vascular shunting away from the involved lung.

◆ Pulmonary angiography currently remains the "gold standard" technique for the diagnosis of PE. There are, however, two main concerns with angiography: (1) reportedly high complication rates and (2) a substantial degree of interobserver variability in study interpretation.

◆ Initial concerns about performing pulmonary angiography were for sudden death from cor pulmonale in patients with elevated right heart (ventricular and pulmonary artery) pressures. Pulmonary angiography was considered contraindicated in patients with very high right heart pressures, although a pressure above which angiography would be contraindicated was never fully defined. The risks of sudden death from pulmonary angiography were placed at approximately 0.1%. This probably was due to increased pulmonary artery pressures following the injection of ionic contrast media in patients with already elevated pressures and compromised right heart function. In a review of 1,434 patients from our institution using low-osmolar contrast agents, no deaths from pulmonary angiography were incurred, suggesting that nonionic contrast media are associated with a relatively lower risk than ionic contrast media.

◆ Interobserver variability occurs mostly with smaller thromboemboli, particularly those involving subsegmental levels. When the emboli are large (as in Figure 7-3B), the interobserver variability is very low.

◆ Helical CT, MRI, and magnetic resonance angiography (MRA) are other methods of imaging of PE that are being evaluated because they provide a noninvasive means of diagnosis in patients who are often quite ill and in whom an invasive procedure should be avoided if possible.

◆ SUGGESTED READING

Hudson ER, Smith TP, McDermott VG, et al. Pulmonary angiography performed with iopamidol: Complications in 1434 patients. Radiology 1996;198:61–65.

Matsumoto AH, Tegtmeyer CJ. Contemporary diagnostic approaches to pulmonary emboli. Radiol Clin North Am 1995;33:167–183.

Newman GE. Pulmonary angiography in pulmonary embolic disease. J Thorac Imag 1989;4:28–39.

CASE 4

Daniel J. Stackhouse

HISTORY

A 51-year-old man with bright red blood per rectum.

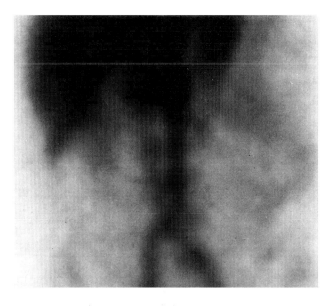

FIGURE 7-4A A Tc-labeled red blood cell nuclear medicine study shows faint accumulation of tracer in the left abdomen.

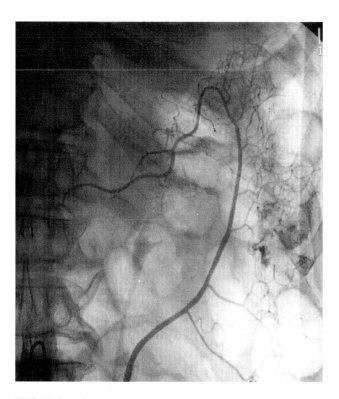

FIGURE 7-4B Arteriogram of the inferior mesenteric artery shows a bleeding site in the descending colon with extravasation of contrast material into the bowel. No abnormal vascularity to suggest tumor vessels or early draining veins to suggest an arteriovenous malformation are seen.

◈ DIFFERENTIAL DIAGNOSIS

A meaningful differential diagnosis can only be generated after the bleeding site is determined, which can be accomplished by endoscopy (frequently unhelpful when bleeding is brisk) by nuclear medicine bleeding studies, or angiography. The following is a differential diagnosis for hemorrhage from a left colon bleeding site (as in the case shown):

◆ **Diverticular hemorrhage**: This cause is the most common etiology of colorectal bleeding (approximately 50% of cases). Diverticula occur more commonly in the left colon, but those that occur in the right colon carry the higher risk of bleeding.

◆ **Angiodysplasia:** Up to 20% of colorectal bleeding is due to these acquired lesions. The angiographic appearance is that of a small tuft of vessels with at least one early draining vein. These findings are not seen in the case illustrated.

◆ **Neoplasm:** Tumors account for about 10% of colorectal bleeding. Tumor vascularity (not present in the case shown) can sometimes be seen at angiography.

◆ **Colitis:** This entity accounts for 5% to 10% of cases of colorectal bleeding. At angiography, prominent opacification of involved segments of colon can often be seen during the capillary phase (not present in the case shown).

◆ **DIAGNOSIS: Hemorrhage due to diverticular disease in the descending colon.**

◆ **KEY FACTS**

CLINICAL

◆ Prompt and adequate hemodynamic stabilization (e.g., placement of large-bore intravenous lines and vascular repletion) of the patient with gastrointestinal (GI) hemorrhage is imperative before diagnostic procedures are started.

◆ Eighty percent of patients with GI bleeding have spontaneous resolution of the hemorrhage without treatment.

◆ It is important to determine whether the source of bleeding is from the upper (i.e., above the ligament of Treitz) or lower GI tract. If gastric lavage contents are clear, a source is presumed to be distal to the pylorus. If the lavage contents are bile stained but without overt evidence of hemorrhage, the source is most likely in the lower GI tract.

◆ Upper or lower endoscopy will frequently identify the bleeding source and provide the initial means of treatment, including cautery, injection of epinephrine, or in the case of variceal bleeding, sclerotherapy or banding.

◆ Substantial nonvariceal upper GI arterial bleeding not responsive to endoscopic therapy is an indication for emergency arteriography.

◆ When the source of lower GI bleeding cannot be determined, a Tc-labeled red blood cell study, which can detect bleeding at a rate of 0.1 ml/min, can be performed to attempt to localize the bleeding site.

RADIOLOGIC

Upper Gastrointestinal Bleeding

◆ Angiography can only identify bleeding occurring at a rate of 1 ml/min, a much faster rate than detectable by tagged red blood cell studies. Extravasation of contrast material into the bowel lumen is seen as pooling of contrast material in the bowel lumen.

◆ Selective injections of the celiac, left gastric, gastroduodenal (if the left gastric injection is negative), and superior mesenteric arteries are performed routinely.

◆ Left gastric artery bleeding sites can be embolized with gelatin sponge pledgets or metal coils because circulation from the gastroepiploic, right gastric, and short gastric arteries provides adequate collateral flow to prevent infarction.

Lower Gastrointestinal Bleeding

◆ Sources of small bowel hemorrhage include ulceration, diverticula, enteritis, neoplasm, angiodysplasia, and aortoenteric fistula.

◆ Sources of colonic hemorrhage include diverticular disease, neoplasm, angiodysplasia, and colitis. Rectal bleeding can be a false localizing sign because the upper GI tract is the source in up to 10% of patients with active rectal bleeding.

◆ During angiographic evaluation of lower GI bleeding, injection of the superior mesenteric artery (SMA) and inferior mesenteric artery (IMA) is performed routinely. If the patient does not have a Foley catheter in place, the IMA should be evaluated before injection of the SMA so that the contrast-filled bladder does not obscure IMA branches.

◆ Lower GI bleeding sites can be treated by injection of vasopressin into the SMA or IMA, causing constriction of smooth muscle in the arterioles and venules.

◆ Vasopressin infusion is contraindicated in patients with history of congestive heart failure, because fluid retention can occur due to the antidiuretic hormone effect of this agent.

◆ After identification of the bleeding site, a trial of vasopressin infusion through the arterial catheter is begun at 0.2 U/minute for 20 minutes. If repeat arteriography shows the bleeding is controlled, the infusion is continued for 12 to 24 hours. If the bleeding is not controlled, the dose is increased to 0.4 U/minute for 20 minutes. If bleeding is then controlled, the infusion is continued for 6 to 12 hours and is decreased by 0.1 U/minute every 6 to 12 hours followed by a saline infusion. If bleeding has then ceased, the catheter is removed.

◆ Bleeding refractory to vasopressin infusion is typically an indication for surgery. However, with the advent of three French coaxial catheter systems, intra-arterial embolization with gelatin sponge pledgets, coils, or polyvinyl alcohol sponge particles can be accomplished in patients who are poor surgical candidates by superselective positioning of the catheter into third- or fourth-order branches. Even though collateral circulation through the most peripheral arcades is left intact, the procedure carries a risk of ischemia and infarction.

◆ **SUGGESTED READING**

Baum S. Angiography of the gastrointestinal bleeder. Radiology 1982;143:569–572.

Kadir S, Ernst CB. Current concepts in angiographic management of gastrointestinal bleeding. Curr Prob Surg 1983;20:287–343.

Keller FS, Rösch J. Embolization for acute gastric hemorrhage. Semin Intervent Radiol 1988;5:25–31.

CASE 5

Glenn E. Newman

HISTORY

A 52-year-old man 1 year status post placement of a left femoral-to-right femoral artery bypass graft for right iliofemoral occlusion. The left femoral pulse is now palpable, but the right femoral artery pulse and the graft pulse are nonpalpable. The right leg is cooler than the left leg.

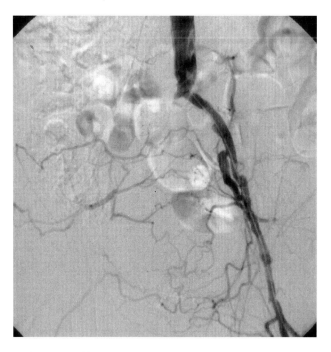

FIGURE 7-5A Pelvic angiogram shows the left iliofemoral arterial system is patent, but the left femoral-to-right femoral graft is thrombosed.

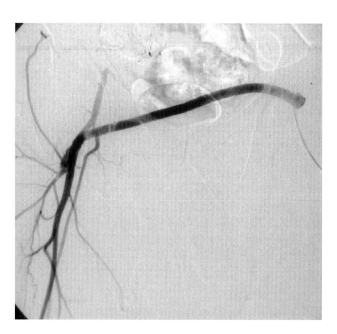

FIGURE 7-5B Pelvic angiogram following urokinase infusion shows successful thrombolysis of the left femoral-to-right femoral graft.

◆ DIFFERENTIAL DIAGNOSIS

- **Acute left iliac artery thrombosis:** This diagnosis could account for the absence of pulses in the graft, but the physical findings of a pulse in the left femoral artery and the opacification of the left femoral artery during angiography are not consistent with this diagnosis.
- **Chronic right iliac artery occlusion and acute graft thrombosis:** This diagnosis adequately accounts for the physical findings and the lack of opacification of the graft prior to thrombolysis.

◆ DIAGNOSIS: Acute thrombosis of left femoral-to-right femoral graft.

◆ KEY FACTS

CLINICAL

- The patency of femoral-femoral grafts is approximately 95% at 5 years. The most important factor is patency of the superficial femoral artery. Failure of femoral-femoral grafts is more often related to progression of outflow (runoff) disease than to progression of inflow (iliac) disease. Another cause of failure is stenosis at the site of graft-arterial anastomosis.
- Femoral-femoral grafts are generally reserved for patients who are at high risk for more extensive surgical arterial reconstruction—e.g., aortofemoral grafting procedures.

RADIOLOGIC

- Diagnostic angiography should be performed to define the presence and extent of "inflow" or "outflow" disease in patients being considered for thrombolytic therapy.

- Thrombolytic therapy is a treatment option in patients (1) with viable extremities and (2) with threatened extremities in whom the rate of progression of ischemia would not preclude a prolonged (8- to 24-hour) thrombolytic infusion. Patients with irreversibly ischemic extremities are not considered candidates for thrombolytic therapy.
- To accomplish a successful thrombolytic infusion, the entire length of the thrombosed graft must be successfully negotiated with a catheter-guidewire infusion system.
- Urokinase is the agent of choice in most institutions. It is usually administered as a bolus (typically a dose of 250,000 units) followed by low-dose (100,000 U/hr) or high-dose (250,000 U/hr) infusion of urokinase into the graft. Serial angiograms are obtained to document results. Infusion is terminated when thrombus is successfully resolved, or when angiography shows no improvement after a 4- to 8-hour infusion.
- The interventionalist must attempt to identify and treat the precipitating lesion responsible for causing graft thrombosis. The treatable causes may be progression of inflow disease (a stenosis proximal to the graft), outflow disease (a stenosis distal to the graft), or a stenosis at the site of anastomosis.

◆ SUGGESTED READING

McNamara TO. Thrombolysis Treatment for Acute Lower Limb Ischemia. In DE Strandness Jr, A van Breda (eds), Vascular Diseases: Surgical and Interventional Therapy. New York: Churchill Livingstone, 1994;355–377.

Welch HJ, Belkin M. Acute Limb Ischemia Resulting from Graft Failure. In DE Strandness Jr, A van Breda (eds), Vascular Diseases: Surgical and Interventional Therapy. New York: Churchill Livingstone, 1994;379–392.

CASE 6

Paul V. Suhocki

HISTORY

A 69-year-old man who was struck in the chest during a motor vehicle accident.

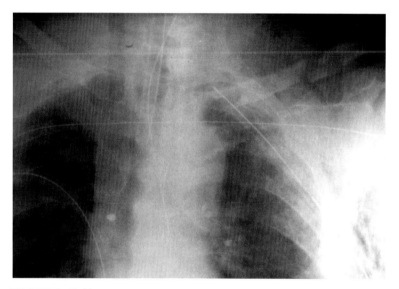

FIGURE 7-6A Anteroposterior chest radiograph. Multiple signs of thoracic trauma are present, including widening of the mediastinal silhouette; deviation of the endotracheal tube to the right; biapical lung opacities; multiple, high thoracic rib fractures; and a left clavicular fracture.

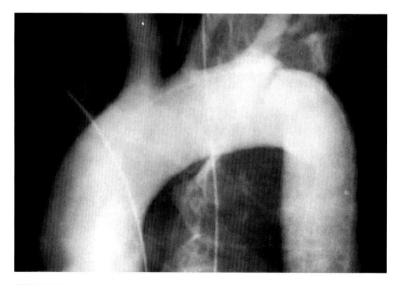

FIGURE 7-6B Aortogram showing linear lucency extends inferiorly from the left upper border of the aorta, just beyond the origin of the left subclavian artery. In this same region, there is a discontinuity ("step off") in the upper contour of the contrast column.

◆ DIFFERENTIAL DIAGNOSIS

- **Aortic tear:** The radiographic findings raise the strong possibility of traumatic tear of the aorta and should prompt the performance of a thoracic aortogram. The abnormalities seen on the aortogram in this case are an indication for emergency surgical repair.
- **Mediastinal widening due to rupture of blood vessels other than the aorta:** The mediastinal widening in the case illustrated could be due to laceration of other blood vessels. However, this is a diagnosis of exclusion that is reached only after angiography has determined whether an aortic injury is present. In the case shown, the angiogram does, in fact, show an aortic injury.
- **Mediastinal widening due to causes other than hematoma:** Mediastinal widening can be caused by a number of conditions other than trauma (e.g., lymphadenopathy, aortic tortuosity). When relatively recent previous radiographs that show an abnormal mediastinal contour are available, such nontraumatic causes should be considered.

◆ DIAGNOSIS: Traumatic tear of the thoracic aorta at the isthmus.

◆ KEY FACTS

CLINICAL

- Only 10% to 20% of patients with traumatic rupture of the aorta survive long enough to come to a hospital. Of those patients who survive long enough to receive medical care, there is a 95% to 97% mortality rate if the aortic rupture is untreated.
- Based on autopsy series, about half of aortic tears are located at the isthmus (distal to the left subclavian artery and proximal to the third intercostal artery). This is the site at which the ligamentum arteriosum attaches the aorta to the left pulmonary artery. The isthmus is the site of aortic laceration in the vast majority (90% to 95%) of patients who survive to reach the hospital.
- About 20% of aortic lacerations involve the ascending aorta. Laceration at this site is nearly always fatal. Less commonly involved sites are the distal thoracic, diaphragmatic, and abdominal aortic segments.
- Multiple tears are seen in 15% to 20% of cases.
- Clinical signs of aortic injury include hypertension in the upper extremities, diminished blood pressure in the lower extremities, and bruits.
- There are several theories for the etiology of aortic tear/transection. One widely accepted hypothesis is that a deceleration injury produces shear and stress at points of maximal fixation of the aorta.
- Emergency surgical repair, usually by placement of a prosthetic aortic graft, is typically indicated. Primary repair (i.e., suturing of the laceration) and patch angioplasty are other, less frequently used, procedures.

RADIOLOGIC

- No single radiographic sign is pathognomonic of aortic rupture. However, a number of chest radiographic findings should strongly raise suspicion of an aortic tear in a trauma patient and should prompt aortography. These include: (1) widened mediastinum, (2) depressed left mainstem bronchus, (3) deviation of the esophagus (deviated nasogastric tube) and trachea at the level of the T4 vertebral body, (4) obscured margins of the aortic arch, (5) left apical opacity ("apical cap"), (6) fracture of any of the first three ribs, (7) widening of a paraspinal line, and (8) widening of the right paratracheal stripe.
- Aortography is usually performed by a transfemoral approach. However, if femoral artery blood pressures are diminished (alone, or in combination with elevated blood pressure in the arms), a brachial artery puncture should be used, because a post-traumatic coarctation may present.
- Aortography remains the gold standard for diagnosis. During aortography, an injection in the left anterior oblique projection should be performed first, followed by a right anterior oblique or lateral projection. The brachiocephalic vessels and region of the descending aorta above the celiac artery should be included in the field of view. An aortic laceration can be missed if only a single projection is used at aortography.
- Most patients develop a pseudoaneurysm at the site of laceration. An intimal tear alone is present in 5% to 10% of cases, seen as a linear lucency on the angiogram.
- Causes of false-positive aortograms, seen in 1% of cases, include ductus diverticulum, aortic aneurysm, atherosclerotic plaque, aortic dissection, and artifacts due to inflow of unopacified blood (i.e., "streaming" artifacts).
- Helical CT of the thoracic aorta is being investigated as a noninvasive means of diagnosis of thoracic aortic injury and has been reported to have 100% sensitivity and 82% specificity. Possible limitations include inadequate evaluation of the ascending aorta (due to cardiac motion artifact), branch artery injury, and subtle aortic intimal tears.

◆ SUGGESTED READING

DelRossi AJ, Cernaianu AC, Madden LD, et al. Traumatic disruptions of the thoracic aorta: Treatment and outcome. Surgery 1990;108:864–870.

Feczko JD, Lynch L, Pless JE, et al. An autopsy case review of 142 nonpenetrating (blunt) injuries of the aorta. J Trauma 1992;33:846–849.

Gavant M, Menke P, Fabian T, et al. Blunt traumatic aortic rupture: Detection with helical CT of the chest. Radiology 1995;197:125–133.

Kodali S, Jamieson WRE, Leia-Stephens M, et al. Traumatic rupture of the thoracic aorta. A 20-year review: 1969–1989. Circulation 1991;84:40–46.

CASE 7

Cynthia S. Payne

HISTORY

A 58-year-old woman with substernal pleuritic chest pain and new dyspnea on exertion. She subsequently experienced an episode of transient hemiplegia following infusion of an intravenous catheter with saline.

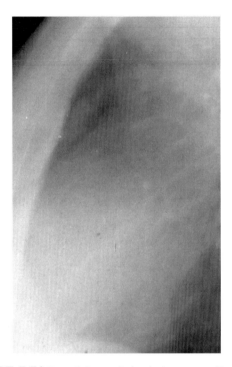

FIGURE 7-7A Lateral chest radiograph shows a curvilinear opacity in the anterior mediastinal compartment. Review of subsequent radiographs showed the lesion to be present on previous studies.

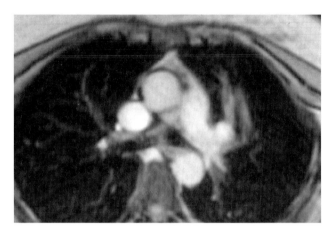

FIGURE 7-7B Gradient echo MRI showing flow within multiple enlarged vessels in the left lung.

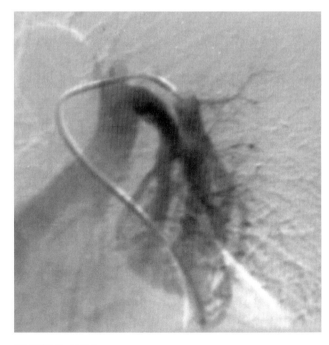

FIGURE 7-7C Angiogram using selective injection of the left upper lobe pulmonary artery shows multiple enlarged vessels supplying a vascular nidus and an early draining vein.

◆ DIFFERENTIAL DIAGNOSIS

More than 95% of all single pulmonary nodules fall into one of the first three categories discussed below.

- **Benign tumor:** A noncalcified, lobulated, well-circumscribed lesion in the periphery of the lung is most likely to represent a hamartoma. Characteristic "popcorn" calcifications and presence of internal fat on CT would strongly support this diagnosis. However, the curvilinear structure on the chest radiograph would be atypical, and the MR and pulmonary angiography findings are not consistent with this diagnosis.
- **Granuloma:** The upper lobe location, well-circumscribed margins, and stability over time may suggest tuberculous or fungal disease. The size and configuration of the lesion seen on the chest radiograph would be unusual for granulomatous disease. Furthermore, the MR and angiography findings are not consistent with this diagnosis.
- **Neoplasm:** The stability over time and well-circumscribed margins on the chest radiograph strongly argue against malignancy. As in the case of the other diagnoses previously mentioned, the MR study and the pulmonary angiogram are not consistent with this diagnosis.
- **Pulmonary arteriovenous malformation (AVM):** The curvilinear opacity seen on the chest radiograph is compatible with the draining vein of an AVM. The presence of flow in multiple enlarged vessels on the gradient echo MRI also suggests an AVM. The diagnosis is definitively established on the pulmonary angiogram that shows enlarged feeding arteries, a vascular nidus, and draining veins.

◆ DIAGNOSIS: Pulmonary arteriovenous malformation.

◆ KEY FACTS

CLINICAL

- Pulmonary AVMs (also called, perhaps more accurately, AV fistulas) can present with hemoptysis, chest pain, hypoxia, and neurologic symptoms (including stroke, transient ischemic attacks, and cerebral abscess formation) from paradoxical emboli.
- Clinical signs include clubbing, cyanosis, polycythemia, chest bruit, and evidence of paradoxical emboli.
- Pulmonary AVMs are usually congenital lesions, although they have been associated with trauma, infection, and prior surgery.
- Pulmonary AVMs are rarely symptomatic if <2 cm in size. Many investigators maintain that treatment is warranted even for asymptomatic lesions <2 cm in size or those having a feeding vessel of ≥3 mm. Increasingly, endovascular therapy using coil or balloon occlusion, rather than surgical ablation, is the treatment of choice.
- The most important clinical association is with hereditary hemorrhagic telangiectasia (HHT) (Osler-Weber-Rendu syndrome). HHT is autosomal dominant with variable penetrance and is characteristically associated with the triad of epistaxis, telangiectasias, and family history of the syndrome. It is estimated that at least one-third of patients with pulmonary AVMs have HHT. However, only approximately 15% of patients with HHT have pulmonary AVMs.

RADIOLOGIC

- More than 95% of patients with pulmonary AVMs have an abnormal chest radiograph.
- Pulmonary AVMs can be classified as simple (i.e., having a single feeding vessel and single draining vein, which is seen in 80% of cases) or complex (i.e., having two or more feeding and/or draining vessels).
- Approximately two-thirds of pulmonary AVMs are solitary lesions.
- Approximately two-thirds of pulmonary AVMs are located in the lower lobes.
- High-resolution CT, MRI, and MRA have shown utility in diagnosis of these lesions.
- Renal and cerebral radiotracer activity during lung perfusion study is a characteristic finding that can be seen due to the right-to-left shunting resulting from pulmonary AVMs. The presence of these findings during a lung perfusion study is a clue to the diagnosis of pulmonary AVM.
- Pulmonary angiography can confirm the diagnosis, classify the type of lesion, and provide the means for endovascular treatment. Permanent occlusion with coils or detachable balloons has a high success rate, with low morbidity and low mortality. The main risk is systemic embolization of coil or balloon during deployment, which is more likely in simple AVMs than in complex AVMs.

◆ SUGGESTED READING

Dinsmore BJ, Gefter WB, Hatabu H, Kressel HY. Pulmonary arteriovenous malformations: Diagnosis by gradient-refocused MR imaging. J Comput Assist Tomogr 1990;14:918–923.

Remy-Jardin M, Wattinne L, Remy J. Transcatheter occlusion of pulmonary arterial circulation and collateral supply: Failures, incidents, and complications. Radiology 1991;180:699–705.

White RI, Lynch-Nyhan A, Terry P, et al. Pulmonary arteriovenous malformations: Techniques and long-term outcome of embolotherapy. Radiology 1988;169:663–669.

CASE 8

Daniel J. Stackhouse

HISTORY

A 36-year-old man with fever, hematuria, and elevated sedimentation rate. He has a history of hepatitis B infection.

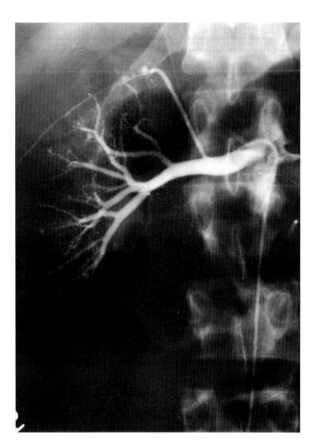

FIGURE 7-8A Renal arteriogram shows multiple small aneurysms.

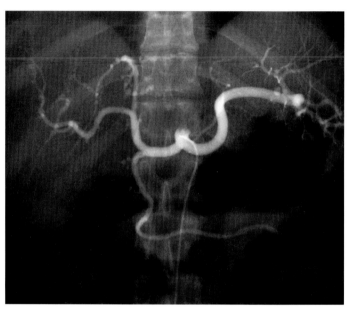

FIGURE 7-8B Celiac arteriogram shows multiple small aneurysms and arterial stenoses.

◆ DIFFERENTIAL DIAGNOSIS

◆ **Polyarteritis nodosa (PAN):** PAN is a necrotizing vasculitis of unknown etiology, which has been associated with prior hepatitis B virus infection. The typical findings consist of multiple small aneurysms in the renal and other abdominal arterial circulation. The clinical history and angiographic findings in the case illustrated make this the most likely diagnosis.

◆ **Vasculitis of intravenous drug abuse:** This entity is also a necrotizing vasculitis, which can have an identical angiographic appearance to PAN. The absence of a history of drug abuse favors an alternative diagnosis, although it must be kept in mind that such a history is often not revealed by the patient.

◆ **Vasculitis associated with connective tissue disorders:** These include a number of connective tissue disorders (e.g., systemic lupus erythematosus, rheumatoid arthritis, and Sjögren's syndrome) that have an angiographic appearance similar to the findings in the case illustrated. The diagnosis is based on clinical and serologic tests and is typically known by the time angiography is performed.

◆ DIAGNOSIS: Polyarteritis nodosa.

◆ KEY FACTS

CLINICAL

◆ PAN is an immune complex–mediated necrotizing vasculitis affecting multiple organ systems.

◆ A 3 to 1 male-to-female predominance has been reported.

◆ PAN can be seen at any age, but the peak incidence is in the fourth and fifth decades.

◆ The clinical symptoms reflect the multisystem involvement and include fever, weight loss, weakness, and malaise. The remainder of symptoms are organ system–specific and vary considerably among patients.

◆ Laboratory findings include elevated erythrocyte sedimentation rate, anemia, and elevated white blood cell count. Rheumatoid factor is present in many patients, and evidence of previous hepatitis B infection is seen in 15%. Elevated circulating immune complexes and hypocomplimentemia strongly suggest the diagnosis.

◆ Renal involvement, often manifested by rapidly progressive renal failure and hypertension, is present in 75% to 85% of PAN patients. Renal abnormalities can include a necrotizing glomerulonephritis, vasculitis, and small renal artery aneurysms.

◆ Neurologic involvement is common but is usually confined to one or more peripheral or cranial nerves. Less commonly, the brain or spinal cord is involved by infarction or hemorrhage.

◆ Gastrointestinal (GI) involvement is seen in 50% of patients and may involve any organ in the GI system. Bowel ischemia and perforation secondary to necrotizing vasculitis can be life-threatening.

◆ Cardiac involvement, including congestive heart failure, myocardial infarction, and pericarditis, is seen in 80% of patients.

◆ Musculoskeletal involvement, including myalgias and a polyarthritis that is clinically similar to rheumatoid arthritis, is also relatively common.

◆ Untreated, the 5-year survival rate is 10% to 15%, with death commonly resulting from hypertension-related complications, cardiac involvement, or complications due to infarction of one or more organs. Treatment with high-dose corticosteroids and cyclophosphamide has resulted in 5-year survival rates of 80%.

RADIOLOGIC

◆ Abnormal renal angiograms are seen in 70% to 80% of PAN patients, usually involving small- and medium-sized arteries, often within intrarenal branches. The major findings (many of which are the result of necrosis and inflammation) include small aneurysms at bifurcations, segmental narrowing or dilation (due to loss of vasomotor control), and arterial occlusions (due to a necrotizing, inflammatory process).

◆ Involvement of the mesenteric arteries occurs in 65% of PAN patients. The findings are generally similar to those seen in the renal arteries.

◆ Appropriate assessment of PAN patients by angiography includes selective renal, celiac, and superior mesenteric injections.

◆ SUGGESTED READING

Citron BP, Halpern M, McCarron M, et al. Necrotizing angiitis associated with drug abuse. N Engl J Med 1970;283:1003–1011.

Cupps TR, Fauci AS. Systemic Necrotizing Vasculitis of the Polyarteritis Nodosa Group. In The Vasculitides. Philadelphia: Saunders, 1981;26–49.

Travers RL, Allison DJ, Brettle RP, Hughes GRV. Polyarteritis nodosa: A clinical angiographic analysis of 17 cases. Semin Arthritis Rheum 1979;8:184–199.

PAN

Renal

Mesenteric – celiac

— SMA

CASE 9

Glenn E. Newman

HISTORY

A 27-year-old woman with a painful mass in the posterior aspect of the distal left thigh. The mass was associated with a thrill and bruit.

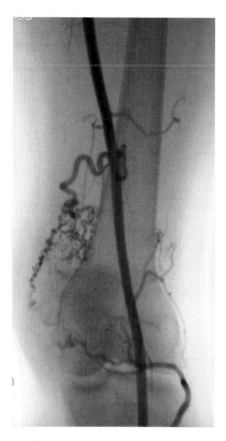

FIGURE 7-9A Early arterial phase of an angiogram shows a vascular lesion predominantly supplied by three arteries arising from the popliteal artery.

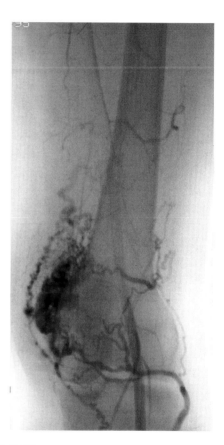

FIGURE 7-9B Slightly later in the arterial phase, early draining veins are seen arising from the lesion.

◆ DIFFERENTIAL DIAGNOSIS

◆ **Arteriovenous (AV) fistula:** An AV fistula consists of a direct communication of a large, identifiable artery draining directly into a vein, without an intervening retiform plexus (nidus). Fistulas can be single (one artery–one vein) or multiple. This diagnosis is incorrect because a nidus is clearly identified in the case illustrated.

◆ **Hemangioma:** This diagnosis is incorrrect because hemangiomas typically appear at angiography as a vascular blush without large feeding arteries or draining veins. However, the lesion in the case illustrated has the appearance of a tangle of vessels (nidus) with discrete feeding arteries and draining veins.

◆ **Peripheral arteriovenous malformation (AVM):** This diagnosis is correct because the lesion shown above has all of the features of an AVM, which are outlined in Case 7.

◆ DIAGNOSIS: Peripheral arteriovenous malformation.

◆ KEY FACTS

CLINICAL

◆ Peripheral AVMs are congenital and are presumed to represent a focal persistence of primitive vascular elements that arise in the first trimester of gestation. Rarely, AVMs are genetic in nature.

◆ AVMs within extremities can have a clinical presentation of a cosmetic deformity, pulsatile mass, or painful lesion. Very large AVMs can produce high-output cardiac failure due to AV shunting. However, AVMs are frequently stable lesions that require no specific therapy.

◆ Some AVMs aggressively expand, necessitating treatment. The primary mechanism of expansion is by enlargment of existing channels and recruitment of new collateral vessels, rather than by cellular proliferation.

RADIOLOGIC

◆ AVMs are generally fed by more than one artery. Peripheral AVMs can have a variable degree of capillary blush.

◆ Large AVMs can contain one or more fistulous sites.

◆ The extent of AVMs can be well defined by cross-sectional imaging studies such as CT, MRI, and MRA, but dynamic flow patterns are best seen on catheter angiography.

◆ AVMs are frequently treated by transcatheter embolization, alone or in conjunction with surgery. On occasion, AVMs are treated by surgery alone, especially when only one or a few feeding arteries, which are directly accessible to surgery, are present.

◆ Transcatheter embolization can be performed using a number of embolic agents. Polyvinyl alcohol particles are frequently used because, depending on the size of the particles chosen, they can be directly deposited within the nidus. Embolization of the arteries feeding the AVM is an undesirable result because it can result in the recruitment of secondary arterial supply to the AVM, necessitating repeat treatments. Furthermore, occlusion of feeding arteries can hamper subsequent efforts at embolization by blocking access of embolic agents to the nidus.

◆ SUGGESTED READING

Riles TS, Rosen RJ. Arteriovenous Fistulae. In DE Strandness Jr, A van Breda (eds), Vascular Diseases: Surgical and Interventional Therapy. New York: Churchill Livingstone, 1994;1109–1114.

Rosen RJ, Riles TS. Arteriovenous Malformations. In DE Strandness Jr, A van Breda (eds), Vascular Diseases: Surgical and Interventional Therapy. New York: Churchill Livingstone, 1994;1121–1137.

CASE 10   *James T.T. Chen*

HISTORY

An 18-year-old woman with exertional dyspnea with chest pain for 18 months.

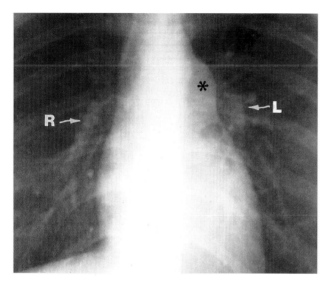

FIGURE 7-10A Frontal chest radiograph. Mild cardiomegaly with dilatation of the pulmonary trunk (*) and left pulmonary artery (L) is seen. The right pulmonary artery (R) is smaller in size than normal. On the lateral radiograph (not shown), mild right ventricular enlargement was seen.

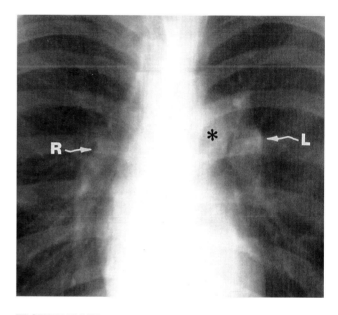

FIGURE 7-10B Frontal chest radiograph in a 12-year-old boy with a similar clinical presentation and the same diagnosis. A striking discrepancy in size of his two pulmonary arteries is seen, with the left (L) being much larger than the right (R). The pulmonary trunk (*) is also dilated.

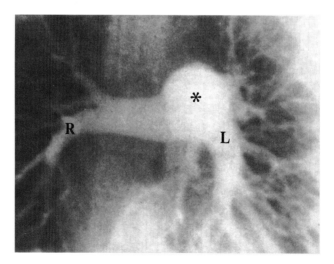

FIGURE 7-10C Pulmonary arteriogram in a third patient, also with the same diagnosis. The late phase of a right ventricular angiogram shows dilatation of the pulmonary trunk (*) and left pulmonary artery (L). The right pulmonary artery (R) is small. The pulmonary blood flow is asymmetric between the two lungs, being greater on the left.

◆ DIFFERENTIAL DIAGNOSIS

◆ **Secundum atrial septal defect (ASD):** Right ventricular enlargement is a feature of an ASD. However, the increase in pulmonary vascularity should be diffuse and symmetric (unlike the cases shown), making this an unlikely diagnosis.

◆ **Right pulmonary artery hypoplasia:** This entity might be considered because of the discrepancy in pulmonary blood flow between the two lungs. However, this diagnosis is unlikely because the right lung is almost always hypoplastic in this disorder, whereas the right lung is normal in the above examples.

◆ **Pulmonary embolism:** This entity can produce asymmetric pulmonary blood flow. However, no emboli are evident on the angiogram.

◆ **Pulmonary artery aneurysm:** This very rare entity can produce a prominent shadow at the confluence of the pulmonary arteries. However, it is an unlikely diagnosis in this case, because the pulmonary blood flow is symmetric in this condition.

◆ **Pulmonary hypertension:** This entity might be a consideration, because in severe cases the right side of the heart is enlarged (in accordance with the findings in Figure 7-10A). However, symmetric prominence of the central pulmonary arteries with diminutive flow peripherally would be seen, unlike the asymmetric vascularity seen in the cases shown above.

◆ **Valvular pulmonary stenosis:** Asymmetric pulmonary blood flow and enlargement of the right ventricle are the hallmarks of this entity and make it the most likely diagnosis.

◆ DIAGNOSIS: Valvular pulmonary stenosis.

◆ KEY FACTS

CLINICAL

◆ Valvular pulmonary stenosis is a relatively common congenital heart disorder. Dyspnea and fatigue are the most common symptoms. The size of the valve orifice in cases of mild to moderate stenosis tends to increase as the patient grows, allowing survival into adulthood.

◆ A loud ejection systolic murmur heard at the upper left sternal border is typical. Electrocardiogram (ECG) findings indicate right ventricular hypertrophy and right axis deviation. Cardiac catheterization shows valvular pulmonary stenosis with a systolic pressure gradient across the pulmonic valve.

◆ A similar ejection systolic murmur in the pulmonary area and ECG evidence of right ventricular hypertrophy can be seen with a secundum ASD. A fixed, split-second heart sound is typical of an ASD, although not invariably present. The two entities are distinguishable by imaging findings (see below).

◆ Echocardiography is usually diagnostic, obviating the need for an invasive procedure such as catheterization. However, catherization is performed for diagnostic purposes when the clinical data and echocardiographic findings are discrepant or, in some cases, for therapeutic purposes—e.g., if balloon angioplasty to improve blood flow across the stenotic valve is a consideration.

RADIOLOGIC

◆ The characteristic radiographic findings of valvular pulmonary stenosis can be explained on the basis of the abnormal hemodynamics.

    a. During systole, the high pressure within the right ventricle is converted into high-velocity flow, creating a forceful jet in the direction of the left pulmonary artery. Dilatation of the main and left pulmonary artery results.

    b. A low-pressure zone can be created immediately lateral to the central axis of the jet stream. Such reduced pressure has a suction effect, facilitating the leftward flow at the expense of right pulmonary flow. The resultant abnormal flow pattern can be shown by chest radiographs, pulmonary angiograms, or perfusion lung scan.

◆ Successful valvulotomy is usually followed promptly by a reversion to the normal flow pattern.

◆ The above-mentioned left lateralized pulmonary blood flow pattern of valvular pulmonary stenosis is distinctly different from the bilateral symmetrical increase in pulmonary vascularity seen in secundum ASD.

◆ SUGGESTED READING

Chen JTT. Essentials of Cardiac Roentgenology. Boston: Little, Brown, 1987;56–58.

Friedberg CK. Diseases of the Heart. Philadelphia: Saunders, 1966;670–671.

Perloff LK. The Clinical Recognition of Congenital Heart Disease (4th ed). Philadelphia: Saunders, 1994.

Steiner RM, Gross GW, Flicker S, et al. Congenital heart disease in the adult patient: The value of plain film chest radiology. J Thorac Imaging 1995;10:1–25.

CASE 11

Tony P. Smith

HISTORY

Two patients with hypertension: patient A, shown in Figure 7-11A, is a 67-year-old man with an abdominal bruit; patient B, shown in Figure 7-11B, is a 37-year-old woman with hypertension of recent onset.

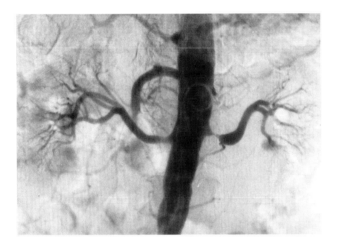

FIGURE 7-11A Catheter angiogram of the abdominal aorta shows a smoothly contoured, tight stenosis of the left renal artery. Mild stenosis of the right renal artery is also present.

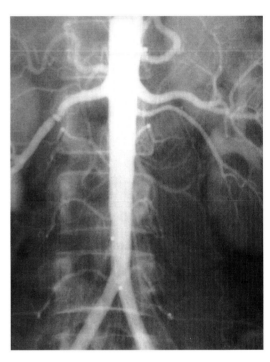

FIGURE 7-11B Catheter angiogram shows a multilobulated ("beaded") appearance of stenosis of the right renal artery.

◆ DIFFERENTIAL DIAGNOSIS

◆ **Patient A:** The findings are typical of atherosclerotic renovascular disease, with a smoothly tapered contour of the stenotic lesion located near the origin of the artery.
◆ **Patient B:** The multilobulated, "beaded" appearance and the fact that the distal main renal artery is involved (rather than the orifice) is typical of fibromuscular dysplasia. Neurofibromatosis is another rare entity that could also produce the same appearance. However, neurofibromatosis would be expected to be associated with other clinical (e.g., cutaneous manifestations) or radiologic findings, which are not present in the case illustrated.

◆ DIAGNOSES: Atherosclerotic renal artery disease (patient A) and fibromuscular renal artery disease (patient B).

◆ KEY FACTS

CLINICAL

◆ The symptomatic clinical presentation of renal artery stenosis is hypertension, renal failure, or both. The emphasis in this discussion is on hypertension.

◆ Approximately 60 million Americans are affected by hypertension. Renovascular hypertension, however, accounts for only a small minority (<5%).

◆ Indications that hypertension may be renovascular in nature include (1) presence of an abdominal or flank bruit (due to renal artery stenosis), (2) increase in serum creatinine levels by 0.5 mg/dl or more following antihypertensive treatment with angiotensin-converting enzyme (ACE) inhibitor therapy, and (3) malignant hypertension (i.e., hypertension that is rapid in onset and refractory to medical therapy).

◆ The diagnosis of renal artery stenosis is then made by radiographic techniques, including nuclear scintigraphy and angiography. Angiography remains the gold standard and has the advantage of visualizing the arteries and permits treatment (i.e., percutaneous transluminal angioplasty [PTA]) during the same examination. Nuclear scintigraphy does not directly visualize the renal arteries but can determine relative perfusion as well as renal function. Other techniques to visualize the renal arteries include CT angiography, MRA, and sonography.

◆ PTA has become the initial treatment of choice in many patients with renovascular hypertension, especially those with hypertension refractory to medical therapy. In particular, PTA has become the treatment of choice for fibromuscular disease.

RADIOLOGIC

◆ Renal artery stenosis is considered hemodynamically significant when there is ≥75% narrowing of the cross-sectional area of the lumen.

◆ In performing renal PTA, it is important to choose the appropriate balloon size. Careful measurements of the "normal" arterial lumen should be made before balloon insertion. When measurements are made from angiograms performed using conventional film-screen techniques, a magnification factor of 10% to 20% can be assumed. It is generally considered acceptable to overdilate the artery by that degree. Measurement programs are available to measure the size of the artery when angiography is performed using digital subtraction technique. In this setting, overdilation by 20% is again acceptable.

◆ During renal PTA, guidewires and catheters should be passed across stenoses carefully and pressures obtained on each side of a stenosis. Although controversy exists about exact values, pressure gradients of >10 mm Hg systolic are generally considered abnormal.

◆ Renal PTA is usually performed after the patient is fully anticoagulated. After placement of the balloon-tipped catheter across the stenosis and dilatation with the balloon, repeat angiography is performed while the guidewire is traversing the stenosis.

◆ If the angioplasty result is radiographically acceptable (e.g., <10% residual stenosis), follow-up pressures can be obtained and the procedure discontinued.

◆ There are multiple reasons for treatment failure (as defined by a poor angiographic result). Treatment of unwanted results must be considered on an individual basis and is often decided by a multidisciplinary team of an internal medicine physician, a surgeon, and the interventional radiologist. Possible undesired outcomes include:

   a. The stenosis is still present. Treatment then often consists of use of either or both a larger balloon and placement of a stent.

   b. A large intimal dissection has resulted. This complication is usually treated by stent placement.

   c. Extravasation of contrast material is seen. In this circumstance, typically the balloon is reinflated to occlude the site of extravasation and emergency surgical repair is performed.

◆ The results of revascularization (whether by surgery or PTA) have been standardized by the Society for Vascular and Interventional Radiology, based on the resultant reduction in blood pressure. Results are categorized according to the diastolic blood pressure (BP_D) after treatment:

Cure	BP_D ≤90 mm Hg without medication
Improvement	90 mm Hg ≤BP_D ≤110 mm Hg with at least a 15% decrease in BP_D after PTA on similar or decreased medications
Failure	All other results

◆ Results and complications reported in the medical literature have been extensively reviewed using the above classification. Although results vary among studies, the average overall cure rate for atherosclerotic disease is 13%, with another 55% improved, and an approximate 9% complication rate. The results for fibromuscular disease are much more encouraging, with a 40% to 45% cure rate and improvement in another 45% of patients. The complication rates are comparable or less than for atherosclerotic lesions.

◆ Controversy still exists over the efficacy of PTA for ostial renal artery lesions (defined as within 5 mm of the aorta). Although such lesions were once thought to be refractory to PTA, the most recent data indicate reasonable success rates (although they are lower than for lesions within the mid-portion of the renal artery). Most investigators agree that successful PTA of ostial stenoses usually also requires stent placement.

◆ SUGGESTED READING

Martin LG, Rees CR, O'Bryant T. Percutaneous Angioplasty of the Renal Arteries. In DE Strandness Jr, A Van Breda (eds), Vascular Diseases: Surgical and Interventional Therapy. New York: Churchill Livingstone, 1994;721–741.

CASE 12

Michael J. Kelley

HISTORY

A 7-month-old with respiratory distress and stridor.

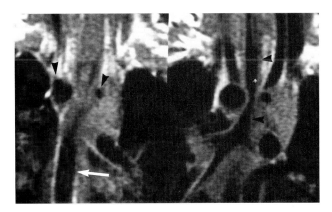

FIGURE 7-12A This is a series of coronal T1-weighted MRIs taken from posterior to anterior through the mediastinum with two-on-one filming. In each figure, the left image is posterior to the right image. On the left image (obtained through the posterior medi-astinum), two vascular channels (arrowheads) are seen on-end in the middle of the image. The vascular channel on the patient's right is the larger of the two. The descending aorta (arrow) is seen in the midline in the posterior half of the image. On a more posterior image (not shown), the two vascular channels were seen connecting to the descending aorta. On the right image, the two vascular channels are seen compressing the trachea (arrowheads). Most of the tracheal compression is by the large right vascular channel.

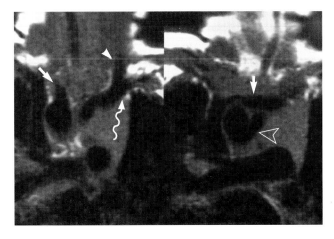

FIGURE 7-12B On these more anterior slices, the left image shows the right common carotid (arrow) artery arising from the right vascular channel and the left common carotid (arrowhead) and left subclavian (curved arrow) arteries arising from the left vascular channel. The trachea is superior, just coming into the field. The right image shows the aortic arch bifurcating into two vascular channels (open arrowhead). The innominate vein is seen coursing just superior to this bifurcation (solid arrow).

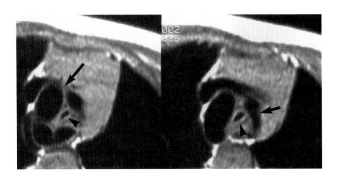

FIGURE 7-12C T1-weighted axial images through the level of the aortic arch. The left image is more caudad than the right image. The large right vascular channel (arrow) is seen on the left image, associated with marked narrowing of the trachea (arrowhead). The small left vascular channel (arrow) is seen best on the right image, again associated with marked tracheal narrowing (arrowhead). The innominate vein is located anterior to the two vascular channels.

◆ DIFFERENTIAL DIAGNOSIS

- **Right arch with aberrant left subclavian artery:** This entity might be considered because a vascular channel is seen coursing to the right of the trachea in the images shown above. However, a left aortic arch is also clearly delineated, making this an incorrect diagnosis.
- **Double aortic arch:** This entity frequently causes tracheal stenosis of the type shown above. In the case illustrated, two vascular channels are clearly seen, one on each side of the trachea. This is the correct diagnosis.

◆ DIAGNOSIS: Double aortic arch.

◆ KEY FACTS

CLINICAL

- The double aortic arch results from a persistence of the theoretical embryologic double arch. The double arch courses on both sides of the trachea and fuses posteriorly to form the descending aorta, which usually descends to the left of the spine. The right component of the double arch is usually larger and more cephalad than the left component. Separate great vessels (a carotid and a subclavian artery) arise from each arch. A separate ductus arteriosus also arises from each arch, but the right ductus arteriosus is usually atretic.
- The double aortic arch usually results in a tight vascular ring which produces upper airway obstruction and dysphagia in early life. This condition requires immediate surgical intervention.

- The most common type of double aortic arch is seen in the case shown above, with two patent arches (type I double aortic arch). In the type II double aortic arch, the left aortic arch is atretic.
- Another form of vascular ring is that of a right aortic arch with an aberrant left subclavian artery. This entity is a more common anomaly than the double aortic arch, but the vascular ring in the right aortic arch with an aberrant left subclavian artery is usually loose and less frequently requires surgical repair.

RADIOLOGIC

- The diagnosis of double aortic arch can readily be made on MRI. Coronal and axial spin echo MRIs are usually necessary to confirm the diagnosis.
- Coronal MRIs best show the presence of two aortic arches and the more cephalad relation of the right arch relative to the dominant left arch.
- Images in the axial plane best show esophageal and tracheal compression secondary to the presence of the double aortic arch.

◆ SUGGESTED READING

Gomes AS, Lois JF, George B, et al. Congenital abnormalities of the aortic arch: MR imaging. Radiology 1987;165:691–695.

Link KM. Cardiovascular MR Imaging: Present Status. Radiology Syllabus. Chicago: Radiological Society of North America, 1990.

Stewart JR, Kincaid OW, Edwards JG. An Atlas of Vascular Rings and Related Malformations of the Aortic Arch System. Springfield, IL: Charles C. Thomas, 1964.

CASE 13

Glenn E. Newman

HISTORY

A 19-year-old physically active man with a history of progressively increasing intermittent claudication involving only the right calf. There was no history of trauma. The right femoral pulse is normal, but the right popliteal and pedal pulses were present only by Doppler examination.

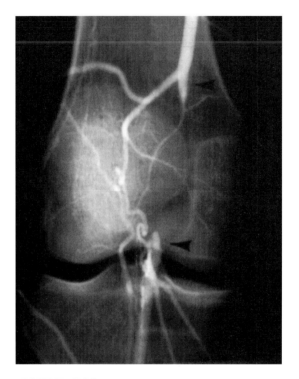

FIGURE 7-13 Angiogram showing occlusion of the popliteal artery (arrowheads) at the level of the popliteal fossa.

◆ DIFFERENTIAL DIAGNOSIS

- **Atherosclerotic occlusion:** An atherosclerotic popliteal occlusion is unlikely in the patient shown above on the basis of age alone. Atherosclerotic occlusions are much more common in older men and more common at Hunter's canal (adductor canal) than at the popliteal level.
- **Thrombosed popliteal aneurysm:** The typical features of popliteal aneurysms are one or more of the following features: claudication (present in the case described above), acute thrombosis, and embolization from the aneurysm. However, popliteal aneurysms are more common with advancing age and would be unusual in a young patient, making this an unlikely diagnosis.
- **Popliteal artery occlusion secondary to popliteal entrapment syndrome:** The young age of the patient shown above, history of vigorous physical activity, presence of claudication, and occlusion of the artery at the level of the popliteal fossa make this the most likely diagnosis.

◆ DIAGNOSIS: Popliteal artery entrapment syndrome.

◆ KEY FACTS

CLINICAL

- Popliteal artery entrapment syndrome is characteristically seen in young athletes with unilateral or bilateral claudication and is seen more commonly in men.
- Classifications of this syndrome are based on the relationship of the popliteal artery to the gastrocnemius muscle attachment to the femur.
- The pulses in patients with this syndrome can be normal, diminished, or absent. Typically, plantar flexion of the foot will diminish or obliterate the pulses.

RADIOLOGIC

- Some degree of medial deviation of the popliteal artery is typically seen at angiography in patients with this syndrome. If the popliteal artery is patent with the leg in the neutral position, provocative (stress) angiography during plantar flexion of the foot will typically show narrowing or occlusion of the artery.
- Angiography can show a stenosis or occlusion when the pulses are diminished or absent, respectively. The occlusion may be chronic on both clinical and angiographic grounds.

◆ SUGGESTED READING

Collins PS, McDonald PT, Lim RC. Popliteal artery entrapment: An evolving syndrome. J Vasc Surg 1989;10:484–489.

Greenwood LH, Hallett JW, Yrizarry JM, et al. The angiographic evaluation of lower extremity arterial disease in the young adult. Cardiovasc Intervent Radiol 1985;8:183–186.

Persky JM, Kempczinski RF, Fowl RJ. Entrapment of the popliteal artery. Surg Gynecol Obstet 1991;173:84–90.

HISTORY

A 15-year-old boy with easy fatiguability, exertional dyspnea, cyanosis, and intermittent chest pain of 4 years' duration.

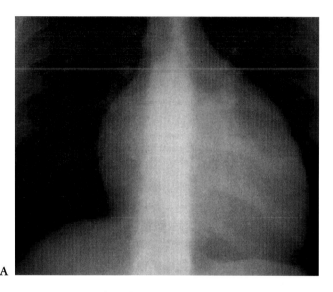

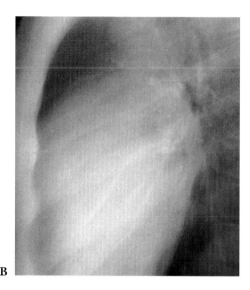

FIGURES 7-14A and 7-14B Frontal (**A**) and lateral (**B**) chest radiographs. Gross cardiomegaly is evident, with severe bilateral pulmonary oligemia. Marked right-sided cardiomegaly is seen without evidence of left-sided involvement. The hilar shadow is small, reflecting the diminutive pulmonary arteries and pulmonary veins.

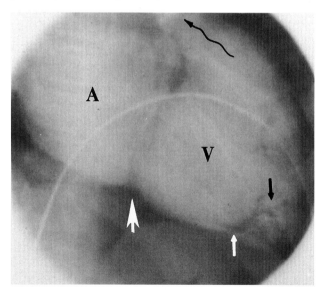

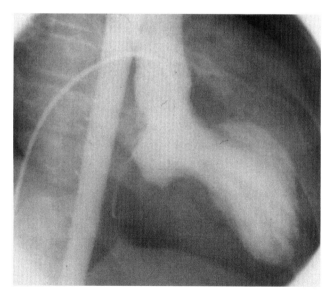

FIGURE 7-14C Right ventriculogram performed at 11 years of age. Prominent dilatation of the right atrium (A) and the right ventricle (V) is seen. The large arrow points to the lower end of the tricuspid annulus. The small arrows point to the site of the displaced leaflets of the tricuspid valve. Between the two white arrows lies the segment of the atrialized right ventricle. The spiral arrow traverses the right ventricular outflow tract toward the pulmonary valve.

FIGURE 7-14D Left ventriculogram. A catheter was inserted from the right atrium, crossing an ASD, through the left atrium to the left ventricle. The opacified left ventricle was smaller than normal and was markedly displaced by the huge right heart to the left and superiorly.

◆ DIFFERENTIAL DIAGNOSIS

◆ **Isolated pulmonary atresia (without a VSD):** The markedly enlarged heart raises this entity as a possible diagnosis. However, without benefit of surgery, patients usually succumb in infancy. The pulmonary outflow tract is also patent in the case shown and would not be expected in pulmonary atresia.

◆ **Tetralogy of Fallot (TOF):** Despite the similarity of pulmonary oligemia and clinical cyanosis in both entities, the heart in patients with TOF would not attain the size shown above because of the presence of a large VSD (a pathway for blood flow when the pulmonary outflow tract is obstructed). Furthermore, the aorta would be expected to be much larger due to the large right-to-left shunt across the VSD found in patients with TOF.

◆ **Cardiomyopathy:** Heart enlargement of the degree shown above can be seen with cardiomyopathy. However, the pulmonary blood flow would not be expected to be diminished.

◆ **Pericardial effusion:** This entity can produce marked cardiomegaly. Large effusions are usually chronic. However, in the case of pericardial effusion, the angiogram would be expected to be normal other than for the presence of an opacity separating the myocardium from the lung (representing the pericardial fluid).

◆ **Ebstein's anomaly:** This is the best diagnosis based on the large right heart and displacement of the tricuspid valve into the right ventricle ("atrialization of the right ventricle").

◆ DIAGNOSIS: Ebstein's anomaly (with severe tricuspid insufficiency and right-to-left shunt across the atrial septum).

◆ KEY FACTS

CLINICAL

◆ Ebstein's anomaly can present in the newborn period (with cyanosis and marked cardiomegaly) or later in childhood, usually with cyanosis, dyspnea, chest pain, or arrhythmias.

◆ Typically, a harsh holosystolic murmur of tricuspid regurgitation is heard at the left lower sternal border. The ECG shows right axis deviation. Cardiac conduction disturbances can also be evident.

◆ Severe tricuspid insufficiency is typically present. The posterior and septal leaflets of the tricuspid valve are displaced into the right ventricle, with atrialization of a portion of the right ventricle. A right-to-left shunt across an ASD or patent foramen ovale can often be seen.

◆ Standard surgical repair involves replacement of the tricuspid valve, plication of the atrialized right ventricle, and closure of an ASD.

RADIOLOGIC

◆ The radiographic findings in Ebstein's anomaly are highly suggestive of the diagnosis, which can often be established definitively by echocardiography.

◆ Gross enlargement of the right ventricle and the right atrium is typical for Ebstein's anomaly because severe tricuspid insufficiency causes considerable right-sided volume overload without a runoff at the ventricular level.

◆ Pulmonary oligemia is caused by (1) marked decrease in forward pulmonary blood flow, (2) severe tricuspid insufficiency, and (3) right-to-left shunting across the atrial septum.

◆ The principal alternative diagnosis to be considered based on the typical clinical and radiographic findings is pulmonary atresia without a VSD.

◆ Cardiomyopathy and pericardial effusion can also give marked cardiomegaly, but without the decreased pulmonary blood flow present in Ebstein's anomaly.

◆ SUGGESTED READING

Chen JTT. Essentials of Cardiac Roentgenology. Boston: Little, Brown, 1987.

Kelley MJ, Jaffe CC, Kleinman CS. Cardiac Imaging in Infants and Children. Philadelphia: Saunders, 1982.

Nugent EW, Plauth WH, Edwards JE, Williams WH. The Pathology, Pathophysiology, Recognition, and Treatment of Congenital Heart Disease. In RC Schlant, RW Alexander (eds), The Heart (8th ed). New York: McGraw-Hill, 1994.

CASE 15

Daniel J. Stackhouse

HISTORY

A 55-year-old patient status post motor vehicle accident in which he was ejected from the car.

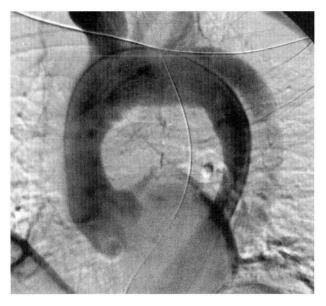

FIGURE 7-15A The contrast-filled ascending aorta and descending aorta are narrowed. A channel parallel to the descending aorta is partially contrast filled. The brachiocephalic arteries are contrast filled and normal in caliber.

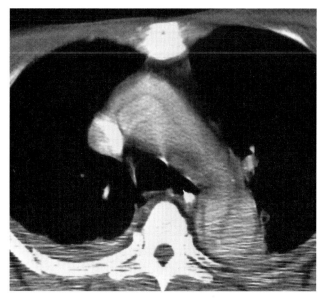

FIGURE 7-15B Contrast-enhanced CT of the aortic arch shows a linear lucency interposed between the two vascular channels. The linear lucency is present in the ascending aorta and the descending aorta.

◈ DIFFERENTIAL DIAGNOSIS

- **DeBakey type I aortic dissection:** This category of dissection involves both the ascending aorta and descending aorta. This is the correct diagnosis.
- **DeBakey type II aortic dissection:** This form of dissection is localized to the ascending aorta and rarely seen at angiography. The descending aorta is clearly involved in the case illustrated, making this an incorrect diagnosis.
- **DeBakey type III aortic dissection:** This form of dissection involves only the descending aorta.

◆**DIAGNOSIS:** Thoracic aortic dissection, DeBakey type I.

◆**KEY FACTS**

CLINICAL

◆ Predisposing factors include hypertension (the main risk factor), pregnancy, collagen vascular disease (e.g., Marfan's syndrome), bicuspid aortic valves, aortic coarctation, mycotic aneurysm, and giant cell arteritis.

◆ The typical presentation is severe chest or back pain (seen in 90%) radiating into the neck, arms, abdomen, or hips. End-organ ischemia such as infarction of the brain or heart can occur when arteries arising from the aorta (e.g., carotid or coronary arteries) are compromised.

◆ Physical findings can include hypertension (70% of cases), murmur of aortic insufficiency (due to extension of the dissection to involve the aortic valve), and asymmetric pulses between upper and lower extremities.

◆ Two schemes used for classification are the Stanford and DeBakey types. Stanford type A includes any dissection involving the ascending aorta; Stanford type B includes all dissections beginning distal to the left subclavian artery. The DeBakey classification is outlined above in the Differential Diagnosis section. Rates for each type are: type I: 51%; type II: 6%; and type III: 43%.

◆ Stanford type A dissections are treated surgically, with replacement of the ascending aorta and, if necessary, the aortic valve. The goal is to prevent dissection of the aortic root and rupture into the pericardium. Stanford type B dissections are repaired when arterial branches are compromised or progressive enlargement of the false lumen to >6 cm occurs. Aggressive control of hypertension is critical to prevent extension of the dissection.

◆ Involvement of major branch vessels should be defined preoperatively by CT or angiography. Surgical repair consists of placement of a mural graft replacement at the site of the intimal tear and obliteration of the false lumen by suturing, taking care to not occlude major arteries arising from the false lumen.

RADIOLOGIC

◆ Twenty-five percent of patients with aortic dissection have normal chest radiographs. Mediastinal widening is the most helpful finding, especially if the mediastinum appeared normal on a previous radiograph. Internal displacement of aortic calcifications from the periphery of the aorta is another finding that should raise suspicion of aortic dissection.

◆ Aortic arch arteriography provides the most detailed information of available diagnostic studies. Features to be evaluated on angiography include:

   a. The true lumen is typically contrast-filled and narrowed due to compression by the false lumen.

   b. The false lumen is also contrast-filled if not thrombosed. The diameter of the false lumen can vary from very thin to a thickness substantially exceeding that of the true lumen.

   c. The intimal flap is seen as a lucency separating the true and false lumens. If the false lumen is thrombosed, the intimal flap represents the wall of the true lumen closest to the thrombus.

   d. The entry/exit points are seen as contrast-filled sites of communication between the true and false lumens. However, exit and entry points are not always present, as when the dissection occurs due to hypertension-related hemorrhage into the vasa vasorum.

   e. Other features to be evaluated include integrity of the coronary arteries and the aortic valve.

◆ False-negative angiograms can occur due to (1) small, focal dissections near the aortic root; (2) a small, thrombosed false lumen that does not appreciably narrow the true lumen; or (3) simultaneous opacification of both lumens in which the intimal flap is not apparent.

◆ CT is the most commonly used screening study for the evaluation of possible aortic dissection. As with angiography, the presence of true and false channels separated by an intimal flap is necessary to make the diagnosis. Secondary signs include clotted blood in a false channel, inward displacement of aortic wall calcifications, and compression of the true lumen. CT can also show pericardial, pleural, and mediastinal hemorrhage, all of which indicate arterial rupture. Limitations of CT include inability to evaluate the aortic valve and coronary arteries. Furthermore, evaluation of branch arteries is limited.

◆ The MRI diagnosis of aortic dissection is based on the fact that flowing blood has different signal characteristics (i.e., "flow void") than thrombus on both spin echo and gradient echo pulse sequences. Aortic flow is best evaluated on gradient echo images. Potential causes of false-positive findings include normal structures that can mimic an intimal flap (e.g., superior pericardial recess or origin of the brachiocephalic arteries) and cardiac motion artifacts.

◆ Transthoracic and transesophageal echocardiography are increasingly used screening methods for diagnosis of aortic dissection. Advantages include their noninvasive nature and identification of complications—e.g., aortic insufficiency, abnormal cardiac wall motion, and presence of pericardial fluid. These techniques are highly sensitive in the detection of thoracic aortic dissection but have the limitation (unlike other methods) of being insensitive to the presence of dissection of the descending aorta.

◆**SUGGESTED READING**

Demos TC, Posniak HV, Marsan RE. CT of aortic dissection. Semin Roentgenol 1989;24:2237.

De Sanctis RW, Doroghazi RM, Austen WG, Buckley MJ. Aortic dissection. N Engl J Med 1987;317:1060–1067.

Fisher ER, Stern EJ, Godwin JD II, et al. Acute aortic dissection: Typical and atypical imaging features. Radiographics 1994;14:1263–1274.

Nienaber C, Kodolitsch Y, Niclas V, et al. The diagnosis of thoracic aortic dissection by noninvasive imaging procedures. N Engl J Med 1993;328:1–9.

CASE 16 · Tony P. Smith

HISTORY

A 67-year-old manual laborer with left arm cramping after exercise and gradual onset of dizziness.

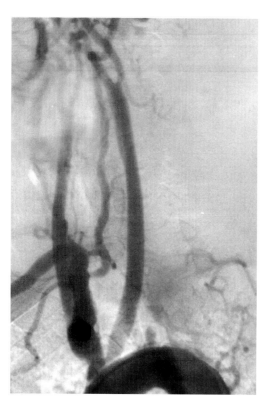

FIGURE 7-16A Early phase of arch angiogram shows occlusion of the left subclavian artery just beyond its origin. The innominate and left common carotid arteries are well opacified, but mild atheromatous narrowing of these arteries is also seen.

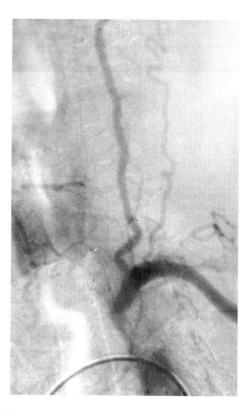

FIGURE 7-16B Late phase of arch angiogram shows opacification of the left subclavian artery via retrograde filling from the left vertebral artery.

◆ DIFFERENTIAL DIAGNOSIS

◆ The etiology of the left subclavian artery occlusion is most likely atherosclerotic disease, particularly given the disease in the other great vessels.

◆ Other reasons for great vessel occlusion include trauma, arteritis (including Takayasu's and radiation therapy), and neurofibromatosis. Because a clinical history of trauma is not given, this is not likely to be the diagnosis in the case shown above. Arteritis and neurofibromatosis usually have the angiographic appearance of smooth, concentric arterial narrowing rather than the abrupt occlusion shown above. Furthermore, the presence of mild changes typical of atheromatous disease in other arteries makes these diagnoses unlikely.

◆ DIAGNOSIS: Left subclavian artery stenosis with retrograde flow in the left vertebral artery ("subclavian steal").

◆ KEY FACTS

CLINICAL

◆ Most patients with retrograde flow in the vertebral artery—i.e., angiographic subclavian steal—are asymptomatic. Symptoms such as arm claudication (as in this case) occur in only about one-third of patients with angiographic findings of steal phenomenon. In a minority of cases, ischemic vertebrobasilar symptoms (e.g., dizziness, vertigo, and visual disturbance) develop in patients in whom these angiographic findings are seen.

◆ The diagnosis is often suspected initially due to a discrepancy in blood pressures between the arms.

◆ Data based on noninvasive studies such as sonography, MRI, and MRA suggest that retrograde flow in the vertebral artery may be more common than initially thought.

RADIOLOGIC

◆ The typical angiographic finding in a patient with subclavian steal is a high-grade stenosis (or occlusion) of the subclavian artery proximal to the origin of the vertebral artery. Retrograde flow in the vertebral artery then provides blood supply to the distal segment of the subclavian artery.

◆ The physiologic basis of neurologic symptoms due to the subclavian steal phenomenon is as follows: Exercise-related increased blood demand in the arm supplied by the affected subclavian artery causes hypoperfusion in the territory of the vertebrobasilar circulation.

◆ Angiographic evaluation of patients with subclavian steal should also include the carotid arteries, especially in patients in whom the symptom complex is difficult to localize to a vascular territory.

◆ Angioplasty has proved safe and effective in symptomatic patients with subclavian steal syndrome. In many centers, angioplasty has become the initial treatment of choice. Ischemia or infarction in the vertebrobasilar territory is a potential complication but is uncommon because the contralateral vertebral artery and carotid circulation almost always provide adequate collateral supply.

◆ SUGGESTED READING

Hebrang A, Maskovic J, Tomac B. Percutaneous transluminal angioplasty of the subclavian arteries: Long-term results in 52 patients. AJR Am J Roentgenol 1991;156:1091–1094.

Hennerici M, Klemm C, Rautenberg W. The subclavian steal phenomenon: A common vascular disorder with rare neurological deficits. Neurology 1988;38:669–673.

[Handwritten notes:] DDx Subclavian steal! Atherosclerosis Trauma Arteritis < Rad Tx, Takayasu's } Smooth Narrowing NF

HISTORY

A 2-year-old asymptomatic girl with a cardiac murmur since birth.

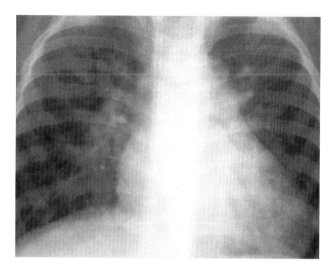

FIGURE 7-17A Frontal chest radiograph shows moderate cardiomegaly with predominantly left-sided enlargement. Generalized dilatation of pulmonary vessels with a normal pulmonary flow pattern is seen. Both the aorta and the pulmonary trunk are dilated.

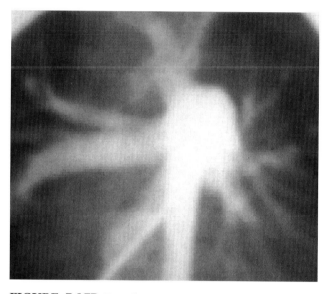

FIGURE 7-17B Frontal angiogram of another patient with the same diagnosis shows a venous catheter extending from the pulmonary trunk into the descending aorta. Following injection of contrast material, sequential opacification was achieved from the aorta to the pulmonary arteries bilaterally.

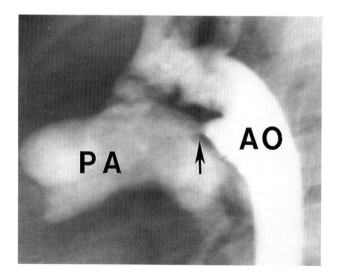

FIGURE 7-17C Lateral aortogram of a 22-year-old man with dyspnea on exertion and the same diagnosis shows sequential opacification of the aorta and the pulmonary trunk through a communicating channel (arrow). (AO = aorta; PA = pulmonary trunk.)

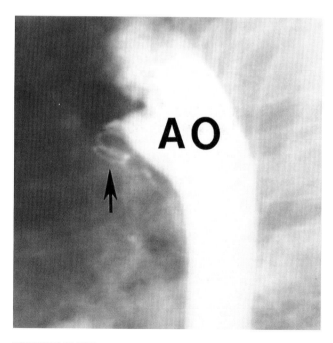

FIGURE 7-17D Repeat aortogram following coil placement (arrow) shows that the communicating channel has been occluded.

◆ DIFFERENTIAL DIAGNOSIS

◆ **Ventricular septal defect (VSD):** VSDs produce biventricular and left atrial enlargement and a normal-sized aorta. At cardiac catheterization, an extracardiac shunt is not seen, unlike the cases shown above.

◆ **Atrial septal defect (ASD):** ASDs produce pure right-sided cardiomegaly with a huge pulmonary trunk and small aortic arch. At catheterization, the left-to-right shunt is seen only at the atrial level, unlike the cases shown here.

◆ **Patent ductus arteriosus (PDA):** This lesion should be considered because it produces cardiomegaly and dilatation of the pulmonary arteries. A communication between the aorta and pulmonary trunk is seen at aortography, as in the cases shown above. This is the correct diagnosis.

◆ DIAGNOSIS: Left-to-right shunt via a patent ductus arteriosus.

◆ KEY FACTS

CLINICAL

◆ Patients with PDA are usually symptomatic in infancy because of congestive heart failure. Older children and adults with PDA tend to be asymptomatic until they develop Eisenmenger's physiology.

◆ Because a left-to-right shunt is present, PDA patients are not cyanotic. A continuous, "machinery-like" mur-

mur is usually heard over the left upper sternal border. The electrocardiographic findings indicate left ventricular and left atrial hypertrophy.

◆ Surgical ligation and division of the ductus is the standard treatment. However, transcatheter occlusion of the ductus is being increasingly performed with success.

RADIOLOGIC

◆ All pulmonary vessels are dilated as an expression of a substantial left-to-right shunt.

◆ In the absence of congestive heart failure or Eisenmenger's physiology, there is usually pure left-sided cardiomegaly with dilatation of both great arteries.

◆ The passage of a catheter from the pulmonary trunk to the descending aorta alone is diagnostic of a PDA. The lesion can be defined further by an aortogram showing the point of communication between the aorta and pulmonary trunk. Furthermore, the aortogram can be performed for therapeutic purposes—i.e., embolization of the PDA.

◆ SUGGESTED READING

Chen JTT. Essentials of Cardiac Roentgenology. Boston: Little, Brown, 1987.

Kelley MJ, Jaffe CC, Kleinman CS. Cardiac Imaging in Infants and Children. Philadelphia: Saunders, 1982.

Nugent EW, Plauth WH, Edwards JE, Williams WH. The Pathology, Pathophysiology, Recognition, and Treatment of Congenital Heart Disease. In RC Schlant, RW Alexander (eds), The Heart (8th ed). New York: McGraw-Hill, 1994.

CASE 18

Michael J. Kelley

HISTORY

A 34-year-old man who was told at the time of a military physical that he had an "abnormal" chest radiograph.

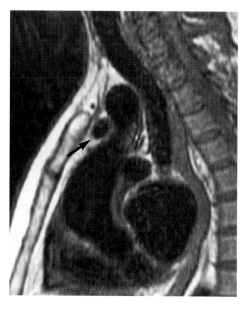

FIGURE 7-18A Sequential sagittal oblique (LAO) T1-weighted images showing the ascending aorta and the proximal aspect of the transverse aortic arch. The ascending aorta has a tortuous configuration with a high transverse aorta located above the brachiocephalic vein (arrow) and the sternum.

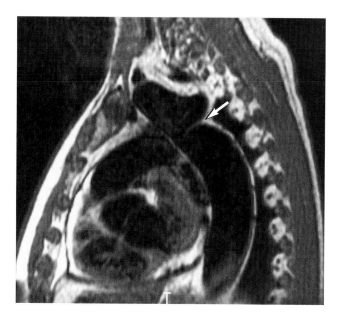

FIGURE 7-18B A well-delineated, shelf-like structure is seen projecting from the posterior wall of the descending aorta (arrow) due to buckling of the aorta. The descending aorta beyond this point is slightly dilated. No enlarged collateral arteries (e.g., intercostal or internal mammary arteries) are noted.

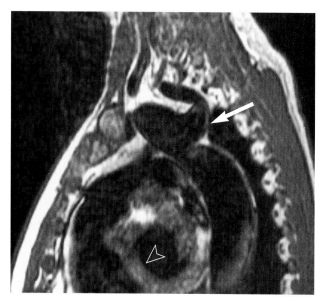

FIGURE 7-18C The left ventricle is normal in size and has normal wall thickness (open arrowhead). The left subclavian artery arises from the previously noted high transverse aorta at the level of the sternoclavicular junction (arrow). Just inferior to the origin of the left subclavian artery, the shelf-like structure is again seen projecting from the posterior aortic wall.

◆ DIFFERENTIAL DIAGNOSIS

- **Aortic coarctation:** In this entity, relative obstruction of aortic flow leads to development of numerous collateral vessels to the descending aorta. This finding is not present in the case shown above, making this diagnosis unlikely.
- **Pseudocoarctation of the aorta:** This entity is characterized by kinking of the aortic arch in the region of the ligamentum arteriosus and elongation of the thoracic aorta, but without formation of collateral vessels because no obstruction to blood flow is present. This diagnosis is most likely based on the imaging findings shown in the case above. In the case shown, the shelf-like structure seen projecting from the aortic wall was due to buckling of the aorta, not a true stenosis.

◆ DIAGNOSIS: Pseudocoarctation of the thoracic aorta.

◆ KEY FACTS

CLINICAL

- Coarctation of the aorta is a common congenital anomaly characterized by a discrete infolding of the posterior wall of the descending thoracic aorta at the level of the ligamentum arteriosus. In the postductal or adult type, this defect is located just distal to the insertion of the ductus arteriosus. Another form of coarctation presents in infancy and is associated with hypoplasia of the aortic arch. The posterior wall infolding is located proximal to the ductus. The location of the coarctation proximal to the ductus is thought to

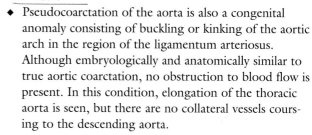

prevent normal flow-stimulated development of the aortic isthmus in utero.

- In both the pediatric and adult forms, aortic obstruction leads to development of collateral vessels to the descending aorta. In addition, coarctation may be associated with a bicuspid aortic value (20% to 30%) or a VSD.
- Pseudocoarctation of the aorta is also a congenital anomaly consisting of buckling or kinking of the aortic arch in the region of the ligamentum arteriosus. Although embryologically and anatomically similar to true aortic coarctation, no obstruction to blood flow is present. In this condition, elongation of the thoracic aorta is seen, but there are no collateral vessels coursing to the descending aorta.

RADIOLOGIC

- Coronal and sagittal left anterior oblique T1-weighted images as well as gradient echo images in similar imaging planes can easily detect (and discriminate between) coarctation and pseudocoarctation of the aorta. Collateral vessels in the intercostal regions and enlarged internal mammary arteries are present in true aortic coarctation but not in pseudocoarctation.

◆ SUGGESTED READING

Gomes AS, Lois JF, George B, et al. Congenital abnormalities of the aortic arch: MR imaging. Radiology 1987;165:691–695.

LePage JR, Szezchenyi E, Ross-Duggan JW. Pseudoarctation of the aorta. Magn Reson Imaging 1988;6:65–68.

Shapiro IL, Bartolome M, Candiolo MD, et al. Pseudoarctation of the aortic arch. Arch Intern Med 1968;122:345–348.

CASE 19

Cynthia S. Payne

HISTORY

A patient with dyspnea, deep venous thrombosis (DVT), and a ventilation-perfusion scan indicating high probability for pulmonary embolism (PE). He is referred for placement of an inferior vena cava (IVC) filter.

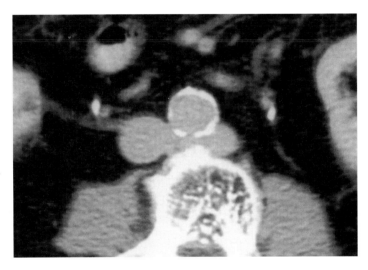

FIGURE 7-19A Noncontrast CT scan at the low lumbar level shows a vessel coursing posterior to the aorta and emptying into the inferior vena cava.

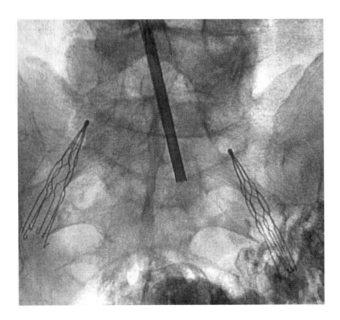

FIGURE 7-19B Radiograph taken after placement of a Greenfield filter in each common iliac vein. The delivery sheath for the filters is seen in the midline.

◆ DIFFERENTIAL DIAGNOSIS

The findings seen in Figure 7-19A indicate a retroaortic left renal vein, a normal variant that occurs in 3% of the population. This finding is important because this renal vein is at the L4 level, instead of the usual L2 level. Failure to note this fact before IVC filter placement could result in inadvertent placement of a filter between the two levels of the renal veins.

◆ DIAGNOSIS: Retroaortic left renal vein.

◆ KEY FACTS

CLINICAL

◆ Indications for placement of an IVC filter for the prevention of PE are:

    a. Contraindication to anticoagulation in a patient with either or both known DVT and PE.

    b. Failure of anticoagulation with recurrent DVT or PE, or a complication of anticoagulation.

    c. Patients at high risk of substantial hemodynamic compromise from even a small PE—e.g., a recent PE with residual clot burden and limited pulmonary reserve.

    d. Prophylaxis in high-risk patients—e.g., before hip replacement or in paraplegic patients. This is done in some centers but is not widely accepted.

◆ Risks of IVC filter placement include:

    a. Thrombosis at the insertion site (5% to 10%).

    b. Injury to the vein used for access or the IVC (which can be lethal).

    c. Filter migration, a rare event if the IVC is measured before placement and the device properly deployed. Long-term migration is not infrequent but usually is caudal to the original placement site.

    d. Filter fracture, a rare event that can occur after prolonged use, potentially penetrating the IVC or adjacent organs.

    e. PE recurrence despite appropriate filter placement (3% to 5%).

    f. IVC occlusion. This occurs in 10% to 20% of cases and is usually asymptomatic, but it can cause marked leg edema.

◆ There are currently six Food and Drug Administration–approved types of filters available.

    a. The first three types are varieties of the Greenfield filter (Medi-Tech): one titanium and two stainless steel versions. The original version is seldom used due to the large sheath required. A new version is deployed over a wire.

The remaining types include:

    b. Simon-Nitinol (Nitinol Medical Technologies, Inc): The small size and malleable nature make this device the only filter that can be deployed from a peripheral vein.

    c. Gianturco-Roehm Bird's Nest (Cook, Inc.): This filter is the only device that can be deployed in an IVC measuring >28 mm. The maximal IVC diameter in which it can be used is 40 mm.

    d. Vena-Tech (Braun).

RADIOLOGIC

◆ Cavography is performed to determine patency of the IVC and iliac veins, IVC size, and position of the renal veins. The presence of thrombus in the iliac vein is an indication to use an entry site through the contralateral iliac vein or the right jugular vein.

◆ An IVC measuring >28 mm is an indication to place filters within each common iliac vein or a bird's nest filter in the IVC.

◆ The top of the filter should be placed about 1 cm below the lowest renal vein. In the case shown above, placement of a filter at a point between the levels of the renal veins could cause left renal vein thrombosis.

◆ All brands of filters can be inserted via either a femoral or jugular vein entry, but individual filters are specifically designed for only one of these approaches (except the bird's nest filter).

◆ Manipulation of a tilted or migrated filter should rarely be performed, and then only by an experienced operator. The treatment when a filter has migrated or severely tilted is placement of a second filter above the first, usually from a jugular approach.

◆ SUGGESTED READING

Greenfield LJ, Proctor MC. Twenty-year clinical experience with the Greenfield filter. Cardiovasc Surg 1995; 3:199–205.

Hicks ME, Dorfman GS. Vena Caval Filters in Vascular Diseases. In DE Strandness Jr, A van Breda (eds), Surgical and Interventional Therapy. New York: Churchill Livingstone, 1994;1017–1044.

Mohan CR, Hoballah JJ, Sharp WJ, et al. Comparative efficacy and complications of vena caval filters. J Vasc Surg 1995;21:235–246.

Wojtowycz M. Handbook of Interventional Radiology and Angiography (2nd ed). St. Louis: Mosby, 1995.

CASE 20

James T.T. Chen

HISTORY

A 7-day-old child with tachypnea, cyanosis, bilateral crackling rales, and a heart murmur. Her cyanosis deepened during feeding.

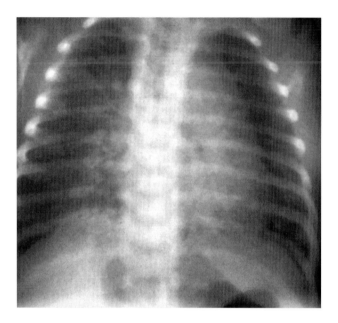

FIGURE 7-20A Frontal chest radiograph shows severe diffuse pulmonary edema with a normal cardiac size.

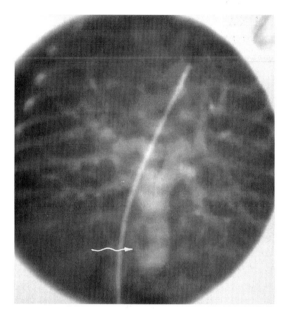

FIGURE 7-20B Frontal view of the venous phase of a pulmonary arteriogram shows that all pulmonary veins from both lungs converge to a common collecting vessel that traverses the diaphragm and extends into the upper abdomen. The vessel becomes markedly constricted (arrow) after turning abruptly toward the liver.

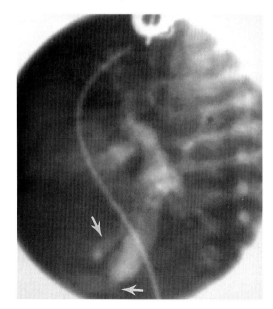

FIGURE 7-20C Lateral view of the same study shows that the common collecting pulmonary vein becomes markedly constricted (horizontal arrow) after turning anteriorly. The smaller inferior vena cava (oblique arrow) appeared to fill indirectly from the common vein.

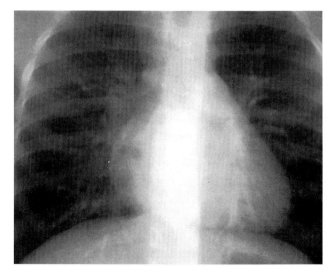

FIGURE 7-20D Seven years after surgical repair, the posteroanterior radiograph is normal.

◆ DIFFERENTIAL DIAGNOSIS

◆ **Hypoplastic left heart syndrome:** This entity is a cause of neonatal cyanotic heart disease and severe pulmonary edema. There are severe left-sided obstructive lesions with a right-to-left shunt at the ductal level and a left-to-right shunt at the atrial level. There may be differential cyanosis with pink arms and blue legs. Three facts make this diagnosis unlikely: (1) the cardiac size is usually markedly enlarged, (2) the pulmonary veins drain normally into the left atrium, and (3) differential cyanosis is often present. None of these features is present in the case shown.

◆ **Left-sided obstructive lesions:** These lesions—e.g., aortic stenosis and coarctation of the aorta—may present in the neonatal period with severe congestive heart failure. However, two facts make this diagnosis unlikely: (1) patients with these lesions are not cyanotic, and (2) the heart is usually markedly enlarged.

◆ **Systemic arteriovenous (AV) fistulae:** These lesions—e.g., huge AV fistulae involving the vein of Galen or the liver—can cause frank congestive heart failure early in life. However, this diagnosis is unlikely for three reasons: (1) patients with these lesions are not cyanotic, (2) the heart is markedly enlarged, and (3) the pulmonary vessels are significantly dilated due to increased blood flow.

◆ **Total anomalous pulmonary venous return:** In this entity, patients are cyanotic (worsening during feeding, as in the case illustrated), have pulmonary edema, and have a normal heart size. These features, along with the pulmonary angiogram findings shown above, make this the correct diagnosis.

◆ DIAGNOSIS: Total anomalous pulmonary venous connection to the portal vein with obstruction.

◆ KEY FACTS

CLINICAL

◆ Neonates with severe congestive heart failure due to this disorder present with cyanosis, tachypnea, and crackling rales. Frequently the rales are loud enough to obscure the cardiac murmur. Because the heart size is normal, newborn respiratory distress syndrome can be mistakenly diagnosed.

◆ Helpful clues to the correct diagnosis include (1) normal heart size, (2) severe pulmonary edema, and (3) deepening cyanosis with feeding.

◆ Without surgical intervention, patients progressively worsen.

◆ Emergency surgical repair is indicated and consists of anastomosis of the pulmonary venous confluence (almost always found just behind the left atrium) to the left atrium. Thereafter, the atrial septal defect is repaired.

RADIOLOGIC

◆ In this disease process, the common collecting pulmonary vein is severely obstructed by both intrinsic stenoses and extrinsic compression at multiple sites—e.g., during passage through the esophageal hiatus and at the level of the capillary bed of the liver.

◆ Immediate definitive diagnosis is indicated in this disease process if a good outcome is to be reached. The radiologist can play a major role by initially suggesting the diagnosis and then confirming it by imaging studies.

◆ The diagnosis can be made by a number of means, including echocardiography, MRI, and angiocardiography.

◆ SUGGESTED READING

Burrows PE, Smallhorn JF, Moes CAF. Congenital Cardiovascular Disease. In CE Putman, CE Ravin (eds), Textbook of Diagnostic Imaging (2nd ed). Philadelphia: Saunders, 1994.

Chen JTT. Essentials of Cardiac Roentgenology. Boston: Little, Brown, 1987.

Kelley MJ, Jaffee CC, Kleinman CS. Cardiac Imaging in Infants and Children. Philadelphia: Saunders, 1982.

Nugent EW, Plauth WH, Edwards JE, Williams WH. The Pathology, Pathophysiology, Recognition, and Treatment of Congenital Heart Disease. In RC Schlant, RW Alexander (eds), The Heart (8th ed). New York: McGraw-Hill, 1994.

CASE 21

James T.T. Chen

HISTORY

A 10-month-old girl with worsening cyanosis since 3 months of age.

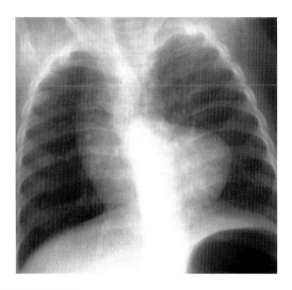

FIGURE 7-21A Frontal chest radiograph shows a boot-shaped cardiac contour. The apex of the heart is tilted upward. The pulmonary trunk area is deeply concave, and the aorta is quite large and is right-sided. The pulmonary vascularity is decreased, with smallness of all vessels and hyperlucent lungs. The overall cardiac size is within normal limits.

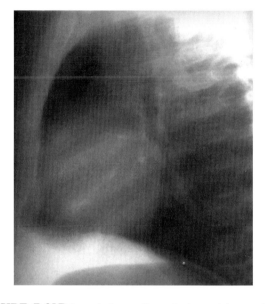

FIGURE 7-21B Lateral chest radiograph shows right ventricular enlargement, decreased pulmonary vascularity, and a very small hilum. The trachea is in the normal position, consistent with a mirror-image type of right-sided aortic arch.

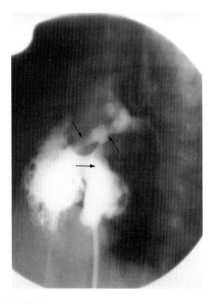

FIGURE 7-21C Early phase of right ventriculogram of another patient with the same diagnosis shows a large right-to-left shunt across a ventricular septal defect (horizontal arrow). The left oblique arrow denotes the severe infundibular pulmonary stenosis, and the right oblique arrow denotes the mild, valvular pulmonary stenosis.

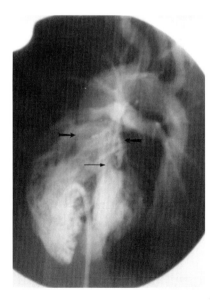

FIGURE 7-21D The late phase of a right ventriculogram shows an overriding, markedly dilated aorta (opposing arrows). The right-to-left shunt through the ventricular septal defect is denoted by the inferior arrow.

◆ DIFFERENTIAL DIAGNOSIS

- **Pseudotruncus arteriosus:** This entity is the most severe form of tetralogy and is impossible to distinguish from tetralogy of Fallot (TOF) on chest radiographs. It has a higher incidence of right-sided aortic arch than TOF. The ventriculograms help to distinguish the two entities because pulmonary atresia (rather than the infundibular pulmonary stenosis shown above) is present in pseudotruncus arteriosus.

- **Ebstein's anomaly:** Ebstein's anomaly might be considered because it presents clinically with cyanosis and has the radiographic finding of decreased pulmonary vascularity. However, the cardiac size is much larger in Ebstein's anomaly than in the cases shown because of considerable volume overload caused by tricuspid insufficiency without a ventricular septal defect (VSD).

- **Pulmonary atresia without a VSD:** As in the case of Ebstein's anomaly, the heart tends to be much bigger in patients with this disease than in the cases shown above because a VSD is not present.

- **Tricuspid atresia:** Flattening of the right atrial border on the posteroanterior view and that of the right ventricular border on the lateral view is usually seen in tricuspid atresia. These findings are not present in the cases shown above.

- **TOF:** The boot-shaped cardiac contour, upward tilt of the heart, and pulmonary concavity are typical of TOF. The VSD and overriding aorta shown on the ventriculogram are characteristic findings.

◆ DIAGNOSIS: Severe tetralogy of Fallot with a right-sided aortic arch.

◆ KEY FACTS

CLINICAL

- Patients with severe TOF usually become symptomatic after 3 or 4 months of life.
- These patients are cyanotic and have a high hematocrit. They characteristically need to squat to decrease their dyspnea. Clubbing of the fingers is typically seen.

RADIOLOGIC

- All pulmonary vessels are small, with hyperlucent lungs. A decrease in pulmonary vascularity is seen routinely, primarily due to a large right-to-left shunt across the VSD.
- The odd shape of the heart is likened to a wooden shoe (*coeur en sabot* is the original description in French).
- Angiocardiography shows (1) severe infundibular pulmonary stenosis (PS); (2) mild valvular PS; (3) large VSD shunting blood right-to-left; (4) hypertrophy of the right ventricle; and (5) an overriding of the aorta, which is dilated. Right-sided aortic arch occurs in 25% to 50% of cases in proportion to the degree of PS.

◆ SUGGESTED READING

Chen JTT. Essentials of Cardiac Roentgenology. Boston: Little, Brown, 1987.

Kelley MJ, Jaffe CC, Kleinman CS. Cardiac Imaging in Infants and Children. Philadelphia: Saunders, 1982.

Nugent EW, Plauth WH, Edwards JE, Williams WH. The Pathology, Pathophysiology, Recognition, and Treatment of Congenital Heart Disease. In RC Schlant, RW Alexander (eds), The Heart (8th ed). New York: McGraw-Hill, 1994.

CASE 22

Michael J. Kelley

HISTORY

An 18-year-old male basketball player with chest pain.

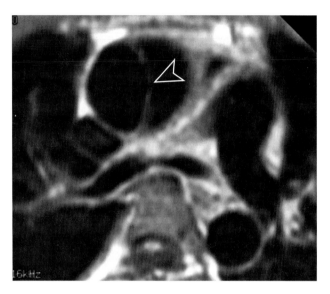

FIGURE 7-22A Axial T1-weighted MRI showing the ascending and descending aorta at the level of the carina. Dilatation of the ascending aorta (diameter approximately 4 cm) is seen, with a discrete flap in the central portion of the lumen (open arrowhead). The descending aorta is of normal diameter and no flap is noted within it.

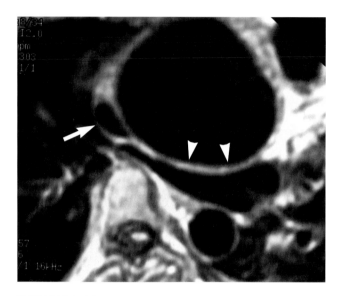

FIGURE 7-22B Axial T1-weighted MRI showing the ascending and descending aorta at the level of the left atrium. Marked dilatation of the ascending aorta is seen at this level, with estimated diameter of 7 cm in the anteroposterior dimension and 8 cm in the transverse dimension. The dilated ascending aorta compresses the left atrium (arrowheads) and the superior vena cava (arrow).

◆ DIFFERENTIAL DIAGNOSIS

Many common conditions can cause a dilated ascending aorta, including lesions that cause turbulence (e.g., aortic stenosis), volume overload (e.g., aortic regurgitation), or pressure overload (e.g., hypertension). However, the finding of an intimal flap within the ascending aorta is direct evidence of aortic dissection as the cause of the aortic dilatation in the case shown above.

◆ DIAGNOSES: Dissection of the ascending thoracic aorta (DeBakey type II, Stanford type A), and probable annuloaortic ectasia (see Case 15 in this chapter).

◆ KEY FACTS

CLINICAL

- Dissection of the thoracic aortic wall is the result of repeated trauma to the arterial media. The most frequent etiology is hypertension. The formation of a hematoma in the media and subsequently the serosa results in loss of support of the intima. A tear can then form in the intima with the false lumen propagating along the media.
- Dissections commonly develop in aortas that have underlying abnormalities of the media, such as cystic medial necrosis, Marfan's syndrome, and annuloaortic ectasia.
- Dissections involving the descending aorta respond well to control of underlying hypertension. Involvement of the ascending aorta constitutes a surgical emergency.
- The following classifications are those used to refer to forms of aortic dissection:
  - a. DeBakey Type I: dissection involves the ascending aorta, transverse arch, and descending aorta
  - b. DeBakey Type II: dissection confined to the ascending aorta
  - c. DeBakey Type III: dissection confined to the descending aorta, distal to the left subclavian artery
  - d. Stanford Type A: dissection involves the ascending aorta (DeBakey I and II)

  - e. Stanford Type B: dissection confined to descending aorta (DeBakey III)
- The ascending aorta (as in the case shown above) is involved in approximately 60% of dissections, and the descending aorta in 40%.

RADIOLOGIC

- In hemodynamically stable patients with suspected or known thoracic aortic disease, such as aortic dissection, MRI is the imaging study of choice. MRI allows the location and extent of the dissection (including involvement of the ascending aorta, descending aorta, or both) to be shown in a noninvasive manner.
- Direct and indirect signs of aortic dissection on MRI are similar to those seen with other imaging techniques. The pathognomonic direct findings are the presence of an intimal flap and a double lumen. Indirect findings include compression of the true lumen, thickening of the aortic wall, aortic regurgitation, and ulceration projecting beyond the aortic wall.
- Dynamic techniques such as gradient echo MRI must be used to assess the aortic valve and exclude pericardial effusion. Slow flow in the false lumen can be difficult to distinguish from partial thrombosis of the false lumen. Phase mapping techniques have been suggested as a way to resolve this question.

◆ SUGGESTED READING

Kersting-Sommerhoff BA, Higgins CB, White RD, et al. Aortic dissection: Sensitivity and specificity of MR imaging. Radiology 1988;166:651–655.

Link KM, Lesko NM. The role of MR imaging in the evaluation of acquired diseases of the thoracic aorta. AJR Am J Roentgenol 1992;158:1115–1125.

Nienaber CA, von Kodolitsch Y, Nicolas V, et al. The diagnosis of thoracic aortic dissection by noninvasive imaging procedures. N Engl J Med 1993;328:1–9.

Nugent EW, Plauth WH, Edwards JE, Williams WH. The Pathology, Pathophysiology, Recognition, and Treatment of Congenital Heart Disease. In RC Schlant, RW Alexander (eds), The Heart (8th ed). New York: McGraw-Hill, 1994.

CASE 23

Paul V. Suhocki

HISTORY

A 46-year-old man with a history of cigarette smoking and coronary artery disease. He has a 2-year history of postprandial abdominal pain.

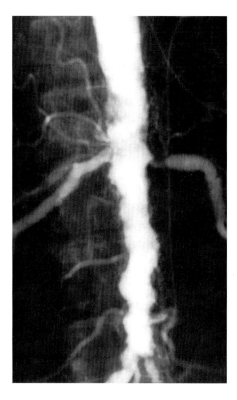

FIGURE 7-23A Anteroposterior view of abdominal aortogram shows multiple sites of narrowing of the aortic lumen as well as stenosis of the left renal artery.

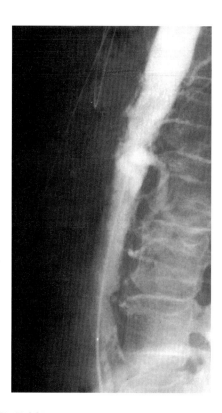

FIGURE 7-23B Lateral view of abdominal aortic angiogram shows occlusion of the proximal segments of the celiac, superior mesenteric, and inferior mesenteric arteries.

◆ DIFFERENTIAL DIAGNOSIS

- **Atherosclerotic disease:** This entity is the most common cause of proximal occlusion of the mesenteric arteries and can cause chronic mesenteric ischemia if two of the three major arteries supplying the bowel are occluded.
- **Abdominal aortic aneurysm:** Mural thrombus in an abdominal aortic aneurysm can narrow the origin of mesenteric arteries or embolize into the vessels, causing an acute mesenteric ischemia. However, the external diameter of the aorta would be expected to be enlarged with a filling defect within an aneurysm. These findings are not seen in the case presented above.
- **Aortic dissection:** The false channel of an aortic dissection can involve the mesenteric artery origins and cause acute mesenteric ischemia (see Case 15). However, in the presence of aortic dissection, two contrast-filled channels or a narrowed true lumen adjacent to a thrombosed false lumen would be expected. Those findings are not present in the case illustrated.
- **Embolic occlusion:** Emboli related to cardiac arrhythmias or myocardial infarction can travel to the mesenteric arteries, resulting in acute mesenteric ischemia. The clinical history of chronic symptoms is not compatible with this diagnosis. Furthermore, the expected findings of multiple branch occlusions or intraluminal filling defects are not present in the case shown above.

◆ DIAGNOSIS: Chronic mesenteric ischemia due to atherosclerotic disease.

◆ KEY FACTS

CLINICAL
- Atherosclerotic occlusion of the vessel origins occurs slowly, usually allowing formation of adequate collateral arterial supply for bowel viability.
- The pancreaticoduodenal arteries are the major source of collateral circulation between the celiac artery and superior mesenteric artery (SMA).
- The marginal artery of Drummond and the arc of Riolan provide collateral circulation between the SMA and the inferior mesenteric artery (IMA).

- The IMA receives collateral supply from the middle and inferior hemorrhoidal arteries, which arise from the internal iliac arteries.
- When two or more of the major mesenteric arteries become occluded near their origin, even the collateral blood supply is affected, and mesenteric ischemia can result.
- Symptoms of abdominal pain due to mesenteric ischemia are often ill-defined and can mimic other disease states—e.g., gastrointestinal malignancy and peptic ulcer disease. The most common complaints are those of weight loss, diarrhea, and abdominal pain. Postprandial pain (usually within 2 hours of eating) is common and can cause the patient to avoiding eating.
- Treatment typically consists of surgical bypass. Percutaneous balloon angioplasty has a high technical success rate but has been shown to be less effective than surgery for long-term symptomatic relief.

RADIOLOGIC
- Abdominal aortography is essential for evaluating the proximal segments of the celiac, superior mesenteric, and inferior mesenteric arteries.
- The diagnosis of chronic mesenteric ischemia is confirmed by the angiographic finding of severe stenosis or occlusion of at least two of the major mesenteric arteries.
- If the proximal segments of the artery are seen to be normal at angiography, selective catheterization is necessary to rule out a mesenteric steal phenomenon caused by a mesenteric arteriovenous fistula or arterial-to-arterial shunts that can be seen when the lower aorta is occluded. Peripheral branch stenoses or occlusions are rarely responsible for ischemia.

◆ SUGGESTED READING

Bakal CW, Sprayregen S, Wolf EL. Radiology in intestinal ischemia. Surg Clin North Am 1992;72:125–141.

Kadir S. Esophago-Gastrointestinal Angiography. In S Kadir (ed), Diagnostic Angiography. Philadelphia: Saunders, 1986;338–376.

Rose SV, Quigley TM, Raker EJ. Revascularization for chronic mesenteric ischemia: Comparison of operative arterial bypass grafting and percutaneous transluminal angioplasty. J Vasc Interv Radiol 6:339-349.

Scholz FJ. Ischemic bowel disease. Radiol Clin North Am 1993;31:1197–1218.

CASE 24
Michael J. Kelley

HISTORY

A 14-year-old acyanotic girl with Down's syndrome.

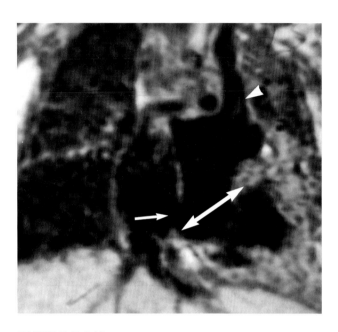

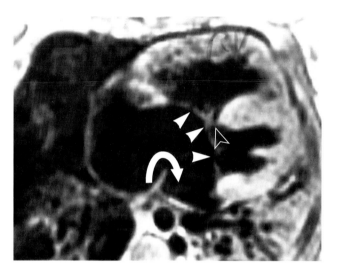

FIGURE 7-24A Coronal T1-weighted image taken through the atria shows an atrial septal defect (arrow) involving the lower portion of the atrial septum (the septum primum). The section is through the level of the atrioventricular (AV) valves, and there appears to be a defect across the atrioventricular valve level as well (double arrow). In the left upper lobe region, a vertical tubular structure with signal flow void is seen that appears to course into the left atrium superiorly (arrowhead). This structure corresponds to a persistent left superior vena cava (SVC).

FIGURE 7-24B Axial T1-weighted image through the ventricles and atria shows a common atrioventricular valve (arrowheads) coursing across the intraventricular septum and a large atrial septal defect (curved arrow). A small ventricular septal defect (open arrowhead) may be present at the level of the atrioventricular valve confluence.

◆ DIFFERENTIAL DIAGNOSIS

◆ Atrial septal defects (ASDs) are commonly classified into three types: sinus venosus, ostium secundum, and ostium primum. The ostium secundum defect is the most common form and occurs in the midseptal region at the fossa ovalis. This entity is the most common type of congenital heart disease in adults. Sinus venosus defects are often associated with anomalous return of the right upper lobe pulmonary vein into the superior vena cava (SVC) or right atrium.

◆ DIAGNOSES: Ostium primum atrial septal defect and persistent left superior vena cava.

◆ KEY FACTS

CLINICAL

◆ The ostium primum ASD is part of the spectrum of arteriovenous (AV) septal defects. It occurs in the central AV region near the confluence of the lower atrium septum, the AV valves, and the membranous ventricular septum. Ostium primum ASD is invariably associated with a cleft in the anterior leaflet of the mitral valve. The defect may be partial (as in this case), intermediate, or complete. A complete defect is associated with a common AV valve and a moderate-to-large VSD. Approximately 40% of children with a complete AV canal have Down's syndrome.

◆ One or more pulmonary veins may connect to the right atrium or its inflow connections (SVC, inferior vena cava, coronary sinus, innominate vein, etc.). The most common supracardiac anomaly is anomalous venous connection of the upper lobe pulmonary vein to the left innominate vein via the left vertical vein. A persistent left SVC occurs with a prevalence of 0.5% and usually drains into the coronary sinus. When it drains into the left atrium (as in the case shown above), the coronary sinus is absent.

RADIOLOGIC

◆ Findings of endocardial cushion defects on MRI include moderate enlargement of the right atrium and right ventricle, but usually the left atrium is normal in size unless severe mitral regurgitation is also present.

◆ On MRI, the ASD can be seen at the level of the AV valves.

◆ Mitral regurgitation can be detected readily on gradient echo MRI. Right ventricular free wall hypertrophy (>1 cm) can be seen in the presence of associated pulmonary hypertension.

◆ SUGGESTED READING

Dinsmore RE, Wismer GL, Guyer D, et al. Magnetic resonance imaging of the intra-atrial septum and atrial septal defects. AJR Am J Roentgenol 1985;145:697–703.

Higgins CB. MRI of Congenital Heart Disease. In CB Higgins (ed), Essentials of Cardiac Radiology and Imaging. Philadelphia: Lippincott, 1992.

Lowell DG, Turner DA, Smith SM, et al. The detection of atrial and ventricular septal defects with electrocardiographically synchronized magnetic resonance imaging. Circulation 1986;73:89–94.

Perloff JK. Congenital heart disease in adults: A new cardiovascular subspecialty. Circulation 1991;84:1881–1890.

CASE 25

Cynthia S. Payne

HISTORY

A middle-aged man previously had undergone percutaneous nephrostomy (PCN) for treatment of renal obstruction due to stricture of a ureteroileal loop anastosmosis. A catheter exchange was attempted to introduce a larger catheter for stricture dilatation. At a point when only a guidewire (and no catheter) was in place, brisk pulsatile bleeding from the PCN tract was seen.

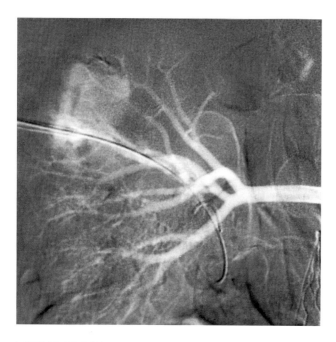

FIGURE 7-25A Images obtained during a renal angiogram show a guidewire entering the upper pole of the right kidney. An extraluminal collection of contrast material is seen adjacent to the guidewire.

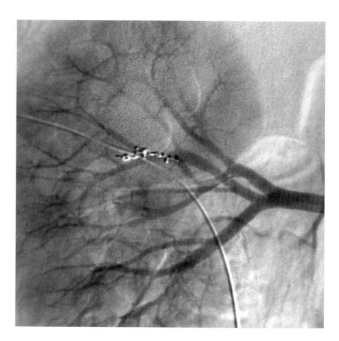

FIGURE 7-25B Renal angiogram performed after embolization of the interlobar artery with microcoils.

◆ DIFFERENTIAL DIAGNOSIS

◆ Brisk bleeding from a PCN site almost invariably is due to arterial injury. The injury can be an arterial tear (which can be accompanied by pseudoaneurysm formation) or arterial transection. If no arterial injury is seen at angiography, considerations include hemorrhage due to an arterial injury that has ceased bleeding, a bleeding diathesis, inadvertent catheter placement through a vascular abnormality such as a tumor, or, less likely, renal vein injury.

◆ DIAGNOSIS: Hemorrhage due to arterial injury.

◆ KEY FACTS

CLINICAL

◆ Indications for PCN include (1) renal or ureteral obstruction, (2) need for access for an interventional procedure (e.g., stone extraction or lithotripsy, stricture dilatation, or to aid retrograde access), (3) renal abscess drainage or direct antibiotic infusion into a site of fungal infection, and (4) urinary diversion (e.g., during treatment of ureteral injuries or hemorrhagic cystitis).

◆ Mild hematuria is seen frequently after placement and is not considered a serious complication. The rate of major complication during PCN placement is <10%. Complications of PCN and nephroureteral catheter placement can include: (1) sepsis, which is the most common complication (seen in 1% to 9% of cases); (2) frank hemorrhage, which can be either acute or delayed in onset; (3) perforation of the renal collecting system (e.g., ureteral injury); (4) inadvertent injury of adjacent organs (usually colon or spleen); or (5) pneumothorax, when the route of entry is not subcostal.

◆ Bleeding can result from (1) renal parenchymal or capsular injury, (2) arterial injury causing transection (as in the case shown), laceration, or formation of a pseudoaneurysm or arteriovenous fistula. Arterial injury typically involves the renal artery, but nonrenal arteries (e.g., the intercostal artery) can also be injured and cause frank hemorrhage.

◆ Proper preprocedure patient management includes (1) assessment of findings from other imaging studies indicating the rationale for the procedure, (2) recording of pertinent recent laboratory studies (e.g., hematocrit, hemoglobin, platelet count, coagulation studies, and renal function studies), (3) establishment of a secure intravenous line, (4) provision of adequate analgesia, and (5) administration of broad-spectrum antibiotics for prophylaxis against gram-negative organisms.

RADIOLOGIC

◆ Either sonography or fluoroscopy is used as guidance for access. If fluoroscopy is used and renal function is normal, the renal collecting system is typically opacified using intravenous contrast administration. Alternatively, a "blind" approach may be taken using anatomic landmarks. Small-gauge needles (20 or 22 g) are usually used for initial access.

◆ Usually an attempt is made to place the needle in a posterior lower pole calyx because there is a relative paucity of arteries in this region ("Brodal's bloodless incision line") compared to the more vascular upper pole. Entry into an upper pole calyx could have contributed to the hemorrhagic complication in the patient shown above. The calyx should be entered end-on to avoid injury to the arcuate arteries traversing the infundibular portion of the calyx. An anterior calyx entry point should be avoided because it makes passage of wires and catheters difficult.

◆ The choice of catheters for drainage procedures varies, but generally an 8 or 10 F, self-retaining, pigtail catheter is used, with the pigtail tip left within the renal pelvis.

◆ When the renal collecting system is infected, caution must be exercised to minimize the amount of air or contrast material used to distend the collecting system so that the risk of sepsis is minimized. If sepsis develops, urine in the renal pelvis is aspirated, catheter placement is completed as quickly as possible, and as necessary, fluid resuscitation and antibiotic administration are started. If the collecting system is infected, any additional procedures are usually deferred until a later time.

◆ Brisk, pulsatile, or nonremitting bleeding from the catheter, tract, or bladder should raise suspicion of vascular injury. The first step in treatment should be tamponade of the bleeding site by the catheter, which may require placement of a larger catheter.

◆ Marked hemorrhage during PCN is an indication for angiography. During the preparation for angiography, large-bore intravenous access should be secured, fluid resuscitation started, blood sent for type and cross match, and urgent consultation with a urologist performed in the event surgery is needed. During angiography, a selective renal angiogram is performed. If the site of hemorrhage is a distal vessel (as in the case shown), embolization should be performed immediately using coils or gelatin sponge (Gelfoam) pledgets. Particulate agents are avoided. In the case illustrated above, microcoils (rather than gelatin foam pledgets or larger coils) were used because permanent occlusion was desired. Distal placement of the coils allows a larger segment of the parent artery to be spared and results in preservation of more of the renal parenchyma.

◆ Injuries to the proximal renal artery or vein are often treated by emergency surgery. Less severe bleeding can sometimes be treated with catheter tamponade alone.

◆ SUGGESTED READING

Castañeda-Zúñiga WR, Tadavarthy SM, Hunter DW, et al. Interventional Uroradiology. Part 1. In WR Zúniga, SM Tadavarthy (eds), Percutaneous Uroradiologic Techniques in Interventional Radiology (2nd ed, vol 2). Baltimore: Williams & Wilkins, 1992;777–989.

Lee WJ, Patel R, Patel S, Illari GP. Emergency percutaneous nephrostomy: Results and complications. J Vasc Interv Radiol 1994;5:135–139.

Wojtowycz M. Handbook of Interventional Radiology and Angiography. St. Louis: Mosby, 1995.

CASE 26

James T.T. Chen

HISTORY

A 10-year-old girl with a history of cyanosis, squatting, and clubbing of fingers since early childhood.

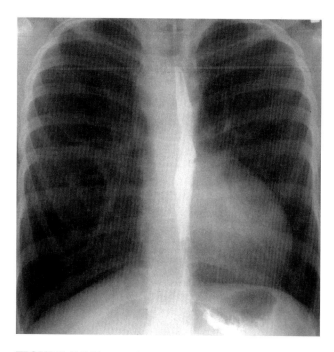

FIGURE 7-26A Frontal chest radiograph following barium swallow. A boot-shaped cardiovascular contour is seen. The aortic arch is on the right side, deviating the trachea and the barium-filled esophagus to the left. The pulmonary blood flow is decreased diffusely, with small pulmonary arteries and veins (numerous small, tortuous vessels in the medial upper lung zones were evident on close inspection, representing bronchial arterial collaterals).

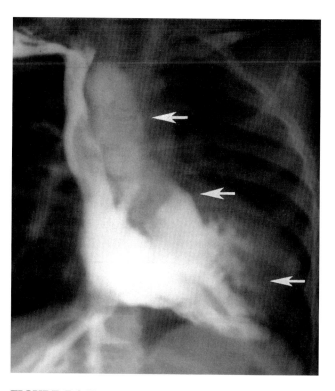

FIGURE 7-26B An angiogram via the right arm vein with opacification of the superior vena cava. Sequential opacification of the superior vena cava, right atrium, and right ventricle is seen. Flow of contrast material ends in a blind pouch (middle arrow) in the right ventricular outflow tract. Contrast material flows across a ventricular septal defect to the left ventricle and into a very large right-sided aorta (upper arrow). The right ventricle appears mildly enlarged and markedly trabeculated (lower arrow).

◆ DIFFERENTIAL DIAGNOSIS

- **Isolated pulmonary atresia with competent tricuspid valve:** This is an unlikely diagnosis in a patient of this age because patients usually succumb shortly after birth.
- **Isolated pulmonary atresia with incompetent tricuspid valve:** This diagnosis might be considered based on the angiogram findings of atresia of the pulmonary outflow tract seen in Figure 7-26B. However, this diagnosis is incorrect for two reasons: first, a ventricular septal defect (VSD) is present in the case shown above, but would not be expected in isolated pulmonary atresia; and second, right ventricle hypertrophy (but not dilatation) is present in the case shown above, whereas marked dilatation of the right ventricle would be expected in isolated pulmonary atresia.
- **Admixture lesions with pulmonary stenosis:** Examples of this category include (1) D-loop transposition of the great arteries with pulmonic stenosis, and (2) double-outlet right ventricle with pulmonic stenosis. These lesions could mimic the present case. It would be difficult to distinguish them on the basis of clinical grounds or plain radiographs, but the echocardiography and cardiac catheterization findings would differ from those in the case illustrated.
- **Pulmonary atresia with VSD:** This is the best diagnosis given the clinical presentation and the radiologic findings of coexistent atresia of the pulmonary outflow tract, a VSD, and right ventricle hypertrophy.

◆ DIAGNOSIS: Pulmonary atresia with ventricular septal defect (severe tetralogy of Fallot).

◆ KEY FACTS

CLINICAL

- The physiology of pulmonary atresia with VSD is essentially that of severe TOF.
- Without surgery, 75% of these patients die within 10 years. Cyanotic spells indicate severe pulmonary stenosis. Complete obstruction can ensue with poor surgical outcome.
- The method of surgical repair depends on whether the branch pulmonary arteries are confluent. Confluent pulmonary arteries can be repaired with a conduit. Nonconfluent arteries may require a palliative shunt or unifocalization (i.e., creation of a common conduct encompassing all the separate pulmonary arteries from both lungs).
- Numerous small and tortuous vessels in both upper lung zones are frequently seen, representing bronchial arterial collateral circulation.

RADIOLOGIC

- The initial chest radiographic findings of pulmonary atresia with VSD are the same as those for severe TOF.
- The *coeur en sabot* ("boot-shaped") cardiovascular configuration is explained by the enlarged right ventricle, which displaces the left ventricle leftward, posteriorly, and superiorly and causes uptilting of the cardiac apex.
- Both infundibular pulmonic stenosis and hypoplasia of pulmonary arteries can also cause a concavity in the region of the pulmonary trunk.
- The large right-to-left shunt via a VSD is responsible for a markedly dilated aorta.
- Severe pulmonary oligemia is caused by the large right-to-left shunt.

◆ SUGGESTED READING

Chen JTT. Essentials of Cardiac Roentgenology. Boston: Little, Brown, 1987.

Kelley MJ, Jaffe CC, Kleinman CS. Cardiac Imaging in Infants and Children. Philadelphia: Saunders, 1982.

Nugent EW, Plauth WH, Edwards JE, Williams WH. The Pathology, Pathophysiology, Recognition, and Treatment of Congenital Heart Disease. In RC Schlant, RW Alexander (eds), The Heart (8th ed). New York: McGraw-Hill, 1994.

HISTORY

A left-handed baseball pitcher with pain and numbness in the left hand and fore-arm when throwing a ball.

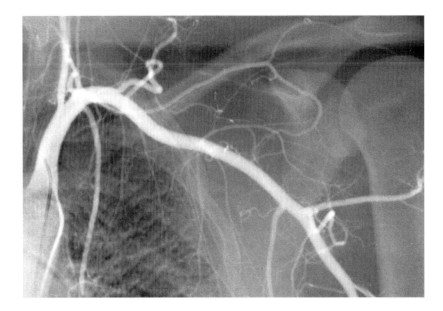

FIGURE 7-27A Selective left subclavian artery angiogram performed with the left arm held in neutral position shows no abnormalities.

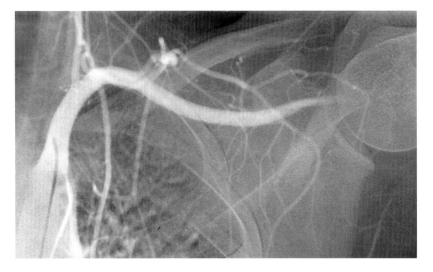

FIGURE 7-27B Repeat angiogram performed a few minutes later with the left arm in abduction shows occlusion of the distal axillary artery.

◆ DIFFERENTIAL DIAGNOSIS

◆ **Thoracic outlet syndrome:** The findings on the second angiogram, if viewed in isolation, could be due to a wide number of entities. However, when the findings of the two angiograms are considered together, the occlusion of the subclavian artery must be explained by arterial compression due to change in the position of the arm. Such compression would most likely be due to arterial compression by adjacent muscle or rib.

◆ DIAGNOSIS: Thoracic outlet syndrome.

◆ KEY FACTS

CLINICAL

◆ The axillary artery is the continuation of the subclavian artery and is defined as the segment extending from the lateral margin of the first rib to the inferior lateral margin of the teres major muscle. Distal to this point, the artery continues as the brachial artery.

◆ Thoracic outlet syndrome results from compression of the nerves and vessels as they course through the upper thorax and shoulder in the region referred to as the "thoracic outlet." These structures can be compressed at several sites (most commonly the interscalene triangle, costoclavicular space, and the pectoralis minor triangle) and by a number of mechanisms, including compression by a rib or fibrous bands. The distal location of the occlusion in the case shown suggests that compression by the pectoralis minor muscle (which became hypertrophied secondary to the repeated arm motions involved in pitching) is the most likely etiology.

◆ More commonly, the subclavian artery is compressed by the first rib or an anomalous cervical rib. The diagnosis is often first suspected based on clinical history and physical findings of diminished pulses or reproducible pain on abduction of the arm.

◆ Thrombosis at the site of arterial compression or distal embolization can rarely cause limb ischemia.

RADIOLOGIC

◆ On occasion, chest radiographs may show a cervical rib as a suspected cause of vascular compromise.

◆ Doppler sonography can serve as a helpful noninvasive study for detection of arterial compression.

◆ Selective angiography of the subclavian artery is indicated when ischemia is a prominent feature and surgery is a consideration. The artery is injected initially with the arm in neutral (adducted) position. The entire arterial supply of the arm should be evaluated for evidence of distal embolization. Thereafter, the arm is hyperabducted and repeat filming performed over the shoulder region.

◆ Angiographic findings in thoracic outlet syndrome include subclavian or axillary artery stenosis or occlusion (occasionally in neutral position rather than during abduction), poststenotic dilatation, arterial displacement, pseudoaneurysm, thrombosis, and distal embolization.

◆ Patients whose symptoms are severe enough to warrant angiographic evaluation are often surgical candidates. The most common surgical approaches include resection of the first rib or a cervical rib, if present, and release of fascial bands surrounding nerves and vessels.

◆ SUGGESTED READING

Fechter JD, Kuschner SH. The thoracic outlet syndrome. Rev Orthop 1993;16:1243–1251.

Kadir S. Diagnostic Angiography. Philadelphia: Saunders, 1986.

Kutz JE, Rowland EB Jr. Vascular compression about the shoulder. Hand Clin 1993;9:131–138.

HISTORY

A newborn boy noted to be extremely cyanotic, tachypneic, and tachycardic. An emergency palliative procedure has been performed.

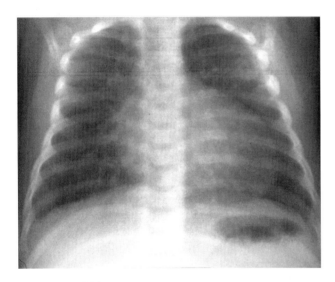

FIGURE 7-28A Frontal chest radiograph. Moderate cardiomegaly and an egg-shaped cardiac contour are seen. The cardiac waist (i.e., superior mediastinum) is narrow. In addition, diffuse and symmetric increase in pulmonary vascularity is seen but no pulmonary edema.

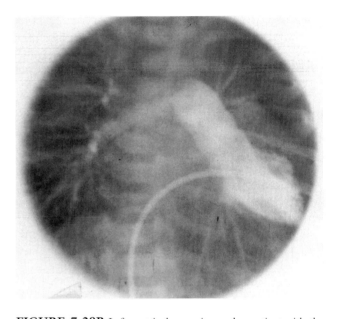

FIGURE 7-28B Left ventriculogram in another patient with the same disorder. The catheter extends from the right atrium across a patent foramen ovale and mitral valve into the left ventricle. The left ventricle is smooth and normal in position and appearance. However, it gives rise to pulmonary arteries through a pulmonary valve which is lower and more medial than normal. There is no evidence of ventricular septal defect or pulmonic stenosis.

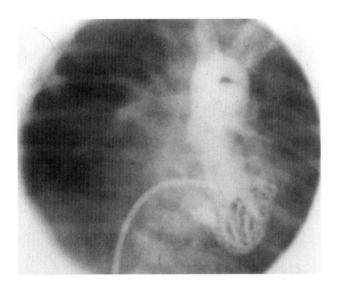

FIGURE 7-28C Right ventriculogram in the same patient as in Figure 7-28B. A normally trabeculated right ventricle is seen in normal position. The right ventricle gives rise to the aorta through an aortic valve which is higher and more medial than normal. When compared with Figure 7-28A, the abnormal position of both great arteries, which tend to overlap anteroposteriorly, can be seen. The sequential opacification of the aorta and of the pulmonary arteries is consistent with the diagnosis of a patent ductus arteriosus.

◆ DIFFERENTIAL DIAGNOSIS

- **Large ventricular septal defect (VSD):** Patients with a large VSD can become dusky when in severe congestive heart failure, but they are not cyanotic. Furthermore, the patients presented here were not in congestive heart failure. Newborns with a VSD do not have increased pulmonary blood flow due to physiologic high pulmonary vascular resistance. Shunting is insignificant until pulmonary resistance falls, but thereafter proceeds in a left-to-right direction. These factors all argue against the diagnosis of a large VSD as the diagnosis in the cases shown.
- **Hypoplastic left heart syndrome:** Patients with this syndrome are also cyanotic neonates, but they are almost always in profound heart failure with pulmonary edema (and do not have increased pulmonary flow, as in the case presented). Furthermore, their hearts tend to be larger than those seen in the cases shown. These factors make this diagnosis unlikely.
- **Total anomalous pulmonary venous connection with obstruction:** These patients are also cyanotic neonates, but they are always in profound heart failure with severe pulmonary edema and have a normal cardiac size.
- **Atrial septal defect (ASD):** This defect can have a variety of clinical presentations, depending on the size and location of the defect. It usually presents late in infancy (unlike the case presented here), with pulmonary overcirculation following a fall in the pulmonary vascular resistance. Furthermore, patients with this disorder do not have a narrow superior mediastinum, because the great vessels are normally related. Finally, patients with ASD are not cyanotic. This is an incorrect diagnosis.
- **D-loop transposition of the great arteries:** This diagnosis is the best choice, given the history and radiographic findings. The characteristic findings are present on the angiogram, confirming the diagnosis.

◆ DIAGNOSIS: D-loop transposition of great arteries (TOGA), patent ductus arteriosus status post–atrial septostomy.

◆ KEY FACTS

CLINICAL

- D-loop transposition of great arteries accounts for 4% of congenital cardiac defects in children.
- D-loop transposition of great arteries is the most common lesion to present with severe cyanosis immediately after birth.

- Infants with an intact ventricular septum are usually severely cyanotic but not in congestive heart failure. The patency of either or both the ductus and the foramen ovale allows for initial survival, but atrial septostomy is required for long-term survival.
- The diagnosis is usually established by echocardiography, which may be sufficient for operative planning; a septostomy may be performed using angiographic or sonographic guidance.
- Current definitive repair is the Jatene procedure, in which the aorta and pulmonary vessels are switched. Previously, Mustard and Senning atrial baffle procedures were performed. These procedures resulted in a systemic right ventricle that eventually failed.

RADIOLOGIC

- Following emergency atrial septostomy, there is increased pulmonary vascularity with moderate cardiomegaly.
- The "egg on the string" appearance of the heart is due to several factors. The right heart is pumping against the high systemic vascular resistance and is enlarged to a greater degree than the left heart. Hence, a globular cardiac contour results. The thymus is absent due to the stress, and the aorta and main pulmonary artery take on a more overlapping configuration.
- For D-loop TOGA, the angiocardiographic findings are usually also well shown by echocardiography. The basic pathologic anatomy is as follows: The aorta arises from the right ventricle and the pulmonary artery arises from the left ventricle. The parallel arrangement of the two circulations is incompatible with life without some kind of communication (either patent foramen ovale, ASD/VSD, or a septostomy).
- The pathophysiology of this entity can be considered as a spectrum with two extremes. On one end, communications between the right and left circulatory pathways are too numerous and too large, resulting in pulmonary plethora, congestive heart failure, and mild cyanosis. On the other end, communications are too small and too few in number, causing pulmonary oligemia and severe cyanosis but not heart failure.

◆ SUGGESTED READING

Chen JTT. Essentials of Cardiac Roentgenology. Boston: Little, Brown, 1987.

Kelley MJ, Jaffe CC, Kleinman CS. Cardiac Imaging in Infants and Children. Philadelphia: Saunders, 1982.

Nugent EW, Plauth WH, Edwards JE, Williams WH. The Pathology, Pathophysiology, Recognition, and Treatment of Congenital Heart Disease. In RC Schlant, RW Alexander (eds), The Heart (8th ed). New York: McGraw-Hill, 1994.

HISTORY

A 24-year-old man with a long history of respiratory difficulty, frequent pulmonary infections, and recent onset of hemoptysis.

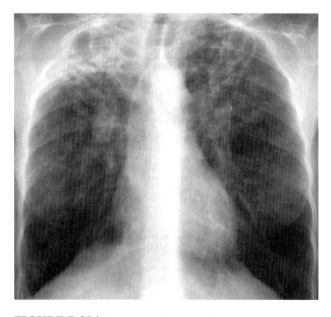

FIGURE 7-29A Posteroanterior chest radiograph shows hyperexpanded lungs, upper lobe fibrobullous change, and diffuse bronchiectasis.

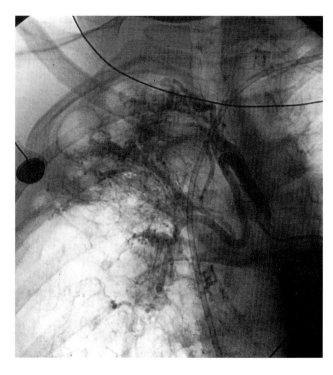

FIGURE 7-29B Angiogram of the bronchial artery shows a hypertrophied, dilated bronchial artery and hypervascularity in the right upper lobe.

◆ DIFFERENTIAL DIAGNOSIS

A wide range of entities can produce the radiographic appearance seen in Figure 7-29A. These entities include:

◆ **Cystic fibrosis:** This is the most likely diagnosis in a young patient with the findings shown in Figure 7-29A, especially given the associated finding of dilated bronchial arteries seen in Figure 7-29B.

◆ **Collagen disorders:** The findings shown above can be seen in some collagen vascular disorders, especially ankylosing spondylitis. However, the presence of bronchiectasis and the absence of skeletal abnormalities are evidence against this diagnosis.

◆ **Tuberculosis (TB) and atypical mycobacterial infections:** TB and atypical mycobacterial infections, such as *Mycobacterium avium* complex, could produce the changes shown in Figure 7-29A (see below).

◆ **Sarcoidosis:** The above findings can be seen in sarcoidosis. However, low lung volumes, rather than the increased lung volumes shown above, would be expected.

◆ **Pneumoconiosis:** The absence of nodularity and conglomerate masses makes this diagnosis less likely.

◆ **Hemoptysis with enlarged bronchial arteries** can be produced by many causes, such as TB, coal worker's pneumoconiosis, bronchiectasis, aspergillosis, carcinoma, and congenital heart disease (due to enlarged collateral vessels). However, the young age of the patient in the case shown above, the lack of a history of appropriate exposure to TB, coal dust, etc., and the radiologic findings shown in Figure 7-29A are most consistent with cystic fibrosis.

◆DIAGNOSIS: Cystic fibrosis with enlarged bronchial arteries.

◆KEY FACTS

CLINICAL

◆ If untreated, severe hemoptysis of any cause has a 50% to 85% mortality rate (although it is probably less in the cystic fibrosis population). Asphyxiation and, less commonly, exsanguination are the major causes of death.

◆ The bronchial arteries usually arise between the T3 and T8 levels, but the sites of origin vary considerably among individuals. Variations in the number of bronchial arteries are also frequently seen, but the common patterns are: (1) two left arteries and one right artery (40%), (2) a single right and single left bronchial artery (30%), and (3) two left and two right arteries (20%). The bronchial arteries may share a common origin with the intercostal arteries (so-called "intercostobronchial trunk").

◆ Systemic arterial supply to the lungs is actually from two sources: bronchial arteries and nonbronchial arteries. The latter source includes branches of the subclavian artery and proximal axillary arteries, including the internal mammary, intercostal, and phrenic arteries. Supply from these sites is common in patients with cystic fibrosis. Theses sites should all be evaluated in the cystic fibrosis patient with hemoptysis.

RADIOLOGIC

◆ Careful angiographic evaluation must be performed before embolization to determine arterial feeding sites of hemoptysis and define anatomic variants. In particular, the angiographer must define the arterial supply to the spinal cord and exclude the presence of large fistulous connections to the pulmonary artery (to protect against inadvertent embolization of the spinal cord and uninvolved segments of lung, respectively).

◆ Generally, only angiography of the bronchial arteries is performed during evaluation of hemoptysis. Angiography of the pulmonary arteries is reserved for cases in which parenchymal necrosis is suspected.

◆ Bronchial arteries and nonbronchial systemic arteries that are responsible for hemorrhage are usually quite enlarged.

◆ The site of hemoptysis is often only generalized to one lung or the other by bronchoscopy, or may be unknown even after angiography. Contrast material extravasation, even in patients with hemoptysis, is very rare. Therefore, embolization is performed whenever technically possible via selective catheterization of all enlarged bronchial arteries and enlarged systemic bronchial collaterals.

◆ Embolization is often the treatment of choice and usually performed with particulate agents, such as polyvinyl alcohol sponge particles. The small size of these particles allows them to be deposited directly in small feeding arteries, lessening the likelihood of occlusion of proximal arteries. The latter consideration is particularly important, because occlusion of only proximal arteries would still allow development of collateral circulation to nonembolized small bleeding arteries but block catheter access and, therefore, prohibit delivery of embolic agent to the bleeding site. The disadvantage of particles is the potential for inadvertent passage of embolic material into the pulmonary arteries or veins through vascular shunts. The latter point underscores the necessity for determining the presence of such shunts prior to embolization.

◆ In one reported series (Remy-Jardin & Remy, 1991), control of approximately 70% of cases of hemoptysis in a series of 257 patients (only one of whom had cystic fibrosis) was reported. However, hemoptysis recurred in 52%. This result reflects the fact that embolization therapy in this circumstance is palliative, treating the symptom (i.e., hemoptysis) rather than the underlying cause.

◆ Embolization therapy for hemoptysis related to cystic fibrosis is generally thought to be effective. Some series report relatively high rates of rehemorrhage, but this complication is generally responsive to repeat embolization therapy.

◆SUGGESTED READING

Cohen AM, Doershuk CF, Stern RC. Bronchial embolization to control hemoptysis in cystic fibrosis. Radiology 1990;175: 401–405.

Mauro MA, Jaques PF, Morris SM. Bronchial artery embolization for control of hemoptysis. Semin Interv Radiol 1992;9:45–51.

Remy-Jardin M, Remy J. Embolization for the Treatment of Hemoptysis. In S Kadir (ed), Current Practice of Interventional Radiology. Philadelphia: Decker, 1991;194–202.

CASE 30

Paul V. Suhocki

HISTORY

A 22-year-old man who sustained a gunshot wound to the left arm and is found to have decreased left arm pulses.

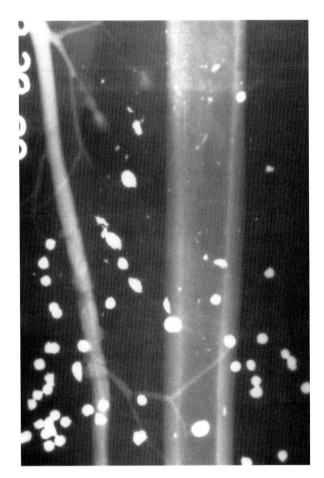

FIGURE 7-30A Left brachial angiogram shows multiple sites of focal narrowing and outpouching of the contrast column and a linear defect in the distal segment of the artery. Branches of the artery terminate abruptly, at which sites extraluminal contrast collections are seen.

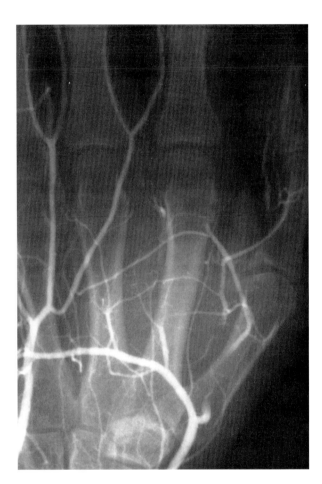

FIGURE 7-30B Several filling defects are seen in the princeps pollicis artery and the proper digital arteries of the first and second digits.

◆ DIFFERENTIAL DIAGNOSIS

◆ **Vasospasm:** Vasospasm can occur after trauma. However, this diagnosis would not account for all of the findings in the brachial artery (e.g., the linear lucency and the extraluminal contrast collections), making this diagnosis by itself incorrect.

◆ **Arterial dissection:** The linear lucency extending along the brachial artery is, in fact, due to arterial dissection. However, this diagnosis alone does not account for all of the findings, including the extraluminal collections and the findings in the digits.

◆ **Arterial injury with distal thromboembolization:** This is the correct diagnosis. The extraluminal contrast collections are due to small sites of arterial hemorrhage. The numerous filling defects in digital arteries are due to thromboembolism distal to the site of intimal injury. The outpouchings are sites of pseudoaneurysm formation.

◆ DIAGNOSIS: Arterial injury with distal thromboembolization.

◆ KEY FACTS

CLINICAL

◆ The clinical signs of an expanding pulsatile mass, diminished blood pressure, or distal limb ischemia in a trauma patient are indications of vascular injury until proven otherwise.

◆ The most reliable clinical sign of arterial injury within a limb is diminished or absent blood pressure. However, in the setting of systemic hypotension, this finding is difficult to evaluate.

◆ Hematoma and vascular occlusion are immediate sequelae of arterial injury. Pseudoaneurysm and AV fistula formation are potential delayed sequelae.

◆ Obvious arterial injuries in an unstable, hypotensive patient are an indication for immediate surgical exploration and repair.

◆ Although most arterial injuries are due to penetrating trauma, injury can also result from nonpenetrating trauma, including stretch injury. The latter is typically seen following joint dislocations (e.g., posterior knee dislocations).

RADIOLOGIC

◆ The role of angiography in the setting of suspected arterial injury is to determine the presence or absence of injury (thereby minimizing the number of unnecessary surgical explorations), define the type of injury, and on occasion, temporize or definitively treat the injury via endovascular therapy.

◆ Typically, two or more angiographic views are obtained to decrease the chance of a false-negative study.

◆ The false-positive rate for angiography is 0% to 4%. False-positive angiograms can be produced by the following causes: (1) arteries seen on-end can be mistaken for pseudoaneurysms, (2) inflow of unopacified blood ("streaming" effect) from collateral arteries can be mistaken for intraluminal thrombus, (3) arterial spasm induced by the catheter, guidewire, or contrast material injection is mistaken for vasospasm related to trauma.

◆ The false-negative rate is 0% to 1.8%. False-negative angiograms can be due to: (1) use of only a single projection, on which a site of injury is obscured by contrast material; (2) wrong choice of contrast material volume (i.e., too little) or injection rate (i.e., too slow); (3) failure to selectively catheterize an artery with a suspected abnormality; and (4) premature termination of the imaging procedure. False-negative studies therefore can be minimized by selective catheterization of the vessel thought to be injured, choice of an injection rate and volume that will completely opacify the vessel, obtaining orthogonal views of the region, and obtaining late images that will show delayed clearance or extravasation of contrast material.

◆ The two most common findings in arterial injury are occlusion and extravasation of contrast material. Arterial occlusion can reflect either intimal injury (and subsequent thrombus formation) or transmural disruption. Other findings that can be seen include the presence of an intimal flap, vasospasm, pseudoaneurysm formation, AV fistula, distal embolization, intramural hematoma, and displacement of vessels by adjacent hematoma.

◆ SUGGESTED READING

Goldberg MC, O'Donnell TF. Acute Ischemia: Upper and Lower Extremity Trauma. In DE Strandness Jr, A Van Breda (eds), Vascular Diseases. New York: Churchill Livingstone, 1994; 399–420.

Kadir S. Arteriography of the Upper Extremities. In S Kadir (ed), Diagnostic Angiography. Philadelphia: Saunders, 1986;172–206.

CHAPTER 8

PEDIATRIC RADIOLOGY

Donald P. Frush, *chapter editor*

Jeffrey B. Betts, George S. Bisset III,
Donald P. Frush, Herman Grossman,
Mark A. Kliewer, Cindy R. Miller,
and Sara M. O'Hara

CASE 1

Donald P. Frush

HISTORY

An 8-year-old boy with pleuritic chest pain and 39°C temperature.

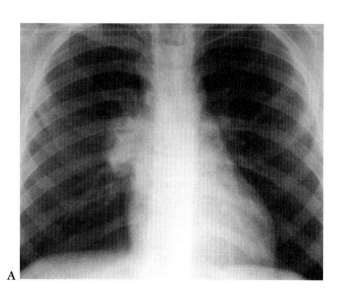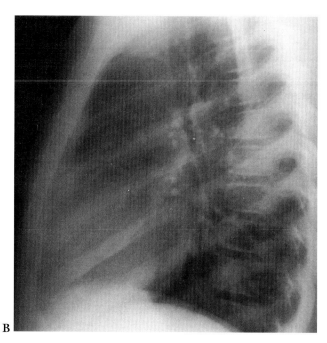

FIGURES 8-1A and 8-1B Frontal (**A**) and lateral (**B**) chest radiographs. There is a well-defined mass in the right lung. Notably, the right hilum is not obscured. This mass is posterior on the lateral view, projected over the upper mid-thoracic spine.

◆ DIFFERENTIAL DIAGNOSIS

◆ **Hilar adenopathy:** This diagnosis is incorrect because the right hilum is seen as separate from the "mass." Therefore, this mass must be anterior or posterior in the right hemithorax.

◆ **Plasma cell granuloma (postinflammatory pseudo-tumor):** Plasma cell granuloma can present as a mass, with calcification in up to 25% of cases. Children are usually asymptomatic or have very minimal symptoms. This is a possible diagnosis in this case, which cannot be excluded on the basis of the radiographs, but it is a relatively rare entity.

◆ **Bronchopulmonary foregut malformation:** Such malformations—e.g., parenchymal bronchogenic cyst or a pulmonary sequestration—are reasonable considerations on the basis of the findings. Cystic adenomatoid malformation is another malformation to be considered, but it rarely presents in older children or adults and is usually hyperlucent. Arteriovenous malformations are usually multiple, with associated enlarged arteries and veins.

◆ **Primary pulmonary malignancy:** Sarcomas and pulmonary blastomas, the most likely primary tumors, could produce these findings, but these lesions are exceedingly rare.

◆ **Metastasis:** This is an unlikely diagnosis because there is no history of malignancy. Furthermore, a single, large metastasis would be unusual.

◆ **Round pneumonia:** Round pneumonia is a very common cause of a pulmonary mass in children. This entity is much more common than a bronchopulmonary foregut malformation.

◆ **Contusion:** This diagnosis is not a reasonable consideration because there is no history of trauma.

◆ **Round atelectasis:** Round atelectasis is a consideration based on the shape of the opacity but is usually basilar in location and is very rare in children.

◆ **Pleural effusion caused by "pseudotumor":** This entity is unlikely because it is usually sharply defined at some aspect in at least one projection.

◆ **Hamartoma:** This diagnosis is a consideration but is usually asymptomatic and is relatively rare.

◆ DIAGNOSIS: Round pneumonia in the superior segment of the right lower lobe.

◆ KEY FACTS

CLINICAL

◆ Almost all pulmonary masses in children are related to infection (e.g., round pneumonia, plasma cell granuloma).

◆ Round pneumonia is a common cause of pulmonary mass in children.

◆ Round pneumonia is rare over 8 years of age.

◆ *Streptococcus pneumoniae* (pneumococcus) is the most common organism responsible for round pneumonia.

◆ Symptoms can be mild or nonspecific early in the clinical course.

◆ With a typical clinical history and recognition of a mass on imaging studies as round pneumonia, antibiotic treatment can be started without further imaging.

◆ In cases in which the clinical information is unclear, a pulmonary mass can be conservatively followed with a repeat chest radiograph in 24 to 48 hours. Round pneumonia will typically become closer in appearance to a lobar pneumonia at that time.

RADIOLOGIC

◆ Round pneumonia is typically a well-defined, mass-like opacity that is usually located in a lower lobe.

◆ Air bronchograms are present initially in a minority of cases.

◆ Calcification is not a feature of this entity.

◆ Pneumonia is initially localized due to immature collateral pathways in children, but eventually becomes a more typical air space disease process (i.e., an ill-defined opacity with air bronchograms).

◆ Adenopathy and pleural effusion are rarely seen with round pneumonia.

◆ SUGGESTED READING

Condon VR. Pneumonia in children. J Thorac Imaging 1991;6:31–44.

Shady K, Siegel MJ, Glazer HS. CT of focal pulmonary masses in childhood. Radiographics 1992;12:505–514.

CASE 2

HISTORY

A 14-month-old boy with a palpable abdominal mass.

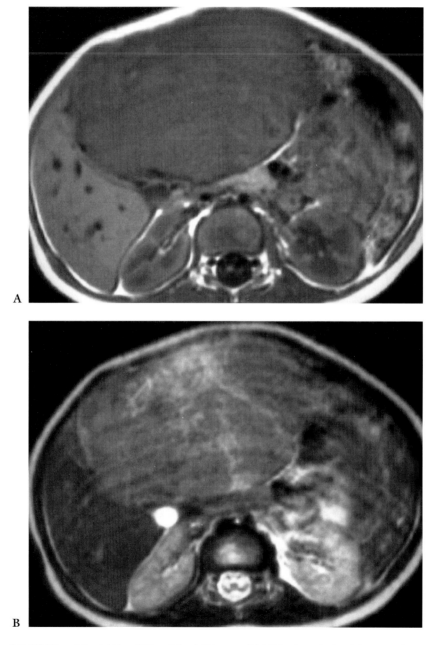

A

B

FIGURES 8-2A and 8-2B T1-weighted (**A**) and T2-weighted (**B**) transaxial MRIs through the abdomen. A heterogenous mass is seen within the left lobe of the liver. The mass displaces the pancreas and inferior vena cava posteriorly and displaces the bowel toward the left.

◆ DIFFERENTIAL DIAGNOSIS

- **Hepatocellular carcinoma:** This diagnosis is unlikely because this neoplasm rarely occurs below the age of 2 years. Furthermore, frequently there is a history of chronic liver disease.
- **Hepatoblastoma:** This is the most common malignant primary liver tumor of childhood, usually occurring before the age of 3 years. The young age of the patient and inhomogeneous appearance of the mass in the present case are consistent with this diagnosis.
- **Mesenchymal hamartoma:** This diagnosis is unlikely because it is rare, cystic, and often exophytic, unlike the case illustrated. The diagnosis is frequently made by prenatal sonography.
- **Hemangioendothelioma:** This entity is the most common symptomatic vascular lesion in infancy and most common mesenchymal tumor of childhood. This diagnosis is unlikely in the case illustrated because it frequently contains large feeding vessels and areas of hypointensity on T1-weighted images, corresponding to fibrosis and hemosiderin deposition.
- **Hepatic adenoma:** These tumors are extremely rare in young children. Furthermore, the lesion frequently contains regions of high signal on T1-weighted images due to fatty change or hemorrhage. This finding is not seen in the case illustrated, further making this diagnosis an unlikely one.

◆ DIAGNOSIS: Hepatoblastoma.

◆ KEY FACTS

CLINICAL
- Hepatoblastoma is probably an infantile form of hepatocellular carcinoma.

- This tumor primarily occurs before the age of 3 years (median age: 1 year).
- A male-to-female predominance between 2 to 1 and 3 to 1 has been reported.
- The tumor is associated with Beckwith-Wiedemann syndrome (i.e., hemihypertrophy and biliary atresia).
- Nearly all patients with this tumor have elevated serum levels of alpha fetoprotein.
- Prognosis is usually good if there are no metastases and the tumor is limited to the liver and is completely resectable.

RADIOLOGIC
- Hepatoblastoma usually presents as a single mass. However, multifocal involvement can sometimes occur.
- On contrast-enhanced CT examination, the mass does not contrast-enhance to a large degree
- This tumor generally has heterogeneous, hyperintense signal on T2-weighted MRI.
- Splaying of hepatic veins around the mass can be seen occasionally.
- The sonographic appearance is that of a hypoechoic mass with displacement of the hepatic arterial and portal venous vessels by the tumor.

◆ SUGGESTED READING

Boechat MI, Kangarloo H, Ortega J, et al. Primary liver tumors in children: Comparison of CT and MR imaging. Radiology 1988;169:727–732.

Finn JP, Hall-Craggs MA, Dicks-Mireaux C, et al. Primary malignant liver tumors in childhood: Assessment of resectability with high field MR and comparison with CT. Pediatr Radiol 1990;21:34–38.

Pobiel RS, Bisset GB. Pictorial essay: Imaging of liver tumors in the infant and child. Pediatr Radiol 1995;25:495–506.

CASE 3

Sara M. O'Hara

HISTORY

A toddler with urinary retention and distended abdomen.

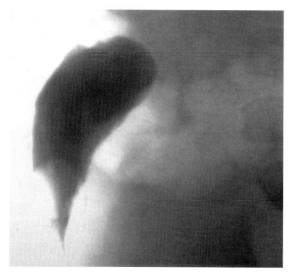

FIGURE 8-3A Lateral spot film from voiding cystourethrogram. The bladder neck is elongated, and the entire bladder is displaced upward and anteriorly out of the pelvis.

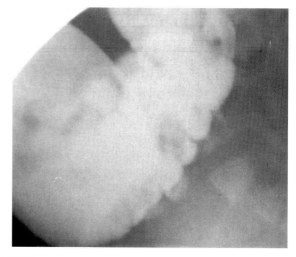

FIGURE 8-3B Lateral spot film from barium enema examination. The rectosigmoid is compressed and displaced anteriorly. No bowel gas or stool is visible in the presacral space.

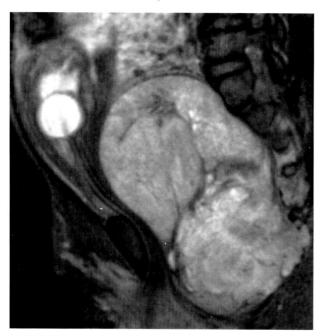

FIGURE 8-3C Sagittal T2-weighted fast spin echo MRI with fat saturation. A mixed-signal intensity mass is present in the presacral region, extending between the sacral segments and into the posterior musculature. The Foley catheter within the bladder is displaced anteriorly and superiorly.

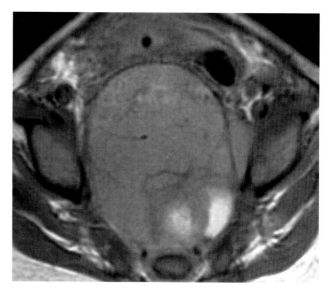

FIGURE 8-3D Axial noncontrast T1-weighted MRI. A predominantly intermediate-signal intensity soft-tissue mass is seen encasing the lower sacrum and displacing the rectum anteriorly and to the left.

◆ DIFFERENTIAL DIAGNOSIS

◆ **Ovarian teratoma:** Any tumorous growth from the ovary could grow to the size shown in this case. However, extension around the sacrum is not a feature typically seen in ovarian tumor, making this an unlikely diagnosis.

◆ **Abscess:** This entity cannot be excluded on the basis of imaging findings alone. However, it is an unlikely diagnosis because the clinical history does not suggest the presence of infectious process.

◆ **Neuroblastoma (or ganglioneuroma):** The location and appearance of the mass are consistent with this diagnosis. However, posterior encasement and direct sacral involvement are not findings that would be expected in pelvic neuroblastoma.

◆ **Sacrococcygeal germ cell tumor (i.e., teratoma):** Teratoma is the best diagnosis, based on the presacral and retrorectal location and, in particular, the encasement of sacral segments.

◆ **Anterior meningocele:** This diagnosis is unlikely because the mass is not cystic.

◆ **Rhabdomyosarcoma:** Because posterior sacral extension would be unusual for rhabdomyosarcoma, this is an unlikely diagnosis.

◆ **Primary bone tumor:** A primary bone tumor is not a likely consideration because there is no bony destruction and sacral involvement in this case is relatively minimal.

◆ **Gastrointestinal duplication:** This diagnosis is unlikely because rectal duplications are very rare and extension to sacrum would not be expected.

◆ DIAGNOSIS: Malignant sacrococcygeal germ cell tumor (teratoma).

◆ KEY FACTS

CLINICAL

◆ Sacrococcygeal teratomas are relatively rare, with an estimated prevalence of 1 in 35,000–40,000 births.

◆ The category of germ cell tumors includes teratomas, choriocarcinomas, embryonal cell carcinomas, yolk sac tumors, and mixed types.

◆ Teratomas are classified as mature, immature, or malignant. Malignancy is rare in mature types.

◆ Treatment consists of chemotherapy and surgical resection.

◆ Early diagnosis and surgical excision is indicated because the incidence of malignant transformation increases with advancing age.

◆ Four types of sacral teratomas have been described, according to the internal and external components of the mass:

Type 1: primarily external to the pelvis
Type 2: predominantly external to the pelvis with intrapelvic component
Type 3: primarily intrapelvic with only a small extrapelvic portion
Type 4: entirely presacral without extrapelvic extension

In general, the greater the intrapelvic component, the greater the likelihood of malignancy.

RADIOLOGIC

◆ Calcification is visible by CT in 50% to 60% of sacrococcygeal teratomas and is more frequent in benign lesions. Amorphous, chunky, punctate, and spiculated calcifications have all been described.

◆ Cystic and fatty components can also be seen within the mass.

◆ Primarily solid lesions are more likely to be malignant. However, the histologic features (i.e., benign or malignant nature) cannot generally be inferred reliably from the imaging characteristics.

◆ Direct invasion of adjacent structures suggests malignant transformation.

◆ Elevated serum alpha-fetoprotein levels are often present and are frequently followed in conjunction with imaging findings as a measure of tumor response.

◆ Presacral masses can coexist with two other entities: anorectal malformations and sacral anomalies, a constellation that is referred to as *Currarino's triad*.

◆ SUGGESTED READING

Prenger EC, Ball WS. Spine and Contents. In DR Kirks (ed), Practical Pediatric Imaging: Diagnostic Radiology of Infants and Children (2nd ed). Boston: Little, Brown, 1991;236–241.

Wells RG, Sty JR. Imaging of sacrococcygeal germ cell tumors. Radiographics 1990;10:701–713.

CASE 4

Mark A. Kliewer

HISTORY

A 15-year-old boy presents with fever, cough, abdominal pain, and diarrhea.

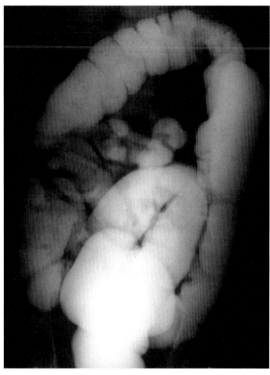

FIGURE 8-4A Barium enema. Luminal narrowing is present, with mucosal irregularity and nodularity in the terminal ileum, cecum, and transverse colon.

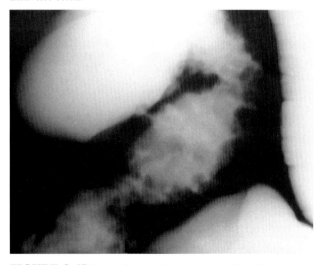

FIGURE 8-4B Image from barium enema coned to the region of the cecum and terminal ileum. The mucosal irregularity and nodularity within the terminal ileum and cecum is seen to better advantage.

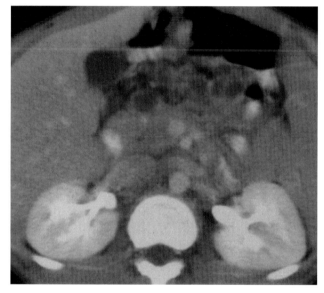

FIGURE 8-4C Contrast-enhanced CT scan of the abdomen. Mesenteric adenopathy is present. Some of the lymph nodes have central low attenuation areas.

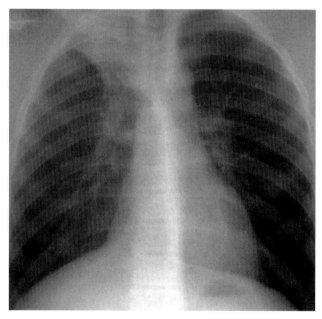

FIGURE 8-4D Frontal radiograph of the chest. Partial collapse of the right upper lobe with elevation of the right hilum is seen.

◆ DIFFERENTIAL DIAGNOSIS

◆ **Crohn's disease:** This diffuse process could cause the barium enema findings but would not explain the findings in the upper abdomen and chest.

◆ **Infectious colitis:** *Salmonella* and *Shigella* enterocolitis and amebiasis can cause abnormalities of the ascending colon. These entities would be unlikely to cause the degree of mucosal ulceration and nodularity seen in the case presented. In addition, they would not explain the findings on the chest radiograph and upper abdomen CT scan.

◆ **Appendicitis:** The inflammatory process resulting from appendicitis can involve the colon and terminal ileum and result in wall thickening. It would be unlikely, however, to cause mucosal destruction.

◆ **Neutropenic colitis:** This diagnosis is not a consideration because the patient is not neutropenic.

◆ **Hemorrhage or ischemic edema:** This entity would not be expected to cause the low attenuation adenopathy and chest radiographic findings.

◆ **Tuberculosis (TB):** This entity provides a unifying diagnosis to explain the constellation of findings in the chest, abdomen, and colon. TB could cause upper lobe disease, fibrosis, and volume loss in the chest, as well as the low attenuation of lymph nodes in the upper abdomen. Furthermore, tuberculous involvement of the colon can mimic Crohn's disease.

◆ DIAGNOSIS: Tuberculosis.

◆ KEY FACTS

CLINICAL

◆ Postprimary TB is rare in children who were infected before 2 years of age. This entity is most commonly seen when initial infection was in adolescence.

◆ Postprimary TB in the lungs can produce fibroreticular or fibronodular opacities in the upper lobes. Superior retraction of the hila, fibrosis of the upper lobes, traction bronchiectasis, volume loss, and focal calcification can result. Cavitation and apical pleural thickening can also be seen. Lymphadenopathy is rare in children with postprimary TB.

◆ In children, similar chest radiographic appearances can be seen with histoplasmosis and atypical mycobacterial infections. Cystic fibrosis can have a similar appearance and distribution but increased lung volumes would be expected.

◆ Gastrointestinal TB in industrialized countries is currently most commonly due to *Mycobacterium tuberculosis*. As a result of improved milk hygiene, *M. bovis* as a gastrointestinal pathogen has been largely controlled.

◆ The most common sites of tuberculous involvement of the gastrointestinal tract are the ileocecal region and the ascending colon.

◆ The clinical symptoms of patients with colonic TB are nonspecific and include diarrhea, abdominal pain, weight loss, and fever.

◆ Colonic TB is commonly seen with either concurrent or prior pulmonary TB, but pulmonary TB need not be present.

◆ Diagnosis of gastrointestinal TB depends on biopsy or segmental resection, because stool examination, cultures, and colonoscopic examinations are frequently nondiagnostic.

RADIOLOGIC

◆ Radiographic findings in children with postprimary pulmonary TB are similar to those seen in adults (postprimary infections are rare in children with normal immune systems) and primarily include a heterogeneous (sometimes cavitary) opacity in the upper lobes. Severe fibrosis can lead to upper lobe volume loss, hilar retraction, and secondary tracheomegaly. Pleural thickening is also common.

◆ Caseous necrosis occurs more often in the mesenteric lymph nodes than the bowel wall. Low attenuation lymph nodes, however, are not unique to TB and can also be found with gonadal metastases, atypical mycobacteria, and lymphoma.

◆ TB involvement of the colon is evident by mucosal ulceration and nodularity, mural rigidity, luminal narrowing, and fistulae. Involvement can be segmental. Occasionally, an intraluminal mass can be identified.

◆ Colonic TB can be radiologically indistinguishable from Crohn's disease. Other potential diagnoses include amebiasis, colonic ischemia, schistosomiasis, and lymphoma. Primary bowel adenocarcinoma can cause a similar picture but is found nearly exclusively in adults.

◆ SUGGESTED READING

Balthazar EJ, Bryk D. Segmental tuberculosis of the distal colon: Radiographic features in 7 cases. Gastrointest Radiol 1980;5:75–80.

Carrera GF, Young S, Lewicki AM. Intestinal tuberculosis. Gastrointest Radiol 1976;1:147–155.

Kuhn JP, Slovis TL, Silverman FN, Kuhns LR. The Neck and Respiratory System. In FN Silverman, JP Kuhn, Caffey's Pediatric X-Ray Diagnosis. St. Louis: Mosby, 1992;511–560.

McAdams HP, Erasmus J, Winter JA. Radiologic manifestations of pulmonary tuberculosis. Radiol Clin North Am 1995;33: 655–678.

Woodring JH, Vandiviere HM, Fried AM, et al. Update: The radiographic features of pulmonary tuberculosis. AJR Am J Roentgenol 1986;146:497–506.

CASE 5

Cindy R. Miller

HISTORY

A 5-year-old boy with a 2-month history of tibial pain and limp.

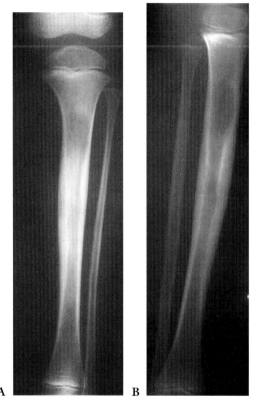

FIGURES 8-5A and 8-5B Frontal (**A**) and lateral (**B**) radiographs of the left tibia. A diaphyseal lesion is present that is lucent and permeative proximally and has sclerosis, cortical thickening, and periosteal reaction more inferiorly.

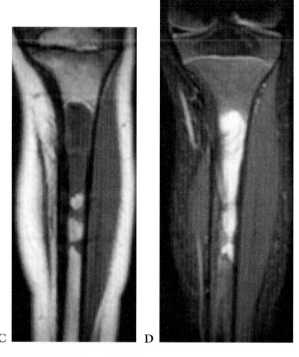

FIGURES 8-5C and 8-5D Noncontrast coronal T1-weighted (**C**) and STIR (relative T2-weighted, fat suppressed) (**D**) images of the left tibia. Abnormal marrow signal is present in the tibial diaphysis on both images. A small region of extraosseous signal abnormality is seen in Figure 8-5D.

◆DIFFERENTIAL DIAGNOSIS

The major considerations in this differential are the small, round, blue cell tumors of childhood. All may present with a permeative pattern and a wide zone of transition.

- **Metastases:** Especially those due to neuroblastoma and rhabdomyosarcoma.
- **Leukemia and lymphoma:** This is a reasonable consideration because the lymphoproliferative malignancies are the most common childhood cancer. Bone abnormalities in leukemia are fairly common (osteoporosis, metaphyseal lucencies, periosteal reaction, sclerotic or lucent lesions, permeative patterns); the involvement is most often multifocal and symmetrical, however. Lymphoma may have an identical appearance.
- **Ewing's sarcoma:** A good consideration based on the history and radiographic findings.
- **Primitive neuroectodermal tumors (PNETs):** Both central nervous system (i.e., medulloblastoma) and non–central nervous system (includes Askin's tumor of the chest wall) types of metastatic PNETs can present with the above history and findings, usually in older children and adolescents.

Considerations other than the small, round, blue cell tumors include:

- **Osteomyelitis:** It may be impossible to differentiate osteomyelitis from Ewing's sarcoma clinically and radiologically.
- **Eosinophilic granuloma:** This entity has a large variety of appearances (classically a lucent defect) that include an aggressive appearance such as this one.

◆DIAGNOSIS: Ewing's sarcoma.

◆KEY FACTS

CLINICAL

- Of the small, round, blue cell tumors discussed above, Ewing's sarcoma and PNET tumors can be very difficult to distinguish clinically, radiographically, and histologically. Electron microscopy may be necessary to demonstrate neural substances or structures not found with Ewing's sarcoma.
- Ewing's sarcoma occurs most commonly in the second half of the first decade of life and the first half of the second decade, a slightly younger age distribution than that of osteosarcoma.
- Males are affected slightly more commonly than females (3 to 2).
- There is a distinct predilection for whites; Ewing's sarcoma is uncommon in Asians and African-Americans.
- The clinical presentation may be identical with that of osteomyelitis, with systemic symptoms of fever, elevated sedimentation rate, and leukocytosis.

- Metastatic spread is most often to other bones and to the lungs, being present in between 10% and 30% of cases at time of diagnosis.
- Poor prognostic indicators include large size (>8 cm), central location, nonresectability, older age, and elevated erythrocyte sedimentation rate and leukocyte count at time of presentation.
- Survival rates have increased significantly with use of preoperative chemotherapy.

RADIOLOGIC

- More than 50% of Ewing's sarcomas arise in the long bones of the extremities, being more common in the lower extremities. The ribs and ilium are the most common flat bones affected. In fact, lesions in the femur account for 23% and those in the ilium for 17% of all cases.
- Lesions are usually metadiaphyseal in location (45%). Diaphyseal lesions are the next most common (33%); metaphyseal lesions are least common (15%).
- Plain films underestimate the extent of bone involved. The most typical pattern is a permeative, lytic pattern accompanied by periosteal reaction. However, other patterns include larger, "moth-eaten" lytic foci, a mixed lytic and sclerotic pattern, bony expansion, and a predominantly sclerotic pattern.
- Ewing's sarcoma of flat bones typically has a large soft-tissue component relative to the osseous component, in contrast to Ewing's sarcoma of long bones.
- MRI is indispensable in evaluating the extent of tumoral involvement of bone, marrow, and soft tissues. There is low signal on T1-weighted images and increased signal on T2-weighted images, except in areas of fibrosis, which will be of low signal. Intravenous contrast material can be used to distinguish tumor from peritumoral edema.
- Both skeletal and adjacent soft tissue components of a Ewing's sarcoma will take up Tc-99m methylene diphosphonate. In addition, bony reaction to the presence of tumor will accumulate the tracer.
- Ewing's sarcoma is gallium-67-citrate avid. Gallium is not accumulated in regions of bony reaction to the presence of tumor.

◆SUGGESTED READING

Dahlin DC, Coventry MB, Scanlon PW. Ewing's sarcoma. A critical analysis of 165 cases. J Bone Joint Surg 1961;43:185–192.

Dehner LP. Primitive neuroectodermal tumor and Ewing's sarcoma. Am J Surg Pathol 1993;17:1–13.

Eggli KD, Quiogue T, Moser RP. Ewing's sarcoma. Radiol Clin North Am 1993;31:325–337.

CASE 6

Donald P. Frush

HISTORY

A 6-year-old girl with fever, cough, and acute stridor.

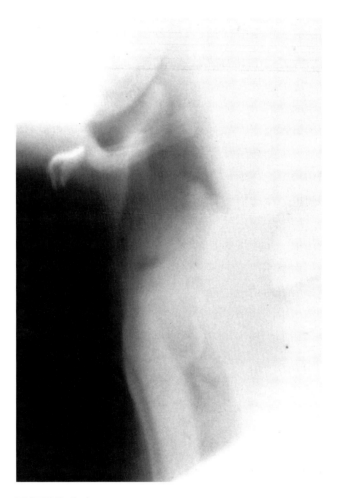

FIGURE 8-6 Lateral airway radiograph. Subtle heterogeneous haziness ("clouding") is seen in the cervical segment of the trachea, along with a curvilinear density in the subglottic trachea.

◆ DIFFERENTIAL DIAGNOSIS

◆ **Tracheal foreign body:** This diagnosis is a possible consideration, but there is no history of aspiration of a foreign body.

◆ **Papilloma:** Papillomas do not usually present with acute stridor and fever; rather, chronic hoarseness is more typical. Furthermore, the opacities in this case are not mass-like, as would be expected with papillomas.

◆ **Tracheal mucus:** This diagnosis is a reasonable consideration that cannot be excluded on the basis of the present study.

◆ **Bacterial tracheitis:** This diagnosis is consistent with the history and radiographic findings.

◆ **Epiglottitis:** The history presented in this case is typical for epiglottitis, but the epiglottis is normal in appearance.

◆ **Croup (laryngotracheobronchitis):** Croup usually occurs in children age 6 months to 3 years, much younger than the child in this case. Furthermore, narrowing of the subglottic trachea ("steeple sign"), which would be expected in croup, is not present.

◆ **Granuloma:** This is an unlikely diagnosis because there is no history of previous tracheal intubation or other trauma.

◆ **Retropharyngeal abscess:** The retropharyngeal soft tissues are normal in this case, excluding the diagnosis of a retropharyngeal abscess as a cause of the stridor.

◆ DIAGNOSIS: Bacterial tracheitis (also known as membranous croup or membranous laryngotracheobronchitis).

◆ KEY FACTS

CLINICAL

◆ Tracheitis is rare compared with other infectious causes of stridor (e.g., retropharyngeal abscess, croup, or epiglottitis).

◆ Acute onset of stridor is typical.

◆ The mean age at presentation is 4 years old, but bacterial tracheitis can be seen at any age.

◆ Prompt recognition is important, because membranes can obstruct the airway acutely.

◆ Infection is bacterial in origin. *Staphyloccus aureus* is the most common agent, but occasionally *Streptococcus pneumoniae* and *Haemophilus influenza* can produce the infection. Tracheitis can also occur as a superinfection following a viral upper airway process.

◆ Flexible endoscopy to confirm the diagnosis is indicated if clinical or radiographic findings suggest tracheitis.

◆ Management includes supportive care (humidification, antibiotics, suctioning). "Elective" intubation may be necessary to protect the airway from obstruction.

RADIOLOGIC

◆ Lateral airway radiographic findings can include "clouding" of trachea, intraluminal tracheal opacities, and wall irregularity.

◆ Occasionally, associated subglottic narrowing can be seen.

◆ The epiglottis and retropharyngeal tissues are normal in tracheitis, distinguishing this entity from other infectious causes of acute stridor in children.

◆ Fifty percent of cases have associated pneumonia.

◆ Importantly, a normal radiograph does not exclude diagnosis of tracheitis.

◆ The major alternative diagnosis based on radiographic findings is tracheal mucus accumulation. The two entities can be indistinguishable on the lateral airway film. Because early treatment of tracheitis is important, this diagnosis should be favored in equivocal cases and treatment begun.

◆ SUGGESTED READING

Eckel H, Widemann B, Damm M, Roth B. Airway endoscopy in the diagnosis and treatment of bacterial tracheitis in children. Int J Pediatr Otorhinolaryngol 1993;27:147–157.

Gallagher P, Myer CM. An approach to the diagnosis and treatment of membranous laryngotracheobronchitis in infants and children. Pediatr Emerg Care 1991;7:337–342.

John SD, Swischuk LE. Stridor and upper airway obstruction in infants and children. Radiographics 1991;12:625–643.

Seigler R. Bacterial tracheitis: Recognition and treatment. J SC Med Assoc 1993;89:83–87.

Walker P, Crysdale W. Croup, epiglottitis, retropharyngeal abscess, and bacterial tracheitis: Evolving patterns of occurrence and care. Int Anesthesiol Clin 1992;30:57–70.

Sara M. O'Hara

HISTORY

A 5-week-old girl with persistent, nonbilious vomiting. There is no history of diarrhea or fever.

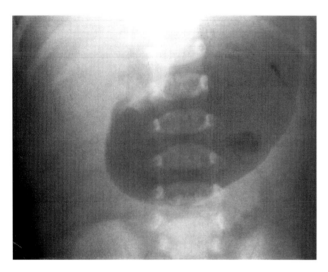

FIGURE 8-7A Anteroposterior abdominal radiograph. The stomach is markedly distended with gas. Minimal bowel gas is seen distally.

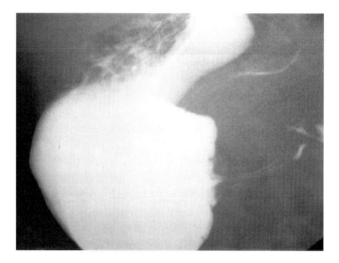

FIGURE 8-7B Upper gastrointestinal series; lateral view of the stomach. A large pool of barium is present in the stomach. Thin lines of barium are visible in an elongated pylorus. Only a very small amount of barium is present in the duodenal bulb.

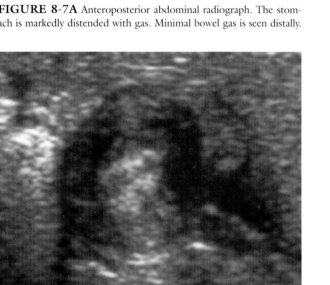

FIGURE 8-7C Transverse sonographic views of the right upper quadrant. The hypoechoic muscularis is thickened (measuring about 6 mm) and surrounds echogenic mucosa.

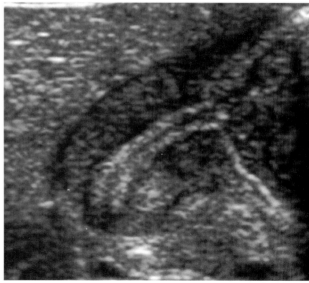

FIGURE 8-7D Longitudinal sonographic views of the right upper quadrant. The pyloric channel is elongated and has a thickened muscularis.

◆ DIFFERENTIAL DIAGNOSIS

◆ **Gastroesophageal reflux:** The patient's history makes this diagnosis a possibility. However, no reflux of contrast material is seen at fluoroscopy. Instead, a pyloric abnormality is visible on upper gastrointestinal series and sonography.

◆ **Pylorospasm:** This is an unlikely diagnosis based on the clinical history and imaging findings. Pylorospasm can be seen in patients who are extremely agitated, dehydrated, or septic, or who have adrenogenital syndrome, none of which appeared in this patient. Furthermore, pylorospasm is unlikely to persist throughout the series of examinations.

◆ **Pyloric channel ulcer:** This entity could account for the delayed gastric emptying and vomiting. However, no ulcer is identified on the imaging studies shown.

◆ **Antral web:** Antral web is another cause of delayed gastric emptying and vomiting. Again, no evidence of an obstructing web is seen on the imaging studies.

◆ **Hypertrophic pyloric stenosis (HPS):** This entity is the best diagnosis based on the history and imaging findings. The sonographic findings of concentric thickening of the pyloric muscularis and elongation of the pyloric channel are typical for this entity. The multiple thin tracks of barium visible in the pyloric channel on the UGI series represent folds of mucosa in a narrowed channel, further evidence of HPS.

◆ **Malrotation with obstruction:** This diagnosis is untenable for a number of reasons. First, in malrotation the site of obstruction is the duodenum, not the pylorus. In the first month of life the obstruction from malrotation is due to midgut volvulus. With malrotation later in infancy and childhood, Ladd bands (peritoneal reflections) cause obstruction and vomiting as they cross the duodenum and fix the malpositioned cecum. Second, volvulus typically presents with bilious vomiting, and nonbilious vomiting is rare.

◆ **Congenital atresia:** Congenital atresia presents clinically much earlier than the patient in the case illustrated. Duodenal atresia is evident at birth with a radiographic "double bubble" due to gas-distended stomach and proximal duodenum. Ileal atresia is evident at birth with distension and vomiting, which is often bilious.

◆ DIAGNOSIS: Hypertrophic pyloric stenosis.

◆ KEY FACTS

CLINICAL
◆ HPS is the most common infantile gastrointestinal abnormality requiring surgery, typically occurring in white boys at a peak age of 4 to 8 weeks.

◆ The clinical presentation is that of nonbilious vomiting, which gradually increases in severity from low-

velocity regurgitation to projectile vomiting. Weight loss, dehydration, and hypochloremic acidosis can occur secondarily. Nonetheless, most patients appear healthy but hungry.

◆ A palpable thickened pylorus ("olive") in the epigastrium is pathognomonic but is usually detectable only by the trained examiner. When an olive is present in the setting of suspected HPS, no preoperative imaging is necessary.

◆ The treatment is pyloromyotomy. Although spontaneous regression of muscular hypertrophy can occur without surgery, nonoperative therapy is difficult to justify given quick, safe, and effective surgical treatment.

◆ A 1981 report in the surgical literature reported an increase in genitourinary abnormalities in children with HPS and recommended routine renal evaluation. More recent studies have not shown such an increased prevalence.

RADIOLOGIC
◆ Plain film findings include (1) gastric distention, (2) mottled retained gastric contents, (3) indentations in gastric wall by hyperperistaltic waves ("caterpillar" stomach), and (4) diminished air beyond the pylorus.

◆ Barium study findings include (1) delayed gastric emptying, (2) string sign through the pyloric channel, (3) double or triple track sign in pyloric channel, (4) "shouldering" in the antrum from muscular hypertrophy, (5) a "beak" sign of contrast material at the pyloric entrance, and (6) indentation on the duodenal bulb by hypertrophied muscularis.

◆ Sonographic findings include an elongated (≥15 mm) pyloric channel and increased thickness (≥3 mm) of the hypoechoic muscle, which are more sensitive than the cross-sectional diameter of the entire pylorus for diagnosis of HPS. A "target" or bull's eye appearance of the pyloric channel is seen on transverse sonographic images. Scanning at a tangent to the pylorus can cause a false-positive examination, because it produces "pseudo-thickening" of the muscularis. So-called "pseudoelongation" of the pyloric channel, another potential cause of false-positive examinations, can result from pylorospasm and use of prostaglandins.

◆ SUGGESTED READING
Blumhagen JD, Maclin L, Krauter D, et al. Sonographic diagnosis of hypertrophic pyloric stenosis. AJR Am J Roentgenol 1988;150: 1367–1370.

Fernbach SK, Morello FP. Renal abnormalities in children with hypertrophic pyloric stenosis—Fact or fallacy? Pediatr Radiol 1993;23:286–288.

Hernanz-Schulman M, Sells L, Ambrosino MM, et al. Hypertrophic pyloric stenosis in the infant without a palpable olive: Accuracy of sonographic diagnosis. Radiology 1994;193:771–776.

O'Keeffe FN, Stansberry SD, Swischuk LE, Hayden CK Jr. Antropyloric muscle thickness at US in infants: What is normal. Radiology 1991;178:827–830.

CASE 8

Cindy R. Miller

HISTORY

A 1-month-old boy with torticollis and a firm mass on the right side of the neck.

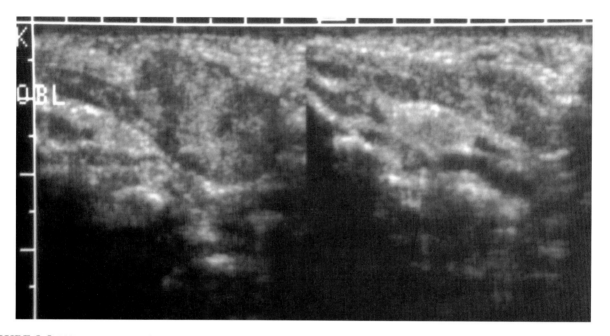

FIGURE 8-8 Oblique sonogram of the right sternocleidomastoid muscle **(left)** and similar view of the left sternocleidomastoid muscle **(right)**. The superior and inferior aspects of the right sternocleidomastoid muscle are normal in appearance. However, there is a well-defined mass that is homogeneous and nearly identical in echotecture to muscle along the course of the sternocleidomastoid muscle. The left sternocleidomastoid muscle is normal in appearance.

◆ DIFFERENTIAL DIAGNOSIS

The differential diagnosis for a mass in this specific location with this clinical history and these sonographic features is very limited. However, a differential diagnosis for a mass in the neck of an infant will be reviewed.

- **Branchial cleft cyst:** This is an unlikely consideration because no cystic components are seen in the mass. These usually arise from the second branchial cleft (occasionally the third). These lesions are typically located anterior to the sternocleidomastoid and may displace it posteriorly. Cysts are also fluctuant and not firm unless inflamed. These lesions usually present later in childhood, often with inflammation.
- **Lymphangioma/hemangioma:** These lesions most often arise from the posterior triangle, dorsal to the sternocleidomastoid. Typically, lymphangiomas/hemangiomas do not displace adjacent structures, but rather insinuate themselves between other structures. Typically, there will be cystic components; those with large cystic components are referred to as *cystic hygromas*. For these reasons, a lymphangioma is not a good consideration.
- **Thyroglossal duct cyst:** The location excludes this diagnosis. These lesions are located in the midline from the base of the tongue to the thyroid (many are in the hyoid bone). As with branchial cleft cysts, imaging shows a purely cystic lesion unless infection or internal hemorrhage has occurred.
- **Adenopathy/adenitis:** Enlarged lymph nodes have a characteristic well-defined, hypoechoic appearance. Furthermore, adenitis is rarely seen in infants under the age of 6 months.
- **Malignancy:** Malignancy is rare at this age. The three most common malignancies seen in the neck in a child are rhabdomyosarcoma, lymphoma, and neuroblastoma. Rhabdomyosarcoma is a consideration in this case because the lesion arises in muscle. The other two lesions are excluded based on the intramuscular location.
- **Ectopic cervical thymus:** This is a solid mass that may not be contiguous with the normal thymus. However, ectopic thymic tissue would be separable from the sternocleidomastoid muscle. Unlike the normal thymus, ectopic thymus can cause airway symptoms but is usually asymptomatic.

Fibromatosis colli: The clinical history of torticollis in a young infant and the sonographic finding of a mass that is isoechoic to muscle are typical of this diagnosis.

◆ DIAGNOSIS: Fibromatosis colli.

◆ KEY FACTS

CLINICAL

- Fibromatosis colli presents as a mass in the sternocleidomastoid 2 or more weeks following birth. Frequently, a history of birth trauma is present.
- Fibromatosis colli typically presents with torticollis, chin pointed away from the side of the palpable mass, and a firm, nontender mass along the course of the sternocleidomastoid.
- Management is typically conservative, with passive range of motion therapy or no therapy.
- The mass usually spontaneously regresses over a 4- to 8-month interval. Only very rarely is surgery required.

RADIOLOGIC

- Sonography is the imaging modality most frequently utilized when fibromatosis colli is suspected. It is convenient because no sedation is necessary. The real-time examination confirms that the lesion moves with the sternocleidomastoid muscle.
- Fibromatosis colli may result in diffuse or focal enlargement of the sternocleidomastoid muscle. It is usually isoechoic to muscle but may have echogenicity slightly greater or less than the muscle.
- Occasionally CT or MRI can be used to image patients with atypical clinical presentations. With both techniques, a well-defined homogeneous mass that is identical in appearance to the normal muscle is seen to follow the course of the sternocleidomastoid muscle. No (or minimal) contrast enhancement is seen. Rarely, there is inhomogeneity following hemorrhage. In these cases, the differential diagnosis should include rhabdomyosarcoma.

◆ SUGGESTED READING

Bloom DA, Applegate K, Laor T, et al. Pediatric case of the day. Radiographics 1996;16:204–206.

Siegel MJ. Pediatric Sonography. New York: Raven, 1991:70–72.

Vazquez E, Enriquez G, Castellote A, et al. US, CT, and MR imaging of neck lesions in children. Radiographics 1995;15:105–122.

CASE 9
Donald P. Frush

HISTORY

A 5-year-old boy with recurrent right lower-lobe pneumonia.

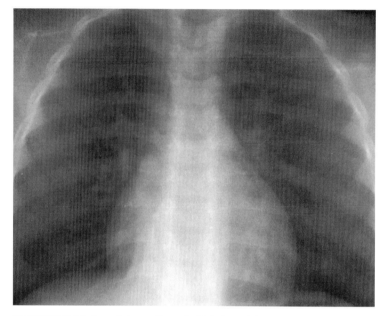

FIGURE 8-9A Frontal chest radiograph. Right lower lobe airspace disease is present.

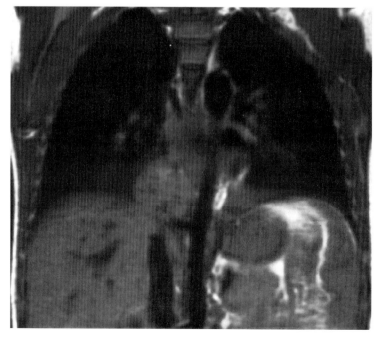

FIGURE 8-9B Coronal T1-weighted noncontrast MRI of the chest in a different patient with the same diagnosis. A posterior paraspinal mass is present, with arterial supply originating directly from the descending thoracic aorta.

◆ DIFFERENTIAL DIAGNOSIS

- **Pulmonary sequestration:** This diagnosis is the most likely, given the history of recurrent infection, lower-lobe location, and systemic arterial supply.
- **Bronchogenic cyst:** This diagnosis is unlikely because a systemic vascular supply would not be expected to be present.
- **Arteriovenous malformation (AVM):** Pulmonary AVMs frequently have an appearance of multiple, mass-like lesions with prominent feeding arteries, which can be of systemic origin. However, the absence of draining veins in the cases illustrated makes AVM an unlikely diagnosis.
- **Recurrent pneumonia/atelectasis from an endobronchial or exobronchial lesion:** The clinical history and chest radiograph are consistent with this diagnosis. Furthermore, a site of recurrent infection can acquire a systemic arterial supply (considered an acquired intralobar sequestration [see below]). However, it is rare in the setting of pneumonia and is not seen with atelectasis. Another form of pneumonia, so-called round pneumonia, is a consideration based on the findings on the chest radiograph in Figure 8-9A but is not compatible with the MRI of the chest in Figure 8-9B.
- **Pulmonary neoplasm:** This is an unlikely diagnosis because these are very rare lesions in children and blood supply from the aorta is not a typical feature.
- **Diaphragmatic hernia/eventration:** The radiographic appearance of this lesion can mimic that of sequestration in some cases, but small diaphragmatic abnormalities are generally clinically silent. Diaphragmatic abnormalities would be expected to be well defined, unlike the appearance of the lesion in Figure 8-9A.

◆ DIAGNOSIS: Pulmonary sequestration (intralobar type).

◆ KEY FACTS

CLINICAL

- The term *sequestration* refers to a nonfunctioning pulmonary parenchymal abnormality that lacks normal tracheobronchial communication and has anomalous systemic (rather than pulmonary) arterial supply. Venous drainage may also be via systemic veins rather than pulmonary veins.
- Traditionally, *intralobar* (i.e., no separate pleura) and *extralobar* (i.e., having a separate pleural investment) types have been distinguished. Sequestration is one of the continuum of bronchopulmonary foregut malformations (variable contribution of anomalies of lung, airway, and vasculature).
- Modes of presentation generally differ according to the age at time of diagnosis.

- In the prenatal period, the diagnosis is based on the finding of an echogenic chest mass at sonography.
- The clinical presentation in the neonatal period consists of respiratory distress.
- In a child (and occasionally an adult), the clinical presentation is that of recurrent pulmonary infections.
- More than half of sequestrations present before adulthood.
- Sequestration can occasionally present in an infant or small child as a murmur and congestive heart failure due to the arteriovenous shunting.
- The intralobar type is the more common type and can be congenital or acquired. Most of these are lower lobe in location, with two-thirds located on the left. Drainage is usually via the pulmonary veins.
- The extralobar type also usually occurs in the lower lobe and is on the left in 90% of cases. Drainage is typically through systemic veins. Fifty percent of cases have associated anomalies (heart disease, diaphragmatic hernias, gastrointestinal and other pulmonary abnormalities). Most extralobar sequestrations are discovered within the first year of life.
- Treatment for all pulmonary sequestrations is surgical excision.

RADIOLOGIC

- The sequestered lung can receive air flow through collateral sources. Therefore, before recurrent infections have occurred, the radiologic appearance can be normal.
- The diagnosis should be considered when persistent or recurrent lower lobe opacity is found.
- Catheter angiography has been replaced by other, non-invasive imaging studies to determine vascular supply. MRI is especially useful for this purpose.
- Helical CT with bolus infusion of contrast material can also be used to diagnose pulmonary sequestration. The systemic vascular supply is well seen.
- Sonography with color Doppler can be used to document arterial supply if a good acoustic window is present to facilitate imaging.

◆ SUGGESTED READING

Felker RE, Tonkin ILD. Imaging of pulmonary sequestration. AJR Am J Roentgenol 1990;154:241–249.

Frush DP, Donnelly LE. Pulmonary sequestration: A new spin with helical CT. AJR Am J Roentgenol 1997;169:679–682.

Kent M. Intralobar pulmonary sequestration. Prog Pediatr Surg 1991;27:894–891.

Kravitz RM. Congenital malformations of the lungs. Pediatr Clin North Am 1994;41:453–472.

Louie HW, Martin SM, Mulder DG. Pulmonary sequestration: 17-year experience at UCLA. Am Surg 1993;59:801–805.

Nicolette LA, Koloske AM, Bartow SA, Murphy S. Intralobar pulmonary sequestration: A clinical and pathological spectrum. J Pediatr Surg 1993;28:802–805.

HISTORY

A full-term infant being evaluated for an abnormality seen on prenatal ultrasound.

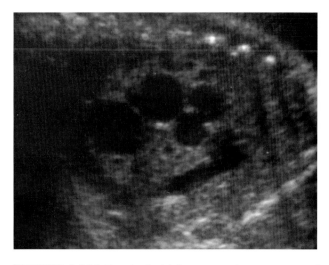

FIGURE 8-10A Longitudinal left upper quadrant sonogram of the fetus. The spine and ribs are in the near field. A subjacent multicystic mass is present.

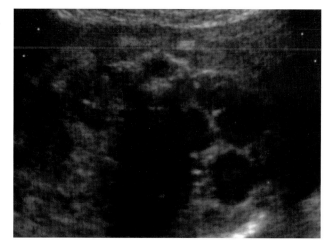

FIGURE 8-10B Transverse left upper quadrant sonogram of the fetus. The spine is present in the midline and produces posterior acoustic shadowing. The relatively hypoechoic right kidney is visible just to the left of the spine. The large multicystic structure seen on the longitudinal image is identified in the contralateral left renal fossa.

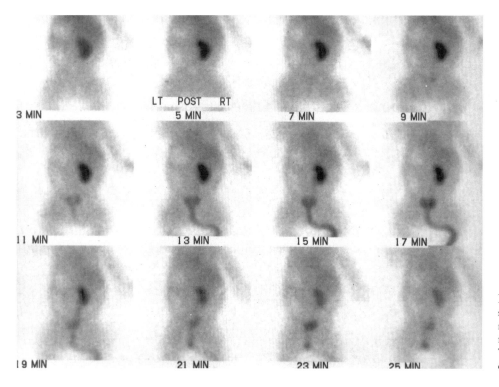

FIGURE 8-10C Posterior renal scintigraphy images from a MAG-3 renal scan performed after birth. No functional left renal tissue is seen. The right kidney functions well. A catheter drains the urinary bladder.

◆ DIFFERENTIAL DIAGNOSIS

◆ **Severe hydronephrosis or obstructed duplication:** This diagnosis is unlikely because the cystic spaces would be expected to communicate, unlike in the case presented. Furthermore, if a distal obstruction was present, a dilated ureter would be expected to be seen.

◆ **Ureteropelvic junction obstruction:** Again, the cystic spaces do not communicate with a centrally located, dilated renal pelvis, making this an unlikely diagnosis.

◆ **Cystic Wilms' tumor or other renal tumor:** Antenatal and congenital renal tumors are rare. Multilocular cystic nephroma is a lesion that could be considered in this case. The presence of a rim of functional renal tissue on nuclear imaging (not present in this case) would make this a more likely diagnosis.

◆ **Multicystic dysplastic kidney (MCDK):** MCDK is the best diagnosis based on the fact that this entity is relatively common, the cysts are interconnecting, and functioning renal tissue is absent on the nuclear medicine study.

◆ DIAGNOSIS: Multicystic dysplastic kidney.

◆ KEY FACTS

CLINICAL

◆ MCDK is the second most common abdominal mass in neonates, second only to hydronephrosis.

◆ MCDK is the most common palpable abdominal mass on the first day of life. An increasing number of cases are now initially seen on prenatal ultrasound and confirmed with additional imaging studies in infancy.

◆ The etiology of MCDK is thought to be atresia of the ureteric bud or failure of the ureteric bud to meet and induce the metanephric blastema in utero.

◆ Approximately one-third of patients with MCDK have contralateral renal abnormalities, most commonly ureteropelvic junction obstruction or reflux.

◆ Because the kidney involved by MCDK is nonfunctional, early detection and treatment of contralateral abnormalities are important to preserve function in the single functioning kidney.

RADIOLOGIC

◆ If the ureter alone is atretic, the hydronephrotic form of MCDK (which is rare) results with a dilated renal pelvis and potentially interconnecting cysts.

◆ More commonly, the entire renal pelvis and proximal ureter are atretic, resulting in the pelvoinfundibular form of MCDK, as seen in the case illustrated here.

◆ Segmental forms of MCDK have also been reported.

◆ Without drainage of urine, the glomeruli become dysplastic and the tubules atrophy, forming variably sized, fluid-filled cysts that do not communicate. There may be a thin rim of cortical tissue with hydronephrosis. In MCDK, the scattered parenchyma is echogenic and not cortical in distribution.

◆ Functional studies of the kidney can be obtained using Tc-99m MAG-3, Tc-99m DTPA (diethylenetriamine pentaacetic acid), or occasionally, other renal agents. Early images or blood flow images can show faint radiotracer activity initially, solely reflecting perfusion of the dysplastic tissue. Delayed images show complete absence of tracer activity in MCDK, as opposed to gradual accumulation of tracer activity in obstructed kidneys.

◆ A small amount of poorly functioning renal tissue is only rarely seen on renal scintigraphy of MCDK.

◆ MCDK is generally accepted to be a benign form of dysplasia. Serial sonographic examinations normally reveal regression of cysts and shrinkage of dysplastic kidney over several years. Rarely, some cysts can enlarge.

◆ A neoplasm arising in a kidney with MCDK is a rare event but should be suspected when a kidney with MCDK enlarges and should prompt surgical removal. Hypertension and infection are other potential complications of MCDK.

◆ SUGGESTED READING

Atiyeh B, Husman D, Baum M. Contralateral renal abnormalities in multicystic dysplastic kidney disease. J Pediatr 1992;122:65–67.

Strife JS, Souza AS, Kirks DR, et al. Multicystic dysplastic kidney in children: US follow-up. Radiology 1993;186:785–788.

Tyrrell PNM, Boivin CM, Burrell DN, et al. Multicystic dysplastic kidney: Another application of Tc-99m MAG3. Clin Radiol 1994;49:400–403.

CASE *11*

Donald P. Frush

HISTORY

An otherwise healthy 1-month-old girl with mild tachypnea.

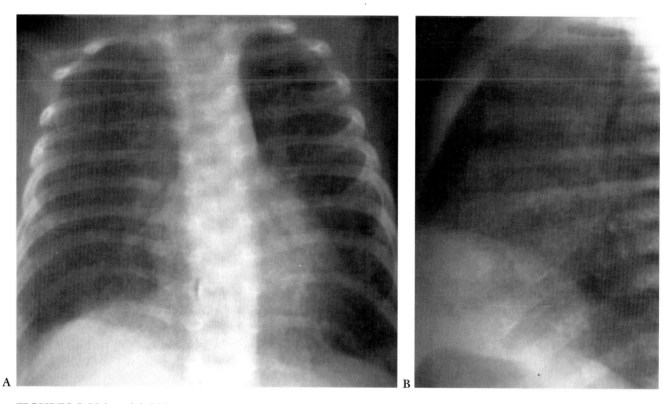

A   B

FIGURES 8-11A and 8-11B Frontal (**A**) and lateral (**B**) chest radiographs. Mild hyperinflation with symmetric aeration is present. Coarse reticular interstitial opacities are seen, but there are no focal opacities. No effusion or adenopathy is present. The heart is normal in size.

◆ DIFFERENTIAL DIAGNOSIS

- **Congestive heart failure:** The heart is not enlarged and there is no pleural effusion, as would be expected with congestive heart failure.
- **Viral pneumonitis:** This diagnosis should be considered on the basis of hyperinflation with interstitial opacities. However, the patient is only minimally symptomatic given the degree of radiographic abnormality, making this diagnosis unlikely.
- *Chlamydia* **pneumonia:** Neonatal conjunctivitis (absent in this case) is frequently, but not invariably, present. The radiographic findings are compatible with this diagnosis.
- **Noncardiac causes of pulmonary edema:** The clinical data in this case (e.g., the absence of sepsis) do not support the diagnosis of noncardiac edema. Primary pulmonary lymphangiectasia, another potential cause of noncardiac pulmonary edema, is usually quite evident earlier in infancy than in the case illustrated, making this diagnosis unlikely.
- **Delayed-onset group B streptococcal pneumonia:** This diagnosis is a possible consideration based on the radiographic findings. However, patients are usually quite ill. The clinical symptoms in the case illustrated, which are minimal, do not support this diagnosis.

◆ DIAGNOSIS: *Chlamydia* pneumonia (congenitally acquired).

◆ KEY FACTS

CLINICAL

- *Chlamydia* pneumonia is a congenitally acquired infection due to *Chlamydia trachomatis*, an obligate intracellular parasite with some features of bacteria.
- A history of neonatal conjunctivitis is present in about 50% of cases. Neonatal rhinitis is another associated feature.

- Symptoms occur beginning at 1 to 3 months, typically at 6 weeks of age.
- Clinical signs include minimal tachypnea, hypoxemia, and mild or absent fever. The radiographic abnormalities are often more impressive than the clinical features.
- Rhinorrhea and "staccato" cough are often present.
- *Chlamydia* is the most common cause of afebrile interstitial pneumonia in infants.
- The diagnosis can be made using a fluorescent antibody test performed on a nasal swab specimen.
- The standard treatment is erythromycin. The infection usually responds well to antibiotic treatment.
- Patients with *Chlamydia* pneumonia have a higher incidence of subsequent chronic respiratory problems compared to the general population.

RADIOLOGIC

- Typical radiologic findings are hyperinflation and coarse, usually diffuse, reticular (occasionally nodular), interstitial opacities.
- Scattered foci of atelectasis can occur and, more rarely, focal ill-defined opacities.
- *Chlamydia trachomatis* pneumonia can have an identical radiologic appearance to that of viral pneumonitis. However, a young age at onset (1 to 2 months), the presence of a staccato cough and rhinorrhea, and only minimal fever and respiratory symptoms strongly favors the diagnosis of *Chlamydia* pneumonia.
- Resolution of radiographic abnormalities typically lags behind clinical improvement.

◆ SUGGESTED READING

Condon VR. Pneumonia in children. J Thorac Imaging 1991;6: 31–44.

Hammerschlag MR. *Chlamydia trachomatis* in children. Pediatr Ann 1994;23:349–353.

Kirks DR. Practical Pediatric Imaging: Diagnostic Radiology of Infants and Children (2nd ed). Boston: Little, Brown, 1991.

CASE 12

Cindy R. Miller

HISTORY

A 2-year-old child who refuses to bear weight.

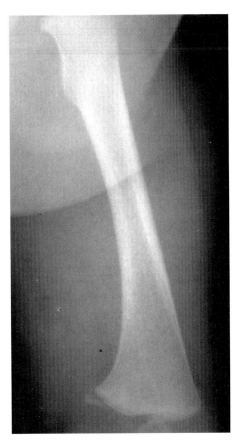

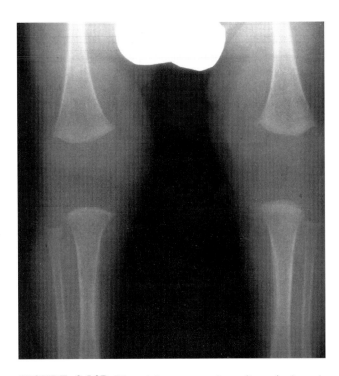

FIGURE 8-12B Bilateral lower extremity radiographs in a 4-month-old child with the same diagnosis. Subtle corner fractures involving the distal left femur and proximal left tibia are present. Periosteal reaction along the medial aspect of both tibial diaphyses is seen.

FIGURE 8-12A Left lower extremity radiograph. A "corner" fracture, synonymous with a "bucket-handle" fracture, is present at the medial aspect of the distal femoral metaphysis.

◆ DIFFERENTIAL DIAGNOSIS

◆ **Nonaccidental trauma (infant and child abuse):** This diagnosis is a likely consideration given the types of fractures in both cases. The clinical information in any individual case is important to rule out other entities that can mimic nonaccidental trauma.

◆ **Accidental trauma:** "Corner" fractures would not be expected to occur from accidental trauma resulting from activities in which a 2-year-old typically engages. Accidental injury is not a consideration for a fracture of this type and location in an infant who has not reached the age of walking (see Figure 8-12B).

◆ **Osteogenesis imperfecta (OI):** The presence of multiple fractures raises this entity as a possible diagnosis. In both cases illustrated above, there was a lack of clinical features (e.g., blue sclerae, deafness, poor dentition) that can be seen in OI.

◆ **Menkes' syndrome:** The clinical history in both of the cases illustrated excludes this diagnosis because patients with this syndrome have mental retardation and die in infancy.

◆ **Metaphyseal irregularity as a normal variant:** This variant is seen at the metaphyses as a "lip" of bone that is continuous with the cortical bone. However, if the lip is not continuous (as in both of the cases illustrated), a fracture is present.

◆ DIAGNOSIS: Child abuse (nonaccidental trauma).

◆ KEY FACTS

CLINICAL

◆ In addition to the multiple types of skeletal injuries seen in the setting of abuse, central nervous system (CNS) injury (e.g., subdural hematoma, diffuse edema, diffuse infarction from hypoxia, and parenchymal hemorrhage) can be present.

◆ The mechanism for these CNS injuries is currently thought to be impact against a soft object in combination with shaking, rather than shaking alone (as was previously thought).

◆ With respect to skeletal injuries, rib fractures are more common in children <1 year old, whereas diaphyseal injuries are more common in those >1 year old. This fact reflects the manner in which the child is typically held during the traumatic event.

◆ Direct blows to the abdomen most frequently result in duodenal hematoma, pancreatitis (with its attendant complications), and hepatic and splenic injuries.

◆ The diagnosis is established with a combination of history (i.e., incompatibility of the reported history in relation to the type and extent of injuries), physical findings (e.g., burns, hand marks, sexual abuse, preretinal hemorrhages), and radiographic findings.

◆ A major diagnostic consideration is OI, in which a family history of fractures, deafness, blue sclerae, and poor dentition can be elicited. If necessary, the diagnosis can be confirmed with a skin biopsy demonstrating a collagen synthesis deficiency.

◆ Another diagnostic consideration is Menkes' syndrome, a rare neurodegenerative disorder due to a defect in copper metabolism, leading to death within the first year of life. These patients have sparse, brittle hair, which accounts for the designation "kinky hair syndrome."

RADIOLOGIC

◆ Child or infant abuse can have CNS, intra-abdominal, or skeletal findings evident on imaging studies. The skeletal manifestations are reviewed below.

◆ Depending on the radiographic projection, a transverse fracture of the metaphysis can appear either as a corner fracture or a "bucket handle" fracture.

◆ Injuries that are highly specific for child abuse include corner fractures and fractures in such unusual locations as the scapulae, sternum, and vertebral posterior elements.

◆ Injuries that are moderately specific for child abuse include fractures of varying ages, complex fractures of the skull, and fractures involving the digits or vertebral bodies.

◆ Spiral fractures are considered injuries having low specificity for likelihood of causation by child abuse. However, suspicion should be raised when such fractures are seen in children who are too young to have engaged in activities that would make an accidental cause likely.

◆ One spiral fracture that should not raise suspicion for child abuse is the "toddler's fracture," a spiral fracture of the distal tibia. As its name implies, this injury is seen in children who are learning to walk. This fracture is not an indication for performing a skeletal survey.

◆ By far, most periosteal reaction in the infant is a normal, physiologic response which is typically seen between 1 and 6 months of age. It is characteristically manifested as a single (or occasionally multiple) thin layer of periosteal reaction on the medial aspect of the femur, tibia, humerus, and radius, and is symmetric in distribution.

◆ Radionuclide bone scan is a complementary method to plain films for detection of injuries due to abuse. A bone scan is particularly sensitive for detection of posterior rib fractures as well as diaphyseal injuries (which may actually be bowing fractures that can be inapparent on plain films).

◆ SUGGESTED READING

Bruce DA, Zimmerman RA. Shaken impact syndrome. Pediatr Ann 1989;18:482–494.

Conway JJ, Collins M, Tanz RR, et al. The role of bone scintigraphy in detecting child abuse. Semin Nucl Med 1993;23:321–333.

Harwood-Nash D. Abuse to the pediatric central nervous system. AJR Am J Roentgenol 1992;13:569–575.

Kleinman PK. Diagnostic imaging in infant abuse. AJR Am J Roentgenol 1990;155:703–712.

CASE 13 *Sara M. O'Hara*

HISTORY

A neonate with low hematocrit following traumatic delivery.

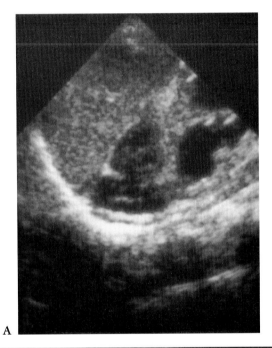

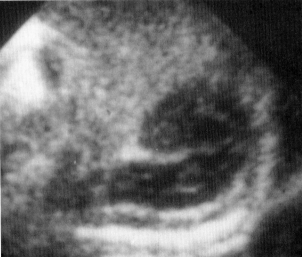

FIGURES 8-13A and 8-13B Longitudinal (A) and transverse (B) views from left upper quadrant sonogram. A structure with heterogeneous echogenicity is seen just superior to the left kidney in the expected location of the left adrenal gland. The limbs of the gland are enlarged but retain their pyramidal shape. Dilatation of the renal collecting system is seen but is an incidental finding.

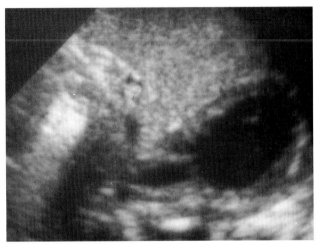

FIGURE 8-13C Transverse sonogram 10 days later. During the period since the initial study, the lesion has become hypoechoic, with an anechoic central region. An echogenic rim which is slightly irregular is evident.

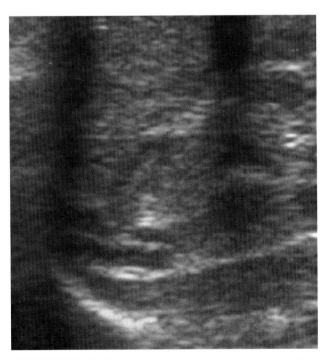

FIGURE 8-13D Transverse sonogram of adrenal gland in a different patient. An adrenal gland in a normal neonate is illustrated for comparison to the previous images. The gland has symmetric, hypoechoic limbs with a central echogenic stripe.

◆DIFFERENTIAL DIAGNOSIS

- **Neuroblastoma:** Congenital neuroblastoma is more often solid than cystic and would not be expected to change from solid to cystic without therapy (chemotherapy or biopsy producing internal hemorrhage). Neuroblastoma also tends to distort the shape of the adrenal gland. For these reasons, this is an unlikely diagnosis.
- **Other retroperitoneal tumors—e.g., lymphangioma, teratoma:** More fluid-filled spaces and calcification are typical of these tumors. They are very rarely located in the retroperitoneum, making them further unlikely considerations in this case.
- **Perinephric abscess:** A phlegmon or abscess could have mixed echogenicity similar to this lesion, but there is no history of infection. Furthermore, rather than a mass adjacent to the adrenal gland (as would be expected in a perinephric abscess), in this case it is the adrenal gland itself that is enlarged and hypoechoic.
- **Congenital adrenal hyperplasia:** This entity should involve the adrenal glands bilaterally. Biochemical abnormalities, which are not present in the case illustrated, are helpful in supporting the diagnosis of congenital adrenal hyperplasia. Therefore, this is an unlikely diagnosis.
- **Adrenal hemorrhage:** This process is the most likely diagnosis in this case based on the mixed echogenicity, retention of shape of the glands, and change in echotexture over a relatively short period of time.

◆DIAGNOSIS: Neonatal adrenal hemorrhage.

◆KEY FACTS

CLINICAL

- Spontaneous adrenal hemorrhage occurs relatively commonly in newborn infants and is occasionally detected in utero.
- Predisposing factors include perinatal stress, traumatic birth, hypoxia, and sepsis. Hemorrhage also occurs with increased frequency in large infants and infants of diabetic mothers.

- Large hemorrhages can present with shock or a palpable mass, while smaller hemorrhages cause mild anemia or jaundice. Biochemical abnormalities are seldom present in either the acute or convalescent phase.
- Adrenal hemorrhage is more common on the left side and is seen bilaterally in approximately 10% of cases.
- Complications are uncommon and include renal vein thrombosis (especially on the left side), secondary infection/abscess, and dystrophic calcification.

RADIOLOGIC

- Solid suprarenal masses in the neonate are most likely to represent either acute adrenal hemorrhage or neuroblastoma. Doppler evaluation of these lesions is helpful, because a hematoma is typically avascular, while a tumor is generally well vascularized.
- At sonography, the hemorrhage is typically initially echogenic, develops mixed echogenicity as the clot retracts, and becomes hypo- or anechoic as it liquefies. Serial sonographic studies documenting rapidly decreasing size exclude neuroblastoma.
- If a suprarenal mass increases in size or does not become more cystic with time, MRI examination should be performed for further evaluation. Even when neuroblastoma is the diagnosis in these infants, the prognosis is generally very good.
- Dystrophic calcifications can be the first radiologic indication of previous adrenal hemorrhage. Adrenal calcification, however, can also be seen in neuroblastoma, ganglioneuroblastoma, Wolman's syndrome, pheochromocytoma, tuberculosis, and adrenal carcinoma.

◆SUGGESTED READING

Dunnick NR. Adrenal imaging: Current status. AJR Am J Roentgenol 1990;154:927–936.

Hendry GMA. Cystic neuroblastoma of the adrenal gland—A potential source of error in ultrasonic diagnosis. Pediatr Radiol 1982;12:204–206.

Westra SJ, Zaninovic AC, Hall TR, et al. Imaging of the adrenal gland in children. Radiographics 1994;14:1323–1340.

HISTORY

A term neonate with mild tachypnea but no cyanosis.

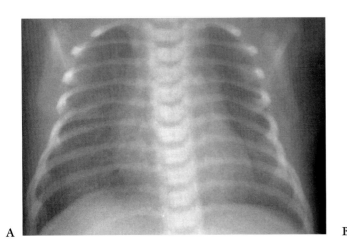

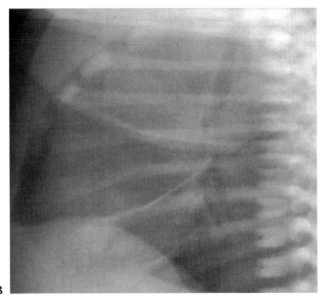

FIGURES 8-14A and 8-14B Frontal (**A**) and lateral (**B**) chest radiograph (2 hours postnatal). Normal lung volumes are present, with streaky hilar opacities, indistinct vascularity, and subpleural and pleural fluid. The heart size is normal.

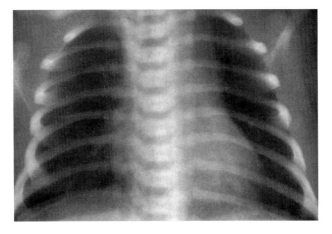

FIGURE 8-14C Frontal chest radiograph (48 hours postnatal). The abnormalities have almost completely resolved.

◆ DIFFERENTIAL DIAGNOSIS

- **Transient tachypnea of the newborn (TTN):** This is the most likely diagnosis in light of the clinical history of mild tachypnea and the rapid resolution of radiologic findings.
- **Respiratory distress due to surfactant deficiency (respiratory distress syndrome, hyaline membrane disease):** This entity is an unlikely diagnosis because, in this condition, the lung volumes are typically reduced (in an infant who is not intubated) and the presence of pleural fluid is very rare. The radiographic pattern with surfactant deficiency is that of a diffuse, fine ("ground glass"), granular appearance, unlike the case illustrated. Furthermore, this entity is seen nearly exclusively in preterm infants.
- **Meconium aspiration:** Generally more patchy opacities (atelectasis) with focal air trapping is seen in this disease process, rather than the streaky opacities seen in the case illustrated.
- **Congestive heart failure:** This is an unlikely diagnosis because the heart size is typically enlarged in congestive heart failure, unlike the case shown here.
- **Neonatal pneumonia:** This entity can initially have a similar radiographic appearance to the case shown here, but pneumonia does not spontaneously resolve in 48 hours. Furthermore, clinical information supporting infection (e.g., prolonged rupture of membranes, maternal fever, infant leukocytosis or leukopenia, infected amniotic fluid) was not present in the case illustrated.

◆ DIAGNOSIS: Transient tachypnea of the newborn (retained fetal lung fluid, wet-lung syndrome, persistent pulmonary edema).

◆ KEY FACTS

CLINICAL

- The radiographic and clinical findings of TTN are due to delayed clearance of fetal lung fluid from the pulmonary interstitium.

- TTN is probably the most common cause of neonatal respiratory distress.
- This entity is slightly more common in males.
- Risk factors for TTN include prolonged labor, cesarean section, precipitous delivery, maternal diabetes, neonatal hypoproteinemia, and maternal administration of hypotonic fluid.
- Tachypnea is present within the first few hours of life. Respiratory distress peaks by 24 hours and is nearly always resolved by 2 to 3 days. Other clinical features include occasional grunting, sternal and intercostal retractions, and mild cyanosis.
- Treatment is conservative and usually consists of an oxygen hood. Antibiotics may be given if it is unclear whether infection is the cause of symptoms.
- Neonatal pneumonia (group B streptococcus), hyaline membrane disease, meconium aspiration, asphyxia, congestive heart failure, and TTN can have similar clinical presentations in the first few hours of life.

RADIOLOGIC

- The radiographic appearance is typically that of streaky, coarse lines, with some haziness. Well-defined focal opacities are rare.
- Lung volumes are normal or increased in TTN, and the heart size is normal.
- Radiographic improvement generally parallels clinical improvement.
- Pulmonary effusions are usually small and are more common on the right.
- Follow-up radiographs are not necessary when the clinical and radiographic presentations are typical.

◆ SUGGESTED READING

Bland RD. Acute Respiratory Distress Syndromes in the Newborn. In AM Rudolph, JIE Hoffman, CD Rudolph (eds), Rudolph's Pediatrics (20th ed). Stamford, CT: Appleton & Lange, 1996;1597–1598.

Kirks DR. Practical Pediatric Imaging: Diagnostic Radiology of Infants and Children (2nd ed). Boston: Little, Brown, 1991.

CASE 15

George S. Bisset III

HISTORY

A 9-year-old boy who was involved as a pedestrian in a motor vehicle accident.

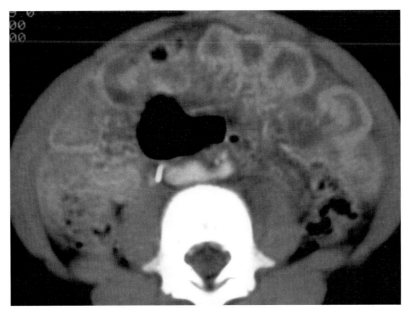

FIGURE 8-15A Contrast-enhanced CT image of the lower abdomen. Diffusely dilated, fluid-filled loops of bowel are seen with abnormal contrast enhancement of the bowel wall. Peritoneal fluid and increased attenuation of mesenteric fat are present. No pneumoperitoneum is present.

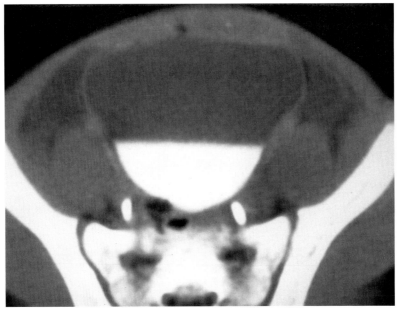

FIGURE 8-15B CT image through the pelvis. A moderate amount of free intraperitoneal fluid is seen lateral to the bladder.

◆ DIFFERENTIAL DIAGNOSIS

◆ **Hypoperfusion complex:** This entity is usually seen in the setting of post-traumatic hypovolemic shock and has the imaging findings of (1) abnormally increased contrast enhancement of the pancreas, kidneys, and bowel wall; (2) fluid-filled bowel loops with free peritoneal fluid; and (3) a small aorta and vena cava due to the reduced blood volume. However, usually more intense contrast enhancement of bowel wall and mesentery is seen than in the present case. The diminished caliber of the major abdominal vessels seen in hypoperfusion complex is not seen in the present case.

◆ **Uncomplicated hemoperitoneum:** This diagnosis is unlikely. Although in the case illustrated there is free intraperitoneal fluid that could be blood (or urine and bile, since these have the same appearance), bowel wall contrast enhancement would not be expected in uncomplicated hemoperitoneum.

◆ **Pancreatic trauma:** This diagnosis is unlikely based on the imaging findings. Pancreatic fractures can be clinically undetected and may present with bowel dilatation secondary to ileus, but the resultant fluid collections would be expected to be retroperitoneal. Furthermore, bowel wall contrast enhancement would not be expected.

◆ **Bowel and mesenteric injury:** This diagnosis is most likely, given the free intraperitoneal fluid and bowel wall contrast enhancement in the setting of a normal caliber aorta and inferior vena cava.

◆ DIAGNOSIS: Bowel perforation (without evidence of pneumoperitoneum).

◆ KEY FACTS

CLINICAL

◆ Either or both substantial bowel and mesenteric trauma are found in 3% to 5% of children who have blunt abdominal trauma.

◆ The clinical signs of bowel injury are nonspecific but include abdominal tenderness and guarding, rebound tenderness, and absent bowel sounds.

◆ Undetected injuries of the bowel result in markedly increased morbidity and mortality.

RADIOLOGIC

◆ The definitive CT signs of bowel perforation are the presence of pneumoperitoneum and extravasated oral contrast material. Pneumoperitoneum occurs in only 30% to 40% of patients and can be subtle. Extravasation of intravenous contrast material is rarely seen.

◆ Typical CT findings include bowel wall thickening, contrast enhancement, and otherwise unexplained peritoneal fluid.

◆ SUGGESTED READING

Bulas DI, Taylor GA, Eichelberger MR. The value of CT in detecting bowel perforation in children after blunt abdominal trauma. AJR Am J Roentgenol 1989;153:561–564.

Gay SB, Sistrom CL. Computed tomographic evaluation of blunt abdominal trauma. Radiol Clin North Am 1992;30:367–388.

Nghiem HV, Jeffrey RB Jr, Mindelzun RE. CT of blunt trauma to the bowel and mesentery. AJR Am J Roentgenol 1993; 160:53–58.

CASE 16

Donald P. Frush

HISTORY

An asymptomatic 8-year-old girl with human immunodeficiency virus (HIV).

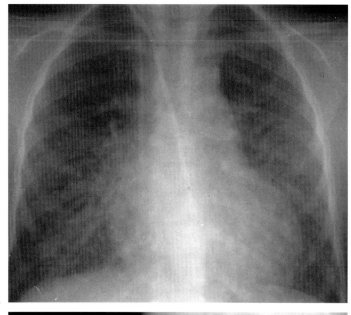

A

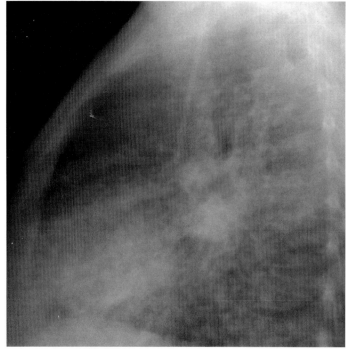

B

FIGURES 8-16A and 8-16B Posteroanterior (**A**) and lateral (**B**) chest radiographs. Diffuse nodular interstitial disease with a basilar predominance is seen. Hilar adenopathy and mild cardiomegaly are also present.

◆DIFFERENTIAL DIAGNOSIS

◆ *Pneumocystis carinii* **pneumonia (PCP):** This diagnosis is an unlikely choice because the patient is asymptomatic. PCP can present with a variety of abnormalities. The most often described are interstitial lung disease (with progression to diffuse airspace disease) and focal consolidation.

◆ **Cytomegalovirus (CMV) pneumonitis:** The radiographic appearance of this disorder is indistinguishable from PCP. As with PCP, CMV pneumonitis would be unusual in an asymptomatic patient.

◆ **Tuberculosis (TB):** Although a miliary pattern can occur with TB (predominately *Mycobacterium avium intracellulare*), the patient would be expected to be symptomatic, with acute, rapidly progressive radiographic changes.

◆ **Lymphocytic interstitial pneumonitis (LIP):** LIP is the best diagnosis in this case because the patient is asymptomatic, and a nodular interstitial disease pattern and hilar adenopathy, common findings in LIP, are present. Heart enlargement can be seen in patients with LIP secondary to HIV cardiomyopathy.

◆ **Other opportunistic infections:** The radiographic pattern may be highly variable. Nodular changes or focal or diffuse airspace disease can be seen. However, the patient would be expected to be symptomatic.

◆ **Other interstitial pneumonitis with fibrosis:** Interstitial disease is common in HIV-positive patients, but the pattern seen in the above patient is more reticular and the lung volumes reduced to a greater degree than would be expected.

◆DIAGNOSIS: Lymphocytic interstitial pneumonitis.

◆KEY FACTS

CLINICAL
◆ Pulmonary manifestations are common in pediatric HIV infection. LIP and PCP are the most common pulmonary disorders.

◆ LIP is a lymphoid response to HIV infection in which lymphoid hypertrophy and plasma cells are found in the alveolar and septal interstitium and in subpleural and peribronchial locations. A more general term for this (and other) patterns of lymphoid hyperplasia is pulmonary lymphoid hyperplasia.

◆ LIP is generally seen in HIV-positive children, but in about 15% of cases is seen in children with other immune-related disorders—e.g., primary immunodeficiencies and renal transplant recipients.

◆ Children with LIP can be relatively asymptomatic. When symptomatic, HIV-positive children are treated initially with adjustment in their antiviral therapy. Other therapy, primarily for non-HIV children, is immune-system mediating agents (i.e., corticosteroids).

◆ Digital clubbing can occur, but hypertrophic pulmonary osteoarthropathy is very unusual.

◆ Bronchoscopy and lavage do not help to establish the diagnosis of LIP. Furthermore, open biopsy is being performed less frequently than in the past for diagnosis. Instead, when typical radiologic changes (see below) develop in an asymptomatic, HIV-positive child, the diagnosis is presumed to be LIP.

◆ There is a strong association of LIP and positive titers to Epstein-Barr virus.

RADIOLOGIC
◆ Diffuse nodular, reticular, or reticulonodular opacities are typically present in the lungs. The changes are chronic and may be stable, worsen slowly, or wax and wane over time.

◆ Adenopathy is very common with LIP, but effusions are rare.

◆ Complications of LIP include pulmonary fibrosis and superimposed bronchiectasis from recurrent infections. Cystic changes have also been reported but are less common in children than adults. As in the adult population, these cystic changes are most often associated with a history of PCP infection.

◆ Focal consolidation, particularly if rapid in onset, is not likely to be due to LIP itself and is usually due to an acute superimposed infection.

◆SUGGESTED READING

Ambrosino MM, Genieser NB, Krasinski K, et al. Opportunistic infections and tumors in immunocompromised children. Radiol Clin North Am 1992;30:639–658.

Berdon WE, Mellins RB, Abramson SJ, Ruzal-Shapiro C. Pediatric HIV infection in its second decade—The changing pattern of lung involvement: Clinical, plain film, and computed tomographic findings. Radiol Clin North Am 1993;31:453–464.

Haller JO, Cohen HL. Pediatric HIV infection: An imaging update. Pediatr Radiol 1994;24:224–230.

CASE 17

Sara M. O'Hara

HISTORY

A 2-year-old boy found to have a palpable abdominal mass at a routine physical examination.

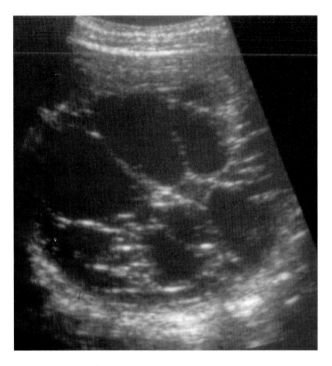

FIGURE 8-17A Longitudinal sonogram of left upper quadrant. A large, septated, cystic mass is present in the left upper abdomen, with sparse parenchyma between noncommunicating, anechoic, fluid-filled spaces.

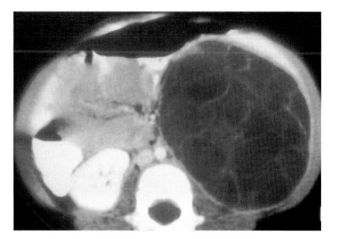

FIGURE 8-17B Contrast-enhanced CT image of the upper abdomen. A multiseptated cystic mass fills the left flank and displaces the aorta and vena cava rightward. The mass is well encapsulated; the septations contrast-enhance mildly. No normal left renal tissue is seen.

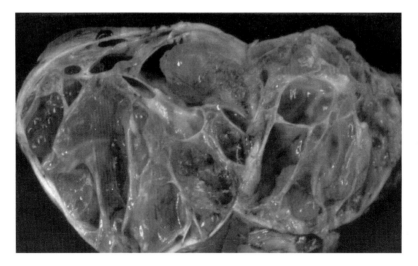

FIGURE 8-17C Gross specimen of the mass following excision. Many noncommunicating cysts are seen, some with paper-thin walls; others have thicker, fibrous-appearing walls.

◆ DIFFERENTIAL DIAGNOSIS

- **Severe hydronephrosis or obstructed duplication:** The cystic spaces would be expected to communicate in these entities and more renal parenchyma should be evident than is seen in the case illustrated. Furthermore, with distal obstruction, a dilated ureter would be expected.
- **Multicystic dysplastic kidney (MCDK):** This diagnosis is a reasonable consideration, but usually more parenchymal tissue is seen between the cysts with MCDK than is seen in this case (see Case 10).
- **Cystic Wilms' tumor:** This diagnosis adequately fits the imaging findings and would be more strongly favored if there were a mass extending into the renal vein or vena cava.
- **Mesoblastic nephroma:** These tumors are typically solid, not cystic, making this an unlikely diagnosis.
- **Clear cell sarcoma, rhabdoid tumor, or renal cell carcinoma:** Cysts may be present in all of these tumors, but there are usually solid components. Renal cell carcinoma, however, is not seen in children of this age.
- **Multilocular cystic nephroma (MLCN):** The clinical presentation of a multicystic renal mass in an otherwise asymptomatic young boy is typical of this entity, making this the most likely diagnosis.

◆ DIAGNOSIS: Multilocular cystic nephroma (without primitive blastemal elements).

◆ KEY FACTS

CLINICAL

- MLCN typically presents as a painless mass in children between 3 months and 4 years of age. Boys are affected twice as often as girls. A second peak in incidence is noted in the third and fourth decade, at which point there is a female-to-male ratio of 8 to 1.
- Rapid development of a mass, hematuria, pain, and infection are less common clinical features.

- These tumors are not familial, nor are they associated with other cystic lesions in abdominal viscera.
- Two histologic patterns are recognized: cystic nephroma, which does not contain blastemal cells in septa, and cystic, partially differentiated nephroblastoma, which has nodular solid elements containing blastemal or other embryonal elements. Both entities are managed in the same manner.
- Lesions are benign but are generally excised because they can be indistinguishable from some malignant renal neoplasms and for relief of mass effect. Local recurrence is rare and is seen with those tumors with primitive blastemal elements.

RADIOLOGIC

- MLCN is typically very large, is well-encapsulated by fibrous tissue, and contains cysts of varying sizes and wall thickness. The walls generally contrast-enhance on CT. The two histologic types of MLCN are indistinguishable radiographically.
- These tumors may be segmental or involve the entire kidney.
- The cyst content is proteinaceous, straw-colored fluid that results in MR signal characteristics, echo texture, and CT-attenuation features similar to water or proteinaceous fluid (unless hemorrhage has occurred). The cyst fluid does not enhance following contrast administration.
- Local invasion or adenopthy is an indication that a mass may be a malignant renal neoplasm rather than MLCN.

◆ SUGGESTED READING

Agrons GA, Wagner BJ, Davidson AJ, et al. Multilocular cystic renal tumor in children: Radiologic–pathologic correlation. Radiographics 1995;15:653–669.

Beckwith JB. Wilms' tumor and other renal tumors of childhood: An update. J Urol 1986;136;320–329.

Kajani N, Rosenberg BF, Bernstein J. Multilocular cystic nephroma. J Urol Pathol 1993;1:33–42.

CASE 18

Cindy R. Miller

HISTORY

A child with short stature and multiple fractures.

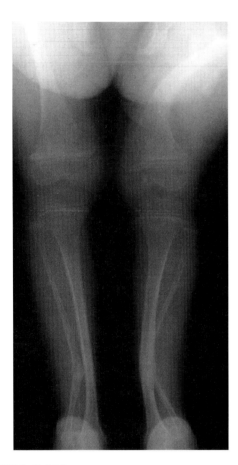

FIGURE 8-18A Anteroposterior view of lower extremities. Marked angulation is seen at the site of an old fracture of the left femur (also present in the right femur but not shown). Additionally, the tibias and fibulas are bowed and gracile.

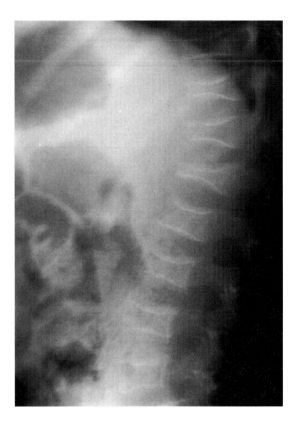

FIGURE 8-18B Lateral view of the spine in another child with the same diagnosis. Multiple compression fractures of the thoracic and lumbar vertebrae are seen.

◆ DIFFERENTIAL DIAGNOSIS

- **Osteogenesis imperfecta (OI):** Osteopenia, multiple fractures, bony deformity, and gracile bones are the classic features of this disorder and are well illustrated in these two patients.
- **Child abuse:** Radiographically, there are several features that distinguish OI from child abuse. With OI, the bones are typically osteopenic, and wormian (intrasutural) bones may be present. Furthermore, the metaphyseal "corner" fractures of child abuse are not seen.

The remaining entities are usually not difficult to differentiate from OI but share the feature of osteopenia, consequently increasing the risk of fracture.

- **Menkes' disease:** This disorder of copper metabolism has radiographic features similar to those of scurvy and child abuse. Metaphyseal spurring, dense metaphyses, and periosteal reaction are features of Menkes' disease that are not seen in OI.
- **Rickets:** Flaring, irregularity of the metaphyses, and widening of the physes are features of rickets that are not seen in OI.
- **Hypophosphatasia:** Patients with hypophosphatasia are severely osteopenic (like patients with OI), but they also have craniosynostosis, lucencies in the distal femurs, and rachitic changes.
- **Homocystinuria:** As in OI, multiple compression fractures of the spine can be seen in homocystinuria. Radiographic manifestations seen in homocystinuria but not OI include epiphyseal flattening and bony spicules extending from the metaphysis into the physis.

◆ DIAGNOSIS: Osteogenesis imperfecta (type 3, Figure 8-18A; type 1, Figure 8-18B).

◆ KEY FACTS

CLINICAL

- A deficiency of type I collagen in OI patients is responsible for the increased bone fragility. Other clinical manifestations include blue sclerae, thin skin, hernias, early vascular calcifications, lax joints, bleeding, cardiac lesions, deafness, and poor dentition.
- Type 1 OI (OI tarda): Despite its name, a small percentage of patients can have fractures at birth. The inheritance pattern is autosomal dominant. All of these patients have blue sclerae. Some have either or both presenile conductive hearing loss and dentinogenesis imperfecta.
- Type 2 OI: This subtype was previously known as OI congenita; the inheritance pattern is usually autosomal recessive. Survival is very short; death results from respiratory insufficiency, cerebral hemorrhage secondary to undermineralization of the skull, or cervical spinal cord compression due to abnormalities of the base of the skull.
- Type 3 OI: Inheritance can be either autosomal dominant or autosomal recessive. Clinical differentiation from type 2 is based on the longer survival for type 3 patients.
- Type 4 OI: This category further subdivides into two subtypes, A and B. In both types, inheritance is autosomal dominant. Subtype A has no dentinogenesis imperfecta or blue sclerae and infrequent fractures. Subtype B may be relatively indistinguishable from type 3 due to a very high frequency of fractures.

RADIOLOGIC

- Type 1 OI: Exuberant callus may be seen about fracture sites. Vertebral bodies may be biconcave, and kyphoscoliosis may result. Neurologic complications may ensue due to basilar invagination.
- Type 2 OI: Long bones are short and broad ("accordion-like") due to multiple, healed fractures. Ribs are thickened and appeared beaded, also due to healed fractures. Marked undermineralization of the skull and multiple compression fractures are typically seen.
- Type 3 OI: There is better mineralization of the calvarium than in type 2. Wormian bones are present at birth. The long bones are not deformed at birth as in type 2, but marked diaphyseal narrowing occurs over time. Severe, progressive bowing deformities of the long bones are typical of type 3. Some type 3 OI patients develop bubbly, cystic changes of the epimetaphyses described as "popcorn" calcifications.

◆ SUGGESTED READING

Ablin DS, Greenspan A, Reinhart MA, et al. Differentiation of child abuse from osteogenesis imperfecta. AJR Am J Roentgenol 1990;154:1035–1046.

Herman TE, McAlister WH. Inherited diseases of bone density in children. Radiol Clin North Am 1991;29:149–164.

CASE 19

Donald P. Frush

HISTORY

A 2-month-old boy with wheezing.

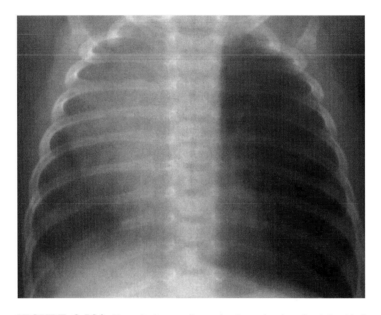

FIGURE 8-19A Frontal chest radiograph. A predominantly right-sided mediastinal mass is present along with hyperinflation of the left lung.

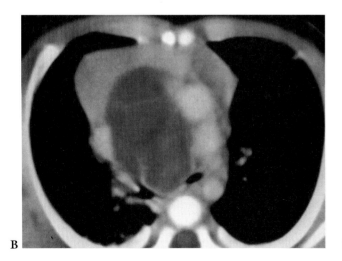

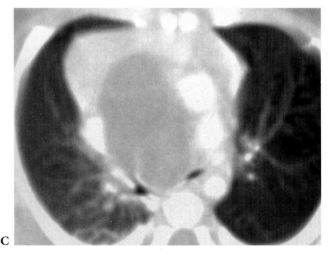

FIGURES 8-19B and 8-19C Contrast-enhanced CT scans of the chest. (**B**) CT image with soft-tissue detail windows. A septated, cystic anterior mediastinal mass is present. (**C**) Same CT slice as in Fig. 8-19B with lung-detail windows. Air trapping is present in the left lung due to narrowing of the left mainstem bronchus by the mass.

◆ DIFFERENTIAL DIAGNOSIS

- **Lymphangioma/hemangioma:** These lesions are cystic masses with a variable amount of solid tissue. Most of intrathoracic lesions extend downward from the neck. These diagnoses cannot be excluded on the basis of the images presented.
- **Teratoma:** These lesions are also cystic mediastinal masses (with occasional calcification and variable solid components), usually located in the anterior mediastinum. This diagnosis is a likely consideration based on the findings presented.
- **Other germ cell tumors:** Such lesions are rare in infancy.
- **Bronchogenic cyst:** This entity is an unlikely diagnosis. When situated in the mediastinum, bronchogenic cysts are typically subcarinal in location rather than in the anterior mediastinum.
- **Esophageal duplication:** This diagnosis is unlikely because esophageal duplications are located in the middle, not anterior, mediastinum.
- **Lymphoma:** This diagnosis is unlikely because lymphomas are usually solid masses that are found in older children and adolescents.
- **Normal thymus:** Normal thymic tissue can have an asymmetric anterior mediastinal distribution, but the normal thymus does not narrow the airway and is not cystic.
- **Thymic cyst:** This diagnosis is unlikely because these lesions are rare in infancy.
- **Abscess/hematoma:** These diagnoses is unlikely because there is no history of infection, instrumentation, trauma, or a bleeding disorder.
- **Aneurysm/dilated ascending aorta:** These diagnoses would be unlikely based on the young age of the patient. Furthermore, dense contrast enhancement of the lesion would be expected if the mass were vascular.

◆ DIAGNOSIS: Cystic teratoma (mature).

◆ KEY FACTS

CLINICAL

- Respiratory distress is a common clinical presentation for neonatal mediastinal masses.
- Teratomas contain tissues derived from all three embryonic cell layers: mesoderm, endoderm, and ectoderm.

- The mediastinum is the third most common location, exceeded only by the pelvis (ovarian/sacrococcygeal) and CNS.
- Most anterior mediastinal teratomas have mature histologic features. Teratomas with mature histologic features are almost always benign. However, teratomas with immature histologic features can be either benign or malignant.
- Cystic teratomas are more likely benign, whereas solid teratomas are more likely malignant.
- Malignant teratomas often have some histologic components of other germ cell tumors, e.g., yolk sac tumors and embryonal cell tumors.
- Exact diagnosis of a cystic mediastinal mass using imaging methods alone can be difficult. Because of this fact and because these lesions can produce life-threatening symptoms and signs (e.g., airway compromise), virtually all masses are removed, if possible.

RADIOLOGIC

- A teratoma can be presumed to be malignant if it is solid, invasive, or metastatic. However, absence of these features is not an indication that the mass is necessarily benign.
- Typical radiographic features of a mediastinal teratoma include a cyst (containing either serous or sebaceous fluid and having occasional thin septations) and presence of fat, calcification, and solid elements. CT or MRI is performed routinely for surgical planning and staging.
- Sonography can show the cystic structure and calcification but is inadequate for showing lesion extent and involvement of adjacent structures (i.e., vessels and airways), which are necessary for surgical planning.

◆ SUGGESTED READING

Lakhoo K, Boyle M, Drake DP. Mediastinal teratomas: Review of 15 pediatric cases. J Pediatr Surg 1993;28:1161–1164.

Nichols CR. Mediastinal germ cell tumors. Clinical features and biologic correlates. Chest 1991;99:472–479.

Quillin SP, Siegel MJ. CT features of benign and malignant teratomas in children. J Comput Assist Tomogr 1992;16:722–726.

Rosado-de-Christenson M, Templeton PA, Moran CA. Mediastinal germ cell tumors: Radiologic and pathologic correlation. Radiographics 1992;12:1013–1030.

CASE 20

Sara M. O'Hara

HISTORY

A 6-month-old boy with renal insufficiency and failure to thrive.

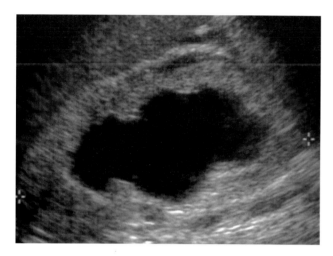

FIGURE 8-20A Longitudinal right upper quadrant sonogram. Marked dilatation of the right collecting system is seen, with preservation of cortical thickness.

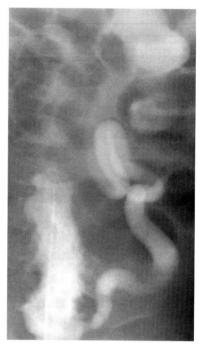

FIGURE 8-20B Anteroposterior view during voiding cytourethrogram. A small-capacity bladder is seen, with pseudodiverticula, muscular hypertrophy, and grade 5 left vesicoureteral reflux.

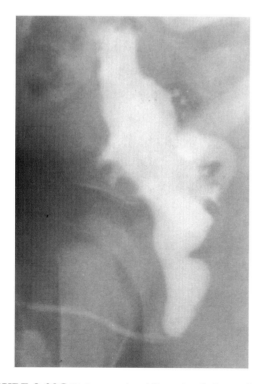

FIGURE 8-20C Right posterior oblique view during voiding. An abrupt caliber change is present in the urethra just distal to the verumontanum. The posterior urethra is markedly dilated. Urine stream was very sluggish.

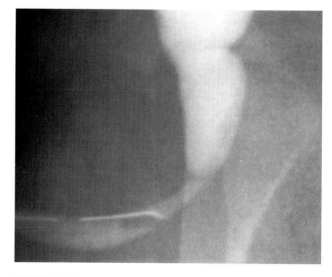

FIGURE 8-20D Right posterior oblique view during retrograde urethrogram. A crescentic filling defect is seen extending from the ventral surface of the urethra at the level of the luminal caliber change seen on the voiding images.

◆ DIFFERENTIAL DIAGNOSIS

- **Neurogenic bladder:** Bladder wall irregularity, thickened muscle bundles, and vertical orientation of the bladder suggest the presence of neurogenic bladder dysfunction. However, urethral abnormalities are not present with an isolated neurogenic bladder.
- **Megaureter:** The dilated, tortuous left ureter seen in this case is similar to primary megaureter. However, the distal ureter in this case does not taper as usually seen in megaureter. Furthermore, the bladder and urethral abnormalities are not explained by this diagnosis.
- **Urethral polyp:** Filling defects in the urethra may cause obstructive symptoms and poor urinary stream, as in this case. Benign fibrovascular polyps typically arise in the region of the verumontanum and prolapse into the prostatic urethra on voiding images. The filling defect in the case illustrated, however, is more web-like and nonmobile.
- **Urethral stricture:** Focal narrowing of the urethra is usually due to previous trauma, scar/inflammatory tissue, or surgery. The retrograde urethrogram (Figure 8-20D) shows that the urethra is actually normal in caliber but contains a filling defect that impedes antegrade urine flow.
- **Posterior urethral valves:** This entity is the best diagnosis, given the posterior urethral filling defect and associated bladder and upper urinary tract findings.

DIAGNOSIS: Posterior urethral valves.

◆ KEY FACTS

CLINICAL

- Posterior urethral valves are the most common cause of urethral obstruction in boys. Early diagnosis and treatment (now sometimes in utero) can help to preserve renal function.
- Boys with urine ascites, hydronephrosis, hydroureter, or poor urinary stream should be evaluated with voiding cystourethrography (VCUG) using steep oblique views of the urethra during voiding to detect the presence of urethral valves.
- Vesicoureteral reflux is common in boys with posterior urethral valves and, when unilateral, may be protective for the contralateral kidney.
- The valve tissue results from abnormal fusion of remnants of the mesonephric duct. In normal circumstances, fusion of the remnants of the mesonephric duct forms the plicae collicularis or mucosal folds in the urethra. However, if this tissue fuses in the midline, a thin flap is formed that acts like a windsock or diaphragm, impeding urine flow.

- The valve tissue is typically very thin and transparent at cystoscopy and may be pushed aside by the cystoscope if not carefully sought. Thereafter, cytoscopic resection/ablation is performed.
- Prognosis is generally good if renal function has not been compromised by prolonged high-grade obstruction, back pressure, and secondary dysplasia.
- A classification of posterior urethral valves (into types 1, 2, and 3 depending on the configuration of the obstructing valve) has been proposed but is not clinically useful.

RADIOLOGIC

- Posterior urethral valves are typically seen on VCUG as a crescentic filling defect within the urine stream just distal to the verumontanum. Occasionally, the valve is not visualized, but its presence is suggested by secondary findings of a dilated posterior urethra with a small-caliber anterior urethra, thickened bladder neck, and muscular hypertrophy of the bladder wall.
- A false-negative VCUG result can occur if the bladder catheter is left in the urethra during voiding images. The catheter then can displace the valve tissue so that a filling defect is not apparent and the urine stream is temporarily improved.
- On sonography, posterior urethral dilation may be measured at rest and during voiding with good predictive value for the diagnosis of valves. A posterior urethral diameter of ≥6 mm on voiding transperineal scans is reported to be 100% sensitive and 89% specific, with a positive predictive value of 88%.
- Compensatory bladder muscle hypertrophy creates pseudodiverticula when contrast material is trapped between thickened muscle bundles, thereby appearing to project beyond the expected lumen of the bladder.
- Vesicoureteral reflux is the most common problem in infants with posterior urethral valves. However, relative obstruction to antegrade flow at the ureterovesical junction may complicate upper tract drainage after valve ablation. The restricted drainage is due to persistent bladder wall thickening and fibrosis which may warrant ureteral reimplantation and bladder augmentation surgery in the postoperative period.

◆ SUGGESTED READING

Cohen HL, Susman M, Haller JO, et al. Posterior urethral valve: Transperineal US for imaging and diagnosis in male infants. Radiology 1994;192:261–264.

Good CD, Vinnicombe SJ, Minty IL, et al. Voiding urethrography in the diagnosis of the posterior urethral valve in male infants [abstract]. Radiology 1995;197:159.

Macpherson R, Leithiser R, Gordon L, Turner W. Posterior urethral valves: An update and review. Radiographics 1986;6:753–791.

CASE 21

George S. Bisset III

HISTORY

A 9-month-old female who presented in the neonatal period with profound cyanosis.

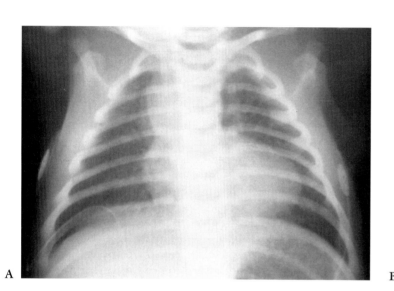

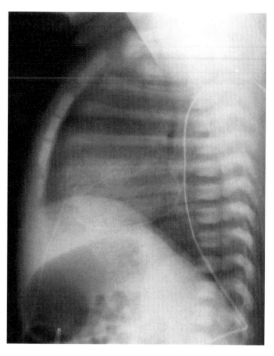

FIGURES 8-21A and 8-21B Frontal and lateral chest radiographs at 1 day of age. The cardiac silhouette is slightly enlarged. The aortic arch is right sided. The pulmonary vascularity is slightly decreased. No bony abnormalities are identified. The main pulmonary artery segment is diminutive.

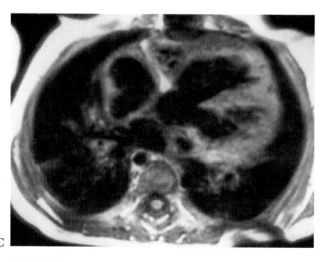

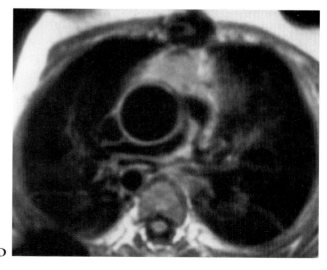

FIGURES 8-21C and 8-21D Axial T1-weighted MR views through the heart at 9 months of age. (**C**) is an axial view through the central cardiac region. A large subaortic ventricular septal defect is noted. Right ventricular hypertrophy is present. The thickness of the right ventricular free wall is equal to that of the left ventricular free wall. (**D**) is an axial view through the pulmonary outflow track. The ascending aorta is moderately enlarged. The aortic arch is right sided. The main pulmonary artery confluence is diminutive. The right and left pulmonary arteries are small and irregular. An artifact related to prior sternotomy for shunt placement is seen in the sternum.

◆ DIFFERENTIAL DIAGNOSIS

- **Isolated pulmonic valve stenosis:** A decrease in pulmonary blood flow would not be expected in the setting of isolated pulmonic valve stenosis (i.e., in the absence of an intracardiac shunt). In this entity, the entirety of blood flow must pass through the lungs. Therefore, the typical finding is a dilated main pulmonary artery with normal flow.

- **Tetralogy of Fallot (TOF):** The combination of a large subaortic ventricular septal defect (VSD), right ventricular hypertrophy, and small pulmonary arteries is typical of this diagnosis. These findings are all present in the case illustrated, making this the most likely diagnosis. The majority of these patients have a left aortic arch, although 25% have a right aortic arch (see Case 21 in Chapter 7).

- **Pulmonary valve atresia with intact ventricular septum:** The presence of cardiomegaly and diminished pulmonary blood flow on the radiographs raises this as a possible diagnosis. However, the presence of a large VSD on the MRI excludes this diagnosis.

- **Ebstein's anomaly:** Patients with Ebstein's anomaly usually present with cyanosis in the neonatal period and have marked right-sided cardiac enlargement (including both the right atrium and right ventricle) and diminished pulmonary blood flow (as a result of severe tricuspid regurgitation and right-to-left shunting across the atrial septum). This diagnosis is unlikely for two reasons: (1) cardiac size is usually (but not invariably) much larger than shown in Figure 8-21A—in particular, the right heart size is increased in Ebstein's anomaly but not in the case shown above; and (2) the MRIs in this case show an aorta overriding a VSD, not a feature of Ebstein's anomaly.

- **Tricuspid atresia:** These patients can present with cardiomegaly and diminished pulmonary blood flow. However, the presence of a normal, thick-walled right ventricular chamber on the MR examination in the case shown makes this an unlikely diagnosis.

◆ DIAGNOSIS: Tetralogy of Fallot with diminutive pulmonary arteries following central shunt.

◆ KEY FACTS

CLINICAL
- The finding of cyanosis with normal or diminished pulmonary vascularity is usually caused by a combination of a ventricular communication and pulmonic stenosis. The exceptions to this rule are Ebstein's anomaly of the tricuspid valve and pulmonary atresia.

- TOF can be associated with pulmonic stenosis at any of four levels: the infundibulum (most common), the pulmonic valve, the pulmonary trunk, or the pulmonary artery branches.

- If pulmonary atresia is present, the entire pulmonary blood flow is through collateral (bronchial) vessels that reach the pulmonary vasculature from the descending thoracic aorta.

- TOF is the most common malformation among cyanotic adults with congenital heart disease.

RADIOLOGIC
- The ascending aorta and aortic knob are prominent in TOF because the aorta receives increased flow from the right-to-left shunt and because of the embryologic defective division of the truncus.

- Cardiac size in TOF is usually normal, although a "boot-shaped" heart can be seen in older infants.

- In the TOF variant, in which there is absence of the pulmonic valve, marked dilatation of the pulmonary trunk and its proximal branches can be seen, frequently resulting in compression of the airway.

- Occasionally, absence of a pulmonary artery branch is seen in TOF, usually involving the left pulmonary artery.

- MRI is a useful tool to determine the size of the pulmonary arteries, which is helpful for preoperative planning and evaluation of growth following a palliative procedure (e.g., after a systemic-arterial shunt). MRI also allows evaluation of important anatomic details—e.g., whether the pulmonary arteries are confluent, which is a factor facilitating surgical repair.

◆ SUGGESTED READING

Bisset GS III. Magnetic resonance imaging of congenital heart disease. Radiol Clin North Am 1991;29:279–291.

Eichenberger AC, von-Schulthess GK. Magnetic resonance imaging of the heart and the great vessels: Morphology, function, and perfusion. Curr Opin Radiol 1992;4:41–47.

Formanek AG, Witcofski RL, D'Souza VJ, et al. MR imaging of the central pulmonary arterial tree in conotruncal malformation. AJR Am J Roentgenol 1986;147:1127–1131.

Kelley MJ, Jaffe CC, Kleinman CS. Cardiac Imaging in Infants and Children. Philadelphia: Saunders, 1982;340–365.

HISTORY

A 2-month-old former premature infant who has spent her entire life in the neonatal intensive care unit.

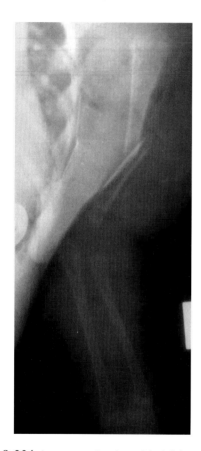

FIGURE 8-22A Anteroposterior view of the left humerus. A fracture of the humeral diaphysis with flaring and irregularity of the metaphyses is seen.

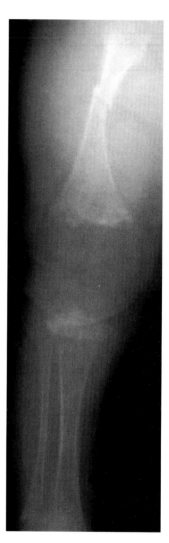

FIGURE 8-22B Anteroposterior view of the right femur. Similar metaphyseal changes are seen in the femur, along with a fracture of its diaphysis.

◆ DIFFERENTIAL DIAGNOSIS

- **Rickets:** The radiographic findings in this case—i.e., metaphyseal flaring and irregularity and insufficiency fractures—are typical of rickets. In premature infants, dietary vitamin D deficiency is the usual etiology.
- **Hypophosphatasia:** This entity, due to deficient activity of alkaline phosphatase, should be considered because the radiographic changes may be virtually indistinguishable from rickets. The distinction is made on the basis of findings of premature cranial synostosis and increased excretion of urinary phosphoethanolamine in hypophosphatasia.
- **Child abuse:** As with rickets, multiple fractures are typically seen. In a child of this age, the fractures may well be diaphyseal. However, mineralization in child abuse will typically be normal (unlike rickets), without metaphyseal flaring. Furthermore, the irregularity of the metaphyses seen in rickets will not be seen in child abuse.
- **Osteogenesis imperfecta (OI):** Like rickets, undermineralization and multiple fractures are seen (see Case 18). However, rickets is not associated with the gracile bones commonly seen in OI. In fact, it is the absence of this characteristic finding that makes OI an unlikely diagnosis in the case shown.

◆ DIAGNOSIS: Rickets.

◆ KEY FACTS

CLINICAL

- Rickets usually presents by 3 to 6 months of age and is almost always diagnosed by age 2 years.
- Clinical manifestations include weakness, tetany, kyphoscoliosis, and craniotabes.
- Nutritional causes can be classified as either secondary to decreased vitamin D synthesis (as can occur in absence of exposure to sunlight, particularly with dark skin) or due to dietary vitamin D deficiency. Premature infants are especially susceptible to rickets from the latter cause. In these children, a diagnosis can be confirmed by finding serum alkaline phosphatase levels >10 times the normal value in adults.
- A variety of intestinal disorders can cause malabsorption of vitamin D and subsequent rickets: pancreatic insufficiency, as might be seen with cystic fibrosis; biliary disease (e.g., biliary atresia); and small-bowel disease, including regional enteritis or short-gut syndrome following resection of diseased bowel.

- A wide spectrum of renal disorders, either glomerular or tubular in nature, can cause rickets. Among the latter is vitamin D–resistant rickets.
- Increased requirement for vitamin D may be responsible for rickets. It may be inherited or acquired (e.g., anticonvulsant therapy, especially phenytoin).
- Rarely, tumors (e.g., giant cell tumor, fibroma, hemangiopericytoma) can cause rickets.

RADIOLOGIC

- The radiographic hallmarks of rickets—metaphyseal flaring, irregularity, and cupping and widening of the physis—reflect lack of mineralization of osteoid that continues to be laid down. These changes occur earliest in the most rapidly growing portions of the bones: the distal femur, proximal and distal tibia and fibula, and distal radius and ulna.
- Changes in the diaphysis occur with more long-standing rickets. These changes include coarsening of the trabecular pattern and greenstick fractures.
- In addition to fractures, enlarged and distorted bones (so-called rachitic rosary) are seen on radiographs.
- The first radiographic sign of healing is reappearance of the provisional zone of calcification.
- In addition to the features noted above, the features of rickets due to X-linked (or familial) hypophosphatemic rickets (due to abnormal transport of phosphate in several sites with resultant hypophosphatemia) include bowing of bones, premature sutural closure, enthesopathy, and biconcave vertebral bodies.
- The radiographic distinction of rickets from hypophosphatasia can be very difficult. Distinguishing features of hypophosphatasia include craniosynostosis and well-defined lucencies of the distal femoral metaphyses and, occasionally, the proximal humeri, epiphyses, and carpal bones.

◆ SUGGESTED READING

Herman TE, McAlister WH. Inherited diseases of bone density in children. Radiol Clin North Am 1991;29:149–164.

Kirks DR. Practical Pediatric Imaging: Diagnostic Radiology of Infants and Children (2nd ed). Boston: Little, Brown, 1991;307–314.

Silverman FN, Kuhn JP (eds). Essentials of Caffey's Pediatric X-Ray Diagnosis. Chicago: Year Book, 1990;895–897.

CASE 23

George S. Bisset III

HISTORY

A 12-year-old boy with a cardiac murmur.

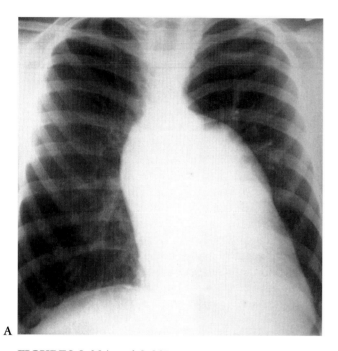
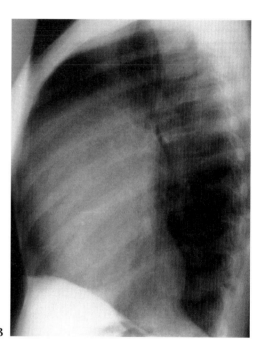

FIGURES 8-23A and 8-23B Frontal and lateral chest radiographs. The left cardiac border has an unusual contour, with increased tissue in both the retrosternal clear space and posteriorly in the location of the left ventricle.

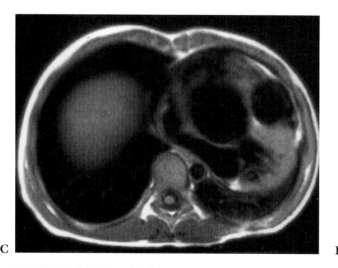
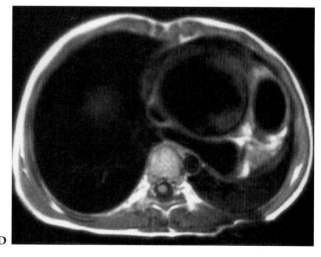

FIGURES 8-23C and 8-23D Axial cardiac-gated T1-weighted MRIs at the level of the aortic valve at (**C**) and just above (**D**) the sinus of Valsalva. Marked enlargement of the ascending aorta above the sinus of Valsalva is seen. The descending aorta is normal in caliber. The left atrium is compressed by the enlarged ascending aorta.

◆ DIFFERENTIAL DIAGNOSIS

◆ **Anterior mediastinal mass:** An anterior mediastinal mass could be suspected because of the frontal chest radiograph findings. However, the lateral radiograph shows that not all of the abnormal density is in the anterior mediastinum; some is also posterior, near the location of the left ventricle. Furthermore, the clinical history (a cardiac murmur) would not be accounted for by the presence of an anterior mediastinal mass. Finally, the MR study shows definitively that a structural cardiovascular lesion is present.

◆ **Ascending aortic aneurysm:** This diagnosis best accounts for the imaging findings. The MR findings explain the unusual appearance of the chest radiograph. The anterior soft tissue is the ascending aortic aneurysm. The left ventricle is enlarged because of aortic regurgitation (not shown).

◆ **Aortic stenosis:** The enlargement of the ascending aorta in this case could potentially be due to the jet effect of aortic stenosis. However, at a point at which the aorta was enlarged to the degree shown in the illustrated case, clinical symptoms and signs (e.g., dyspnea, exertional chest pain, syncope, or an apical systolic ejection murmur) would be expected to be quite evident.

◆ DIAGNOSIS: Ascending aortic aneurysm in Marfan's syndrome.

◆ KEY FACTS

CLINICAL

◆ Aneurysms of the ascending aorta are rare in children but are much more common in adults (in whom the most common etiology is atherosclerotic disease).

◆ Ascending aortic aneurysms in children are usually due to genetic disease (Marfan's syndrome, cutis laxa, pseudoxanthoma elasticum, Ehlers-Danlos syndrome, homocystinuria, osteogenesis imperfecta, Noonan's syndrome, or Turner's syndrome).

• In Marfan's syndrome, an abnormality of the elastic media is present ("cystic medial necrosis" is a term that has been used, although it is a misnomer because necrosis is not present). Other major cardiac anomalies in Marfan's syndrome are aortic and mitral insufficiency, as well as dissection of the aneurysm.

• Ehlers-Danlos syndrome represents a group of related collagen disorders. Hyperelasticity and joint laxity are typical clinical features.

• In homocystinuria, mental retardation is present, unlike in the case illustrated.

• OI type 1 is associated with aortic group dilatation. A clinical history of fractures or blue sclera (not present in the case illustrated) is typically present.

◆ Repair of the ascending aorta usually is performed for an aneurysm of 6.0 cm in the adolescent or adult. Aortic surgery or aortic valve or mitral valve replacement is rarely necessary before adolescence in Marfan's syndrome.

RADIOLOGIC

◆ Although plain films are sometimes the initial imaging technique for detection of ascending aortic aneurysm, they have little value in the follow-up of these patients.

◆ Echocardiography is a helpful noninvasive tool for determining the dimensions of the ascending aortic aneurysm, the presence of valvular regurgitation, and evaluating left ventricular function.

◆ MRI is recommended in situations where the acoustic window is limited (including Marfan's syndrome, where pectus deformity may limit evaluation) and in patients with known dilation of the ascending aorta and acute chest pain (in whom aortic dissection is suspected).

◆ MRI for evaluation of ascending aortic aneurysm should be performed using a combination of transaxial, coronal, and sagittal cardiac-gated T1-weighted sequences. Bright-blood (gradient-recall) pulse sequences may also be helpful, particularly in a cine mode.

◆ Catheter angiography can give much of the same information; however, there is increased risk of aortic injury in a patient with a known aortic aneurysm or suspected dissection.

◆ SUGGESTED READING

Bank ER. Magnetic resonance of congenital cardiovascular disease. Radiol Clin North Am 1993;3:553–572.

Bisset GS. Magnetic resonance imaging of congenital heart disease in the pediatric patient. Radiol Clin North Am 1991;29:279–291.

Fellows KE, Weinberg PM, Baffa JM, Hoffman EA. Evaluation of congenital heart disease with MR imaging: Current incoming attractions. AJR Am J Roentgenol 1992;159:925–931.

Pierpont MEM, Mollor JH. Cardiac Manifestations of Genetic Disease. In GC Emmanovilides, HD Allen, TA Reimenschneider, HP Gutgesell (eds), Moss and Adam's Heart Disease in Infants, Children, and Adolescents Including the Fetus and Young Adult (5th ed). Baltimore: Williams & Wilkins, 1995;1486–1520.

CASE 24
Cindy R. Miller

HISTORY

A 7-year-old white boy with right hip pain and a limp with no clinical or laboratory findings suggesting further infection.

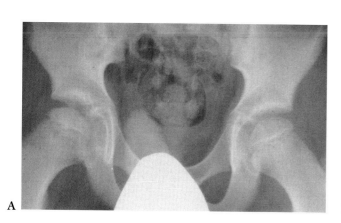

A

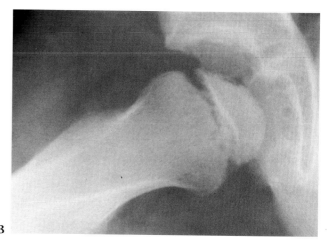

B

FIGURES 8-24A and 8-24B Anteroposterior view of the pelvis (**A**) and frog leg lateral view of the right hip (**B**). The right femoral head is reduced in height, has subtle increased density compared to the left, and on the frog leg lateral view, is seen to have a subchondral lucency, all findings of avascular necrosis.

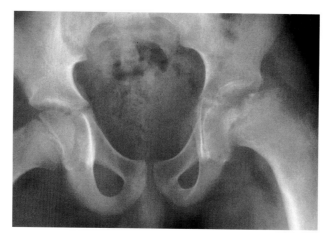

FIGURE 8-24C Anteroposterior view of the pelvis in another boy with the same diagnosis. Marked reduction in height, sclerosis and fragmentation, coxa magna (a sequelum of avascular necrosis), and incomplete covering of the femoral head by the acetabulum are seen.

◆ DIFFERENTIAL DIAGNOSIS

Differential diagnosis for avascular necrosis of the hip in a child includes:

- **Legg-Calvé-Perthes disease (Legg-Perthes disease):** This diagnosis is possible given the patient's age and findings of avascular necrosis.
- **Sickle cell anemia:** This diagnosis is not likely because the child is white. Other bony changes associated with sickle cell hemoglobinopathies including sclerosis, "bone-within-bone" appearance in the femurs, and periosteal reaction (from acute infarction or, less commonly, osteomyelitis) are not present.
- **Trauma:** The absence of a history of trauma makes this an unlikely diagnosis.
- **Osteomyelitis:** Osteomyelitis can cause changes that mimic avascular necrosis, but clinical and laboratory features consistent with infection are usually present. Osteomyelitis can be distinguished from avascular necrosis by a bone scan that shows increased radiotracer activity in all phases of a three-phase scan (unless there is loss of vascular supply due to mechanical factors such as infectious synovitis).
- **Gaucher's disease:** Osteonecrosis can occur in Gaucher's disease, but other stigmata of Gaucher's disease, including expanded medullary cavities with a thin cortex, osteopenia, and absence of normal metaphyseal widening, are not present in the cases shown.
- **Corticosteroid use:** Corticosteroid use can cause avascular necrosis, but such history is absent here.

Diagnostic considerations for fragmented epiphyses include:

- **Hypothyroidism:** This diagnosis is not likely because both femoral heads in hypothyroidism are fragmented at the onset of ossification. The left femoral head shown in Figure 8-24C is not fragmented.
- **Multiple epiphyseal dysplasia:** With age, the epiphyseal fragments often coalesce and resemble the coxa magna appearance seen in Figure 8-24C. However, this diagnosis is not likely as it is also usually bilateral and symmetric.
- **Legg-Calvé-Perthes disease:** In advanced stages of this disease, fragmented epiphyses can be seen. Unlike the two entities previously mentioned, findings are usually unilateral, making it a realistic diagnostic possibility. Furthermore, it is the only entity on both differential diagnosis lists (i.e., as a cause of both fragmented epiphyses and avascular necrosis of the hip), making it the most likely diagnosis.

◆ DIAGNOSIS: Legg-Calvé-Perthes (or Legg-Perthes) disease.

◆ KEY FACTS

CLINICAL

- Legg-Perthes is most common in white boys. The age range is 3 to 12 years, but most cases occur between the ages of 5 and 8 years. The male-to-female ratio is 4 to 1.

- Bilateral abnormalities are present in about 10% of cases. Symptoms and signs include a limp, pain, thigh and buttock atrophy, and limited internal rotation. Pain may be centered about either or both the hip and groin or referred to the knee.
- Older age at onset of symptoms and female gender are associated with a worse prognosis.
- Most children with Legg-Perthes remain symptom free after the acute event for decades even though radiographic changes including coxa magna and flattening of the femoral head persist.

RADIOLOGIC

- The plain film findings in the first few weeks after symptom onset may be widening of the joint space medially and lateral displacement of the femoral head, reflective of edema of either or both the acetabular fossa tissues, and a small joint effusion.
- Several pathophysiologic explanations have been invoked to explain the increased density of the femoral head. For example, sclerosis may be due to a combination of decreased demineralization (due to decreased blood supply) and increased new bone formation (during a stage of revascularization). Alternatively, the increased density may be only apparent, compared to disease-related osteopenia in the femoral neck.
- The "crescent sign" appears following the sclerotic phase and reflects fracture of the softened, avascular femoral head. It usually begins laterally and is more easily detected with a frog leg lateral view.
- A large area of collapse of the femoral head, extensive subchondral lucency, lateral epiphyseal extrusion, and calcification lateral to the femoral head are radiographic signs associated with poor prognosis.
- Proper scintigraphic assessment necessitates meticulous technique, using pinhole collimation. Whether bone scan or MRI is more sensitive for detection of the early changes of avascular necrosis is still a point of controversy.
- The scintigraphic pattern depends on whether the predominant means of repair is recanalization or neovascularization. With recanalization, radiotracer activity is first seen laterally; with neovascularization, radiotracer activity proceeds superiorly from the physis.
- MRI is particularly valuable in assessing articular cartilage. However, the loss of marrow signal in the femoral head seen in Legg-Perthes disease is nonspecific and can be seen in tumor, trauma, and edema from other causes.

◆ SUGGESTED READING

Cardinal E, White SJ. Imaging pediatric hip disorders and residual dysplasia of adult hips. Curr Opin Radiol 1992;4:83–89.

Conway JJ. A scintigraphic classification of Legg-Calvé-Perthes disease. Semin Nucl Med 1993;23:274–295.

Mandell GA, Harcke HT, Kumar SJ. Avascular necrosis and related conditions. Top Magn Reson Imaging 1991;4:31–44.

HISTORY

A previously healthy 3-year-old boy with 2 days of enuresis, dysuria, and hematuria.

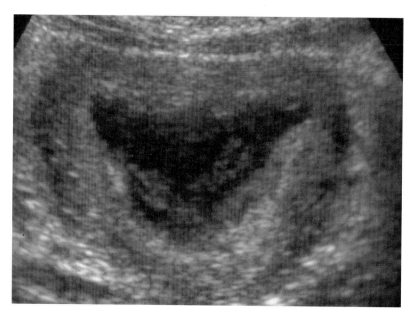

FIGURE 8-25A Transverse pelvic sonogram. Concentric thickening of the bladder wall is seen with more focal thickening posteriorly. Echogenic debris is seen within the bladder lumen.

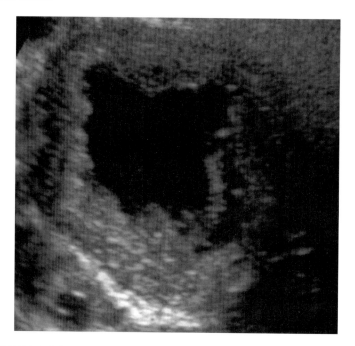

FIGURE 8-25B Longitudinal pelvic sonogram. The irregular wall thickening and intraluminal echogenic debris are again seen. An intraluminal band of material extends anteriorly from the posteroinferior wall of the bladder.

◆ DIFFERENTIAL DIAGNOSIS

- **Neurogenic bladder:** Patients with neurogenic bladder frequently have bladder wall thickening, heavily trabeculated bladder muscle, and debris related to intermittent catheterization. The case illustrated above had no history of bladder dysfunction. The acute onset of symptoms is also not consistent with the history of neurogenic bladder.

- **Augmented bladder:** Cystoplasty, using a part of the gastrointestinal tract, is a common surgical method used to augment bladder capacity that results in an irregularly shaped outer contour of the bladder. The bladder in this case has a smooth outer contour (even though the inner contour is undulating), inconsistent with the diagnosis of augmented bladder.

- **Rhabdomyosarcoma:** This diagnosis is a consideration because the bladder wall is thickened. Bladder sarcoma typically appears as a focal mural mass or region of thickening and can project into the bladder lumen as a polypoid mass (botryiodes configuration). If the mass ulcerates or hemorrhages, echogenic material may be seen in the urine at sonography. However, diffuse bladder wall involvement is uncommon in bladder sarcoma, as is the acute onset of symptoms.

- **Eosinophilic cystitis:** This uncommon entity could cause a similar sonographic appearance or produce polypoid lesions projecting into the bladder lumen. Peripheral eosinophilia (not present in this case) and a negative urine culture are diagnostic.

- **Hemorrhagic cystitis:** The signs, symptoms, and sonogram are consistent with this general diagnosis, which has a number of different causes. There is no history of recurrent skin or pulmonary infection to support a diagnosis of cystitis of chronic granulomatous disease. A history of chemotherapy treatments, which would raise the diagnosis of cytoxan-related cystitis, is not present. No bleeding disorder, trauma, or radiation therapy that might serve as a cause of hemorrhage is reported in this patient. By exclusion, therefore, infection is the most likely cause in this case based on the clinical information.

◆ DIAGNOSIS: Hemorrhagic viral cystitis.

◆ KEY FACTS

CLINICAL

- Acute cystitis with hemorrhage is a fairly common entity in childhood, usually discovered during evaluation for acute onset of gross hematuria, dysuria, frequency, and urgency. Suprapubic pain, fever, and enuresis are less common complaints. In the absence of bacteriuria, adenovirus (types 11 and 21) is the most common causative agent. Varicella and cytomegalovirus cystitis are less common forms.

- An antecedent upper respiratory tract infection may be associated in the minority of cases.

- Virus can be isolated from urine specimens. Alternatively, the presence of virus is inferred from the acute and convalescent serum neutralizing antibody titers. The diagnosis is often presumptive and made on clinical grounds.

- The illness is usually self-limited and lasts a few days to a few weeks. Treatment is supportive, with emphasis on good hydration.

- Other genitourinary tract anomalies and neoplasms must be excluded when symptoms persist.

- Unlike bacterial cystitis, which is more common in females and thought to result from retrograde transurethral spread, viral cystitis has no gender predilection and is likely caused by hematogenous spread.

RADIOLOGIC

- Bladder wall thickening and irregularity, decreased bladder capacity, pseudotumoral masses in the bladder, and particulate debris in patients with hemorrhagic cystitis can be seen by x-ray voiding cystourethrography, intravenous urography, ultrasound, and even CT and MRI.

- At sonography, circumferential wall thickening and inflammatory changes can be accompanied by focal mass-like lesions.

- Filling defects or masses within the bladder sometimes raise the suspicion of neoplasm. In the correct clinical setting, further work-up (e.g., cystoscopy with biopsy) is not needed, as the pseudomass will resolve in 2 to 3 weeks. Repeat imaging during the convalescent phase will document a return to a normal bladder configuration. Pathologic specimens from bladder biopsies performed during the acute phase can be difficult to interpret and may lead to unnecessary surgery.

- In contrast to the circumferential bladder wall thickening seen in cystitis, bladder neoplasms in children tend to be focal, either located in the trigone (75%) or the dome of the bladder (25%). Other conditions that may occur focally in the bladder include inflammation related to appendicitis, Crohn's disease, or pelvic inflammatory disease, impacted ureterovesical junction stones, and ureteroceles.

◆ SUGGESTED READING

Belman AB. Genitourinary Infections. In PP Kelalis, LR King, AB Belman (eds), Clinical Pediatric Urology (2nd ed). Philadelphia: Saunders, 1985;235–250.

Mufson MA, Belshe RB, Horrigan TJ, Zollar LM. Cause of acute hemorrhagic cystitis in children. Am J Dis Child 1973;126:605–609.

Rosenberg HK, Eggli KD, Zerin JM, et al. Benign cystitis in children mimicking rhabdomyosarcoma. J Ultrasound Med 1994;13:921–932.

CASE 26

Jeffrey B. Betts and
Herman Grossman

HISTORY

A 4-week-old, 32-week-gestation neonate with feeding intolerance and guaiac-positive stools.

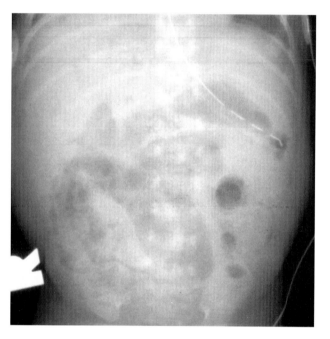

FIGURE 8-26A Supine anteroposterior radiograph of the abdomen. Cystic (right lower quadrant) and crescentic (left lower quadrant) lucencies are present within the bowel wall, representing submucosal and subserosal pneumatosis, respectively.

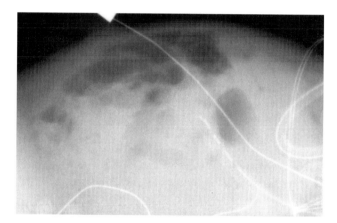

FIGURE 8-26B Cross-table supine radiograph of the abdomen. Pneumatosis and a triangle of free air, anteriorly and just subjacent to the abdominal wall, are seen. A linear lucency in the anterior aspect of the liver is present, representing portal venous gas.

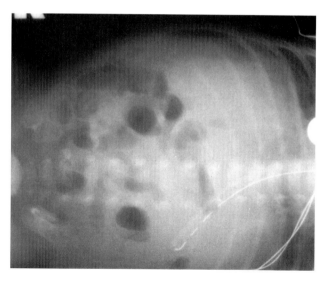

FIGURE 8-26C Left side-down decubital radiograph of the abdomen. Pneumoperitoneum is seen along the lateral margin of the liver.

◆ DIFFERENTIAL DIAGNOSIS

- **Malrotation with midgut volvulus:** This entity is seen in the neonatal period and can cause volvulus, pneumatosis, and perforation. A history of vomiting (typically bilious) is nearly always present, unlike the case shown.
- **Meconium ileus:** This entity is almost always seen in cystic fibrosis; however, pneumatosis is infrequent, and a soap-bubble appearance of the intraluminal contents in the right lower quadrant due to inspissated meconium is usually present.
- **Malrotation with Ladd's bands:** This entity can cause bowel obstruction, ischemia, pneumatosis, and perforation, but it does not usually present in the neonatal period or with distal obstruction.
- **Bowel atresia:** Atresia also presents in the immediate neonatal period. However, bowel dilation is typically much more severe than in the case illustrated. Air would not be expected in the rectum.
- **Meconium plug syndrome:** This entity is rarely seen in preterm children. Pneumatosis is not typical.
- **Small left colon:** This entity usually causes obstruction in the newborn period but is an unlikely diagnosis because pneumatosis is not typically present.
- **Hirschsprung's disease:** This may be considered because it typically presents in the neonatal period, with failure to pass stool in the first 24- to 36-hour period. However, pneumatosis is rare in the absence of enterocolitis, a complication seen beginning several weeks after birth.

Other disorders of peristalsis include:

- **Sepsis/hypoxemia/hypotension:** These entities can cause ileus, bowel wall ischemia, and pneumatosis, but the case presented did not have features indicative of these entities—e.g., cardiovascular collapse or history of respiratory difficulty or infection.
- **Necrotizing enterocolitis (NEC):** This entity is the best diagnosis, based on the history of prematurity, feeding intolerance, guaiac-positive stools, and the plain-film findings of pneumatosis, portal venous gas, and bowel perforation.

◆ DIAGNOSIS: Necrotizing enterocolitis.

◆ KEY FACTS

CLINICAL

- NEC is a result of intestinal mucosal injury with breakdown of the mucosal protective barrier, allowing bacterial proliferation and mural invasion. Abnormal peristalsis is also frequently a contributing factor.
- Approximately 80% of NEC cases occur in premature infants, usually between 3 and 6 days of life during initiation (or advancement) of feeds.
- NEC affects 1% to 5% of all neonates admitted to the intensive care nursery, and about 12% of premature infants weighing <1500 g.
- NEC is associated with hypoxia, stress, ischemia, and infection. Term infants with NEC usually have a severe underlying disease—e.g., mechanical bowel obstruction or congenital heart disease (leading to embolus) or indwelling catheters (e.g., umbilical vascular catheters).
- Clinical features involve the cardiorespiratory system (e.g., apnea, tachypnea/tachycardia, hypotension, lethargy), gastrointestinal system (gastric retention with feeding residuals, vomiting, abdominal distention, bloody stools), and peritonitis in cases of bowel perforation.
- Clinical indications for surgery (consisting of resection of necrotic bowel) include intraperitoneal free air, peritonitis, shock, persistent metabolic acidosis, and disseminated intravascular coagulation.
- Patients with NEC are at increased long-term risk of bowel strictures and adhesions (usually at the splenic flexure) and short-gut syndrome with severe malabsorption.

RADIOLOGIC

- The most common radiologic sign is small bowel distention (secondary to persistent ileus), often localized to the right lower quadrant with a dilated, featureless loop of bowel.
- Pneumatosis intestinalis (gas within the bowel wall, commonly in the ileum and colon) is the second most common (but most sign specific). Two appearances are distinguished: a curvilinear, "target" appearance (due to subserosal air); and a bubbly or cystic appearance (due to submucosal air).
- Intermittent portal venous gas, less common radiographically than pneumatosis, can sometimes be seen at sonography.
- In patients with NEC, repeat anteroposterior and cross-table lateral radiographs should be obtained every 6 to 8 hours to look for intraperitoneal air.
- After initial radiographic improvement, follow-up films are initially performed every 12 to 24 hours, with longer intervals as clinical symptoms diminish.
- Pneumoperitoneum secondary to perforation (best seen on a cross-table lateral radiograph) is the only absolute radiologic indication for surgical intervention. Outlining of the falciform ligament by air may be the only sign of bowel perforation on a supine abdominal radiograph.
- Rarely, bowel perforation can occur without evidence of free air. In these cases, a gasless abdomen or ascites can be seen. Surgery is then performed on the basis of compelling clinical evidence (e.g., shock, acidosis, peritonitis, or disseminated intravascular coagulation) rather than definite radiographic evidence of worsening.
- Contrast enemas are contraindicated because of the risk of perforation and intraperitoneal spillage of fecal material.

◆ SUGGESTED READING

Cox TD, Winters WD, Holterman MJ, et al. Neonatal bowel ischemia attributable to an umbilical arteriovenous fistula: Imaging findings. AJR Am J Roentgenol 1995;165:940–942.

Daneman A, Woodward S, de Silva M. The radiology of neonatal necrotizing enterocolitis (NEC). Pediatr Radiol 1978;7:70–77.

Robinson AE, Grossman H, Brumley GW. Pneumatosis intestinalis in the neonate. AJR Am J Roentgenol 1972;120:333–341.

HISTORY

A 36-hour-old neonate with failure to pass meconium. Visual inspection of the anus revealed no abnormalities.

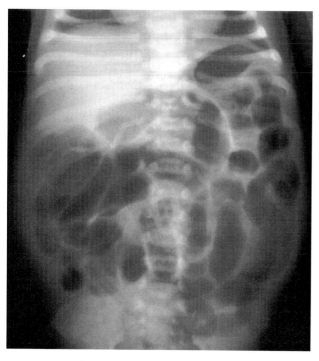

FIGURE 8-27A Supine anteroposterior abdominal radiograph. Dilatation of both large and small bowel, due to obstruction, is present.

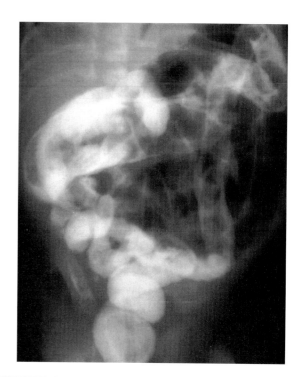

FIGURE 8-27B Oblique abdominal radiograph during barium enema. The colon is narrowed, beginning at the mid–transverse colon and proceeding distally.

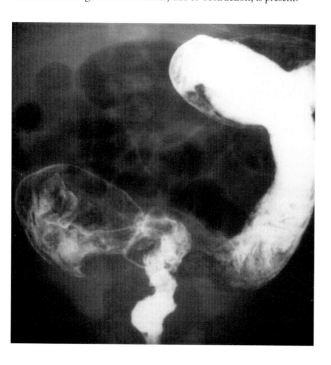

FIGURE 8-27C Another patient with the same disorder. Supine anteroposterior abdominal radiograph following evacuation of contrast material. Spasm of the rectosigmoid is present, with substantial retention of barium.

◆ DIFFERENTIAL DIAGNOSIS

◆ **Meconium plug syndrome:** Contrast material should clearly outline extensive tubular filling defects (meconium plugs) in meconium plug syndrome, which is not seen in the case illustrated.

◆ **Small left colon syndrome:** This entity is a consideration because of the obstruction and a relatively small left colon. A history of maternal diabetes would increase the likelihood of small left colon syndrome.

◆ **Anal atresia:** Absence of an anus would be expected on physical examination. Therefore, this is an incorrect diagnosis in the cases shown.

◆ **Colon atresia:** This very rare entity is diagnosed by a contrast enema showing atresia, not seen in the case shown.

◆ **Meconium ileus:** The history given for this patient raises the possibility of meconium ileus, but bilious vomiting is often present. Barium enema often shows a small, unused colon, unlike that in the cases presented here.

◆ **Ileal atresia:** The history and radiographic evidence of distal obstruction make this a possible diagnosis. However, bilious vomiting is typically present, which is not seen in the case illustrated.

◆ **Hirschsprung's disease (aganglionosis):** This diagnosis is a reasonable consideration given the history of failure to pass meconium and colonic obstruction. Although Hirschsprung's disease usually involves only a short segment of colon, a rare form of the disease can involve a long segment. The radiographic findings of rectosigmoid spasm and narrowing (Figure 8-27C) is seen in short-segment disease.

◆ DIAGNOSIS: Hirschsprung's disease.

◆ KEY FACTS

CLINICAL

◆ Hirschsprung's disease is the most common cause of bowel obstruction in the neonate, usually presenting with obstruction or intermittent diarrhea and constipation.

◆ Symptoms usually date from birth, with a failure to pass meconium during the first 24 hours of life and often bilious vomiting.

◆ The etiology of Hirschsprung's disease is thought to be an arrest of the craniocaudal migration of neuroblasts, producing an absence of ganglion cells in myenteric and submucosal plexus. This results in a hypertonic state with failure of relaxation of the aganglionic segment.

◆ Patients are usually term infants. An association with Down's syndrome (trisomy 21) has been described.

◆ The diagnosis of Hirschsprung's disease is important to establish quickly. Complications include pneumatosis, perforation, and enterocolitis (presumably due to ischemia of the bowel caused by stasis and distention of colon proximal to the obstruction).

◆ A 50% mortality rate by 1 year of age is reported in untreated cases.

◆ Four pathologic types have been described: ultra-short-segment disease (however, the true existence of this entity is in question), short-segment disease (80%), long-segment disease (15%), and total colonic Hirschsprung's disease (5%).

◆ Contemporary diagnosis in the neonate and young child is by suction biopsy, which has replaced barium enema as the principal means of diagnosis. Suction biopsy is less sensitive in older children and therefore more reliance is placed on contrast enema evaluation in these children.

RADIOLOGIC

◆ In the neonate, radiographs show dilated large and small bowel, which suggest a distal obstruction. In neonates, the plain film distinction between dilated small bowel and colon may be impossible. Distal obstruction is suggested by a more extensive amount of dilated bowel.

◆ Definitive radiologic diagnosis of Hirschsprung's disease at any age requires a contrast enema performed with meticulous technique. Filling should be performed with the patient in the lateral position, because a transition zone is best shown on this view. The colon is not prepared with cleansing enemas because cleansing can obscure the transition zone.

◆ A transition zone can be very subtle (or absent) in the newborn because colon proximal to the aganglionic segment has not yet become dilated. The transition zone must be distinguished from a focal colonic contraction, which will eventually resolve, leaving a normal caliber lumen. A transition (to more normal colon) in the proximal colon, as in the case shown above, may indicate Hirschsprung's disease of the long-segment type.

◆ Overhead radiographs at the completion of colonic filling with contrast material and after evacuation may show an abnormal rectosigmoid index (i.e., the maximum diameter of the rectum is less than the maximum diameter of the sigmoid colon).

◆ Patients with Hirschsprung's disease usually have a substantial amount of retained barium after 24 hours. Homogeneous mixing of barium with stool on delayed films is also highly suggestive of Hirschsprung's disease.

◆ SUGGESTED READING

Doig CM. Hirschsprung disease and mimicking conditions. Dig Dis 1994;12:106–116.

Rosenfield NS, Ablow RC, Markowitz RI, et al. Hirschsprung disease: Accuracy of the barium enema examination. Radiology 1984;150:393–400.

Teitelbaum DH. Hirschsprung disease in children. Curr Opin Pediatr 1995;7:316–322.

CASE 28

Donald P. Frush

HISTORY

A 1-month-old infant who presented at birth with pneumonia but has remained tachypneic after resolution of the infection.

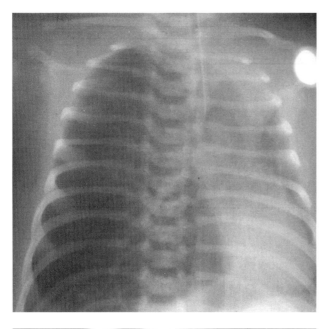

FIGURE 8-28A Anteroposterior chest radiograph. A hyperlucent and hyperinflated right lung is seen with marked leftward mediastinal shift.

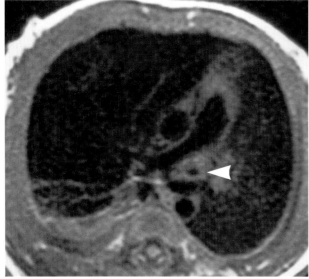

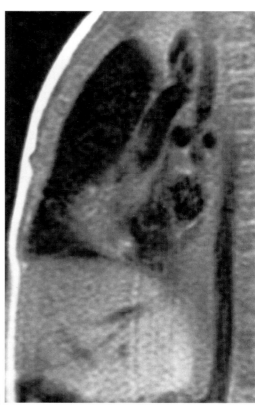

FIGURES 8-28B and 8-28C Cardiac-gated T1-weighted MRIs of the heart. **(B)** Axial MRI. A vessel originates from the right pulmonary artery and travels dorsal to the trachea. The trachea (arrowhead) is displaced to the left and narrowed. Air trapping is present in the right lung as well as collapse of the right lower lobe (which was not present when the chest radiograph was taken). **(C)** Sagittal MRI at the location of the trachea. The aberrant vessel is seen to lie dorsal to the trachea, which is compressed by the vessel.

◈ DIFFERENTIAL DIAGNOSIS

◆ **Pulmonary sling (aberrant origin of left pulmonary artery from the right pulmonary artery):** The finding of an aberrant vessel arising from the left pulmonary artery and coursing posterior to the trachea is characteristic of this diagnosis. Either air trapping, atelectasis, or both can be present. Atelectasis was an intermittent finding in the case illustrated. This is the correct diagnosis.

◆ **Vascular rings causing airway compression:**
(a) Double aorta arch or circumflex aorta: This lesion can cause stridor, but unlike the case illustrated, aeration would be expected to be symmetric. Furthermore, a right arch is not seen on the plain film in the case illustrated. (b) Right arch with anomalous left subclavian artery and ligamentum arteriosum: This anomaly should be considered because it can cause respiratory symptoms, as in the case illustrated. However, the MRI study shows that it is the left pulmonary artery, and not the subclavian artery, that has an anomalous origin. (c) Left aortic arch with aberrant right subclavian artery: The same reasoning as for (b) applies to this diagnosis.

◆ **Tracheal compression by the brachiocephalic artery:** This vascular anomaly can cause stridor, usually evident by 6 months of age. However, in this anomaly, the compression is by a vessel that is anterior to the trachea (unlike the case illustrated) and the pulmonary arteries are normal. The affected infant may outgrow the airway compromise, but occasionally an arteriopexy is needed to relieve significant compromise that produces clinical symptoms.

◆ **Other anatomic causes:** The trachea can be compressed by enlargement or midline position of the aorta, pulmonary arteries, or left atrium. The descending aorta is normally positioned in the present case. Furthermore, no enlargement of cardiovascular structures is seen in this case. None of these causes are likely explanations for the findings in the case shown.

◈ DIAGNOSIS: Aberrant left pulmonary artery (pulmonary artery sling).

◈ KEY FACTS
CLINICAL
◆ Vascular "rings" and "slings" often produce respiratory symptoms, chiefly stridor, in infants and small children (occasionally as apnea during feeding). Dysphagia is more common in older children and adults with these vascular anomalies.

◆ Bronchoscopy performed to evaluate stridor can provide the first evidence of a vascular anomaly by showing an extrinsic, pulsatile mass compressing the trachea.

◆ Rings and slings are often associated with tracheomalacia. The infant may outgrow the tracheal deficiency after vascular repair, but airway reconstruction may be necessary if compromise is significant.

◆ A pulmonary sling is one of the rarer of the vascular anomalies with airway compromise. There can be a spectrum of associated tracheal anomalies, including tracheomalacia, complete cartilaginous rings, stenosis, aberrant origins of bronchi, and atresias. The surgeon performing the vascular repair must take into consideration the potential need for airway reconstruction.

◆ Pulmonary sling is occasionally associated with structural cardiac disease, usually tetralogy of Fallot.

RADIOLOGIC
◆ MRI is the best diagnostic tool for showing the vascular anomaly and secondary airway compromise with vascular rings and slings. MRI is especially useful in older children in whom the sonographic window for optimal echocardiography is more limited.

◆ When the diagnosis is thought likely on clinical grounds, MRI can replace barium swallow as the diagnostic study of choice because more detailed operative information of the vascular anatomy and airway is available on MRI.

◆ High-resolution transaxial and supplemental sagittal and oblique coronal (in the plane of the trachea) MR images give excellent anatomic detail of the vascular and airway structures in patients with a pulmonary sling.

◈ SUGGESTED READING
Berdon WE, Baker DH. Vascular anomalies and the infant lung: Rings, slings and other things. Semin Roentgenol 1972;7:39–64.
Bisset GS. Magnetic resonance imaging of congenital heart disease in the pediatric patient. Radiol Clin North Am 1991;29:279–291.
Bisset GS, Strife JL, Kirks DR, et al. Vascular slings: Magnetic resonance imaging. AJR Am J Roentgenol 1987;149:251–256.
Donnelly LF, Strife JL, Bisset GS. The spectrum of extrinsic lower airway compression in children: MR imaging. AJR Am J Roentgenol 1997;168:59–62.
Weinberg PM. Aortic Arch Anomalies. In GC Emmanovilides, HD Allen, TA Reimenschneider, HP Gutgesell (eds), Moss and Adam's Heart Disease in Infants, Children, and Adolescents Including the Fetus and Young Adult (5th ed). Baltimore: Williams & Wilkins, 1995;810–837.

CHAPTER 9

ULTRASOUND

Mark A. Kliewer, *chapter editor*

Sheri L. Albers, James D. Bowie,
Barbara A. Carroll, Katrina Glazebrook,
Barbara S. Hertzberg, and Mark A. Kliewer

C ASE 1

James D. Bowie

H ISTORY

A 26-year-old pregnant woman who by examination is small for gestational age.

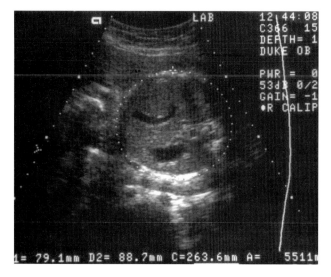

FIGURE 9-1A Transverse sonogram of the abdominal circumference in a 35-week fetus. The fetus appeared normal, but the abdominal circumference (AC) measured at the first percentile (or minus 2.56 standard deviations) for the gestational age (35.3 weeks) as determined by an earlier study in the first trimester. The fetal weight as calculated from sonographic measurements (EFW) was at the third percentile for the gestational age.

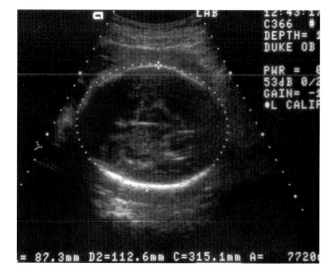

FIGURE 9-1B Transverse sonogram of the head circumference in the same fetus. The head appears larger than the abdomen and the femur length to abdominal circumference (FL:AC) ratio is 23.9, which is elevated (22.5 is considered an upper limit of normal).

◆ DIFFERENTIAL DIAGNOSIS

◆ **Key measurements:** At times, the various routine measurements of the fetus (femur length, biparietal diameter, head circumference, and abdominal circumference) can vary a great deal from each other. The critical step is to look for key measurements (abdominal circumference [AC] and sonographic measurements) to fall below a significant threshold. This can only be done with reasonable certainty when the gestational age has been determined by a prior ultrasound before 24–26 weeks or there is good clinical proof of gestational age (e.g., ovulation induction).

◆ **Abdominal circumference:** A smaller than expected AC can be a result of technical error, fetal diaphragmatic hernia, or gastroschisis. The most common cause is that the fetus is smaller than average.

◆ **Estimated fetal weight (EFW):** The EFW is a calculation generated from routine measurements. The measurements used will vary with the formula chosen, but usually the head circumference, femur length, and AC are used. Small fetal weights are seen in a variety of circumstances. If seen early in pregnancy, the possibility of an early intrauterine infection or a chromosomal abnormality should be considered.

◆ DIAGNOSIS: Small for gestational age fetus at risk for intrauterine growth retardation (IUGR).

◆ KEY FACTS

DEFINITION

◆ IUGR remains an ill-defined grouping of a variety of disorders afflicting the fetus and newborn. No good clinical definition of this condition exists.

◆ IUGR has become defined as small for gestational age (SGA). SGA babies are born below the tenth percentile for gestational age and represent a heterogeneous group including normal babies, babies with severe intrauterine infections and chromosomal abnormalities, and babies born to mothers with various placental vascular disorders.

◆ It is inherently the case that using sonographic measurements to identify SGA babies will falsely identify many normal babies as being at risk for IUGR.

CLINICAL

◆ IUGR babies are at significantly greater risk for perinatal morbidity and mortality.

◆ Identifying the cause of IUGR is often difficult, but critical in the management of these fetuses. Acute and convalescent TORCH titers and genetic amniocentesis are helpful in early or severe IUGR.

◆ Monitoring of maternal blood pressure and related disorders is valuable in other cases.

RADIOLOGIC

◆ Sonography is largely a screening test for SGA fetuses. To some extent, ultrasound provides a diagnosis for certain congenital abnormalities and can also give useful information about placental resistance via umbilical artery Doppler.

◆ The most useful screening measurement is the AC, which, if below the tenth percentile, raises the suspicion for SGA. Despite the relatively high sensitivity, the specificity is low and the predictive value of a positive test is also low.

◆ The EFW is somewhat less sensitive, but because of a higher specificity, it has a much higher predictive value for a positive test.

◆ SUGGESTED READING

Benson CB, Boswell SB, Brown DL, et al. Improved prediction of intrauterine growth retardation with use of multiple parameters. Radiology 1988;168:7–12.

Benson CB, Doubilet PM. Doppler criteria for intrauterine growth retardation: Predictive values. J Ultrasound Med 1988;7:655–659.

Crane JP, Beaver HA, Cheung SW. Antenatal ultrasound findings in fetal triploidy syndrome. J Ultrasound Med 1985;4:519–524.

Hadlock FP. Sonographic estimation of fetal age and weight. Radiol Clin North Am 1990;28:39–50.

Selbing A, Wichman K, Ryden G. Screening for detection of intrauterine growth retardation by means of ultrasound. Acta Obstet Gynecol Scand 1984;63:543–548.

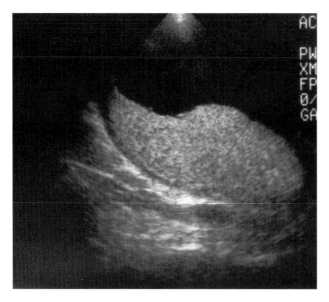
HISTORY

A 32-year-old woman who by examination is "large for dates."

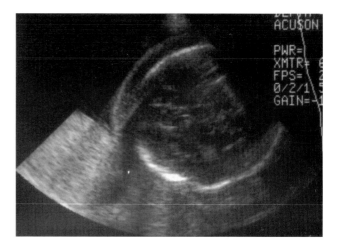

FIGURE 9-2B Transverse sonogram of the fetal head. There is marked thickening of the skin over the fetal head.

FIGURE 9-2A Longitudinal sonogram of the placenta. There is slight thickening of the placenta, with a large pocket of amniotic fluid.

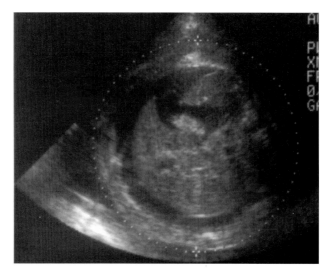

FIGURE 9-2C Transverse sonogram of the fetal body. There is fetal ascites outlining the liver and spleen. There is also skin edema.

◆ DIFFERENTIAL DIAGNOSIS

◆ **Placental enlargement:** This is one manifestation of hydrops. It is also seen with intrauterine infections and certain chromosomal abnormalities (triploidy most commonly) and in some patients with diabetes.

◆ **Polyhydramnios:** This is another manifestation of hydrops. It is also seen in a large number of conditions, including twins, diabetic mothers, and various fetal abnormalities including high gastrointestinal obstructions, central nervous system abnormalities, cardiac abnormalities (both structural and arrhythmias), and in a host of miscellaneous conditions including certain types of limb-shortening syndromes. Many cases of polyhydramnios have no known cause.

◆ **Skin edema:** This is a common feature of hydrops. A similar appearance is seen in lymphangiectasia, which is often present in association with cystic hygromas. Infants of diabetic mothers with severe macrosomia are often mistaken for babies with skin edema.

◆ **Fluid collections:** Collections of fluid within the fetus are frequently seen as an indicator of hydrops. Isolated fluid collections can be seen as a result of local inflammation, obstruction, or unknown mechanisms in conditions other than hydrops. For example, obstruction of the thoracic duct can lead to pleural fluid, and meconium peritonitis can lead to peritoneal fluid, as can rupture of an obstructed bladder or ureter.

◆ DIAGNOSIS: Hydrops fetalis of undetermined etiology.

◆ KEY FACTS

CLINICAL

◆ Most hydrops is still a result of an immune reaction between the fetus and the mother. Rh incompatibility is no longer the most common cause of these in Western nations.

◆ Rhogam is given routinely to Rh-negative mothers in situations of potential Rh exposure.

◆ Alpha-thalassemia is an important cause of hydrops in Asia.

◆ Nonimmune fetal hydrops (NIFH) has a 50% to 95% mortality.

◆ Clinical work-up for hydrops fetalis includes blood type and Rh, antibody screen, VDRL, Kleihauer-Betke test for fetal cells, acute and convalescent TORCH titers, and, in some cases, maternal hemoglobin electrophoresis.

◆ Careful sonographic examination of the fetus, cord, and placenta is essential.

RADIOLOGIC

◆ The diagnosis of hydrops is made when some combination of the following findings are observed: placental thickening, polyhydramnios, dilatation of the umbilical vein, pericardial fluid, pleural fluid, ascites, and subcutaneous edema. It is not clear what the earliest indicator of hydrops is or how many or which signs are the most specific. In general, if any one sign is present, early hydrops should be in the differential diagnosis unless there is another well-documented explanation for the abnormality. When three or more of the findings are present, it is highly likely that hydrops is the appropriate diagnosis.

◆ The task of the sonologist in hydrops is to either guide for percutaneous umbilical blood sampling (PUBS) or to investigate the intrauterine contents carefully for an identifiable cause of NIFH. NIFH has too many causes to list in detail, and hence careful examination of the entire intrauterine contents is necessary. A rough grouping of these conditions is as follows:

◆ Structural cardiac defects. Also consider trisomy 13 and 18 if these are seen.

◆ Fetal arrhythmia. Either very fast or very slow. Look for arteriovenous block and consider an autoimmune process in the mother.

◆ Fetal infections. These are usually detected by serum titers, but focal fluid collections and abdominal calcifications might suggest this as a possibility.

◆ Peripheral shunts. (1) Placental tumors such as chorioangiomas, if near the cord insertion or large, may cause fetal hydrops. (2) Vein of Galen aneurysm, when large, may be associated with hydrops. (3) Acardiac twin. In this rare condition, one fetus supplies blood to a partial twin via placental vessels.

◆ Masses restricting blood return to the heart. (1) Cystic adenomatoid malformation of the fetal lung. (2) Mediastinal teratoma.

◆ SUGGESTED READING

Fleischer AC, Killam AP, Boehm, FH, et al. Hydrops fetalis: Sonographic evaluation and clinical implications. Radiology 1981;141:163–168.

Hoddick WK, Mahony BS, Callen PW, Filly RA. Placental thickness. J Ultrasound Med 1985;4:479–482.

HISTORY

A 29-year-old woman who by examination is small for gestational age.

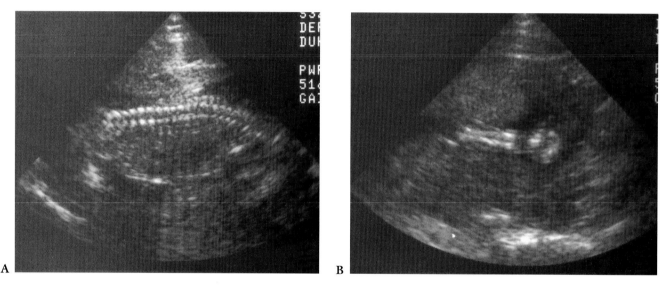

A   **B**

FIGURES 9-3A and 9-3B (**A**) Longitudinal sonogram of the fetal spine. (**B**) Longitudinal sonogram of the fetal limb. In both figures, there is marked absence of amniotic fluid, with crowding of fetal parts, increased contact of fetal structures with the uterine wall, and loss of definition of the fetus.

◆ DIFFERENTIAL DIAGNOSIS

- **Oligohydramnios:** The appearance is characteristic for oligohydramnios with little else to consider. The real issue is the cause of the oligohydramnios.
- **Abdominal pregnancy:** One feature of a rare abdominal pregnancy is the lack of amniotic fluid. This is variable and can be simply a manifestation of the unusual distribution of amniotic fluid. More typically, the fetus is in an extended position and the fetal limbs are spread rather than crowded. The diagnosis in this condition is made by tracing the myometrium from the cervix.

◆ DIAGNOSIS: Oligohydramnios from premature rupture of membranes, not clinically suspected.

◆ KEY FACTS

CLINICAL

- Fetal renal function becomes the primary determinant of amniotic fluid volume at about the eighteenth week of pregnancy.
- Normal amniotic fluid volume increases steadily until about 32 to 34 weeks of pregnancy, then decreases slightly until 42 weeks, then decreases more rapidly.
- The normal variability of amniotic fluid volume at any gestational age is high.
- Amniotic fluid volume is approximately 125 to 300 ml at 16 weeks and 400 to 2000 ml at 32 weeks.
- Clinically, oligohydramnios is suspected if the fundal height is ≥4 cm less than expected or fails to grow appropriately by serial examination.
- Clinically, oligohydramnios is defined as <300 ml of fluid at term.
- Oligohydramnios in the second trimester has a poor prognosis and is associated with fetal pulmonary hypoplasia.
- Causes for oligohydramnios include:

  - Ruptured membranes: Perhaps the most common, but usually clinically apparent.
  - Fetal distress: Including IUGR, but oligohydramnios may appear before IUGR is detected and also as an independent indicator of fetal distress.
  - Fetal death: Cardiac motion should be looked for in every case.
  - Postmaturity: Oligohydramnios does not diagnose this state but is confirmatory and indicates a possible poor outcome.

- Fetal renal abnormalities: These require that renal excretion into the amniotic fluid be reduced in volume or electrolyte content. The most common are complete bladder outlet obstruction, renal agenesis, obstruction of one kidney (usually a ureteropelvic junction obstruction [UPJ]), or multicystic dysplasia (MCD) with an abnormal contralateral kidney (UPJ, MCD, or agenesis).

RADIOLOGIC

- Diagnosis of oligohydramnios can be made by inspection. This subjective impression has been shown to be as good as objective measurements. The appearance of poor fetal definition, increased contact of the fetus with the uterine wall, crowding of fetal parts, and lack of fluid are consistent with this diagnosis.
- Some observers have looked for the largest single pocket of fluid and have measured either the volume or the greatest vertical diameter. When the latter is <2 cm, oligohydramnios is present.
- The amniotic fluid index is commonly used. This index measures the largest vertical diameter of the pockets of fluid in each of the four quadrants of the uterus and takes their sum. The number is looked up in a gestational age-adjusted table. Generally, any number <5 is consistent with oligohydramnios.
- The use of color Doppler in oligohydramnios before attempting to withdraw fluid will reveal that what appears to be a small pocket of fluid in many cases is actually the umbilical cord.
- A phenomenon called first-trimester oligohydramnios has been described. This is a misnomer. The term refers to a gestational sac that is small for the occupying embryo and suggests a poor prognosis.

◆ SUGGESTED READING

Bromley B, Harlow BL, Laboda LA, et al. Small sac size in the first trimester: A predictor of poor fetal outcome. Radiology 1991;178:375–377.

Goldstein RB, Filly RA. Sonographic estimation of amniotic fluid volume: Subjective assessment versus pocket measurements. J Ultrasound Med 1988;7:363–369.

Moore TR, Cayle JE. The amniotic fluid index in normal human pregnancy. Am J Obstet Gynecol 1990;162:1168–1173.

Queenan JT, Thompson W, Whitfield CR, et al. Amniotic fluid volumes in normal pregnancies. Am J Obstet Gynecol 1972;114:34–38.

Seeds, AE. Current concepts of amniotic fluid dynamics. Am J Obstet Gynecol 1980;138:575–586.

James D. Bowie

HISTORY

A 29-year-old pregnant woman referred for a routine fetal ultrasound.

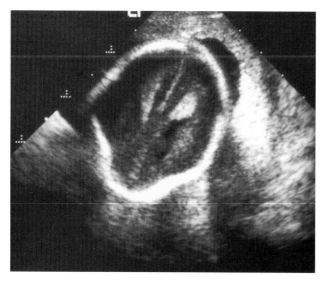

FIGURE 9-4A Transverse sonogram of the fetal head. There is an unusual shape to the frontal portion of the fetal skull. This is often called a "lemon" sign. Note also that the cerebral ventricles are normal in size.

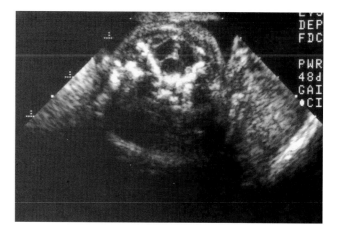

FIGURE 9-4B Transverse sonogram of the fetal head. There is a small posterior fossa with distortion of the cerebellar hemispheres. This is often called a "banana" sign.

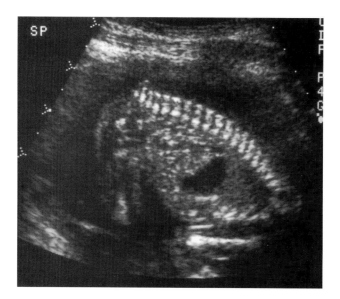

FIGURE 9-4C Longitudinal sonogram of the fetal spine. There is a single, very small, echogenic focus posterior to the last ossification centers of the distal fetal spine (left side of image).

◈ DIFFERENTIAL DIAGNOSIS

◆ **Chiari II malformation:** This is by far the most likely diagnosis. False-positive "lemon" signs occur with some frequency, but false-positive "banana" signs have not been reported.

◆ **Meningocele:** This is the likely reason for the small echogenic focus at the distal spine, but a skin lesion such as a hemangioma could have a similar appearance.

◆ **Sacrococcygeal teratomas:** These may occur in the distal spine, but they are not so directly posterior because they originate anterior to the spine. Furthermore, they tend to be much larger.

◈ DIAGNOSIS: Chiari II malformation with small sacral meningocele.

◈ KEY FACTS

CLINICAL

◆ Chiari II malformation is characterized by a small posterior fossa with downward displacement of the brainstem, resulting in protrusion of the tonsils and vermis below the cisterna magna.

◆ Secondary features seen prenatally include meningocele or encephalocele in about 90% of cases and partial or complete absence of the corpus callosum in about 40% of cases.

◆ Hydrocephalus is commonly seen by sonography as the first indication of Chiari II, but it is not always present early as in this case.

◆ Many of the CT or MRI features of this condition, such as a large massa intermedia, polymicrogyria, beaking of the tectal plate, hydromelia, and syringomelia, have not been described as prenatal sonographic features of Chiari II.

◆ Periconceptional intake of 0.4 mg of folic acid significantly reduces the risk of neural tube defects.

◆ Overall prognosis for a myelomeningocele diagnosed in utero depends on the presence and type of other abnormalities. Approximately 50% to 80% of fetuses have other abnormalities.

◆ Most deaths in patients with an isolated myelomeningocele are the result of the hindbrain dysfunction associated with Chiari II malformation. About 15% of patients die by the age of 10.

◆ About 30% of survivors have IQs >100. About 30% have IQs <80. About one-third have hindbrain dysfunction.

◆ Ninety percent of neonatal survivors require ventriculoperitoneal shunts. About half of these shunts must be revised by age 6. About one-third require two shunt revisions and a fifth three or more.

◆ Almost 100% of survivors have some loss of motor function. Urinary incontinence is common.

RADIOLOGIC

◆ The lemon sign has been said to be a specific finding of Chiari II malformations, but it is also seen in normals. This is especially true for milder degrees of frontal bone contour abnormalities.

◆ The degree of severity of the posterior fossa deformity (the banana sign) correlates with the degree of hydrocephaly.

◆ Both the degree and prevalence of hydrocephaly increases with gestational age.

◆ The absence of ventriculomegaly prior to 24 weeks does not exclude either meningocele or Chiari II.

◈ SUGGESTED READING

Babcock CJ, Goldstein RB, Barth RA, et al. Prevalence of ventriculomegaly in association with myelomeningocele and severity of posterior fossa deformity. Radiology 1994;190:703–707.

Filly RA. The "lemon" sign: A clinical perspective. Radiology 1998; 167:573–575.

Filly RA, Cardoza JD, Goldstein RB, Barkovich AJ. Detection of fetal central nervous system anomalies: A practical level of effort for a routine sonogram. Radiology 1989;172:403–408.

Nelson MD, Bracchi M, Naidich TP, McLone DG. The natural history of repaired myelomeningocele. Radiographics 1988;8:695–706.

Nicolaides KH, Campbell S, Gabbe SG, et al. Ultrasound screening for spina bifida: Cranial and cerebellar signs. Lancet 1986;2:72–73.

Werler MM, Shapiro S, Mitchell AA. Periconceptional folic acid exposure and risk of occurrent neural tube defects. JAMA 1993;269:1257–1261.

CASE 5

James D. Bowie

HISTORY

A 51-year-old woman presents to the emergency room with weight loss, loss of appetite, and vague abdominal pain.

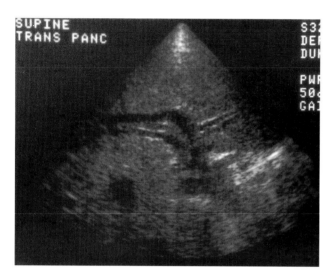

FIGURE 9-5A Transverse sonogram of the liver. This view shows a portion of the liver with parallel tubular structures present. This is the typical appearance of dilated intrahepatic bile ducts.

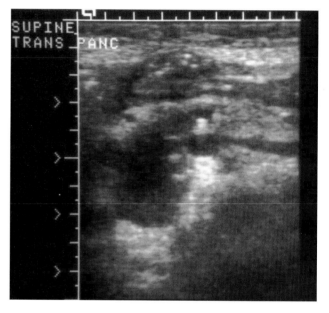

FIGURE 9-5B Transverse sonogram of the epigastrium. This image shows portions of the pancreas. In the head of the pancreas there is a hypoechoic mass. In addition, a single calcification is seen in the body of the pancreas.

◆ DIFFERENTIAL DIAGNOSIS

- **Dilated intrahepatic bile ducts:** These have a relatively specific pattern. On occasion, very large hepatic arteries can produce a similar appearance. This is sometimes seen with alcoholic cirrhosis or portal hypertension. Color Doppler imaging is useful for excluding this unusual possibility. Compared to portal veins, bile ducts may demonstrate posterior acoustical enhancement because bile is noncellular and not moving.
- **A mass in the head of the pancreas:** This could be associated with either pancreatitis (acute or chronic) or carcinoma of the pancreas.
- **A single calcification of the pancreas:** This diagnosis is not helpful. Multiple calcifications, especially in the pancreatic ducts, are strongly suggestive of chronic pancreatitis. Microcystic adenomas of the pancreas often contain calcifications, but many other pancreatic tumors, including islet cell tumors, may also calcify.

◆ DIAGNOSIS: Pancreatic abscess in a patient with recurrent and chronic pancreatitis.

◆ KEY FACTS

CLINICAL

- Pancreatic lithiasis occurs in 20% to 40% of patients with chronic pancreatitis and is highly associated with alcohol-induced pancreatitis. These are true stones lying within the ductal system of the pancreas.
- Calcification of the mass is rare in ductal adenocarcinoma, but calcifications in the pancreas may occur in as many as 25% of patients.
- A pseudocyst is distinguished from an acute fluid collection by the presence of a well-defined wall.
- Pancreatic abscesses likely arise in areas of necrosis. If the necrosis is limited or no longer present, it is called an *abscess.* If there is moderate to severe pancreatic necrosis, this is called *infected pancreatic necrosis.*
- One in four patients with acute pancreatitis will have a severe case. Of these, half will have a complication and a third will die. Eighty percent of the deaths result from infection.
- The mortality for infected pancreatic necrosis is twice that for pancreatic abscess and three times that of sterile necrosis.

RADIOLOGIC

- Infected pancreatic pseudocysts tend to have more internal echoes than noninfected pseudocysts.
- The most common sonographic features of chronic pancreatitis are inhomogeneity, focal or diffuse enlargement, focal bright echoes, pseudocysts, and focal masses in the head of the pancreas. The last feature occurs in about 7% of cases. The pancreatic duct may be enlarged and beaded. The common bile duct is often enlarged as well.
- A little over half of the patients with chronic pancreatitis have dilated extrahepatic bile ducts, and about three-fourths of these have coincident dilated intrahepatic bile ducts. Most of the patients with dilated bile ducts have a dilated pancreatic duct and a mass in the pancreatic head. From 25% to 50% of patients with chronic pancreatitis will have a normal sonogram.
- Pancreatic carcinoma is typically seen as a hypoechoic mass or focal enlargement of the pancreas. The diagnosis is usually made by a percutaneous biopsy.

◆ SUGGESTED READING

Alpern MB, Sandler MA, Kellman GM, Madrazo BL. Chronic pancreatitis: Ultrasonic features. Radiology 1985;155:215–219.

Bradley EL. The Necessity for a Clinical Classification of Acute Pancreatitis: The Atlanta System. In Acute Pancreatitis: Diagnosis and Therapy. New York: Raven, 1994;27–32.

Bressler EL, Rubin JM, McCracken S. Sonographic parallel channel sign: A reappraisal. Radiology 1987;164:343–346.

Condad MR, Landay MJ, Janes JO. Sonographic "parallel channel" sign of biliary tree enlargement in mild to moderate obstructive jaundice. AJR Am J Roentgenol 1978;130:279–286.

Huntington DK, Hill MC, Steinberg W. Biliary tract dilatation in chronic pancreatitis: CT and sonographic findings. Radiology 1989;172:47–50.

Lee CM, Chang-Chien CS, Lin DY, et al. The real time ultrasonography of pancreatic pseudocyst: Comparison of infected and noninfected pseudocysts. J Clin Ultrasound 1988;16:393–398.

Ralls PW, Mayekawa DS, Lee KP, et al. The use of color Doppler sonography to distinguish dilated intrahepatic ducts from vascular structures. AJR Am J Roentgenol 1989;152:291–292.

Wing VW, Laing FC, Jeffrey RB, Guyon J. Sonographic differentiation of enlarged hepatic arteries from dilated intrahepatic bile ducts. AJR Am J Roentgenol 1985;145:57–61.

CASE 6

Mark A. Kliewer

A 35-year-old woman presents with vague right upper quadrant pain.

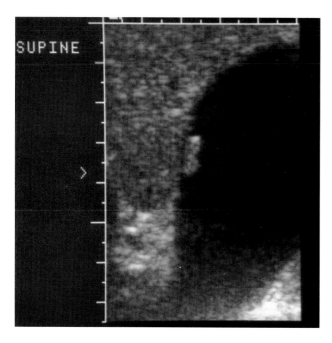

FIGURE 9-6A Longitudinal sonogram of the gallbladder fossa. Attached to the gallbladder wall is a small echogenic mass. This mass does not cause significant ring down or shadowing artifacts.

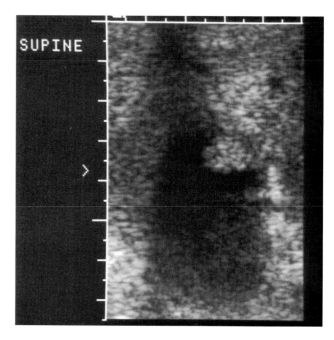

FIGURE 9-6B High-resolution sonogram of this same location. High-resolution image reveals the lobular contour of the gallbladder wall mass.

◆ DIFFERENTIAL DIAGNOSIS

- **Gallstone:** A gallstone is unlikely because the abnormality is adherent to the wall and nonmobile, and because of the absence of posterior acoustical shadowing.
- **Cholesterol polyp:** These polyps are common intraluminal masses that are most often multiple. The polyps tend to be small, usually <5 mm in size, and almost always <1 cm in size. They are not associated with acoustical shadowing.
- **Adenoma or papilloma:** These lesions are almost always singular and are much less common than cholesterol polyps. These masses can be sessile and broad based (adenomas) or pedunculated and lobulated (papillary adenomas). Masses are usually <1 cm.
- **Primary gallbladder carcinoma:** Carcinomas are most often seen as a large, solid mass replacing the gallbladder in the gallbladder fossa. Occasionally, in earlier stages focal intraluminal masses are seen, but these are usually >1 cm in size. Associated findings include wall calcification, biliary duct dilatation, gallstones (80%), and evidence for metastatic spread, particularly to the liver.
- **Tumefactive sludge:** This echogenic bile is not usually adherent to the wall but rather shifts location as the patient is repositioned.

◆ DIAGNOSIS: Cholesterol polyp.

◆ KEY FACTS

CLINICAL
- Cholesterolosis results from the accumulation of cholesterol within the wall of the gallbladder. This accumulation can either be diffuse or polypoid.

- Cholesterol nodules can stud the mucosal surface, producing the so-called "strawberry gallbladder" seen pathologically.
- Cholesterolosis is equally common in men and women. The etiology is uncertain.

RADIOLOGIC
- Intraluminal masses are commonly seen during gallbladder ultrasound. Fortunately, the majority of these are cholesterol polyps that are benign.
- Sonographically, cholesterol polyps are most commonly multiple and small. Most of these benign polypoid masses in the gallbladder are <1 cm. Those masses that are ≥1 cm warrant follow-up imaging in 6 months to document any change or growth of the lesion. Lesions that are significantly >1 cm may require surgery.
- Cholesterol polyps are nonmobile intraluminal masses that are firmly adherent to the wall. They do not cause acoustic shadowing. Such polyps can be hypo- or hyperechoic, though most, in our experience, are hyperechoic.

◆ SUGGESTED READING

Jutras JA. Hyperplastic cholecystoses. AJR Am J Roentgenol 1960; 83:795–827.

Middleton WD. Gallbladder. In BB Goldberg (ed), Textbook of Abdominal Ultrasound. Baltimore: Williams & Wilkins, 1993;116–145.

Price RJ, Stewart ET, Foley WD, Dodds WJ. Sonography of polypoid cholesterolosis. AJR Am J Roentgenol 1982;139:1197–1198.

Ruhe AH, Zachman JP, Mulder BD, Rime AE. Cholesterol polyps of the gallbladder: Ultrasound demonstration. J Clin Ultrasound 1979;7:386–388.

HISTORY

A 53-year-old man presents with acute abdominal pain and vomiting.

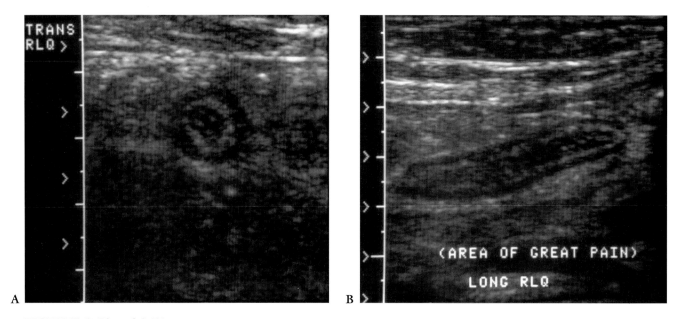

FIGURES 9-7A and 9-7B (A) Transverse sonogram of the right lower quadrant. (B) Longitudinal sonogram of the same area in the right lower quadrant. The transducer was placed over the area of greatest tenderness. Longitudinal and transverse images demonstrate a noncompressible, tubular structure measuring 11 mm in diameter. The rounded end of the structure is clearly identifiable. The structure demonstrates a hyperechoic inner layer and a surrounding, peripheral hypoechoic layer. The patient was particularly tender over this structure.

◆DIFFERENTIAL DIAGNOSIS

- **Normal appendix:** The normal appendix should have a diameter of ≤5 to 6 mm and should be compressible. In addition, there should be no evidence of inflammatory changes in the periappendiceal fat.
- **Crohn's disease:** Hypoechoic, uniform thickening of the bowel wall in the terminal ileum would surround compressed echogenic mucosa centrally. Furthermore, the terminal ileum would not have a blind end.
- **Appendicitis:** This is the best diagnosis for a rigid tubular structure located in the right lower quadrant at the site of maximal tenderness. The diameter measurement from the outer wall to the outer wall of the structure exceeds 6 mm. The structure is noncompressible and blind-ended. On the longitudinal view, a region of increased echogenicity surrounding the appendix suggests inflammation in the periappendiceal fat.
- **Mesenteric adenitis:** With this disease process, enlarged lymph nodes and mural thickening of the terminal ileum will be evident. Peristalsis should also be present in the terminal ileum. Inflamed lymph nodes would be unlikely to have such a smooth tubular contour, or the layering of hyperechoic and hypoechoic strata that constitute the gut signature.
- **Pelvic inflammatory disease (PID):** Though PID is a possible pitfall, findings should be located more in the pelvis than the right lower quadrant. A hydrosalpinx would not have the same echopattern as the bowel.

◆DIAGNOSIS: Appendicitis.

◆KEY FACTS

CLINICAL

- Though the clinical suspicion of appendicitis is correct in 70% of patients with this disease, the clinical picture can be confusing. As a result, surgeons have long accepted a removal rate of normal appendices between 15% and 33%.
- Young women can be particularly difficult to diagnose because of the similarity of symptoms between appendicitis, PID, and ovarian torsion.

RADIOLOGIC

- The technique of examination requires using high-frequency, linear transducers (5 or 7 MHz). The sonologist applies graded compression with the transducer and moves from the right upper quadrant to the right lower quadrant following the right colon inferiorly. Alternatively, the iliac vessels can be identified in the groin and followed superiorly.
- The patient can often direct attention to pathology by localizing pain. Be alert to areas of maximal tenderness.
- The goal is to compress the inflamed appendix against the posterior abdominal wall or the psoas muscles.
- An inflamed appendix is noncompressible and has a diameter of ≥6 mm.
- A fecalith may be seen within the appendix and may be associated with acoustical shadowing.
- Look also for periappendiceal fluid, abscess, or an inflammatory mass. The circumferential echogenic mucosal layer of the appendix may be disrupted when perforation occurs. The periappendiceal fat may be echogenic, indicating inflammatory involvement.
- Increased Doppler signal (blood flow) can be found both within and surrounding the inflamed appendix.

◆SUGGESTED READING

Jeffrey RB, Laing FC, Lewis FR. Acute appendicitis: High-resolution real-time US findings. Radiology 1987;163:11–14.

Kliewer MA. Abdominal Sonography. In CE Ravin, C Cooper, RA Leder (eds), Review of Radiology (2nd ed). Philadelphia: Saunders, 1994;389–401.

Laing FC. Ultrasonography of the acute abdomen. Radiol Clin North Am 1992;30:389–404.

Puylaert JBCM. Acute appendicitis: US evaluation using graded compression. Radiology 1986;158:355–360.

Puylaert JBCM. Mesenteric adenitis and acute terminal ileitis: US evaluation using graded compression. Radiology 1986;161:691–695.

Quillin SP, Siegel MJ. Color Doppler US of children with acute lower abdominal pain. Radiographics 1993;13:1281–1293.

HISTORY

A 32-year-old pregnant woman presents with a discrepancy in her size and dates.

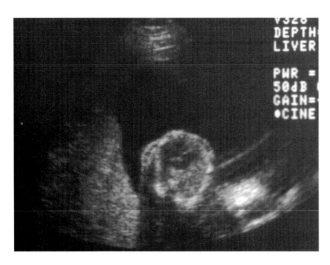

FIGURE 9-8A Transverse sonogram of twin A. A cross-sectional image through the thorax of twin A demonstrates a large amount of fluid surrounding this twin.

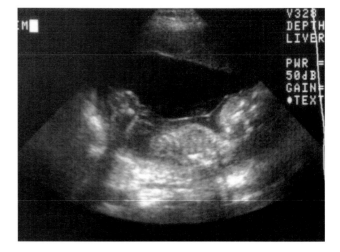

FIGURE 9-8B Longitudinal sonogram of twin B. Twin B lies adjacent to the uterine wall. Anterior to the fetus, a thin membrane is seen which is closely adherent to the contours of the fetal body and head. A minimal amount of amniotic fluid is seen surrounding this fetus.

◆DIFFERENTIAL DIAGNOSIS

◆ **Monoamniotic, monochorionic twinning:** When no separating membrane is seen, the possibility that the twins occupy the same amniotic sac must be considered. In this case, the separating membrane can be seen, although it closely covers portions of twin B.

◆ **Twin transfusion syndrome:** This condition usually results in a small, anemic twin and a hydropic co-twin. Severe fluid discrepancies can occur, as in this case.

◆ **Stuck twin phenomenon:** The phenomenon results from severe fluid discrepancy between twins in different gestational sacs. The stuck twin is rendered immobile within its oligohydramniotic sac.

◆DIAGNOSIS: Stuck twin phenomenon.

◆KEY FACTS

CLINICAL

◆ The stuck twin phenomenon results when there is a severe amniotic fluid discrepancy between the two gestational sacs. The fetus in the severely oligohydramniotic sac appears attached to the uterine wall and will not change location with patient repositioning. Moreover, this twin's movements are restricted.

◆ The co-twin is frequently seen in a polyhydramniotic sac.

◆ Frequently there is a discrepancy in fetal growth.

◆ The stuck twin phenomenon may be a consequence of the twin transfusion syndrome, but the transfusion syndrome is not a necessary precondition.

◆ Both twins have a poor prognosis. Most pregnancies result in the death of both fetuses. Presentation after 26 weeks, however, has been associated with improved survival.

RADIOLOGIC

◆ It is often difficult to identify the separating membranes in the stuck twin phenomenon. This can cause confusion with monoamniotic twinning. The membrane should be sought at the ends of the fetus, particularly as it comes off the head. Occasionally, the membrane can be seen as a thin echogenic sheet covering the normal folds and recesses of the fetal body.

◆ The relative immobility of the fetus in the oligohydramniotic sac can be demonstrated by repositioning the mother.

◆ A careful search for structural abnormalities of both fetuses should be made.

◆ The fetus in the polyhydramniotic sac should be inspected carefully for evidence of hydrops.

◆ Doppler tracings obtained in umbilical cords may provide evidence of the twin transfusion syndrome, although Doppler findings may not be distinguishable from severe growth discrepancies.

◆SUGGESTED READING

Bruner JP, Rosemond RL. Twin-to-twin transfusion syndrome: A subset of the twin oligohydramnios-polyhydramnios sequence. Am J Obstet Gynecol 1993;169:925–930.

Chescheir NC, Seeks JW. Polyhydramnios and oligohydramnios in twin gestations. Obstet Gynecol 1988;71:882–884.

Harrison SD, Cyr DR, Patten RM, Mack LA. Twin growth problems: Causes and sonographic analysis. Semin Ultrasound CT MRI 1993;14:56–67.

Mahony BS, Filly RA, Callen PW. Amnionicity and chorionicity in twin pregnancies: Prediction using ultrasound. Radiology 1985;155:205–209.

Nyberg DA, Finberg HJ. The Placenta, Placental Membranes, and Umbilical Cord. In DA Nyberg, BS Mahony, DH Pretorius (eds), Diagnostic Ultrasound of Fetal Anomalies. Chicago: Year Book, 1990;623–675.

Pretorius DH, Manchester D, Barkin S, et al. Doppler ultrasound of twin transfusion syndrome. J Ultrasound Med 1988;7:117–124.

Weiner CP, Ludomirski A. Diagnosis, pathophysiology, and treatment of chronic twin-to-twin transfusion syndrome. Fetal Diagn Ther 1994;9:283–290.

CASE 9

Mark A. Kliewer

HISTORY

A 26-year-old woman presents for routine obstetric ultrasound.

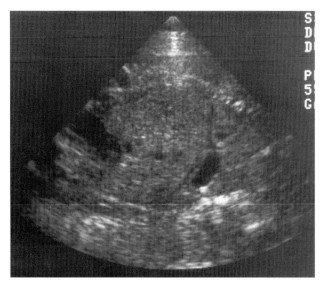

FIGURE 9-9A Longitudinal sonogram of the fetal body, cephalic presentation. The fetal thorax is on the right of the image and the fetal abdomen on the left. The hypoechoic arc of the diaphragm is apparently disrupted. Superior to the diaphragm and posterior to the heart, there is a rounded, fluid-filled structure that most likely represents the stomach.

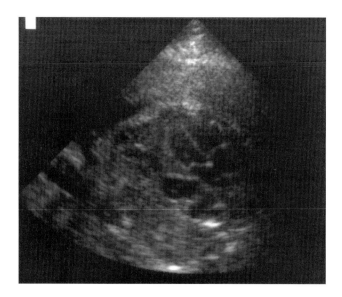

FIGURE 9-9B Transverse sonogram through the fetal chest at the level of the heart demonstrates the fluid-filled structure adjacent to the heart. In this cephalic presentation, the heart is on the right side of the fetal body, indicating displacement from its normal position.

◆ DIFFERENTIAL DIAGNOSIS

- **Cystic adenomatoid malformation:** This entity is typically seen as multiple large cysts or an echogenic mass. Occasionally it can occur with a diaphragmatic hernia.
- **Congenital diaphragmatic hernia (CDH):** A hernia of this type is a likely possibility given the displacement of the stomach into the chest and the apparent discontinuity of the hypoechoic diaphragm.
- **Bronchogenic and esophageal duplication cyst:** It is possible that the fluid-filled structure in the left chest could be a foregut abnormality; however, the stomach is not present in its expected location.
- **Cystic teratoma:** These are typically complex masses with cystic and solid components arising in the mediastinum.
- **Eventration of the diaphragm:** It is difficult to exclude eventration with certainty considering how difficult it is to demonstrate the full contour of the diaphragm in the normal fetus.

◆ DIAGNOSIS: Congenital diaphragmatic hernia.

◆ KEY FACTS

CLINICAL

- Herniation of bowel or solid organs can occur through defects in the diaphragm that form from incomplete closure during embryologic development. Most are Bochdalek defects, which occur posteriorly, usually on the left side.
- Bowel herniating through the left-sided defect will cause displacement of thoracic structures, particularly the heart, to the right.
- When hernias occur on the right side, the liver may be involved.
- Patients sometimes present because their fundal size is greater than their dates. This results when there is associated polyhydramnios, which most often develops in the third trimester.

- More than half of babies with CDH will have an associated anomaly. These anomalies can involve the heart, genitourinary system, the central nervous system, and the gastrointestinal tract. The diaphragmatic hernia can be part of a larger syndrome, such as the trisomy syndromes.
- There is a high mortality rate for infants born with diaphragmatic hernias resulting primarily from pulmonary hypoplasia.

RADIOLOGIC

- Sonographic diagnosis depends on the demonstration of bowel in the fetal thorax. On a true transverse image, the heart should never be at the same level as the stomach. Occasionally, hepatic, portal, and mesenteric blood vessels will be displaced toward the defect. The stomach will not be located in its expected left upper quadrant position, and the abdomen can appear scaphoid due to the relocation of bowel from the abdomen to the thorax.
- Intrathoracic structures are usually displaced to the right with left-sided lesions. The heart, in particular, will be found on the right side. Occasionally, the diaphragm can be inspected directly and a defect identified. The motion of the two hemidiaphragms can be compared during fetal breathing for evidence of dissynchronous motion.
- Polyhydramnios frequently complicates the pregnancy.
- The sonologist should always look for other evidence of fetal abnormality, including other structural anomalies and intrauterine growth retardation.

◆ SUGGESTED READING

Chinn DH, Filly RA, Callen PW, et al. Congenital diaphragmatic hernia diagnosed prenatally by ultrasound. Radiology 1983;148:119–123.

Comstock CH. The antenatal diagnosis of diaphragmatic anomalies. J Ultrasound Med 1986;5:391–396.

May DA, Barth RA, Yeager S, et al. Perinatal and postnatal chest sonography. Radiol Clin North Am 1993;31:499–516.

Morin L, Crombleholme TM, D'Alton ME. Prenatal diagnosis and management of fetal thoracic lesions. Semin Perinatol 1994;18:228–253.

CASE 10

Barbara S. Hertzberg

HISTORY

A 28-year-old woman has vaginal bleeding and a positive beta-human chorionic gonadotropin (β-HCG) level.

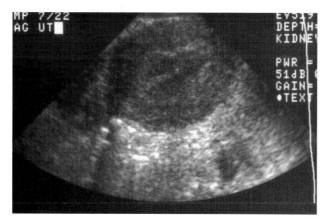

FIGURE 9-10A Sagittal endovaginal sonogram of the uterus. There is no evidence of an intrauterine pregnancy. The endometrial stripe is normal.

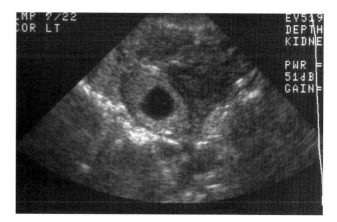

FIGURE 9-10B Coronal endovaginal sonogram of the left adnexa. An echogenic ring surrounds a rounded fluid collection in the left adnexa, consistent with an "adnexal ring sign."

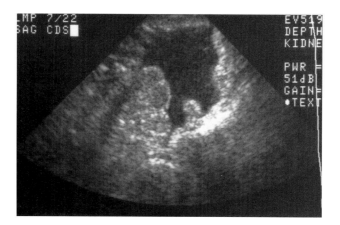

FIGURE 9-10C Sagittal endovaginal sonogram of the pelvic cul-de-sac. Echogenic free fluid surrounds loops of bowel in the cul-de-sac, due to hemoperitoneum.

◆ DIFFERENTIAL DIAGNOSIS

The differential diagnosis includes conditions found in patients with a positive serum β-HCG but no ultrasound evidence of an intrauterine pregnancy:

- **Early intrauterine pregnancy:** This is unlikely because there are abnormal findings in both the adnexa and the cul-de-sac.
- **Spontaneous abortion:** This condition is also unlikely because of the abnormalities in the adnexa and the cul-de-sac.
- **Gestational trophoblastic disease:** This disease is unlikely because the endometrial stripe is normal. There is no evidence of an echogenic intrauterine mass with multiple internal cysts, the finding usually seen in patients with gestational trophoblastic disease.
- **Ectopic pregnancy:** This is the best diagnosis because demonstration of an "adnexal ring sign" in conjunction with sonographically demonstrable hemoperitoneum is highly suggestive of ectopic pregnancy in a patient with a positive β-HCG and no intrauterine pregnancy.

◆ DIAGNOSIS: Left ectopic pregnancy.

◆ KEY FACTS

CLINICAL

- The spectrum of clinical symptoms ranges from pelvic pain and vaginal bleeding (often clinically indistinguishable from spontaneous abortion) to catastrophic intra-abdominal hemorrhage.
- A β-HCG is necessary to interpret the ultrasound findings: a negative serum β-HCG effectively excludes an ectopic pregnancy.
- The "classic clinical triad" suggesting ectopic pregnancy is amenorrhea, pain, and palpable adnexal mass. This triad, however, is often not present.
- All women with positive β-HCG should be considered at risk for ectopic pregnancy. The following groups are at especially high risk: history of pelvic inflammatory disease, intrauterine contraceptive device, prior ectopic pregnancy, tubal reconstructive surgery, prior tubal ligation, or in vitro fertilization.
- A minority of patients with ectopic pregnancy are critically ill and hemodynamically unstable due to massive intra-abdominal hemorrhage. They require rapid fluid resuscitation and immediate laparotomy, and there may be no time for ultrasound imaging in this group.

RADIOLOGIC

- Ultrasound is the imaging procedure of choice in the patient with a suspected ectopic pregnancy.
- One of the main goals of ultrasound is to assess whether there is an intrauterine pregnancy. An intrauterine pregnancy and a coexistent ectopic pregnancy is a rare entity, so if an intrauterine pregnancy is documented, it is generally considered safe to assume there is no ectopic pregnancy.
- An intrauterine pregnancy can be diagnosed based on the demonstration of at least one of the following ultrasound findings: (1) intrauterine embryo with cardiac activity, (2) intrauterine yolk sac, and (3) intrauterine gestational sac. An intrauterine gestational sac must be distinguished from a pseudogestational sac of an ectopic pregnancy because ectopic pregnancies can frequently be associated with fluid collections within the uterus. Demonstration of either a "double decidual sac sign" or an "intradecidual sign," in which the uterine cavity is shown to be separate from the developing gestational sac, indicates the presence of an intrauterine gestational sac.
- The only ultrasound finding 100% diagnostic of ectopic pregnancy is identification of an extrauterine embryo with cardiac activity.
- The adnexal ring sign, produced when echogenic trophoblastic tissue grows on the inner surface of the fallopian tube around the developing gestational sac, is the next most reliable sign of ectopic pregnancy. Other adnexal findings include pelvic and tubal hematomas. These can assume a wide variety of ultrasound appearances depending on the stage of the hematoma.
- In the appropriate setting, fluid in the cul-de-sac should also raise the level of concern for ectopic pregnancy, particularly if it contains low-level echoes suggesting the presence of blood.
- A negative pelvic ultrasound (empty uterus, normal-appearing ovaries, no adnexal masses, and no free fluid in the cul-de-sac) does not exclude an ectopic pregnancy.

◆ SUGGESTED READING

Filly RA. Ectopic pregnancy: The role of sonography. Radiology 1987;162:661–668.

Hertzberg BS. Ultrasound evaluation for ectopic pregnancy. Radiologist 1994;1:11–18.

Nyberg DA, Hughes MP, Mack LA, Wang KY. Extrauterine findings of ectopic pregnancy at transvaginal US: Importance of echogenic fluid. Radiology 1991;178:823–826.

Parvey RH, Maklad N. Pitfalls in the transvaginal sonographic diagnosis of ectopic pregnancy. J Ultrasound Med 1993;3:139–144.

CASE 11

Barbara S. Hertzberg

HISTORY

A 38-year-old pregnant woman presents with third-trimester bleeding.

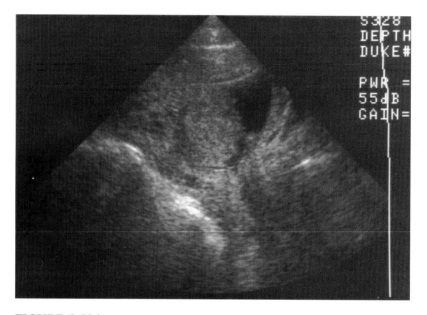

FIGURE 9-11A Midline sagittal transabdominal sonogram of the lower uterus and cervix. There is a posterior placenta. The lower edge of the placenta overlies the endocervical canal.

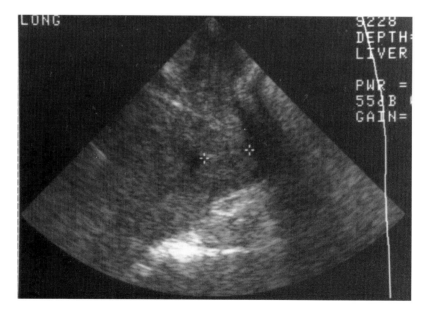

FIGURE 9-11B Transperineal sonogram of the lower uterus and cervix. The transperineal image confirms the presence of placental tissue covering the endocervical canal. (The endocervical canal is delineated by electronic measurement calipers.)

◆ DIFFERENTIAL DIAGNOSIS

Placenta previa should be considered whenever placental tissue overlies the region of the cervix at ultrasonography. False-positive diagnoses of placenta previa are common and must be considered prior to making a definitive diagnosis.

- **False-positive due to distended urinary bladder:** This is unlikely, because the bladder does not appear distended on the ultrasound images.
- **False-positive due to uterine contraction:** A contraction is unlikely because there is no evidence of a lower uterine contraction on either of the images. A uterine contraction might be associated with an elongated cervix that is distorted in its overall appearance. The cervix in this patient is normal in length and configuration.
- **Subchorionic hematoma overlying the cervix:** This condition would be possible if the hematoma were imaged in an acute stage, because the sonographic pattern of an acute hematoma can be remarkably similar to that of placental tissue. It may be possible to appreciate a subtle difference in the echo pattern of the hematoma versus the echo pattern of placental tissue. At times, the distinction is only made at the time of follow-up sonography because a subchorionic hematoma will show evolution in its appearance.
- **Fibroid overlying cervix:** Such a fibroid is unlikely because the tissue overlying the cervix is continuous with placental tissue and does not have a sonographic pattern typical for a leiomyoma.
- **Complete placenta previa:** This is the best diagnosis because placental tissue completely overlies the internal os.

◆ DIAGNOSIS: Complete placenta previa.

◆ KEY FACTS

CLINICAL

- Painless vaginal bleeding is the clinical hallmark of placenta previa. Bleeding most commonly occurs in the third trimester but can also occur during the second trimester.
- Vaginal delivery can result in disastrous complications, including either or both maternal and fetal death due to massive bleeding.
- A cesarean section is required in patients with complete placenta previa. Some patients with milder degrees of placenta previa can deliver vaginally.
- There is a high association between placenta previa and abnormalities of placental attachment, such as placenta accreta, increta, and percreta. Cesarean hysterectomy may be necessary in some patients with these disorders.

RADIOLOGIC

- Ultrasound is the imaging method of choice for placental localization.
- It is necessary to see both the lower edge of the placenta and the cervix to assess placenta previa accurately. Visualization of just the lower edge of the placenta excludes a placenta previa due to the main mass of the placenta but does not exclude an accessory lobe of the placenta overlying the cervix.
- Ultrasound for placenta previa should be done with an empty urinary bladder. If the bladder is full and ultrasound suggests placenta previa, scanning should be repeated after voiding.
- If the cervix cannot be seen using a transabdominal approach, alternate methods such as transperineal or endovaginal scanning can be attempted. In most cases, endovaginal scanning can be avoided by using transperineal scanning. If endovaginal scanning is done, it should be performed with caution, because bleeding is a well-recognized complication of manual examination of the cervix in patients with placenta previa. Nevertheless, a substantial risk from endovaginal imaging has not been documented in patients with placenta previa.
- Grading systems for placenta previa vary from institution to institution, so it is important that the radiologist and clinician be aware of the meaning of the terminology used.
- In general, complete placenta previa refers to the situation in which placental tissue is implanted on both sides of the internal cervical os, completely covering the os. Complete placenta previa can be subdivided into *central complete previa*, in which the placenta is centered over the cervix, and *asymmetric complete placenta previa*, in which the placenta is not centered over the cervix but a margin of placental tissue is implanted on both sides of the os.
- *Partial placenta previa* refers to the situation when placental tissue covers a portion of the internal cervical os, but not the entire os. *Marginal placenta previa* covers part of the cervix without involving the os. It is frequently difficult to distinguish between marginal and partial placenta previa.

◆ SUGGESTED READING

Artis AA, Bowie JD, Rosenberg ER, Rauch RF. The fallacy of placental migration: Effect of sonographic techniques. AJR Am J Roentgenol 1985;144:79–81.

Hertzberg BS, Bowie JD, Carroll BA, Kliewer MA. Diagnosis of placenta previa during the third trimester: Role of transperineal sonography. AJR Am J Roentgenol 1992;159:83–87.

Leerentveld RA, Gilberts EC, Arnold MJ, Wladimiroff JW. Accuracy and safety of transvaginal sonographic placental localization. Obstet Gynecol 1990;76:759–762.

CASE 12

Barbara S. Hertzberg

HISTORY

A 38-year-old woman referred for obstetric ultrasound at 27 menstrual weeks.

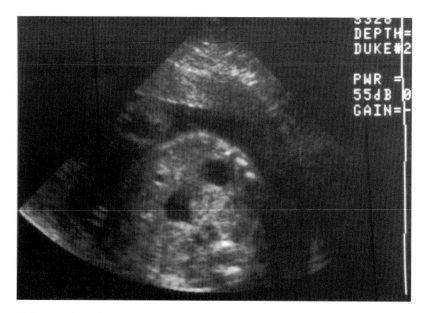

FIGURE 9-12A Axial sonogram through the fetal abdomen. There are two rounded, fluid-filled structures in the mid-abdomen. The more laterally located structure corresponds to the fetal stomach. The second cystic structure, located just to the right of midline, is abnormal. The combination of findings is consistent with the "double bubble" sign.

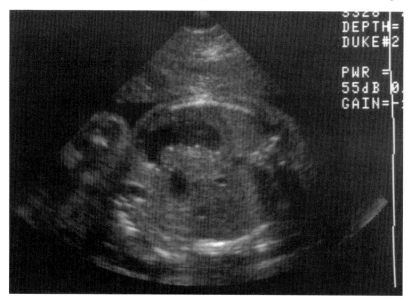

FIGURE 9-12B Oblique sonogram through the fetal abdomen. The two "bubbles" demonstrated in Figure 9-12A are now seen to connect, assuming a configuration typical for the stomach emptying into a dilated duodenal bulb.

◆ DIFFERENTIAL DIAGNOSIS

The "double bubble" sign implies duodenal obstruction, but it must be distinguished from other sources of extra cysts in the fetal abdomen.

◆ **Normal stomach, imaged twice due to oblique scan plane:** This is not simply a normal stomach because Figure 9-12B demonstrates a configuration consistent with the gastric antrum and pylorus emptying into a dilated duodenal bulb.

◆ **Splenic cyst:** This would be unlikely because the extra cyst is located in the right, not the left upper quadrant.

◆ **Bowel duplication cyst:** This is a possibility except that the extra cyst is in an ideal location for a dilated duodenal bulb.

◆ **Choledochal cyst:** This entity would be consistent with the appearance in Figure 9-12A, as the location of the second cyst is appropriate for a choledochal cyst. However, it is not consistent with Figure 9-12B because of the connection between the stomach and the second cyst. A choledochal cyst would not connect to the fetal stomach.

◆ **Renal cyst:** Because of the location of the extra cyst, a renal cyst would be unlikely.

◆ **Dilated duodenal bulb owing to duodenal atresia:** This is the likely diagnosis based on the appearance and location of the two abdominal cysts, in conjunction with sonographic demonstration of fetal stomach emptying into dilated duodenal bulb. At real-time evaluation, peristalsis was observed, further confirming a bowel etiology.

◆ DIAGNOSIS: Duodenal atresia.

◆ KEY FACTS

CLINICAL

◆ Duodenal atresia is the most common type of congenital small bowel obstruction.

◆ The likely etiology is failure to recanalize the duodenal lumen during the tenth to eleventh week of gestation.

◆ There is a high incidence of associated anomalies in fetuses with duodenal atresia. These include esophageal atresia, congenital heart disease, imperforate anus, other small bowel atresias, biliary atresia, renal anomalies, and vertebral anomalies.

◆ Because 20% to 30% of fetuses with duodenal atresia also have trisomy 21, chromosomal analysis should be offered when duodenal atresia is suspected.

RADIOLOGIC

◆ The fluid-filled double bubble sign seen in utero is analogous to the gas-filled double bubble sign seen on postpartum radiographs of infants with duodenal atresia.

◆ The bubbles comprising the double bubble sign consist of an overdistended stomach in the left upper quadrant and a dilated duodenal bulb in the right upper quadrant.

◆ Polyhydramnios is common.

◆ The double bubble sign is not specific for duodenal atresia but can occur secondary to any obstructive process at the level of the duodenum. Among the other possible causes are annular pancreas, duodenal web, duodenal stenosis, and obstruction due to an intestinal duplication.

◆ Many fetuses with duodenal atresia have a completely normal ultrasound, without polyhydramnios or the double bubble sign, until the late second or early third trimester.

◆ SUGGESTED READING

Gross BH, Filly RA. Potential for a normal fetal stomach to simulate the sonographic "double bubble" sign. Can Assoc Radiol J 1982;33:39–40.

Hertzberg BS. Sonography of the fetal gastrointestinal tract: Anatomic variants, diagnostic pitfalls, and abnormalities. AJR Am J Roentgenol 1994;162:1175–1182.

Nelson LH, Clark CE, Fishburne JI, et al. Value of serial sonography in the in utero detection of duodenal atresia. Obstet Gynecol 1982;59:657–660.

HISTORY

A 55-year-old woman presents with a palpable pulsatile abdominal mass.

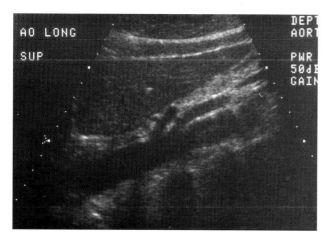

FIGURE 9-13A Sagittal sonogram of the upper abdomen. The upper and mid-abdominal aorta appears normal without evidence of an aneurysm. The celiac axis and superior mesenteric artery are seen arising from the aorta.

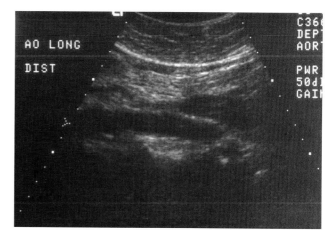

FIGURE 9-13B Sagittal sonogram of the lower abdomen. The lower abdominal aorta also appears normal without evidence of an aneurysm. There is a soft-tissue mass immediately anterior to the inferior portion of the aorta.

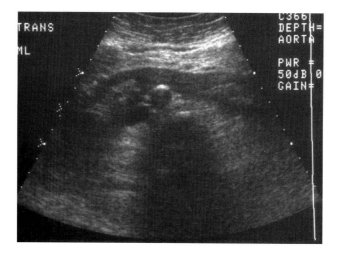

FIGURE 9-13C Transverse sonogram of the lower abdomen. The soft-tissue mass seen anterior to the aorta crosses the midline and extends laterally.

◆DIFFERENTIAL DIAGNOSIS

◆ **Adenopathy/lymphoma:** Patients with lymphoma and retroperitoneal or mesenteric adenopathy could present with the soft-tissue mass seen in Figure 9-13B, but it would not be expected to have the configuration seen laterally on Figure 9-13C.

◆ **Other primary retroperitoneal neoplasm:** Again, this could explain the configuration in Figure 9-13B but not the configuration in Figure 9-13C.

◆ **Retroperitoneal fibrosis:** This is likely to be more circumferential than the soft-tissue mass shown in Figure 9-13B. It does not explain the configuration in Figure 9-13C.

◆ **Horseshoe kidney:** This is the best diagnosis. The soft-tissue mass seen anterior to the aorta corresponds to the isthmus of a horseshoe kidney. The explanation for the palpable pulsatile abdominal mass at physical examination is pulsations transmitted from the aorta to the isthmus of the horseshoe kidney.

◆DIAGNOSIS: Horseshoe kidney.

◆KEY FACTS

CLINICAL

◆ The horseshoe kidney is a congenital renal fusion anomaly, in which the lower poles of both kidneys are joined by a fibrous or parenchymal band.

◆ Horseshoe kidneys are a common entity, occurring in between 1 in 400 to 500 births.

◆ Horseshoe kidneys are more susceptible to trauma compared to normally located kidneys.

◆ Due to urinary stasis from draping of the ureters over the kidneys, there is an increased incidence of stones and infection.

◆ Multiple renal arteries and ectopic renal arteries are common.

◆ Patients with a horseshoe kidney are not uncommonly referred to ultrasound for evaluation of a pulsatile abdominal mass, as in this case.

RADIOLOGIC

◆ Abnormal renal orientation is common in patients with horseshoe kidney. The renal pelvis is frequently directed more anteriorly than usual.

◆ The horseshoe kidney is typically found in a relatively low position, either in the lower abdomen or the upper pelvis. A possible explanation for the low position of the horseshoe kidney is that normal ascent of the kidney is prevented by the inferior mesenteric artery.

◆ The fused lower renal poles are commonly found at the level of the L4–L5 vertebrae.

◆ At sonography, a soft-tissue mass may be seen anterior to the abdominal aorta. The lower poles of the kidneys can sometimes be followed into the mass by scanning in an oblique plane. The upper portions of the kidneys are not usually in their typical locations in the flanks but are relatively low in position.

◆ In many cases, the isthmus of parenchymal or fibrous tissue connecting the two sides of the horseshoe kidney cannot be seen by ultrasound, due to overlying bowel gas. When this occurs, sonography may miss the diagnosis.

◆SUGGESTED READING

Mindell HJ, Kupic EA. Horseshoe kidney: Ultrasonic demonstration. AJR Am J Roentgenol 1977;129:526–527.

Trackler RT, Resnick ML, Leopold GR. Pelvic horseshoe kidney: Ultrasound findings and case report. J Clin Ultrasound 1978;6:51–52.

CASE 14

Barbara A. Carroll

HISTORY

A 39-year-old man presents with a 2-year history of back pain and a bone scan that shows left renal obstruction. Physical exam demonstrates a questionable left testicular mass.

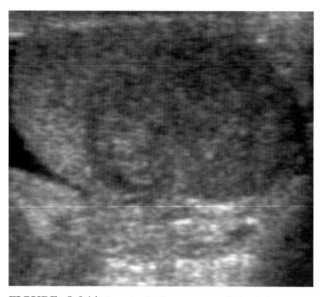

FIGURE 9-14A Longitudinal sonogram of the left scrotum demonstrates a relatively well-circumscribed, homogeneous, hypoechoic, 3-cm mass involving the lower part of the testis.

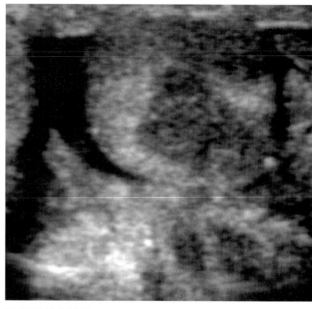

FIGURE 9-14B Transverse sonogram of the left scrotum reveals that this hypoechoic mass envelops the region of the mediastinum testis. A small hydrocele is present.

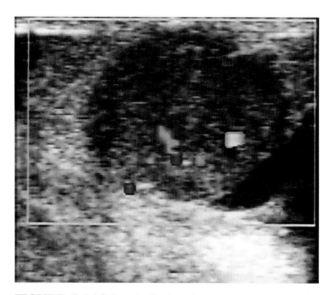

FIGURE 9-14C Longitudinal testicular sonogram with color Doppler. The hypoechoic testicular mass has increased blood flow compared to the adjacent normal testis. (See Color Plate 1.)

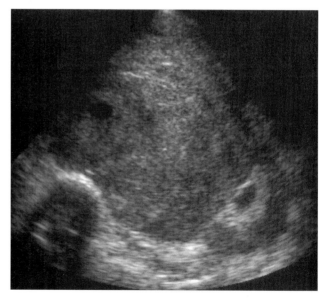

FIGURE 9-14D Transverse mid-abdominal sonogram at the level of the kidneys. A large retroperitoneal mass encasing the abdominal aorta and displacing it away from the spine is seen. Mild pelvocaliectasis of the left kidney is also seen.

◆ DIFFERENTIAL DIAGNOSIS

◆ **Lymphoma:** Non-Hodgkin's lymphoma is a possibility because of the large hypoechoic retroperitoneal mass and a focal testicular mass. However, the majority of malignant lymphomas manifest as diffuse testicular involvement with enlargement of the testis.

◆ **Metastatic disease:** Nonlymphomatous metastases to the testis are uncommon, representing no more than 5% of all testicular neoplasms. The most frequent primary sites are the lung and prostate. Metastases are most common during the fifth and sixth decades and are more frequent than primary germ cell tumors after age 50. Metastatic lesions are commonly multiple and are bilateral in 15% of cases.

◆ **Primary testicular neoplasm:** This is the best diagnosis from the standpoints of sonographic findings and clinical likelihood.

◆ **Infarction:** Testicular infarction may appear as either a focal hypoechoic mass or a diffusely hypoechoic testis of normal size. However, color Doppler would not be expected to show increased flow in the area of an infarct and the gland should not be enlarged.

◆ **Sarcoidosis:** Genital involvement is uncommon, occurring in <1% of patients with systemic sarcoidosis. Differentiation from a neoplasm is difficult. Occasionally, calcific foci with acoustic shadowing may be seen.

◆ DIAGNOSIS: Testicular seminoma with rare elements of choriocarcinoma metastatic to the retroperitoneum.

◆ KEY FACTS

CLINICAL

◆ Seminoma is the most common single-cell–type testicular neoplasm in adults, accounting for 40% to 50% of germ cell neoplasms.

◆ Seminomas are more common in the slightly older age group, demonstrating a peak incidence in the fourth and fifth decades. They are less aggressive than other germ cell tumors, although 25% of patients will have metastases at the time of diagnosis.

◆ Seminomas are relatively radiotherapy and chemotherapy sensitive.

◆ Seminomas are the most common tumors to originate in cryptorchid testes. An increased risk of developing a seminoma remains even after orcheopexy.

◆ Mixed germ cell tumors are the second most common testicular malignancy after seminoma, constituting 40% of all germ cell neoplasms.

◆ Choriocarcinoma is a rare germ cell tumor. However, 23% of mixed germ cell tumors contain some small component of choriocarcinoma.

◆ Choriocarcinomas secrete circulating chorionic gonadotropins and may produce gynecomastia.

RADIOLOGIC

◆ Seminomas are characteristically homogeneous, round or oval in shape, and hypoechoic.

◆ Sonographic features of seminomas parallel their relatively homogeneous histologic features.

◆ Seminomas may appear to be relatively well encapsulated or may be poorly marginated. They may be isolated or involve the entire testicle.

◆ Virtually all hypoechoic, focal solid testicular masses should be considered potential neoplasms unless there is compelling clinical evidence to the contrary.

◆ Color Doppler ultrasound cannot distinguish focal neoplasms from inflammatory lesions. However, color Doppler may be helpful in depicting subtle infiltrative lesions. Furthermore, the absence of power and color Doppler flow in a large hypoechoic mass using optimized flow settings is suggestive of an infarct.

◆ SUGGESTED READING

Horstman WG, Melson GL, Middleton WD, Andriole GL. Testicular tumors: Findings with color Doppler US. Radiology 1992;185:733–737.

Luker GD, Siegel MJ. Pediatric testicular tumors: Evaluation with gray-scale and color Doppler US. Radiology 1994;191:561–564.

Schwerk WB, Schwerk WN, Rodeck G. Testicular tumors: Prospective analysis of real-time US patterns and abdominal staging. Radiology 1987;164:369–374.

Stewart R, Carroll BA. The Scrotum. In CM Rumack, ST Wilson, JW Charboneau (eds), Diagnostic Ultrasound (Vol 1). St. Louis: Mosby–Year Book, 1991;565–589.

Subramanyam BR, Horii SC, Hilton S. Diffuse testicular disease: Sonographic features and significance. AJR Am J Roentgenol 1986;145:1221–1224.

CASE 15

Barbara A. Carroll

HISTORY

A 62-year-old man presents with a pulsatile mass and bruit in the right groin 2 days after coronary angioplasty via the right femoral artery.

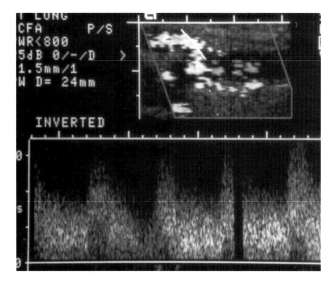

FIGURE 9-15A A duplex sonogram of the right common femoral artery in the longitudinal plane at the level of the catheterization puncture. There is a disturbed arterial flow pattern with increased end-diastolic flow (a low resistance arterial waveform) and marked spectral broadening ("turbulence").

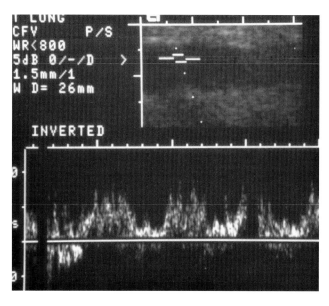

FIGURE 9-15B A duplex sonogram of the right common femoral vein at the same level. There is pulsatile, high-velocity venous flow.

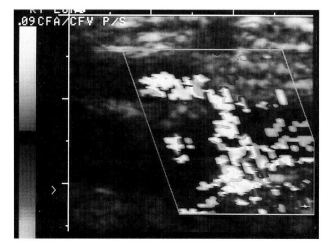

FIGURE 9-15C A color Doppler sonogram in the region of the puncture. A color Doppler "bruit" is manifested as scattered color Doppler pixels in the soft tissues surrounding the femoral artery and vein. (See Color Plate 2.)

◆ DIFFERENTIAL DIAGNOSIS

- **Arterial stenosis:** A stenosis of the femoral artery could cause increased diastolic flow, loss of high resistance, arterial waveform, and color Doppler bruit, but it should not alter the venous waveforms.
- **Arterial dissection:** A dissection or flap may have features similar to atherosclerotic narrowing, but no venous waveform changes should occur.
- **Venous stenosis:** A narrowed and stenotic vein may cause high-velocity venous flow, but no arterial changes.
- **Arteriovenous fistula (AVF):** This is the best diagnosis because it explains both the arterial and venous waveform changes.

◆ DIAGNOSIS: Femoral arteriovenous fistula.

◆ KEY FACTS

CLINICAL

- An AVF resulting from arterial puncture and catheterization is a less common complication than a pseudoaneurysm.
- An AVF is an abnormal communication between the arterial and venous systems that creates a shunt from the high-resistance arterial system into the low-resistance venous system.
- An AVF is caused by simultaneous puncture of the adjacent artery and vein and by simultaneous arterial and venous catheterization.
- An AVF is manifest clinically by a continous bruit or thrill in the region of trauma.
- An AVF may be asymptomatic or can produce localized symptoms, including pain, claudication distal to the AVF secondary to decreased arterial flow, and venous stasis due to increased venous pressure. Systemic symptoms such as high-output congestive heart failure and angina may also result.
- An asymptomatic AVF does not require treatment and may resolve spontaneously.
- Surgical treatment or ultrasound-guided compression/repair may be necessary.
- An AVF may coexist with a postcatheterization pseudoaneurysm.

RADIOLOGIC

- The classic arterial pattern is high diastolic flow (a low resistance waveform) with spectral broadening just proximal to the fistula.
- The classic venous pattern is increased flow velocity with pulsatile disturbed waveforms near the fistula.
- Color Doppler signal in the soft tissues surrounding the AVF is caused by the transmitted thrill from disturbed flow.
- A visible tract of flow connecting the artery and vein may be seen, especially with color Doppler.
- There is often decreased arterial flow distal to the fistula.
- Some AVFs may not demonstrate all of these features.

◆ SUGGESTED READING

Coley BD, Roberts AC, Fellmeth BD, et al. Postangiographic femoral artery pseudoaneurysms: Further experience with US-guided compression repair. Radiology 1995;194:307–311.

Igidbashian VN, Mitchell DG, Middleton WD, et al. Iatrogenic femoral arteriovenous fistula: Diagnosis with color Doppler imaging. Radiology 1989;170:749–752.

Robidoux MA, Hertzberg BS, Carroll BA, Hedgepeth CA. Color flow and image-directed Doppler ultrasound evaluation of iatrogenic arteriovenous fistulas in the groin. J Clin Ultrasound 1990;18:463–469.

CASE 16

Barbara A. Carroll

HISTORY

A 62-year-old man presents with a pulsatile right groin mass 24 hours after coronary angioplasty via the right femoral artery.

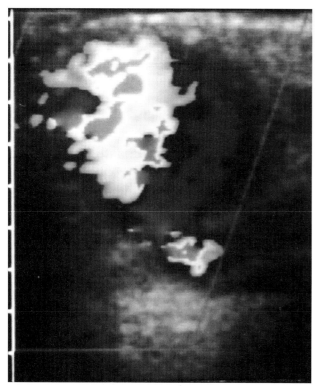

FIGURE 9-16A A transverse color Doppler sonogram of the right groin in the region of the visible catheterization puncture site demonstrates a "yin-yang" appearance of swirling bidirectional color flow within a hypoechoic mass. The short "neck" of flow can be seen between the mass and the common femoral artery. (See Color Plate 3.)

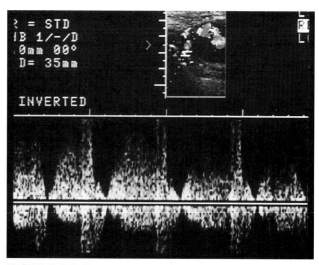

FIGURE 9-16B Pulsed Doppler spectral waveform in the region of the "neck" shows a "to-and-fro" waveform. (See Color Plate 4.)

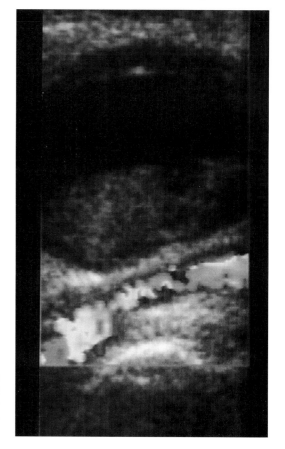

FIGURE 9-16C A longitudinal color Doppler sonogram of the right groin following ultrasound-guided compression repair shows no flow within the mass, which now contains a layer of echogenic material. Flow is maintained in the underlying common femoral artery. (See Color Plate 5.)

◆ DIFFERENTIAL DIAGNOSIS

◆ **Postcatheterization hematoma:** Hematomas in the region of a puncture site can produce an anechoic or hypoechoic mass. This mass may contain flecks of color due to transmitted pulsations from the adjacent femoral artery. However, pulsed Doppler evaluation will not reveal a "to-and-fro" arterial waveform.

◆ **Arteriovenous fistula (AVF):** The localized intense soft-tissue bruit associated with an AVF may sometimes mimic this color Doppler flow pattern. However, the pulsed Doppler waveforms within the adjacent artery and vein should demonstrate characteristics consistent with an AVF.

◆ **Hyperplastic lymph nodes:** The increased flow in hyperplastic lymph nodes can produce a very vascular mass on color Doppler ultrasound. However, no neck connecting the hyperplastic lymph node to the femoral artery will be observed, and the flow within the node will not have a "yin-yang" appearance.

◆ **Inguinal hernia:** Particulate material within ascites in an inguinal hernia sac may produce a similar swirling color flow pattern. Pulsed Doppler evaluation will show that these swirling color changes are associated with transmitted motion from respiration and abdominal peristaltic activity rather than vascular pulsations.

◆ **Arterial pseudoaneurysm:** This is the best diagnosis considering the pulsatile swirling blood flow in the mass and the waveform in the "neck" connecting the artery to the pseudoaneurysm.

◆ **DIAGNOSIS:** **Femoral artery pseudoaneurysm with successful ultrasound-guided compression repair.**

◆ KEY FACTS

CLINICAL

◆ A femoral artery pseudoaneurysm is an increasingly common complication of therapeutic catheterization procedures, including percutaneous transluminal coronary angioplasty and stenting.

◆ Occurrence rates as high as 6% have been reported. Pseudoaneurysms can produce complications including hemorrhage, pain, neuropathy, infection, local skin ischemia, peripheral embolization, and even frank rupture leading to exsanguination.

◆ Factors that lead to pseudoaneurysm development include large catheters and sheaths, use of anticoagulant or thrombolytic agents during and following the procedure, simultaneous arterial and venous catheterizations, and suboptimal postprocedural compression.

◆ Pseudoaneurysms are not true aneurysms. They develop a fibrous capsule but do not have a complete arterial wall surrounding them.

◆ Pseudoaneurysms present as pulsatile masses near the arterial puncture site. Audible systolic bruits are frequently heard but are not always present.

◆ Pseudoaneurysms must be distinguished from overlying hematomas with transmitted pulsations.

◆ Pseudoaneurysms may coexist with AVFs.

◆ Although the natural history of pseudoaneurysms is variable, spontaneous thrombosis is common. Unfortunately, there is no way of discerning which pseudoaneurysms will thrombose based on their ultrasound appearance.

◆ Traditional therapy for pseudoaneurysms has been surgical intervention. However, many pseudoaneurysms thrombose spontaneously. Furthermore, nonsurgical ultrasound-guided compression repair (UGCR) has been found to be a very successful interventional technique.

◆ UGCR is slightly more effective in nonanticoagulated patients; however, successful repair can be achieved in patients with anticoagulation. Reversal of anticoagulation before UGCR is nevertheless recommended. The age of the pseudoaneurysm does not appear to affect the ability to compress and thrombose the lesion adequately.

◆ Contraindications to UCGR include overlying skin ischemia or skin infection, peripheral vascular compromise, location of the pseudoaneurysm above the inguinal ligament, and inability to compress the pseudoaneurysm without simultaneous occlusion of the underlying artery.

◆ Complications of UCGR are uncommon; they include arterial occlusion, peripheral embolization, pseudoaneurysm rupture, and thrombosis of the adjacent common femoral vein.

RADIOLOGIC

◆ Pseudoaneurysms demonstrate a characteristic appearance on both color Doppler and pulsed Doppler ultrasound. Color Doppler demonstrates the neck of the pseudoaneurysm, which connects the pseudoaneurysm with the underlying femoral artery. During early systole, a color Doppler jet of blood flow into the pseudoaneurysm is seen. During the remainder of the cardiac cycle, eddy currents of color Doppler flow swirl around within the pseudoaneurysm and flow exits the pseudoaneurysm through the neck. The internal appearance of a pseudoaneurysm is frequently likened to the yin-yang sign, with equal parts of the pseudoaneurysm cavity filled with antegrade and retrograde swirling blood flow.

◆ To-and-fro pulsed Doppler waveforms are localized to the region of the pseudoaneurysm neck.

◆ Pseudoaneurysms may be multiple and create a "string-of-beads" appearance.

◆ SUGGESTED READING

Abu-Yousef MM, Wiese JA, Shamma AR. The "to-and-fro" sign: Duplex Doppler evidence of femoral artery pseudoaneurysm. AJR Am J Roentgenol 1988;150:632–634.

Coley BD, Roberts AC, Fellmeth BD, et al. Postangiographic femoral artery pseudoaneurysms: Further experience with US-guided compression repair. Radiology 1995;194:307–311.

Mitchell DG, Needleman L, Bezzi M, et al. Femoral artery pseudoaneurysm: Diagnosis with conventional duplex and color Doppler US. Radiology 1987;165:687–690.

HISTORY

A 67-year-old woman presents with a history of intermittent left upper extremity weakness and numbness. On physical examination there is a right carotid bruit.

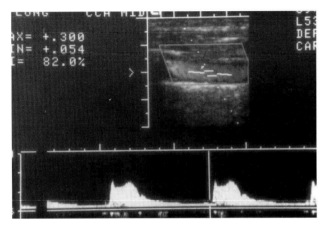

FIGURE 9-17A A duplex sonogram of the right common carotid artery demonstrates very low peak systolic and end diastolic velocities, 30 cm/sec and 5 cm/sec, respectively.

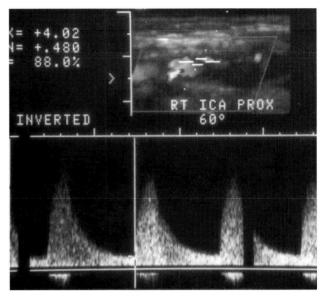

FIGURE 9-17B A duplex sonogram of the right internal carotid artery in the region of a visible hypoechoic plaque demonstrates a markedly elevated peak systolic velocity and an elevated end diastolic velocity, measuring 402 cm/sec and 48 cm/sec, respectively.

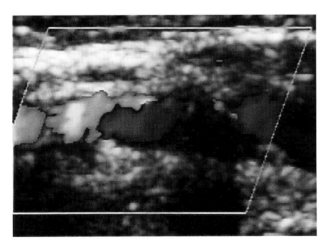

FIGURE 9-17C A color Doppler sonogram of the right internal carotid artery demonstrates an extremely high-grade stenosis with flow disturbance and a relatively hypoechoic plaque. Tiny areas of slow reversed flow are seen within the hypoechoic plaque, a finding that can be suggestive of plaque ulceration. (See Color Plate 6.)

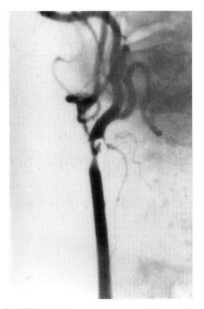

FIGURE 9-17D A right common carotid arteriogram demonstrates a markedly narrowed long segment stenosis involving the proximal internal carotid artery as well as the external carotid artery. Plaque ulceration is also present.

◆ DIFFERENTIAL DIAGNOSIS

◆ **Carotid dissection:** Dissections are less common than atherosclerotic plaque in the seventh decade. However, dissections should be considered as a cause of carotid stenosis or occlusion in younger patients, particularly those with a history of trauma, and in those with no atherosclerotic risk factors and a relative paucity of visible plaque.

◆ **Carotid stenosis:** This is the best diagnosis considering the age of the patient, the intraluminal lesions, and the focal velocity elevation.

◆ **Spurious velocity elevations due to contralateral stenosis:** Collateral shunting of blood to the circle of Willis on the side opposite a high-grade carotid stenosis can result in spuriously elevated velocities disproportionate to the amount of visible vessel narrowing. In this case, there was no evidence for a contralateral lesion, and the color Doppler clearly shows a large intraluminal filling defect associated with the areas of high velocity in the internal carotid artery.

◆ **Suboptimal Doppler angle:** If the angle theta used to obtain velocity values exceeds 70 degrees, spurious results may be obtained that are not representative of true flow velocity. In this case, the Doppler angle theta is 60 degrees, which is an acceptable Doppler angle. Ideally, the Doppler angle should not exceed 60 degrees.

◆ DIAGNOSIS: <90% diameter stenosis of the proximal internal carotid artery with plaque ulceration.

◆ KEY FACTS

CLINICAL

◆ Stroke caused by atherosclerotic disease is the third leading cause of death in the United States.

◆ Approximately 50% of these strokes are caused by atherosclerotic disease located within 2 cm of the carotid bifurcation.

◆ Carotid sonography using duplex ultrasound has become a valuable, noninvasive screening technique to determine which patients have potentially "operable" lesions.

◆ Carotid endarterectomy is now thought to be highly beneficial for symptomatic patients who have a 70% to 99% diameter stenosis involving the internal carotid artery.

◆ Ongoing investigations suggest that patients with an asymptomatic >80% diameter stenosis who are scheduled to undergo cardiopulmonary bypass may also derive benefit from endarterectomy.

◆ Other ongoing research suggests that endarterectomy may be of benefit for asymptomatic patients with a >60% diameter internal carotid artery stenosis.

◆ Ultrasound screening allows selection of appropriate patients for angiography before surgery. There are some instances in which surgery can be performed without angiography.

RADIOLOGIC

◆ Pulsed Doppler spectral analysis and color Doppler ultrasound are approximately of equal accuracy for diagnosing >50% diameter stenoses (>90% accuracy).

◆ The hallmark of a high-grade stenosis is a progressive increase in peak systolic and end diastolic velocities beginning at approximately 50% diameter stenosis and continuing until one reaches a preocclusive stenosis (>95% diameter), at which time the peak systolic and end diastolic velocities decrease precipitously.

◆ Peak systolic velocities >225 to 250 cm/sec are usually associated with a >70% diameter stenosis. End diastolic velocities >80 cm/sec are usually associated with the same degree of stenosis. Velocity ratios comparing the peak systolic or peak end diastolic velocities in the internal carotid artery in the region of the stenosis versus those in the more proximal common carotid artery may also be of value.

◆ Color Doppler ultrasound allows one to display blood flow information in real time over a selected area. Stationary soft-tissue structures that lack phase or frequency shifts associated with flowing blood receive an amplitude gray scale value, while the flowing blood in the vessels receives a color assignment dependent on the direction of blood flow relative to the Doppler transducer, as well as the Doppler angle and the velocity of the flowing blood.

◆ Color Doppler is helpful as an initial screen during the carotid examination to pinpoint areas of vascular narrowing and abnormal flow for subsequent pulsed Doppler interrogation.

◆ Carotid plaque characterization is a controversial topic; however, plaque such as the one seen in this case, which is heterogeneous and hypoechoic and contains areas of low velocity disturbed flow within the plaque, is frequently associated with ulceration.

◆ With an extremely high-grade stenosis or occlusion of the internal carotid artery, flow in the proximal common carotid artery may become damped with relatively low peak systolic and end diastolic velocity readings.

◆ SUGGESTED READING

Carroll BA. Carotid sonography. Radiology 1991;178:303–313.

Executive Committee for the Asymptomatic Carotid Atherosclerosis Study. Endarterectomy for asymptomatic carotid artery stenosis. JAMA 1995;273:1421–1428.

Gardner DJ, Gosink BB, Kallman CE. Internal carotid artery dissections: Duplex ultrasound imaging. J Ultrasound Med 1991;10:607–614.

Mitchell DG. Color Doppler imaging: Principles, limitations, and artifacts. Radiology 1990;177:1–10.

North American Symptomatic Carotid Endarterectomy Trial Collaborators. Beneficial effect of carotid endarterectomy in symptomatic patients with high-grade stenosis. N Engl J Med 1991;325:445–453.

Polak JF, Dobkin GR, O'Leary DH, et al. Internal carotid artery stenosis: Accuracy and reproducibility of color-Doppler-assisted duplex imaging. Radiology 1989;173:793–798.

Schwartz LB, Bridgman AH, Kieffer RW, et al. Asymptomatic carotid artery stenosis and stroke in patients undergoing cardiopulmonary bypass. J Vasc Surg 1995;21:146–153.

CASE 18 *James D. Bowie*

HISTORY

A 26-year-old woman referred for fetal ultrasound because of uncertainty about her dates.

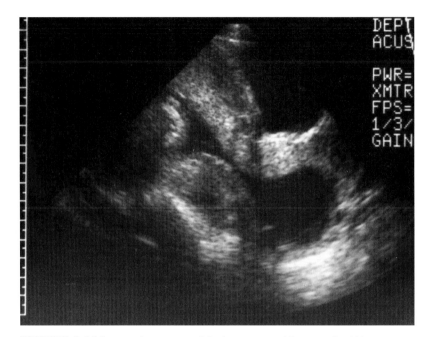

FIGURE 9-18A Sagittal sonogram of the lower uterus. There is a fluid-like structure that extends from the amniotic cavity through the cervix into the upper vagina.

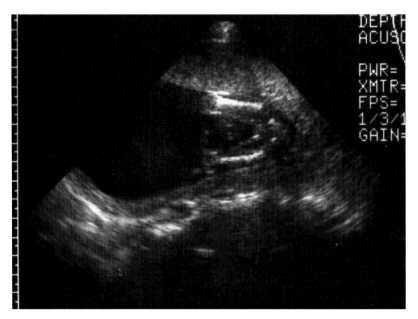

FIGURE 9-18B Transverse sonogram of the upper uterus. This view shows a normal amount of amniotic fluid in the upper uterus.

◆ DIFFERENTIAL DIAGNOSIS

- **"Hourglass membranes":** This term refers to the presence of fluid in the upper vagina as a result of herniation of the amniotic membranes through the cervix. The sonographic finding is characteristic, and few conditions mimic this appearance. The important thing to recognize is the location of the uterine cervix.
- **Nabothian cyst:** A very large nabothian cyst can have a similar appearance. In this case, the cervix is normal.

◆ DIAGNOSIS: Incompetent cervix with herniation of the amnion into the upper vagina, often referred to as "hourglass membranes."

◆ KEY FACTS

CLINICAL

- Preterm labor continues to be a major cause of perinatal death and morbidity.
- The patients are often without symptoms and do not have a history of premature delivery.
- There is no universally accepted treatment for this condition once it has progressed to this point. Various regimens have been suggested including: (1) doing nothing, (2) bed rest in the Trendelenburg position with tocolytic agents, and (3) cerclage for some patients.

RADIOLOGIC

- Routine images should be obtained of the cervix from 15 to 30 weeks of gestation. Ideally, these are done with an empty bladder. Often the transabdominal approach is adequate, but transperineal and endovaginal imaging may be needed in some cases. It is wise to examine the patient with a transabdominal scan before any endovaginal imaging to exclude the possibility of hourglass membranes.

- The normal cervix is about as high as it is wide. Measurements are taken of the length of the endocervical canal from the internal to the external os. This length should exceed 3 cm up to about 30 weeks.
- The normal endocervical canal can be hypoechoic or echogenic. A hypoechoic endocervical canal should not be mistaken for cervical incompetence.
- Myometrial contractions can give the appearance of an elongated endocervical canal. Measurements of the length of the endocervical canal should not be taken when a contraction distorts this area.
- The cervix can change in length during the course of an examination. Generally, the shortest measurement is most representative of the true clinical state. Also, "funneling" of the cervix is sometimes intermittent. The clinical consequences of intermittent funneling are the same in a cervix that consistently remains funneled—that is, there is a significant increase in risk for preterm labor and delivery of a premature infant.

◆ SUGGESTED READING

Andersen HF. Transvaginal and transabdominal ultrasonography of the uterine cervix during pregnancy. J Clin Ultrasound 1991;19:77–83.

Bowie JD, Andreotti RF, Rosenberg ER. Sonographic appearance of the uterine cervix in pregnancy: The vertical cervix. AJR Am J Roentgenol 1983;140:737–740.

Hertzberg BH, Bowie JD, Weber TM, et al. Sonography of the cervix during the third trimester of pregnancy: Value of the transperineal approach. AJR Am J Roentgenol 1991;157:73–76.

Mahony BS, Nyberg DA, Luthy DA, et al. Translabial ultrasound of the third-trimester uterine cervix: Correlation with digital examination. J Ultrasound Med 1990;9:717–723.

McGahan JP, Phillips HE, Bowen MS. Prolapse of the amniotic sac ("hourglass membranes"). Radiology 1981;140:463–466.

Parulekar SG, Kiwi R. Dynamic incompetent cervix uteri: Sonographic observations. J Ultrasound Med 1988;7:481–485.

Sarti DA, Sample WF, Hobel CJ, Staisch KJ. Ultrasonic visualization of a dilated cervix during pregnancy. Radiology 1979; 130:417–420.

CASE 19

Barbara S. Hertzberg

HISTORY

A 47-year-old man presents with intermittent episodes of right flank discomfort.

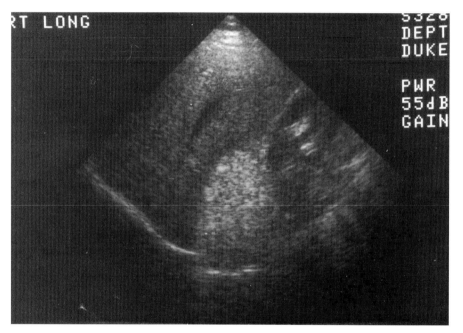

FIGURE 9-19 Longitudinal sonogram of the right upper quadrant. An echogenic mass is seen, posteroinferior to the liver and immediately superior to the kidney. Behind the mass, the diaphragm appears to be interrupted and displaced posteriorly.

◈ DIFFERENTIAL DIAGNOSIS

- **Adrenal hemorrhage:** Acute hemorrhage could cause a mass of markedly increased echogenicity, but it would not result in the apparent discontinuity and posterior displacement of the diaphragm behind the mass.
- **Renal angiomyolipoma:** This hamartomatous mass is possible, although it appears more suprarenal rather than originating from the kidney.
- **Retroperitoneal fat-containing mass such as a liposarcoma:** It would be unlikely for anatomic fat to be as well defined as this mass or be localized solely to the suprarenal area.
- **Adrenal myelolipoma:** This is the most likely diagnosis because the apparent discontinuity and posterior displacement of the diaphragm is due to a "speed propagation artifact." This occurs because the speed of ultrasound is slower in fatty masses than in many other soft tissues, resulting in misregistration of the location and apparent posterior displacement of the diaphragm immediately behind the fatty mass.
- **Adrenal carcinoma with acute hemorrhage:** This could result in an echogenic mass in a suprarenal location, but it would be unlikely to cause discontinuity and posterior displacement of the diaphragm behind the mass.

◈ DIAGNOSIS: Adrenal myelolipoma.

◈ KEY FACTS

CLINICAL

- An adrenal myelolipoma is an uncommon, benign, nonfunctioning hamartomatous adrenal mass that contains both fatty and bone marrow elements.
- Many patients with adrenal myelolipomas are asymptomatic, but some present with pain or discomfort.

Discomfort can be secondary to hemorrhage, necrosis, or pressure on surrounding structures.

- They are most common in the fourth to sixth decades of life, and they occur with approximately equal frequency in men and women.
- These lesions span a variety of sizes, ranging from microscopic to 30 cm or more in diameter.

RADIOLOGIC

- The ultrasound appearance depends on the relative quantities of the various tissue components.
- Many myelolipomas are markedly echogenic on ultrasound. This is considered the most characteristic appearance and is more likely to be seen when there is a high fat content.
- If the fat content is relatively low, a hypoechoic or heterogeneous mass may result.
- In some cases the "speed propagation artifact" is subtle, seen only in certain scan planes, or not seen at all. Inability to demonstrate this particular artifact does not exclude an adrenal myelolipoma.
- Even in the presence of a "speed propagation artifact," the diagnosis should be confirmed with a CT scan. The CT can confirm the presence of both fatty components as well as the adrenal origin of the mass.
- Adjacent retroperitoneal fat may mask a small adrenal myelolipoma.

◈ SUGGESTED READING

Musante F, Derchi LE, Zappasodi F, et al. Myelolipoma of the adrenal gland: Sonographic and CT features. AJR Am J Roentgenol 1988;151:961–964.

Vick CW, Zeman RK, Mannes E, et al. Adrenal myelolipoma: CT and ultrasound findings. Urol Radiol 1984;6:7–13.

CASE 20 *Barbara S. Hertzberg*

HISTORY

A 32-year-old pregnant woman has an elevated serum alpha-fetoprotein.

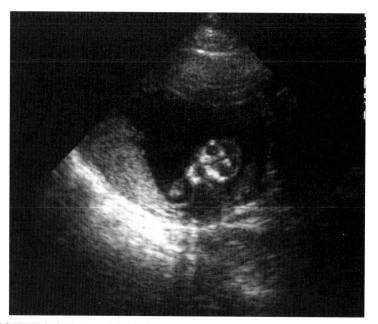

FIGURE 9-20A Transabdominal coronal sonogram of the fetal head. The brain and calvarium are not seen above the level of the orbits. Only a small amount of disordered soft tissue is identified.

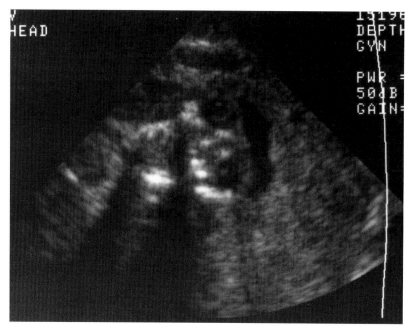

FIGURE 9-20B Endovaginal sonogram of the fetal head. Endovaginal sonogram confirms the absence of calvarium and brain above the level of the orbits.

◆ DIFFERENTIAL DIAGNOSIS

The differential diagnosis includes congenital malformations characterized by absence or decreased prominence of the calvarium:

- **Amniotic band syndrome:** This diagnosis is possible but unlikely because there is no evidence of intrauterine membranes. Additionally, the loss of the cranial vault is complete and symmetric, as opposed to amniotic band syndrome in which it is typically incomplete and asymmetric. Finally, additional lesions characteristic of amniotic band syndrome such as amputated limbs and atypical abdominal wall defects are not seen.
- **Severe microcephaly:** It could resemble this case if the calvarium is not recognized because of its diminutive size. Microcephaly is unlikely, however, because the images demonstrate complete absence of the calvarium, rather than a small calvarium.
- **Exencephaly:** Absence of the calvarium is consistent with exencephaly, but a larger amount of abnormally developed brain tissue would be seen in exencephaly.
- **Osteogenesis imperfecta:** This is a consideration because it is associated with marked underminerilization of the cranium. It is unlikely, however, because the underlying brain tissue would be normal in quantity and have a normal sonographic pattern.
- **Anencephaly:** This is the best diagnosis because of the combination of complete symmetric absence of the calvarium in conjunction with absence of normal brain tissue above the level of the orbits.

◆ DIAGNOSIS: Anencephaly.

◆ KEY FACTS

CLINICAL
- Anencephaly is a neural tube defect characterized by absence of the fetal cranium and cerebral hemispheres.
- Despite the implications of literal translation of the term *anencephaly*, there is not a complete absence of brain and head. Functioning neural tissue and calvarial structures are almost always present at the base of the skull.
- The disorder is uniformly fatal. Most affected infants die in utero or within a few days of birth.
- Anencephaly is often associated with additional defects, including spine anomalies, facial clefts, cardiovascular anomalies, and urinary tract malformations.

- After birth of one fetus with a neural tube defect, the risk of recurrence in a subsequent pregnancy is approximately 3% to 5%.

RADIOLOGIC
- Ultrasound changes in anencephaly are dramatic, so the detection rate approaches 100% by the early second trimester.
- If the fetal head is low in the pelvis, directly abutting the uterine wall or cervix, the diagnosis may not be immediately obvious by transabdominal sonography. In such a case, the abnormality should still be perceived when the examiner is unable to obtain a biparietal diameter in the conventional scan plane. Endovaginal or transperineal sonography can then be used to confirm the diagnosis.
- The combination of lack of cranial vault and of normal brain tissue above the level of the orbits results in a fetal head pattern that has been termed "frog-like."
- Identification of disorganized soft tissue above the level of the orbits does not exclude anencephaly. Such soft tissue is frequently seen due to the presence of angiomatous stroma. It tends to be most prominent when anencephaly is detected early in the pregnancy.
- Though additional anomalies occur in up to 50% of affected fetuses, detection of these lesions is not usually considered a critical component of the ultrasound study since anencephaly is uniformly fatal.
- Polyhydramnios is identified in many but not all cases.
- Exencephaly is considered an embryologic precursor to anencephaly. It is characterized by complete or partial absence of the calvarium, in association with a large amount of abnormally developed brain tissue. Absence of the calvarium in exencephaly is postulated to expose the brain to repeated trauma and amniotic fluid, leading to eventual brain destruction and anencephaly.

◆ SUGGESTED READING
Goldstein RB, Filly RA. Prenatal diagnosis of anencephaly: Spectrum of sonographic appearances and distinction from the amniotic band syndrome. AJR Am J Roentgenol 1988;151:1547–1550.

Goldstein RB, Filly RA, Callen PW. Sonography of anencephaly: Pitfalls in early diagnosis. J Clin Ultrasound 1989;17:397–402.

Hendricks SK, Cyr DR, Nyberg DA. Exencephaly—Clinical and ultrasonic correlation to anencephaly. Obstet Gynecol 1988;72:898–901.

Stumpf DA, Cranford RE, Elias S, et al. The infant with anencephaly. N Engl J Med 1990;322:669–674.

Wilkins-Haug L, Freedman W. Progression of exencephaly to anencephaly in the human fetus—An ultrasound perspective. Prenat Diag 1991;11:227–233.

CASE 21

Mark A. Kliewer

HISTORY

A 57-year-old man presents with fever, abdominal pain, and vomiting.

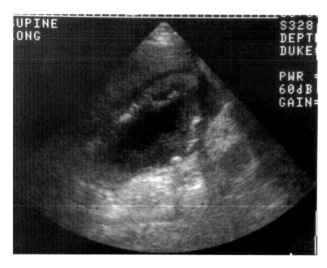

FIGURE 9-21A Longitudinal sonogram of the gallbladder fossa. The wall of the gallbladder is abnormally thick and irregular. Within the wall there are echogenic foci that cause acoustical shadowing.

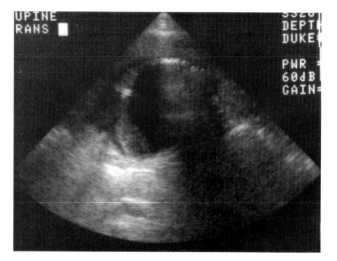

FIGURE 9-21B Transverse sonogram of this same area. The echogenic foci are again seen within the wall of the gallbladder. Posterior to these echogenic foci, a curtain of "dirty" shadowing is produced by acoustic noise.

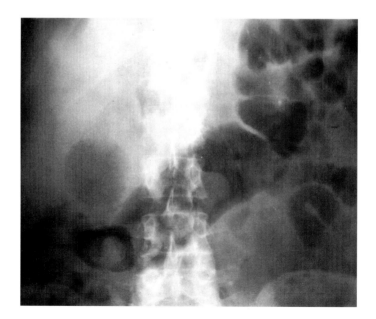

FIGURE 9-21C Plain radiograph of the upper abdomen. An unusual rounded lucency is noted in the right upper quadrant, above the hepatic flexure of the colon. Inferior to this, there is an additional discrete curvilinear lucency.

◆ DIFFERENTIAL DIAGNOSIS

◆ **Emphysematous cholecystitis:** This is a good possibility because of the presence of brightly echogenic foci within the wall and within the lumen of the gallbladder. The acoustic noise and ring-down posterior to these foci suggests the presence of gas.

◆ **Porcelain gallbladder:** The calcified wall in this condition would be expected to produce cleaner shadows without the reverberation artifacts seen in this case.

◆ **Gallbladder full of stones:** The echogenic foci in this case appear to be located in the wall of the gallbladder itself. Intraluminal gallstones would be expected to be separated from the wall by a crescent of bile, thus producing the wall-echo-shadow sign.

◆ **Bowel gas:** A loop of bowel can be displaced into the gallbladder fossa, especially after cholecystectomy. One would expect to find, however, the gut signature typical of bowel wall, and also continuity with an adjacent loop of bowel.

◆ DIAGNOSIS: Emphysematous cholecystitis.

◆ KEY FACTS

CLINICAL

◆ Emphysematous cholecystitis is an unusual variant of acute cholecystitis caused by gas-forming bacteria.

◆ This is a particularly fulminant type of infection that is five times more likely to result in gallbladder perforation.

◆ There is a male predilection (unlike more typical acute cholecystitis), and it is most often seen in the elderly.

◆ There is a strong association with diabetes mellitus.

◆ Patients often have a deceptively mild clinical presentation.

RADIOLOGIC

◆ Sonographic features of emphysematous cholecystitis depend on the relative amounts of intraluminal and intramural gas.

◆ Intraluminal gas is seen as an interface of highly reflective echoes. Posterior to this line, acoustic noise and ring-down reverberation are seen.

◆ Intramural gas can be located within the thickened, edematous gallbladder wall. This gas is often seen as a broken line of echoes (dots and dashes) that have distal reverberation artifacts. Occasionally, these echoes can be seen to float up to a nondependent portion of the gallbladder. This has been referred to as the *effervescent gallbladder.*

◆ Because of the seriousness of the diagnosis, additional imaging is indicated to confirm the suspicion of emphysematous cholecystitis. Plain film radiography, and especially CT, can confirm the presence of air.

◆ SUGGESTED READING

Bloom RA, Libson E, Lebensart PD, et al. The ultrasound spectrum of emphysematous cholecystitis. J Clin Ultrasound 1989;17: 251–256.

Hunter ND, MacIntosh PK. Acute emphysematous cholecystitis: An ultrasonic diagnosis. AJR Am J Roentgenol 1980;134:592–593.

Nemcek AA Jr, Gore RM, Vogelzang RL, Grant M. The effervescent gallbladder: A sonographic sign of emphysematous cholecystitis. AJR Am J Roentgenol 1988;150:575–577.

Parulekar SG. Sonographic findings in acute emphysematous cholecystitis. Radiology 1982;145:117–119.

HISTORY

A 62-year-old man presents with abdominal pain.

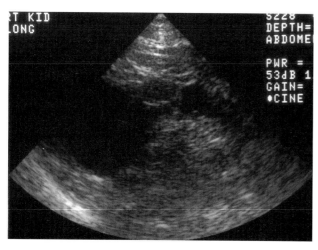

FIGURE 9-22A Longitudinal sonogram of the right kidney. A hypoechoic mass is seen in the upper pole of the right kidney which has mild increased through-transmission and a few low-level internal echoes. A "beak" sign is identified anterolaterally, suggesting a slower growing and less aggressive lesion.

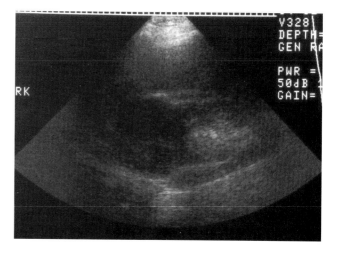

FIGURE 9-22B Longitudinal sonogram of the right kidney obtained approximately 1 month later. The mass has developed increased internal echogenicity.

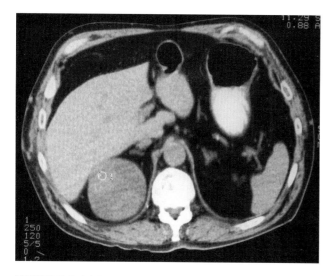

FIGURE 9-22C Noncontrast CT through the upper pole of the right kidney. The time interval from the most recent ultrasound is approximately 16 months. The mass demonstrates variable attenuation. Measurement of attenuation values suggests soft tissue elements (+32 Hounsfield units [HU]).

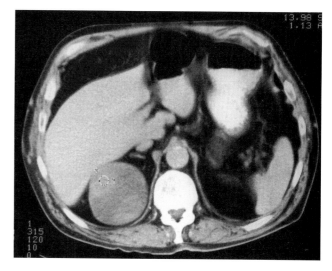

FIGURE 9-22D Contrast-enhanced CT through the upper pole of the right kidney. Comparing attenuation values from precontrast to postcontrast images reveals significant enhancement (+55 HU). Portions of a thickened, irregular wall are identified anteromedially.

◆ DIFFERENTIAL DIAGNOSIS

◆ **Simple renal cyst:** The mass does not meet strict sonographic criteria for a simple cyst, which must be anechoic, demonstrate increased through-transmission, and have a well-defined back wall.

◆ **Hemorrhagic or infected renal cyst:** This is a possibility because of the predominantly cystic nature of the lesion, which has low-level internal echoes, only moderate through-transmission, an imperceptible wall, and relatively smooth margination.

◆ **Renal abscess:** This diagnosis is possible because of reduced through-transmission and internal echoes. The patient should have an elevated white blood cell count and localized flank pain. The ultrasound and CT appearance of an abscess does depend on the time at which it is studied, but usually more inflammatory changes are evident in both the kidney and the perinephric space.

◆ **Renal cell carcinoma:** This is the most likely diagnosis because of the variable attenuation, areas of irregular wall thickening, and demonstration of significant contrast enhancement (>10 HU increase).

◆ DIAGNOSIS: Renal cell carcinoma developing in the wall of a cyst.

◆ KEY FACTS

CLINICAL

◆ Renal cell carcinomas account for >90% of all cancers in the kidney.

◆ The class triad of hematuria, abdominal mass, and pain is an uncommon presentation. Microhematuria is absent in up to 40% of cases. A more common presentation includes fever, malaise, anemia, weight loss, or a paraneoplastic process. Detection is frequently incidental.

◆ These tumors are most frequent in the sixth and seventh decades, although recently an increased incidence in younger females and adolescents has been noted. The male-to-female ratio is approximately 2 to 1.

◆ Larger neoplasms (>10 cm) frequently are locally invasive or have metastasized at the time of diagnosis. Small neoplasms (≤3 cm) uncommonly present with metastases.

◆ Renal cell carcinoma commonly metastasizes to the lung, ipsilateral renal hilar lymph nodes, and para-aortic/paracaval lymph nodes. There may also be direct extension to the perinephric and paranephric spaces. Invasion of the major renal veins and the inferior vena cava is common. Osseous metastases are usually lytic and expansile.

RADIOLOGIC

◆ A cystic mass is considered a simple cyst by ultrasound if it is:

 ◆ Rounded, smoothly marginated, intraparenchymal, or exophytic with a smooth, thin, or imperceptible wall

 ◆ Anechoic (a few, thin smooth septations are acceptable)

 ◆ Characterized by increased through-transmission of sound

◆ By CT, a simple cyst will be rounded, smoothly marginated, intraparenchymal or exophytic, and have a smooth, thin, or imperceptible wall. Attenuation values should be uniformly those of water (−10 to +20 HU), and there should be no evidence of enhancement on immediate postcontrast images (≤10 HU increase).

◆ Renal cysts can be categorized according to the Bozniak criteria as follows:

Category I: Simple uncomplicated benign cyst. These lesions need no further radiologic work-up.

Category II: Minimally complicated renal cyst with specific radiologic findings that are of concern. They include all cysts with one or more fine septations; cysts with thin, fine calcifications within the wall or septae; and cysts that are high in attenuation (>+20 HU). These cysts must not demonstrate postcontrast enhancement. They are benign and do not require surgery.

Category III: Cysts with features also seen with malignant lesions. These features include thickened, irregular walls or septae; thickened, irregular calcifications within the walls or septae; some enhancement on postcontrast imaging. These cysts require surgical intervention.

Category IV: Cysts that are clearly malignant. These masses will have irregular margins, vascular elements, solid tissue, and areas of necrosis. Some will be neoplasms that have grown adjacent to or in the wall of a simple cyst. These cysts require surgical intervention.

◆ By CT, renal cell carcinomas demonstrate some or all of the following: variable attenuation, thickened wall, irregular septae, soft-tissue components, significant enhancement (>10 HU increase) on postcontrast imaging, irregular margins on the parenchymal interface, calcifications, hemorrhage, renal vein and inferior vena cava invasion, perinephric invasion, lymphadenopathy, and metastases.

◆ SUGGESTED READING

Bosniak MA. The current radiologic approach to renal cysts. Radiology 1986;158:1–10.

Dunnick NR. Renal lesions: Great strides in imaging. Radiology 1992;182:305–306.

McClennan BL, Deyoe LA. The imaging evaluation of renal cell carcinoma: Diagnosis and staging. Radiol Clin North Am 1994;32:55–69.

Yamashita Y, Watanabe O, Miyazaki T, et al. Cystic renal cell carcinoma: Imaging findings with pathologic correlation. Acta Radiol 1994;35:19–24.

HISTORY

A 56-year-old woman 5 days status post renal transplantation presents with increasing creatinine and no urine output.

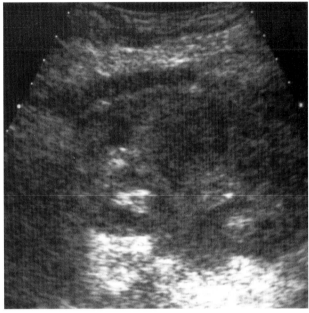

FIGURE 9-23A Longitudinal sonogram of the right iliac fossa renal allograft demonstrates heterogeneous internal architecture without evidence of renal obstruction. There is a small perinephric fluid collection anteriorly.

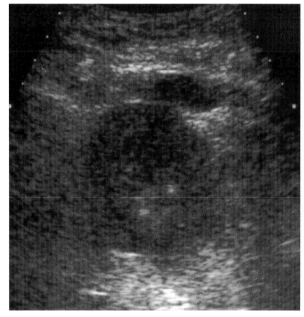

FIGURE 9-23B Transverse sonogram of the right renal allograft in its mid portion demonstrates no evidence of postrenal obstruction. The small anterior fluid collection is again noted.

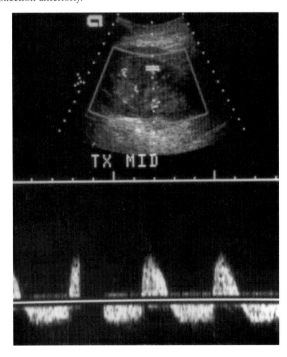

FIGURE 9-23C Duplex Doppler ultrasound obtained from an interlobar vessel of the mid portion of the renal allograft demonstrates reversed end diastolic arterial flow. No flow is identified in the renal vein.

◆ DIFFERENTIAL DIAGNOSIS

◆ **Acute transplant rejection:** In acute transplant rejection, venous flow should be present. However, this condition cannot be distinguished reliably from acute tubular necrosis.

◆ **Severe acute tubular necrosis:** Acute tubular necrosis and acute graft rejection have a similar appearance, and both occur frequently in the first few days to 1 week post transplant. Acute tubular necrosis would also show venous flow.

◆ **Subcapsular hematoma:** Subcapsular hemorrhage can produce a Page kidney effect; however, there is no evidence of a large subcapsular hematoma.

◆ **Renal vein thrombosis:** This is the best diagnosis given the Doppler arterial waveform and the conspicuous absence of venous flow.

◆ DIAGNOSIS: Renal vein thrombosis.

◆ KEY FACTS

CLINICAL

◆ Causes of renal allograft dysfunction are myriad, including acute rejection, acute tubular necrosis, drug toxicity, obstruction, infection, subcapsular hematoma, and vascular complications.

◆ The normal renal allograft is similar to the normal native kidney in that it has a low resistance vascular system requiring perfusion throughout the cardiac cycle (i.e., both systolic and diastolic flow).

◆ Renal blood flow changes reflect the relative severity of disease by increased resistance to allograft perfusion. The more severe the renal disease, the greater the increase in resistance to arterial flow.

◆ Vascular complications are frequent events following renal transplantation. Renal artery stenosis, arterial or venous thrombosis, arteriovenous fistulas, and pseudoaneurysms may all occur. Duplex and color Doppler ultrasound have proven useful for detecting the presence of flow as well as vascular abnormalities. Whereas renal artery stenosis/occlusion in renal transplants occurs in anywhere from 1.6% to 16% of allografts, renal vein thrombosis as a cause of acute renal failure is uncommon.

◆ The main role of diagnostic imaging in the immediate post-transplant period is to exclude renal obstruction, evaluate the presence of arterial and venous flow, assess the presence or absence of peritransplant fluid collections, and guide renal biopsies and fluid drainages.

RADIOLOGIC

◆ The image findings in this renal allograft are nonspecific. The internal parenchymal texture is very heterogeneous, consistent with any number of causes of renal transplant dysfunction. There is no evidence of obstruction or a subcapsular hematoma.

◆ Increased resistance to allograft perfusion is reflected by a disproportionate decrease in diastolic flow. This results in an elevation of the arterial:

$$\text{RI (Resistive index} = \frac{A - B}{A})$$

and

$$\text{PI (Pulsatility index} = \frac{A - B}{\text{time averaged mean velocity}})$$

where A = peak systolic velocity and B = end diastolic velocity.

◆ Reversed end diastolic flow indicates markedly increased resistance to renal allograft perfusion. This nonspecific finding does not allow one to distinguish between acute tubular necrosis and acute rejection. However, combined abnormally elevated arterial resistance and absence of venous flow is extremely suggestive of acute renal vein thrombosis as a cause of renal dysfunction.

◆ Occasionally, very slow venous flow may mimic renal vein thrombosis. In the absence of color Doppler flow, the use of power or amplitude Doppler to direct subsequent pulsed Doppler spectral analyses may alleviate these diagnostic problems.

◆ While ultrasound can document the presence of arterial and venous flow and assess for obstruction and peritransplant fluid collections, the Doppler arterial waveforms are not sufficient for distinguishing between different causes of transplant dysfunction, many of which produce an increased RI. In most instances, if the clinical situation is not diagnostic of the cause of renal dysfunction, a biopsy will be necessary. Ultrasound provides a valuable service in guiding renal transplant biopsies, particularly for avoiding extrarenal vessels.

◆ SUGGESTED READING

Genkins SM, Sanfilippo FP, Carroll BA. Duplex Doppler sonography of renal transplants: Lack of sensitivity and specificity in establishing pathologic diagnosis. AJR Am J Roentgenol 1989;152: 535–539.

Grenier N, Douws C, Morel D, et al. Detection of vascular complications in renal allografts with color Doppler flow imaging. Radiology 1991;178:217–223.

Kaveggia LP, Perrella RR, Grant EG, et al. Duplex Doppler sonography in renal allografts: The significance of reversed flow in diastole. AJR Am J Roentgenol 1990;155:295–298.

Reuther G, Wanjura D, Bauer H. Acute renal vein thrombosis in renal allografts: Detection with duplex Doppler US. Radiology 1989;170:557–558.

HISTORY

A 27-year-old pregnant woman is referred for an elevated maternal serum alpha fetoprotein level at 16 menstrual weeks.

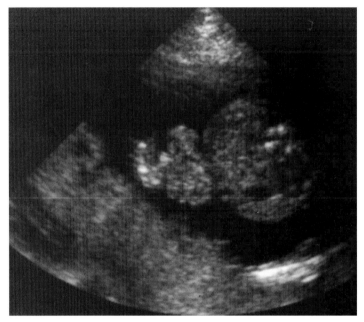

FIGURE 9-24A Transverse sonogram at the level of the fetal abdomen. A lobulated and echogenic mass is seen contiguous with the fetal abdomen. This mass is not obviously contained within a membrane.

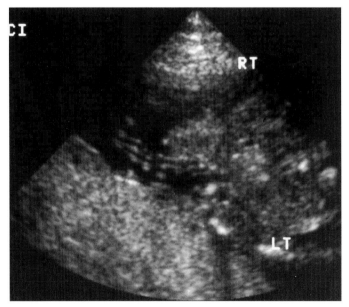

FIGURE 9-24B Transverse sonogram at the level of the umbilical cord insertion into the fetal abdomen. The umbilical cord insertion is seen separate from and medial to the mass. No bowel dilatation is seen within the abdomen.

◆ DIFFERENTIAL DIAGNOSIS

◆ **Omphalocele:** This is a possibility, but to be the correct diagnosis the mass should be surrounded by a membrane and the cord insertion should be into the mass, not to one side of it. The abdominal wall defect tends to be large in omphalocele, and the mass may contain liver. Ascites can be found in the fetal abdomen.

◆ **Gastroschisis:** This is the most likely possibility because of the eccentric location of the mass, the insertion of the cord adjacent to the mass, the absence of a limiting membrane, and the echogenicity and lobulation of the mass resulting from the conglomeration of bowel loops that are possibly thick walled.

◆ **Limb-body wall complex:** This is characterized by severe and widespread abnormalities, which can include eviscerated liver, cranial and extremity defects, and scoliosis. Eviscerated organs are often entangled with membranes.

◆ **Pentalogy of Cantrell:** This is an unlikely diagnosis given that the pentalogy is defined by the presence of an omphalocele, ectopic cordis, diaphragmatic hernia, cardiac malformation, and sternal cleft.

◆ **Cloacal extrophy:** This is less likely as it is diagnosed on the basis of the failure to identify a normal urinary bladder and splaying of the pubic rami. There are often additional genitourinary abnormalities.

◆ **Amniotic band syndrome:** This diagnosis is suggested by an unusual collection of abnormalities that could include abdominal wall defects, limb reduction abnormalities or amputations, eccentric cephaloceles, and a cleft lip. The absence of associated membranes also argues against this diagnosis.

◆ DIAGNOSIS: Gastroschisis.

◆ KEY FACTS

CLINICAL

◆ The etiology of gastroschisis has been attributed to abnormal involution of the right umbilical vein and to omphalomesenteric artery disruption.

◆ Though this defect was once thought to mandate a cesarean section, many obstetricians now perform vaginal delivery, at least for subsets of these fetuses.

◆ Most cases occur sporadically, although there are reports of familial recurrence.

◆ Most cases come to attention because of an abnormally elevated maternal serum alpha fetoprotein level.

◆ Gastroschisis is not usually associated with chromosomal abnormality or other malformations.

RADIOLOGIC

◆ The diagnosis is based on the presence of an abdominal wall defect from which a mass protrudes that is not covered by a membrane. The defect is usually to the right of the umbilical cord, and ascites is not typically present in the fetal abdominal cavity.

◆ Though a systematic search for other abnormalities should be performed, fetuses with gastroschisis usually do not have additional structural abnormalities.

◆ In most cases, bowel alone is eviscerated, though portions of the genitourinary system can also be involved in the defect. Some reports have suggested that liver can rarely be involved, though these reports have been contested.

◆ Usually the task of the sonographer is to distinguish gastroschisis from omphalocele. The two most telling features of gastroschisis are its paramedian location (lateral to the umbilical insertion) and the absence of a limiting membrane. In contrast, an omphalocele is encased by a membrane and occurs at the umbilical cord insertion such that the cord inserts directly into the mass.

◆ The extruded bowel can become thick walled and matted. Furthermore, the mass can become encased by fibrous bands.

◆ Fetuses may develop evidence of bowel wall thickening, bowel obstruction, and perforation. Meconium peritonitis is suspected when there are abdominal calcifications or pseudocysts. Ischemic injury to the bowel can occur.

◆ Intrauterine growth retardation is a frequent complication.

◆ SUGGESTED READING

Bair JH, Russ PD, Pretorius DH, et al. Fetal omphalocele and gastroschisis: A review of 24 cases. AJR Am J Roentgenol 1986;147:1047–1051.

DeVries PA. The pathogenesis of gastroschisis and omphalocele. J Pediatr Surg 1980;15:245–251.

Kirk EP, Wah R. Obstetric management of the fetus with omphalocele or gastroschisis: A review and report of 112 cases. Am J Obstet Gynecol 1983;146:512–518.

Lindfors KK, McGahan JP, Walter JP. Fetal omphalocele and gastroschisis: Pitfalls in sonographic diagnosis. AJR Am J Roentgenol 1986;147:797–800.

Nelson PA, Bowie JD, Filston HC, et al. Sonographic diagnosis of omphalocele in utero. AJR Am J Roentgenol 1981;138:1178–1180.

Stringer MD, Brereton RJ, Wright VM. Controversies in the management of gastroschisis: A study of 40 patients. Arch Dis Child 1991;66:34–36.

CHAPTER 10

NUCLEAR MEDICINE

R. Edward Coleman, *chapter editor*

Salvador Borges-Neto, R. Edward Coleman,
Rosalie J. Hagge, Michael W. Hanson, Sara M. O'Hara,
Robert R. Reiman, Jr., and Robert H. Wilkinson, Jr.

CASE 1

R. Edward Coleman

HISTORY

A 54-year-old woman with left knee pain.

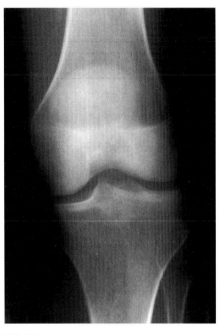

FIGURE 10-1A Anteroposterior view of the left knee obtained at time of presentation. No evidence for a fracture is seen on the radiograph.

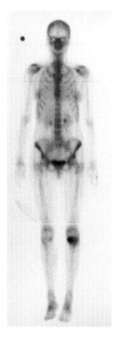

FIGURE 10-1B Anterior whole body images of a bone scan obtained 2 hours after the intravenous administration of Tc-99m methylene diphosphate. A focal area of abnormal accumulation is present in the proximal left tibia.

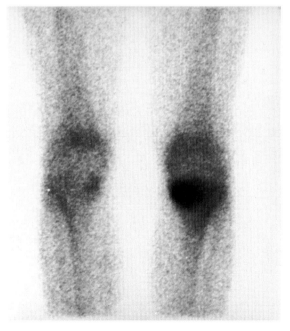

FIGURE 10-1C Anterior image of the knees. A region of increased radiotracer activity is present in the left tibial plateau, with greater accumulation medially than laterally.

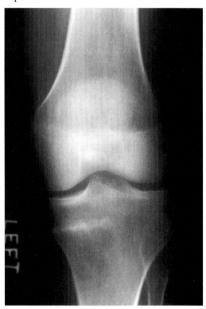

FIGURE 10-1D Anteroposterior view of the left knee obtained 1 month after the initial radiograph and bone scan. A linear region of sclerosis has developed in the medial left tibial metaphysis.

◆ DIFFERENTIAL DIAGNOSIS

- **Metastatic disease:** This is an unlikely diagnosis because of the absence of a primary malignancy and because only a single abnormality is present. Multiple abnormalities would be expected with metastatic disease.
- **Osteosarcoma:** This tumor usually occurs in the 10- to 25-year-old age range and is apparent radiographically at the time of presentation, making this an unlikely diagnosis.
- **Insufficiency fracture:** This is the best diagnosis because initial radiographs commonly are normal in the face of an abnormal bone scan, with development of sclerosis at the fracture site demonstrable on radiographs a few weeks later.
- **Osteomyelitis:** This diagnosis is unlikely because the patient is older than most patients with osteomyelitis and because of the absence of a predisposing factor. Furthermore, at least some radiographic abnormality would be expected in osteomyelitis.
- **Degenerative joint disease:** This diagnosis is unlikely because the bone scan abnormality is not in the joint space but in the tibial metaphysis. Furthermore, the radiograph does not demonstrate changes of degenerative joint disease.

◆ DIAGNOSIS: Insufficiency fracture.

◆ KEY FACTS

CLINICAL
- Musculoskeletal injury accounts for 15% to 20% of emergency department visits and 30% of patient visits in routine orthopedic practice.
- Physical examination and plain film radiography of the site of injury are typically performed at the time of presentation.

- Insufficiency fractures occur when bones weakened by osteoporosis or other metabolic bone disease are placed under normal stress.
- Stress fractures occur when normal bones are exposed to abnormal stress of a repetitive type.
- Pathologic fractures occur when bones weakened by tumor involvement are exposed to normal stress.

RADIOLOGIC
- Radiographic studies are often initially normal at the time of development of an insufficiency fracture or a stress fracture. In fact, abnormalities may not be present until 1 to 2 weeks later.
- If pain is considered to be of osseous origin and the plain radiographs are normal, a radionuclide bone scan is the next imaging modality that is generally used to evaluate possible fracture. The bone scan will typically be abnormal at that time.
- On a three-phase bone scan, acute fractures demonstrate increased perfusion on the dynamic phase, poorly defined abnormal radiotracer accumulation on the blood pool images, and focal abnormal accumulation on delayed images.
- MRI can demonstrate cortical and marrow changes associated with fracture.
- Insufficiency fractures in elderly patients with osteoporosis can mimic metastatic disease on plain films.

◆ SUGGESTED READING
Holder LE. Clinical radionuclide bone imaging. Radiology 1990;176:607–614.

Holder LE. Bone scintigraphy in skeletal trauma. Radiol Clin North Am 1993;31:739–781.

Martin P. Basic principles of nuclear medicine techniques for detection and evaluation of trauma and sports medicine injuries. Semin Nucl Med 1988;18:90–112.

HISTORY

A 4-year-old child with a history of recurrent urinary tract infections.

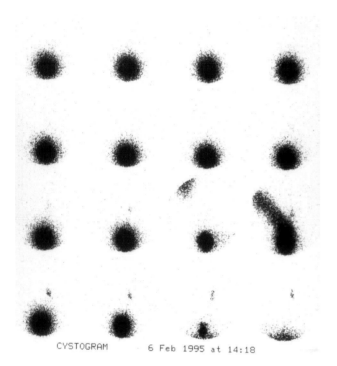

CYSTOGRAM   6 Feb 1995 at 14:18

FIGURE 10-2A Posterior images from radionuclide cystogram. Sequential images were obtained during bladder filling and voiding, with motion evident on frames 11 and 12 while the patient was being moved from supine to sitting position on the bed pan. Radiotracer activity is visible in the right ureter and collecting system at maximal bladder capacity on the bottom two rows of images. This activity increases in intensity as the patient voids. No radiotracer activity is seen on the left side above the level of the bladder.

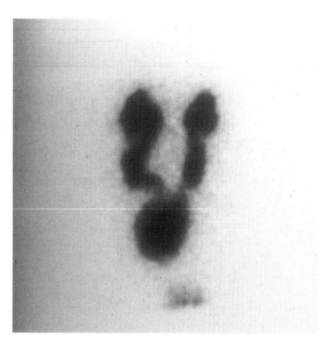

FIGURE 10-2B Single-frame posterior image from a radionuclide cystogram in another patient with the same diagnosis. Intense radiotracer activity is visible in both renal collecting systems, greater on the left side.

◆ DIFFERENTIAL DIAGNOSIS

◆ **Neurogenic bladder:** High grades of vesicoureteral reflux can be seen in patients with neurogenic bladder, often at relatively low bladder volumes. However, in both of the cases illustrated, the patients were able to void voluntarily to complete bladder emptying, which is inconsistent with the diagnosis of neurogenic bladder.

◆ **Unilateral hydronephrosis:** This entity is typically seen in the setting of obstruction and is evaluated by an antegrade study. However, the radionuclide cystogram, performed in the cases illustrated, is a retrograde examination undertaken to detect vesicoureteral reflux.

◆ **Contamination from voided radionuclide material:** Such contamination pools around the external genitalia. In the cases illustrated, the distribution on voiding conforms to the shape of the ureter and intrarenal collecting system.

◆ **Vesicoureteral reflux:** This is the best diagnosis for the cases illustrated. The radiotracer activity in the ureters in these patients is due to vesicoureteral reflux before and during voiding. Many different grades of vesicoureteral reflux are demonstrated in these two examinations: grades 2 (Figure 10-2A, right ureter), 3 (Figure 10-2B, right ureter), and 4 (Figure 10-2B, left ureter).

◆ DIAGNOSIS: Vesicoureteral reflux.

◆ KEY FACTS

CLINICAL

◆ The overall prevalence of vesicoureteral reflux is <1% in the general population. However, 35% of children with urinary tract infections have vesicoureteral reflux, and 25% to 50% of asymptomatic siblings also have vesicoureteral reflux.

◆ Vesicoureteral reflux spontaneously resolves in approximately 80% of cases.

◆ Patients with vesicoureteral reflux are treated with prophylactic antibiotics and re-evaluated with annual cystograms. The goal of therapy is to avoid pyelonephritis, which can leading to renal scarring. However, vesicoureteral reflux alone, without superimposed infection, is also believed to damage nephrons. Therefore, early surgery is recommended for some cases of severe reflux, even in the absence of infection, to prevent renal insufficiency.

RADIOLOGIC

◆ The most appropriate means of evaluating pediatric urinary tract infections is a matter of controversy. Most physicians agree that the first cystogram in boys should be an x-ray voiding cystogram, in order to evaluate the urethra. In girls, a radionuclide cystogram is adequate, especially when combined with sonography, which provides adequate anatomic assessment.

◆ The classification of vesicoureteral reflux is as follows:
Grade 1: Reflux into the ureter only
Grade 2: Reflux reaching the renal pelvis and calyces, without calyceal dilation
Grade 3: Reflux reaching the calyces, with mild calyceal dilation
Grade 4: Reflux reaching the calyces, with marked calyceal dilation
Grade 5: Progressive calyceal dilation and ureteral tortuosity

◆ Advantages of radionuclide cystography include

◆ Approximately 1/100th radiation exposure compared with x-ray voiding cystogram

◆ Continuous imaging during bladder filling and voiding, unlike noncontinuous imaging using intermittent fluoroscopy with x-ray voiding cystourethrogram (VCUG).

◆ Radionuclide cystography technique: The radiopharmaceutical is instilled into the bladder, which is gradually filled with saline via a gravity drip. Imaging continues during bladder filling and voiding.

◆ Filling the bladder to maximum capacity is important for optimal sensitivity. Inadequate bladder filling can produce false-negative examinations. Furthermore, reflux tends to occur at increasingly higher bladder volumes with advancing age as patients outgrow the abnormality.

◆ SUGGESTED READING

Heyman S. Radionuclide Renal Scans in Pediatrics. In LM Freeman, H Weissmann (eds), Nuclear Medicine Annual. New York: Raven, 1989;179–224.

Heyman S. Radionuclide Studies of the Genitourinary Tract. In JH Miller, MJ Gelfand (eds), Pediatric Nuclear Imaging. Philadelphia: Saunders, 1994;195–251.

Majd M. Urinary Tract Infections in Children. In BL McClennan (ed), Syllabus: A Categorical Course in Genitourinary Radiology. Oak Brook, IL: RSNA, 1994;63–70.

CASE 3

Salvador Borges-Neto

HISTORY

A 76-year-old woman with a history of coronary artery disease, hypertension, elevated serum lipids, and atrial fibrillation presents with increasing shortness of breath.

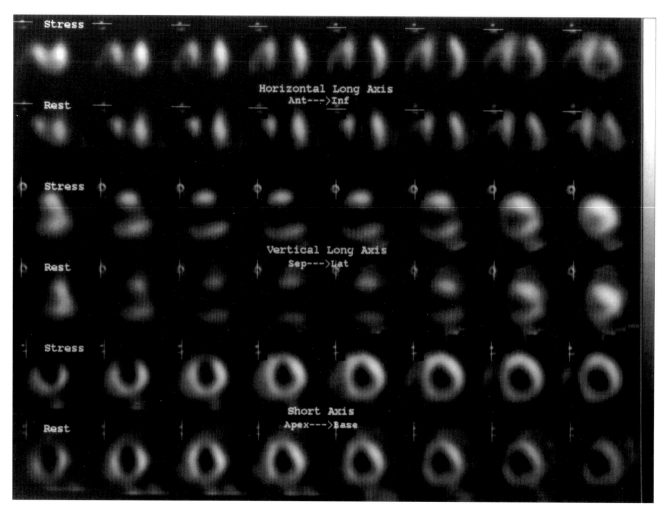

FIGURE 10-3 Stress (Tc-99m sestamibi) and rest (Tl-201) single-photon emission computed tomography myocardial perfusion images displayed in the horizontal long axis (**top 2 rows**), vertical long axis (**middle 2 rows**), and short axis views (**bottom 2 rows**). The stress perfusion images show an area of markedly decreased perfusion involving the low anterior, anteroapical, anteroseptal, and inferoapical regions. The rest perfusion images also show decreased activity in the same areas. The extent and severity of the perfusion defects are essentially the same on the stress and rest perfusion images.

◆ DIFFERENTIAL DIAGNOSIS

- **Myocardial infarction without stress-induced ischemia:** This is the best diagnosis based on the presence of a fixed perfusion defect with essentially no change in the extent and severity of the perfusion abnormalities between rest and stress studies.
- **Myocardial ischemia without infarction:** This diagnosis is made when a perfusion defect induced by stress is not present on the rest study. This is not the situation in the case illustrated.
- **Myocardial infarction and stress-induced ischemia:** This diagnosis is made when a stress-induced perfusion abnormality incompletely or only partially normalizes on the rest images.
- **Nonischemic cardiomyopathy:** Large perfusion defects either or both at rest and during stress are typically absent in nonischemic cardiomyopathy. The large defects that are present in this study make this diagnosis unlikely. Furthermore, left ventricular dilatation is a prominent feature of this entity but is not seen in the present study.

◆ DIAGNOSIS: Myocardial infarction without stress-induced ischemia.

◆ KEY FACTS

CLINICAL

- Several risk factors are known to predispose to coronary artery disease, including age, family history, hypertension, smoking, and diabetes.
- Patients with coronary artery disease may present with symptoms such as either or both angina and shortness of breath. However, silent ischemia is a well-recognized entity, particularly in diabetic patients. Such patients can have arterial occlusion and infarction in the absence of symptoms.
- Myocardial infarction with coexistent low left-ventricular ejection fraction is associated with a poor prognosis.

RADIOLOGIC

- Myocardial perfusion studies are performed to determine the severity and extent of myocardial ischemia and infarction and assess prognosis.

- Tl-201 and Tc-99m sestamibi are myocardial perfusion radiotracers that distribute in proportion to blood flow. There is a good correlation between myocardial perfusion defect size and actual infarct size.
- Tc-99m pyrophosphate and In-111 antimyosin are myocardial infarct imaging radiotracers. These radiotracers are infarct-avid, localizing in infarcted myocardium. However, these radiotracers are used infrequently because the information provided using studies with these agents can be obtained from other tests.
- On perfusion imaging, myocardial infarction is typically seen as one or more persistent defects on both rest and exercise studies. However, areas of persistent defects at 4 hours on the redistribution Tl-201 study can decrease or resolve (indicating myocardial viability) after reinjection or on 24-hour redistribution images.
- Large perfusion defects are associated with poor left ventricular function and poor prognosis.
- The term *hibernating myocardium* refers to regions of wall motion abnormality or ventricular dysfunction that improve on perfusion images at 24-hour redistribution or reinjection Tl-201 studies. Foci of hibernating myocardium are thought to result from chronic reduction in coronary artery blood flow and represent areas of impaired function with reversible myocardial damage.
- The gold standard study for myocardial viability is positron emission tomography (PET) imaging with F-18 fluorodeoxyglucose (FDG) and N-13 ammonia. Approximately 25% of areas with fixed perfusion defects on Tl-201 studies are found to be viable on FDG studies.

◆ SUGGESTED READING

Bonow RO, Dilsizian V. Thallium-201 for assessment of myocardial viability. Semin Nucl Med 1991;21:230–241.

Palmer EL, Scott JA, Strauss HW. Practical Nuclear Medicine. Philadelphia: Saunders, 1992;71–120.

Verani MS. Tl-201 myocardial perfusion imaging. Curr Opin Radiol 1991;3:797–809.

CASE 4

Salvador Borges-Neto

HISTORY

A 49-year-old woman who underwent complete thyroidectomy for papillary carcinoma of the thyroid. A metastasis to a left superior jugular node was found at surgery but not resected. An I-131 whole body scan was performed to evaluate for residual thyroid tissue and metastases after the patient developed hypothyroidism.

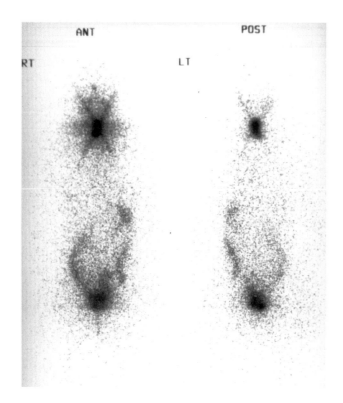

FIGURE 10-4A I-131 total body scans in the anterior (**left image**) and posterior (**right image**) projections obtained at 48 hours after the oral administration of 5 mCi of I-131 sodium iodide. A prominent region of radiotracer accumulation is seen within the neck. The star pattern that is seen in the neck region is caused by septal penetration of the collimator by the high energy photons (364 keV). Normal activity is present in the salivary glands, stomach, bladder, and bowel.

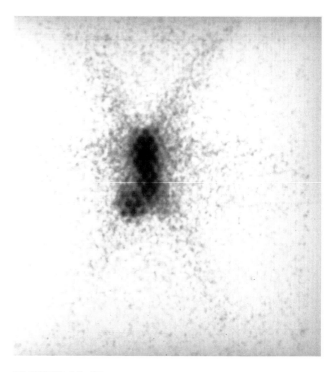

FIGURE 10-4B Anterior magnification view of the neck. The region of radiotracer accumulation in the neck is actually seen to consist of two foci. The larger focus is in the midline. Another smaller focus is present along the right lower border of the larger focus. The very small photopenic regions within each focus of radiotracer accumulation are due to attenuation of activity by the lead collimator. The star pattern mentioned in Figure 10-4A is seen again.

◆ DIFFERENTIAL DIAGNOSIS

◆ **Solely residual thyroid tissue:** The presence of residual thyroid tissue alone could produce the larger, midline focus of radiotracer accumulation but would not account for the smaller focus to the right of midline. Furthermore, it is known that residual metastatic disease was left at the time of surgery. Therefore, this diagnosis is incorrect.

◆ **Functioning thyroid metastatic disease alone:** This diagnosis is incorrect because it would not account for the large midline focus, which is at the expected site of the thyroid gland. In addition, it is quite unusual to have no residual thyroid tissue remaining after attempted total thyroidectomy.

◆ **Residual thyroid tissue and functioning metastasis:** This diagnosis would account for both foci of radiotracer accumulation and is the most likely consideration.

◆ **Swallowed radioiodine:** Radioiodine that is swallowed can often be seen in the esophagus. This artifarct is prevented by having the patient ingest small amounts of food and fluids. However, the radiotracer activity would be expected to be seen only in the midline. This diagnosis is incorrect because it would not account for the small focus of radiotracer accumulation to the right of midline.

◆ **Residual thyroid tissue in the neck with metastatic spread to the abdomen and pelvis:** The radiotracer activity in the abdomen and pelvis in the case illustrated is that which is normally seen on I-131 total body scans, due to excretion into the stomach, colon, and bladder. This radiotracer activity does not represent metastasis.

◆ DIAGNOSIS: Residual functioning thyroid tissue and functioning metastasis.

◆ KEY FACTS

CLINICAL

◆ Thyroid cancers are rarely of a single cell type and are designated by the predominant histologic type.

◆ Three types of carcinoma—well-differentiated papillary carcinoma, follicular carcinoma, and mixed papillary-follicular carcinoma—comprise about 75% of all primary thyroid malignancies.

◆ Anaplastic and poorly differentiated thyroid carcinomas comprise 20% of all thyroid malignancies and occur primarily in elderly patients.

◆ Medullary thyroid carcinoma constitutes approximately 5% of all primary thyroid cancers and can be associated with other endocrine lesions such as pheochromocy-

toma as part of a multiple endocrine neoplasia syndrome.

◆ In well-differentiated thyroid cancers, the overall prognosis is good, with a 5-year survival rate of >95% in properly treated patients.

◆ Well-differentiated papillary carcinoma tends to metastasize to local lymph nodes in the neck, whereas follicular carcinoma tends to spread hematogenously, producing metastases in lungs and bone.

◆ When evaluating patients with well-differentiated thyroid cancer using I-131 sodium iodide, it is important to stop thyroid replacement therapy and allow thyroid-stimulating hormone (TSH) levels to elevate before administration of radiotracer for a total body scan. The resultant high TSH levels stimulate any remaining thyroid tissue or functioning metastases and increase detection of these sites on imaging studies.

◆ Elevation of endogenous TSH takes approximately 4 to 6 weeks to occur after a total thyroidectomy or after cessation of exogenous thyroxin.

RADIOLOGIC

◆ Normal radiotracer accumulation of I-131 occurs within the salivary glands, stomach, bladder, and bowel.

◆ To optimize the tumor-to-background ratio, imaging should be performed 48 or 72 hours after administration of I-131.

◆ The usual dose of I-131 administered for whole body imaging for the detection of metastatic differentiated thyroid cancer is 5 to 10 mCi.

◆ Tl-201 can be used to image functioning metastases from well-differentiated thyroid carcinoma. An advantage of Tl-201 over I-131 is that the patients do not need to be in a hypothyroid state for the Tl-201 to detect metastatic foci.

◆ Medullary and anaplastic thyroid cancers rarely, if ever, concentrate I-131.

◆ Significant residual thyroid tissue can produce a star pattern that is caused by septal penetration of the collimator by the high energy photons. The star pattern is less likely to result from accumulation in thyroid cancer because the accumulation in functioning thyroid cancer is usually less than in normal thyroid gland.

◆ SUGGESTED READING

Hurley JR, Becker DV. Treatment of Thyroid Carcinoma with Radioiodine. In A Gottschalk, PB Hoffer, EJ Potchen (eds), Diagnostic Nuclear Medicine. Baltimore: Williams & Wilkins, 1988;792–814.

Mettler FA, Guiberteau MJ. Essentials of Nuclear Medicine Imaging. Philadelphia: Saunders, 1991;87–93.

HISTORY

A 50-year-old man with a history of coronary artery disease and atypical chest pain 6 months after angioplasty of the right coronary artery. Repeat coronary angiography (not shown) revealed stenosis of the left anterior descending coronary artery.

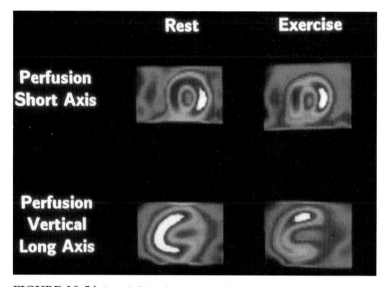

FIGURE 10-5A Rest **(left)** and exercise **(right)** midventricular slices from Tc-99m sestamibi perfusion study displayed in short axis **(top row)** and vertical long axis **(bottom row)** views. The rest perfusion images show a focal area of decreased activity present in the posterobasal wall (6 o'clock position on the short axis view). Stress perfusion images show an area of severe decrease in perfusion involving the inferior, anterior, and apical regions.

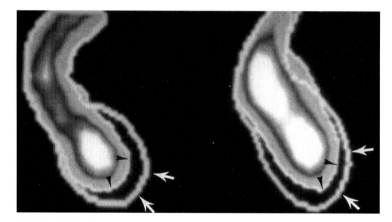

FIGURE 10-5B Rest **(left)** and exercise **(right)** first-pass radionuclide angiography images are shown using an anterior projection. The left ventricle is the rounded structure at the bottom of the image, and the aorta is the curvilinear structure in the middle of the image. The systolic (arrowheads) and diastolic (arrows) contours are shown. The resting first-pass study shows mild akinesis of the inferior-posterobasal wall. The exercise first-pass images show severe hypokinesis of the anterior and apical regions and now mild hypokinesis of the posterobasal region. The left ventricle dilates during exercise with an increase in end systolic volume and decrease in ejection fraction from 41% to 37%.

◆ DIFFERENTIAL DIAGNOSIS

◆ **Myocardial infarction without stress-induced ischemia:** The inferior wall motion abnormality at rest is consistent with previous infarction. Myocardial infarction without exercise-induced ischemia would be seen on a perfusion study as a fixed perfusion defect with no significant change between rest and stress studies. However, the changes in perfusion and function from rest to exercise, development of new wall motion abnormalities, and decrease in ejection fraction with exercise indicate that ischemia is also present.

◆ **Myocardial ischemia without infarction:** Myocardial ischemia alone would produce a stress-induced perfusion defect (typically in the apical, inferior, and anterior walls of the left ventricle) against the background of a relatively normal resting study. Alternatively, ischemia could be seen as exercise-induced wall motion abnormalities on the first-pass study in the anterior and apical regions. However, the resting study in this patient is not normal; the presence of a fixed perfusion defect and resting wall motion abnormality in the inferior wall indicate previous infarction.

◆ **Myocardial infarction and stress-induced ischemia:** This diagnosis is made when a resting perfusion defect is present that accentuates (i.e., increases in either or both severity and extent) during exercise. Typically, the wall motion study shows a wall motion abnormality at rest that worsens during exercise. All these findings are present in this case, making this consideration the best diagnosis.

◆ **Nonischemic cardiomyopathy:** In the case illustrated, multiple perfusion defects and a new focal wall motion abnormality are induced by exercise. These findings would not be expected in nonischemic cardiomyopathy.

◆ **Valvular heart disease:** This entity is not commonly associated with perfusion defects and focal wall motion abnormalities. Therefore, valvular heart disease alone (without ischemic heart disease) is an unlikely diagnosis.

◆ DIAGNOSIS: Myocardial infarction and stress-induced ischemia.

◆ KEY FACTS

CLINICAL

◆ Atherosclerotic coronary artery disease is the most common cause of cardiovascular disability and death in the United States.

◆ Elevated total serum cholesterol and low-density lipoproteins are involved in the development of atherosclerosis and are markers of high-risk patients. Other risk factors are age, genetic predisposition, hypertension, smoking, and diabetes.

◆ High-density lipoproteins play an equally important protective role against the development of atherosclerotic coronary artery disease.

◆ Atherosclerosis is a chronic process that occurs over decades. However, most acute ischemic syndromes such as infarction and unstable angina are precipitated by plaque ulceration, intimal hemorrhage, and thrombosis.

◆ Advanced stages of coronary artery disease can remain clinically silent, particularly in diabetic patients. Silent ischemic episodes have the same prognostic importance as episodes associated with chest pain.

◆ The most sensitive procedure for determining coronary artery stenosis location and extent is coronary angiography, but myocardial ischemia can be detected noninvasively by either or both myocardial perfusion and left ventricular function studies.

◆ Indications for radionuclide stress testing include evaluation of chest pain, determination of severity and extent of disease, and prognostic assessment.

◆ Patients with multiple perfusion defects (more than three segments) and low left ventricular ejection fraction (LVEF) during exercise (<40%) have a poor prognosis.

◆ Left ventricular exercise ejection fraction provides about 80% of the prognostic information obtained from radionuclide angiography.

◆ Patients with low ejection fraction during exercise are more likely to benefit from revascularization.

RADIOLOGIC

◆ Tc-99m–labeled myocardial perfusion radiotracers such as Tc-99m sestamibi allow assessment of myocardial perfusion and left ventricular function with a single injection of radiopharmaceutical. Ventricular function studies can be performed with either a first-pass study or gated images of the perfused myocardium.

◆ If both the perfusion and functional studies are normal, significant coronary artery disease is extremely unlikely.

◆ If both tests are abnormal, the likelihood of significant coronary artery disease is very high, even if the disease prevalence is low.

◆ Myocardial perfusion and left ventricular function studies provide different, independent types of diagnostic information.

◆ Another method for performing ventricular function studies is to label the blood pool with Tc-99m albumin or Tc-99m red blood cells and to gate the acquisition to the electrocardiogram. This technique is referred to as a gated blood pool study or MUGA study.

◆ SUGGESTED READING

Borges-Neto S, Coleman RE. Radionuclide ventricular function analysis. Radiol Clin North Am 1993;31:817–830.

Borges-Neto S, Coleman RE, Potts JM, Jones RH. Perfusion and function at rest and treadmill exercise using technetium-99m sestamibi: Comparison of one- and two-day protocols in normal volunteers. J Nucl Med 1990;31:1128–1132.

Borges-Neto S, Coleman RE, Potts JM, Jones RH. Combined exercise radionuclide angiocardiography and single photon emission computer tomography perfusion studies for assessment of coronary artery disease. Semin Nucl Med 1991;21:223–229.

CASE 6

Robert H. Wilkinson, Jr.

HISTORY

A 77-year-old Englishman with progressive swelling and deformity of legs and right upper arm. He has also noted increasing frequency of headaches and increasing hat size over several years. Laboratory studies include an elevated alkaline phosphatase level and normal acid phosphatase and prostate-specific antigen values.

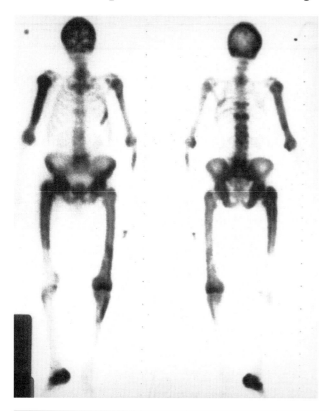

FIGURE 10-6A Anterior (**left**) and posterior (**right**) images of a whole body bone scan obtained after the intravenous administration of Tc-99m methylene diphosphonate. Markedly abnormal regions of increased radiotracer bone uptake are noted within the axial and appendicular skeleton.

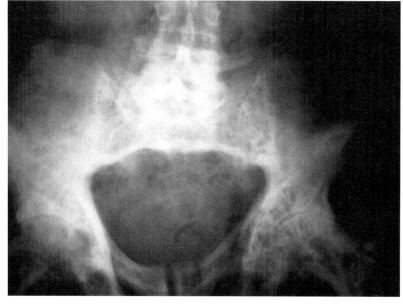

FIGURE 10-6B Anteroposterior radiograph of the pelvis revealing bony expansion, sclerosis, and cortical thickening.

◆ DIFFERENTIAL DIAGNOSIS

◆ **Paget's disease of bone:** The pattern seen on the radionuclide bone scan is that of regions of markedly increased bone tracer accumulation with an expanded appearance to the entire bone. These features are typical of Paget's disease, the most likely diagnosis.

◆ **Metastases:** Metastases can simulate lesions of Paget's bone disease. The advanced degree of tracer accumulation and expanded bone appearance seen in this case are atypical even for advanced prostate, breast, or lung carcinoma. This diagnosis is an unlikely consideration.

◆ **Fractures:** The expanded bone and diffuse tracer accumulation make fractures unlikely considerations.

◆ **Osteomyelitis:** Regions of intense tracer accumulation can be seen in osteomyelitis, but the clinical setting, the diffuse nature of the abnormalities, and the expansile changes seen on the radiograph make this diagnosis highly unlikely.

◆ **Fibrous dysplasia:** Polyostotic fibrous dysplasia can produce increased tracer accumulation in multiple bones, as is seen in this case. However, the history of progressive bony expansion late in life and the radiographic findings make this diagnosis unlikely.

◆ DIAGNOSIS: Paget's disease of bone.

◆ KEY FACTS

CLINICAL

◆ Paget's disease is most commonly encountered in Eastern and Western Europe (with the exception of Scandinavia), with a prevalence of 3.5% to 4.5% and with a 3 to 2 male-to-female predominance.

◆ The etiology of Paget's disease is not known definitively. Slow virus inoculation early in life is one hypothesis that has been strongly considered.

◆ Progression of Paget's disease can be classified into three stages: (1) bone resorption, (2) mixed bone resorption and deformation, and (3) decline in resorption accompanied by a decrease in irregularity and fibrosis.

◆ The prevalence of fractures in Paget's disease is reported to be 8% to 18%, based on retrospective series.

◆ Sarcomatous degeneration of pagetoid bone can occur and can be solitary or multicentric.

◆ Elevated cardiac output is seen in some patients with Paget's disease due to the increased vascularity of acute pagetoid bone.

RADIOLOGIC

◆ On radiographs, vertebrae appear enlarged and deformed; the scapulae and pelvic bones appear expanded and thickened; the skull enlarges with basilar flattening and cortical thickening; and the long bones bow and develop cortical thickening.

◆ The degree of radiotracer accumulation in pagetoid bone is variable.

◆ The radionuclide study is reported to be more sensitive than radiographs: 5% to 20% of patients have abnormal bone scans and normal radiographs, compared to 1% with abnormal radiographs and normal radionuclide bone scan.

◆ Bone scan findings do not correlate well with the severity of bone pain in Paget's disease.

◆ Reduced accumulation of In-111–labeled leukocytes and of Tc-99m sulfur colloid has been reported to occur in Paget's disease.

◆ Photopenic regions can be seen in pagetoid bone in instances of sarcomatous degeneration, most likely due to proliferation of nonosteoblastic tissue.

◆ A photopenic area in a bone scan that occurs in a radiographically evident region of Paget's disease can represent either early disease or sarcomatous degeneration.

◆ Ga-67 may be useful for sarcoma detection. In one small study, slightly more than half of Paget's disease patients with sarcomas and a focal photopenic area on bone scan were found to have increased Ga-67 accumulation at the site of the sarcoma. Another small series found the Ga-67 scan to be less sensitive.

◆ SUGGESTED READING

Altman RD. Paget's Disease of Bone. In FL Coe, MJ Favus (eds), Disorders of Bone and Mineral Metabolism. New York: Raven, 1992;1027–1061.

Boudreau RJ, Lisbona R, Hadjipavtou A. Observations on serial radionuclide blood flow studies in Paget's disease. J Nucl Med 1983;24:880–885.

Smith J, Bitet JF, Yeh SJ. Bone sarcomas in Paget's disease: A study of 85 patients. Radiology 1984;152:583–590.

CASE 7

Robert H. Wilkinson, Jr.

HISTORY

The bone scans of three patients are presented. Patient A is a 67-year-old man with an elevated prostate-specific antigen value of 86 ng/ml and biopsy-proven prostate cancer. Patient B is a 69-year-old man with a history of prostate carcinoma and a borderline normal prostate specific antigen value of 6 ng/ml. Patient C is a 71-year-old woman with a history of stage IV breast carcinoma. A different diagnosis is possible in each of the cases.

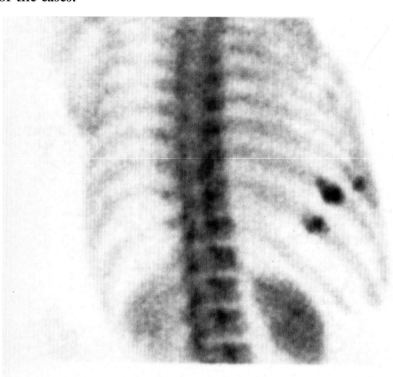

FIGURE 10-7B Patient B: right posterior oblique view of the chest shows foci of increased radiotracer accumulation in adjacent ribs in a "string-of-pearls" pattern.

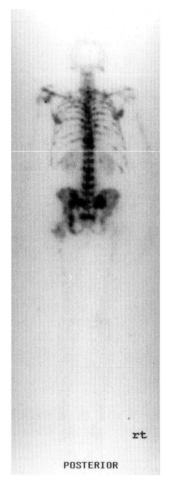

FIGURE 10-7A Patient A: posterior image from total body bone imaging study. Multiple foci of abnormally increased bone radiotracer accumulation are seen in the axial and proximal appendicular skeleton.

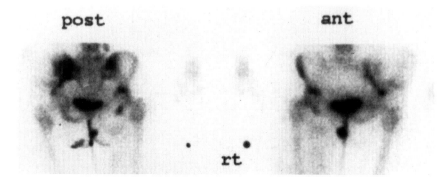

FIGURE 10-7C Patient C: anterior and posterior pelvis images. A mixed pattern of abnormal foci of abnormally increased and decreased radiotracer accumulation is seen in the left ilium.

◆ DIFFERENTIAL DIAGNOSIS

◆ **Metastases:** Bone metastases can appear on bone scans as any or all of the following: multiple foci of increased radiotracer accumulation (Figure 10-7A), increased or decreased radiotracer accumulation (Figure 10-7C), and normal bone radiotracer accumulation. The pattern and location of the abnormalities in Figures 10-7A and 10-7C make bone metastases the most likely consideration.

◆ **Pathologic fractures:** Pathologic fractures can be solitary or multiple and usually occur in metastatic bone lesions that are subject to stress or trauma. Bone metastases in weight-bearing regions are particularly susceptible to fracture.

◆ **Multiple benign fractures:** The pattern, location, and clinical history are important in distinguishing benign fractures from metastatic disease. Some patterns of fractures (e.g., the string-of-pearls appearance in Figure 10-7B) are typical of benign fractures. This is the diagnosis in patient B.

◆ **Degenerative joint disease/arthritides:** These processes occur at joints and can be difficult to distinguish from metastases. Concomitant benign arthropathic disease can occur in patients with metastatic disease, but the pattern of nonarticular bone abnormalities in all three patients shown above makes benign arthropathic disease alone unlikely.

◆ DIAGNOSIS: Patients A and C: multiple bone metastases; patient B: benign rib fractures.

◆ KEY FACTS

CLINICAL

◆ The likelihood of bone metastases depends on the primary tumor (e.g., most primary bone tumors rarely metastasize) and stage of disease.

◆ The lifetime risk of developing breast cancer in American women is reported to be approximately 11%, and over one-half of breast cancers occur in women after the age of 65 years. In autopsy series of women with metastatic breast carcinoma, the frequency of bone metastases has been reported to be between 44% and 71%.

◆ The digital rectal examination and serum prostate-specific antigen (PSA) test are currently the recommended screening procedures for prostate carcinoma. Approximately one-third of men over the age of 50 years harbor foci of prostatic carcinoma without clinical evidence of disease.

◆ Approximately 80% of patients with detectable prostate carcinoma and distant metastases are found to have bone metastases.

RADIOLOGIC

◆ The majority of metastatic bone tumors appear as focal regions of increased radiotracer accumulation on radionuclide bone scan. However, photopenic foci can be seen in malignancies such as breast, lung, renal, and anaplastic carcinomas; neuroblastoma; and multiple myeloma.

◆ Soft-tissue neoplasms can invade bone and produce increased radiotracer uptake or a photopenic focus, which usually has a rim of increased radiotracer accumulation.

◆ Benign bone conditions that can appear photopenic include bone infarction, bone resection, very early osteomyelitis, radiation-induced bone changes, and histiocytosis X.

◆ Skeletal involvement from multiple myeloma, plasmacytoma, neuroblastoma, and eosinophilic granuloma can produce normal, increased, or decreased radiotracer accumulation.

◆ Particular care must be taken in evaluating the radionuclide bone imaging study of a patient with bone metastases during the first 4 to 6 months after starting chemotherapy, because a disparity between the clinical/radiologic status and findings on radionuclide bone scan can be seen. These patients can improve clinically and have a decrease in number and size of bone lesions on radiographs but no change or apparent worsening of lesions (the so-called flare phenomenon) on the radionuclide bone imaging study. This pattern change presumably reflects healing of lesions and is most commonly reported in bone metastases from a primary breast or prostate tumor. Following further healing of bone lesions after this initial period, the radionuclide bone study reflects the clinical and radiologic status more accurately.

◆ Patients with a PSA value of <10 ng/ml during their initial evaluation for prostate carcinoma have a very low likelihood of having a positive radionuclide bone imaging study for metastases.

◆ The likelihood of a solitary bone scan lesion being a metastasis is reported to range from 10% (in adults) to 60% (in children).

◆ In the presence of a known primary malignancy, approximately 10% to 20% of solitary rib lesions on bone scans are metastases. On the other hand, focal rib lesions having a string-of-pearls pattern are highly likely to be benign rib fractures.

◆ Correlation with radiographs or other imaging studies is often useful to confirm the presence of bone metastases in patients with bone scan abnormalities. In the presence of an abnormal radionuclide bone scan, a normal radiograph actually makes a bone metastasis a likely consideration by excluding other possible causes.

◆ SUGGESTED READING

Hanks GE, Myers CE, Scardino PT. Cancer of the Prostate. In VT DeVita Jr, S Hellman, SA Rosenberg (eds), Cancer—Principles and Practice of Oncology (4th ed). Philadelphia: Lippincott, 1993;1073–1113.

Janicek MJ, Hayes DF, Kaplan WD. Healing flare in skeletal metastases from breast cancer. Radiology 1994;192:201–204.

O'Connor MK, Brown ML, Hung JC, Hayostek RJ. The art of bone scintigraphy—Technical aspects. J Nucl Med 1991;32:2332–2341.

HISTORY

A 75-year-old man being treated for hypercalcemia.

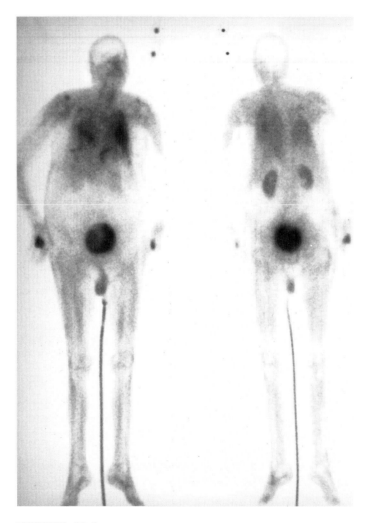

FIGURE 10-8 Anterior (left) and posterior (right) images from a radionuclide bone scan obtained 2 hours after administration of 20 mCi of Tc-99m methylene diphosphonate. Abnormal accumulation of radiotracer is present in the lungs and in the stomach as a result of the hypercalcemia. However, no radiotracer accumulation is seen in the bones. Normal renal and bladder radiotracer accumulation are seen, as well as a small focus of activity at the injection site in the right hand.

◆DIFFERENTIAL DIAGNOSIS

◆ **Administration of incorrect radiopharmaceutical:** This diagnosis is unlikely because no radiopharmaceutical has the pattern of distribution seen in this patient.

◆ **Presence of excess aluminum ion:** Contamination of Tc-99m methylene diphosphonate (MDP) with aluminum ion from the eluate or the presence of high plasma aluminum levels in patients taking aluminum hydroxide antacids can alter the biodistribution of radiopharmaceutical. However, these conditions cause increased uptake in the liver and kidney and not the lung accumulation seen in the case illustrated.

◆ **Effect of therapy for hypercalcemia:** The patient shown above was receiving intravenously administered etidronate for treatment of hypercalcemia. Etidronate (hydroxyethylidene diphosphonic acid [EHDP]) inhibits the formation, growth, and dissolution of hydroxyapatite crystals. This agent can cause the lack of radiopharmaceutical accumulation within bones, as shown above.

◆ **Premature imaging:** Images obtained immediately after administration of Tc-99m MDP will typically show blood pool activity, prominent soft-tissue activity, and some bone accumulation. However, accumulation in the lungs would not be expected, making this diagnosis unlikely.

◆ **Iron overload:** This diagnosis might be considered because in iron overload conditions such as occur in hemochromatosis or following multiple blood transfusions, the accumulation of Tc-99m MDP into bone is diminished and renal excretion is increased. However, pulmonary deposition of the radiotracer would not be expected.

◆DIAGNOSIS: Hypercalcemia with etidronate therapy.

◆KEY FACTS

CLINICAL

◆ Hypercalcemia can occur secondary to a number of entities, including hyperparathyroidism, metastatic skeletal disease, hyperthyroidism, and sarcoidosis.

◆ Biphosphonates such as etidronate and pamidronate are used to treat the hypercalcemia of malignancy because of their effect on bone turnover. The biphosphonates interact with the hydroxyapatite crystal, inhibiting bone resorption, and may impair osteoclast

function. These agents are also used to treat Paget's disease and heterotopic ossification and may have a role in treating osteoporosis.

◆ Radionuclide bone scans in patients with hypercalcemia and elevated calcium phosphorus products frequently show abnormal localization of the radiopharmaceutical in the lungs, stomach, and kidneys, reflecting the acid-base changes that occur in these tissues. Furthermore, these are the sites of metastatic calcification that can occur in these patients.

◆ The effect of biphosphonates on Tc-99m MDP bone scans is variable. The biphosphonate used and the method of administration (oral or intravenous) may make a difference in the effect on the bone scan. Some studies report difficulty in interpretation of radionuclide bone scans of patients undergoing biphosphonate therapy, whereas other studies have shown no effect on the sensitivity of the bone scan.

RADIOLOGIC

◆ A Tc-99m MDP bone scan that shows poor bone uptake and prominent soft-tissue accumulation usually results from a radiopharmaceutical preparation problem, with excess Tc-99m pertechnetate in the preparation. The excess pertechnetate is manifested by radiotracer accumulation in the thyroid and stomach.

◆ The clue to the diagnosis in the patient shown above is accumulation of the Tc-99m MDP in the lungs, which occurs with hypercalcemia. In a patient with accumulation of Tc-99m MDP in the lungs, associated bone scan findings should be considered as possibly related to hypercalcemia or its treatment.

◆ Radionuclide bone scans usually provide diagnostic information in patients receiving biphosphonates, but as noted above, this agent can affect the scan. The effect of this therapy needs to be taken into account when interpreting the images.

◆SUGGESTED READING

Chong WK, Cunningham DA. Case Report: Intravenous etidronate as a cause of poor uptake on bone scanning, with a review of the literature. Clin Radiol 1991;44:268–270.

Pecherstorfer M, Schilling T, Janisch S, et al. Effect of clodronate treatment on bone scintigraphy in metastatic breast cancer. J Nucl Med 1993;34:1039–1044.

Sahni M, Guenther HL, Fleisch H, et al. Biphosphonates act on rate of bone resorption through mediation of osteoblasts. J Clin Invest 1993;91:2004–2011.

CASE 9

Sara M. O'Hara

HISTORY

A 6-week-old girl with jaundice, total bilirubin of 19.8 mg/dl, and a conjugated bilirubin of 7.8 mg/dl.

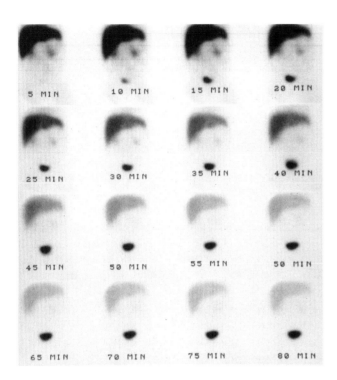

FIGURE 10-9A Anterior images of a diisopropyliminodiacetic acid scan obtained immediately after injection. Good extraction of the radiopharmaceutical by the hepatocytes is seen, with prompt clearance of the blood pool. Homogenous radiotracer activity is present throughout the liver. Tracer activity is identified in both kidneys and the bladder. However, the central bile ducts, gastrointestinal tract, and gallbladder have not accumulated the radiotracer. This pattern persisted on 24-hour delayed films.

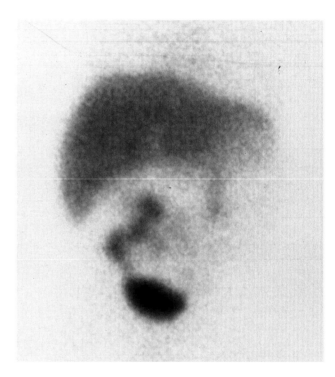

FIGURE 10-9B Follow-up study 1 month later. In the interim since the previous study, the patient has undergone a Kasai procedure (portoenterostomy). Anterior image obtained 3.5 hours after injection. Radiopharmaceutical is again distributed homogeneously throughout the liver parenchyma. Gastrointestinal activity is now identified in the mid-abdomen, partially superimposed over the lower pole of the right kidney.

◆ DIFFERENTIAL DIAGNOSIS

- **Idiopathic neonatal hepatitis:** Jaundice and bile stasis are features of idiopathic neonatal hepatitis, but the biliary system is patent (unlike the case illustrated). Hepatic uptake and blood pool clearance of radiotracer can be delayed in neonatal hepatitis, and the degree of delay reflects the severity of hepatocyte damage.
- **Choledochal cyst:** The absence of visualization of the proximal ducts or an actual cyst makes this diagnosis unlikely.
- **Biliary atresia:** This is the best diagnosis because good hepatocyte extraction of radiopharmaceutical is seen in the absence of visible intrahepatic bile ducts or gastrointestinal (GI) activity, even on 24-hour images.
- **Bile plug syndrome:** This rare condition results in conjugated hyperbilirubinemia due to obstruction of the common bile duct by inspissated bile/secretions. Sepsis, hemolytic disorders, dehydration, total parenteral nutrition, and cystic fibrosis are predisposing conditions. Careful ultrasound examination to exclude echogenic, nonshadowing bile plugs within the dilated biliary tree is necessary to distinguish this condition from biliary atresia.
- **Arteriohepatic dysplasia (Alagille syndrome):** This syndrome is characterized by typical dysmorphic facies, pulmonary artery stenosis, and hepatic ductular hypoplasia. Distinction from true biliary atresia can be difficult if the other components of the syndrome are not recognized.

◆ DIAGNOSIS: Biliary atresia.

◆ KEY FACTS

CLINICAL

- Hyperbilirubinemia is a common problem in neonates and infants. Unconjugated hyperbilirubinemia, in which <15% of the total bilirubin is conjugated (or "direct," which is the nomenclature used on laboratory reports) is most often due to physiologic jaundice of the newborn, breast milk jaundice, or erythroblastosis fetalis. In conjugated hyperbilirubinemia, where at least 30% of the bilirubin is conjugated, a search for causes of obstructive jaundice is necessary. The most common causes of obstructive jaundice are included in the differential diagnosis listed above.
- Biliary atresia is the most common cause of extrahepatic cholestasis in infants. The incidence ranges from 1 in 8,000 to 1 in 10,000 live births.
- Distinction between idiopathic neonatal hepatitis, a nonsurgical disease, and biliary atresia, a surgical disease, is important within the first 3 months of life. The Kasai procedure (or portoenterostomy) is performed using a Roux-en-Y loop of intestine to bypass the hypoplastic or absent biliary duct segments. The surgical success rate varies according to patient age at the time of surgery. The procedure is 90% effective in patients <2 months of age, but only 17% effective in patients >3 months of age.

RADIOLOGIC

- DISIDA (diisopropyliminodiacetic acid, disofenin) and mebrofenin (trimethyl-bromo-IDA) have the highest extraction rate by hepatocytes and shortest transit time of the IDA derivatives. Between 5% and 15% of the disofenin is excreted via the kidneys in normal subjects. Dynamic image acquisition immediately after radiopharmaceutical injection is helpful to determine hepatocyte extraction and hepatocyte function. Static images performed over the next 1 to 2 hours with delayed images taken up to 24 hours are generally required.
- Pretreatment with oral phenobarbital (5 mg/kg/day for 5 days) is recommended to improve bile flow. With phenobarbital pretreatment, biliary scintigraphy is approximately 95% accurate in determining biliary patency in infants <3 months of age.
- Progressive hepatocyte damage and hepatic cirrhosis occur in the setting of untreated biliary atresia and in persistent neonatal hepatitis. The two diseases can be indistinguishable in patients >3 months of age.

◆ SUGGESTED READING

Kasai M, Suzuke H, Ohashi E, et al. Technique and results of operative management of biliary atresia. World J Surg 1978;2:571–580.

Paltiel HJ. Imaging of neonatal cholestasis. Semin Ultrasound CT MR 1994;15:290–305.

Treves ST, Jones AG, Markisz J. Liver and Spleen. In ST Treves (ed), Pediatric Nuclear Medicine. New York: Springer, 1995;466–495.

Wells RG, Sty JR. Radionuclide Imaging of the Liver, Biliary System, and Spleen. In JH Miller, MJ Gelfand (eds), Pediatric Nuclear Imaging. Philadelphia: Saunders, 1994;103–156.

CASE 10

Michael W. Hanson

HISTORY

A 68-year-old man with a history of Crohn's disease of the terminal ileum and colon presents with a 3-day history of nausea and right upper quadrant pain radiating posteriorly to the back. The pain is worsened by eating.

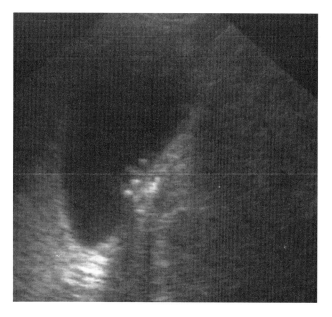

FIGURE 10-10A Ultrasound shows small gallstones in the gallbladder with mild thickening of the gallbladder wall. There is no pericholecystic fluid. The common bile duct appears normal.

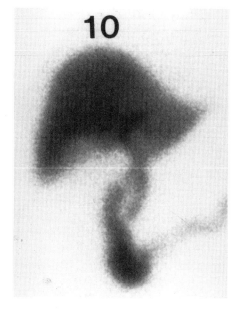

FIGURE 10-10B Hepatobiliary imaging study at 10 minutes. There is good hepatic extraction of Tc-99m disofenin with good visualization of the hepatic parenchyma. Radiotracer in the common bile duct and the duodenum indicates patency of the common bile duct.

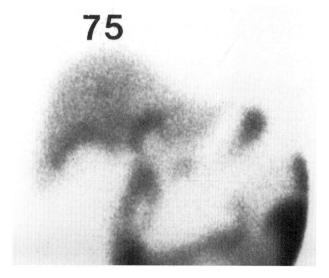

FIGURE 10-10C Hepatobiliary imaging study at 75 minutes. Persistent radiotracer is seen in the common bile duct and within small bowel. No radiotracer is present in the gallbladder, but a region of relatively increased radiotracer is seen within the liver parenchyma along the gallbladder fossa.

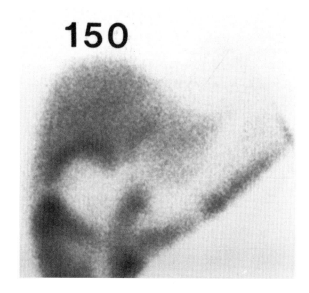

FIGURE 10-10D Hepatobiliary imaging study at 150 minutes. The gallbladder is not visualized. A persistent region of prominent radiotracer accumulation exists in the liver parenchyma, consistent with pericholecystic hepatic uptake of Tc-99m disofenin.

◆ DIFFERENTIAL DIAGNOSIS

◆ **Acute pancreatitis:** This process presents with abdominal pain and can be seen in patients with Crohn's disease. An elevated serum amylase is usually present. Hepatobiliary imaging studies are normal unless pancreatitis is due to underlying hepatobiliary disease. This diagnosis is therefore unlikely.

◆ **Acalculous cholecystitis:** Acute inflammation of the gallbladder can occur in the absence of cholelithiasis, most often as a complication of severe underlying illnesses (e.g., burns, trauma, sepsis, and following major surgery) associated with bile stasis. The benign clinical features and sonographic finding of gallstones make this diagnosis unlikely.

◆ **Common bile duct obstruction:** Approximately 10% to 15% of patients with cholelithiasis will pass a gallstone into the common bile duct (CBD), from which it can (1) pass into the duodenum, (2) remain without producing symptoms, or (3) obstruct the CBD. The presence of radiotracer in the CBD and the duodenum by 10 minutes essentially excludes CBD obstruction.

◆ **Chronic cholecystitis:** Patients with chronic cholecystitis frequently have gallstones and gallbladder wall thickening, and can have repeated bouts of biliary colic without cystic duct obstruction. The most frequent abnormal finding on scintigraphy is delayed visualization of the gallbladder beyond 1 hour, but imaging is normal frequently. Scintigraphy is generally an ineffective study in the evaluation of chronic cholecystitis, except to exclude a superimposed acute cystic duct obstruction. The majority of patients with only chronic cholecystitis would be expected to have visualization of the gallbladder by 180 minutes, making this diagnosis unlikely in the case illustrated.

◆ **Acute cholecystitis:** This entity typically has the presentation of right upper quadrant pain and tenderness with fever and leukocytosis. It often begins as an attack of biliary colic that progressively worsens and is associated with anorexia, nausea, and, commonly, emesis. With cystic duct obstruction, bile does not flow into or out of the gallbladder (as in the case presented above). The imaging findings in this case make this the most likely diagnosis.

◈ DIAGNOSIS: Cholelithiasis with acute cholecystitis.

◈ KEY FACTS

CLINICAL

◆ Patients with Crohn's disease are at increased risk for development of cholelithiasis (due to altered bile salt absorption) and acute cholecystitis.

◆ Acute cholecystitis is most commonly caused by acute occlusion of the cystic duct by a gallstone.

◆ Seventy-five percent of patients with acute cholecystitis respond to medical therapy, of whom 25% have recurrent acute cholecystitis within 1 year. Another 25% of patients treated conservatively develop a major complication, such as empyema, hydrops, gangrene, emphysematous cholecystitis, perforation of the gallbladder, or gallstone ileus. Therefore, early surgical therapy is the preferred treatment.

◆ As expected, patients with suspected empyema, emphysematous cholecystitis, or perforated gallbladder require more urgent surgical intervention than those with uncomplicated acute cholecystitis. It is important to search for evidence of these complications at the time of imaging.

◆ Perforation of the gallbladder has an estimated 30% mortality rate. These patients can have sudden transient relief of right upper quadrant pain as the distended gallbladder decompresses but then develop generalized signs of peritonitis.

RADIOLOGIC

◆ The diagnosis of acute cholecystitis can be confidently excluded on the basis of a normal hepatobiliary imaging study (negative predictive value of 98%).

◆ False-positive hepatobiliary scans can be seen in the following settings: alcoholism, total parenteral nutrition or prolonged fasting, within 2 hours of eating, and in severe intercurrent illnesses.

◆ Radiotracer in the duodenum or pericholecystic hepatic uptake of radiotracer (the "rim sign") can be mistaken for gallbladder uptake, resulting in a false-negative interpretation. The finding of pericholecystic hepatic uptake of radiotracer is important to recognize. It is present in 57% of patients with gangrenous cholecystitis and 31% of patients with perforated gallbladder.

◆ Potential mechanisms by which pericholecystic hepatic uptake occurs include hyperemia with increased delivery and extraction of radiotracer along the gallbladder fossa, focal hepatic cellular injury with impaired excretion of radiotracer, and mechanical obstruction with focally delayed clearance of radiotracer.

◆ If the gallbladder is not seen by 30 to 45 minutes but there is radiotracer in the small bowel, the study can be shortened from 4 to 2 hours by giving intravenous morphine sulfate (0.04 mg/kg; maximum 4 mg). Morphine sulfate contracts the sphincter of Oddi and redirects bile flow into the gallbladder if the cystic duct is patent. The study can be stopped when the gallbladder is filled or at 2 hours (whichever occurs first).

◈ SUGGESTED READING

Grossman SJ, Joyce JM. Hepatobiliary imaging. Emerg Med Clin North Am 1991;9:853–874.

Krishnamurthy GT, Turner FE. Pharmacokinetics and clinical application of technetium-99m-labeled hepatobiliary agents. Semin Nucl Med 1990;2:130–149.

Watson A, Kalff V. Hepatobiliary imaging. Curr Opin Radiol 1991;3:851–858.

CASE 11

Michael W. Hanson

HISTORY

A 59-year-old man with melena 48 hours prior to developing brisk, bright red rectal bleeding. Upper and lower GI endoscopy failed to show a bleeding source. A Tc-99m sodium pertechnetate-labeled red blood cell imaging study was obtained, followed by selective abdominal arteriography.

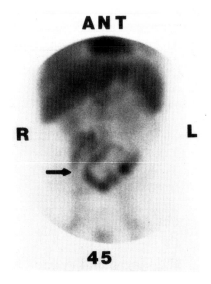

FIGURE 10-11A Anterior abdominal blood pool images at 45 minutes. Expected radiotracer is seen in the cardiac blood pool, liver, and spleen. Major abdominal vasculature and both kidneys are seen faintly. Moderately intense abnormal radiotracer accumulation is seen in the mid abdomen, the pattern of which conforms to the mid-portion of the small bowel, most likely the jejunum (arrow).

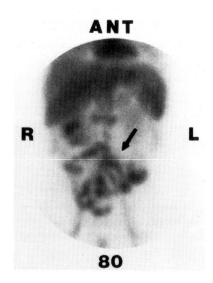

FIGURE 10-11B Anterior abdominal blood pool images at 80 minutes. The pattern of abnormal radiotracer accumulation now conforms to multiple bowel loops in the mid and distal segments of the small bowel (arrow).

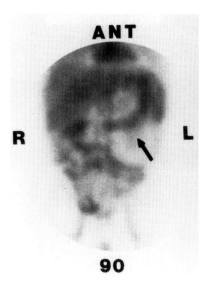

FIGURE 10-11C Anterior abdominal blood pool images at 90 minutes show further abnormal radiotracer accumulation in small bowel loops. Abnormal radiotracer is now seen in the transverse colon and the splenic flexure (arrow).

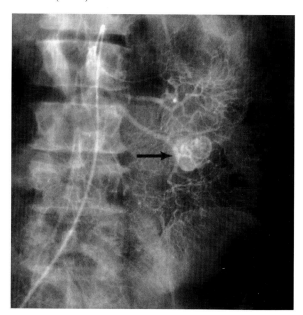

FIGURE 10-11D Selective arteriogram of the superior mesenteric artery. A brisk bleeding site is seen during the late arterial phase of the arteriogram in the left upper quadrant (arrow), proximal to the mid-jejunum.

◆ DIFFERENTIAL DIAGNOSIS

◆ **Abdominal aortic aneurysm:** An abdominal aortic aneurysm can have focally increased radiotracer on blood pool imaging. This is an unlikely diagnosis because it is generally seen early and does not change in shape or location during the study.

◆ **Free Tc-99m pertechnetate in the bowel:** Free Tc-99m sodium pertechnetate can be present on reinjection of tagged red blood cells. Pertechnetate is normally secreted by gastric mucosa. The stomach will be visualized, and during the latter part of the study, some of the normally secreted pertechnetate can occasionally enter small bowel. However, the intensity of radiotracer activity within bowel is usually faint and moves only minimally, making this an unlikely diagnosis in this case.

◆ **Inflammatory bowel disease:** Inflammatory bowel disease can produce a positive gastrointestinal (GI) bleeding scan by two mechanisms: (1) active bleeding, and (2) blood pool accumulation of radiotracer at sites of inflammation, even in the absence of active bleeding (in which case the sites remain static during the study). The latter possibility is unlikely in the case shown because the abnormal radiotracer accumulation in the case presented above is seen to progress through the small bowel.

◆ **Active bleeding originating in the colon:** Unless retrograde movement of radiotracer from the cecum into the terminal ileum occurs, radiotracer activity in the small bowel is generally not seen after hemorrhage from a colonic bleeding source. The findings in the patient shown are therefore unlikely to be due to an active bleeding site originating in the colon.

◆ **Active small bowel bleeding:** Active small bowel hemorrhage can usually be distinguished from that arising in large bowel and further localized to the proximal, mid–, or distal small bowel. The findings of this case make the diagnosis of a mid–small bowel (jejunal) bleeding site the most likely diagnosis.

◆ DIAGNOSIS: Acute mid-jejunal gastrointestinal hemorrhage.

◆ KEY FACTS

CLINICAL

◆ The presence of melena usually denotes bleeding from the esophagus, stomach, or duodenum, but lesions in the jejunum, ileum, and the ascending colon can cause melena, depending on the transit time of blood within the GI tract.

◆ Hematochezia generally signifies a bleeding site from a source distal to the ligament of Treitz, but rapid hemorrhage from the esophagus, stomach, or duodenum with rapid peristalsis can also produce bright red rectal bleeding.

◆ Initial attempts to localize a GI bleeding site should include nasogastric tube insertion, esophagogastroduodenoscopy, sigmoidoscopy, and colonoscopy (which is impaired when the lumen of the colon is obscured by large amounts of brisk bleeding).

◆ Peptic ulceration, erosive gastritis, variceal bleeding, and Mallory-Weiss syndrome account for 90% of all cases of upper GI hemorrhage in which a definite cause is found.

RADIOLOGIC

◆ The primary purpose of the scintigraphic GI bleeding study is to localize an active bleeding site to serve as a guide before selective abdominal angiography.

◆ In general, the rate of bleeding required for scintigraphic detection of GI bleeding is less than that required for detection by angiography. Therefore, if the scintigraphic GI bleeding study is negative, angiography is not indicated.

◆ Evaluation for GI bleeding by scintigraphy can be performed using sulfur colloid. The major disadvantage of this technique is rapid removal of the sulfur colloid by the liver, spleen, and bone marrow. Active bleeding must occur within minutes of radiotracer injection if the bleeding site is to be shown.

◆ Because GI bleeding is often intermittent, the labeled red blood cell technique is the preferred method for scintigraphic evaluation. Imaging is performed for a minimum of 2 hours, allowing a reasonable time for bleeding to occur.

◆ GI bleeding study findings are evaluated best by reviewing the images in a dynamic cine display (obtained at a rate of 1 frame per minute), which increases conspicuity of radiotracer movement compared to sequential static images by making subtle findings more apparent. Dynamic display should be a routine part of the imaging protocol.

◆ SUGGESTED READING

Alavi A, McLean G. Radioisotopic Detection and Localization of Gastrointestinal Bleeding: A Combined Endoscopic, Angiographic and Scintigraphic Approach. In LM Freeman, HS Weissmann (eds), Nuclear Medicine Annual 1980. New York: Raven, 1980.

Bunker SR, Lull RJ, Tanasescu DE, et al. Scintigraphy of gastrointestinal hemorrhage. Superiority of Tc-99m red blood cells over Tc-99m sulfur colloid. AJR Am J Roentgenol 1984:143: 543–548.

Winzelberg GG. The Versatility of Tc-99m Red Blood Cell Pool Imaging in Demonstrating Bleeding Sites. In LM Freeman, HS Weissmann (eds), Nuclear Medicine Annual 1985. New York: Raven, 1985.

CASE 12

R. Edward Coleman

HISTORY

A 43-year-old woman presents with a history of multiple hepatic masses.

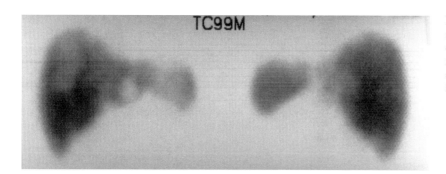

FIGURE 10-12A Anterior (**left**) and posterior (**right**) images of the liver and spleen obtained after the intravenous administration of 4 mCi of Tc-99m sulfur colloid. Multiple large focal areas of decreased activity are seen in the right and left lobes of the liver.

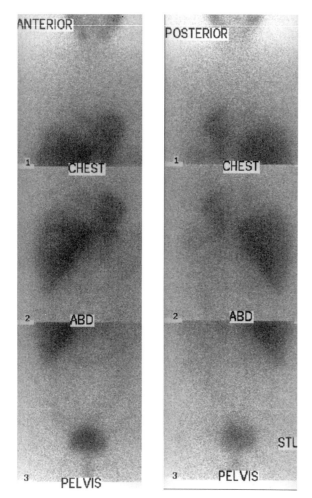

FIGURE 10-12B Anterior (**left**) and posterior (**right**) images obtained 24 hours after the intravenous administration of 2 mCi of I-131 meta-iodobenzylguanidine. Focal areas of decreased activity are present in the right and left lobes of the liver. Normal accumulation of radiotracer is noted in the left ventricular myocardium.

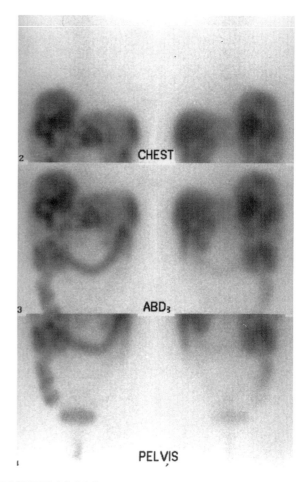

FIGURE 10-12C Anterior (**left**) and posterior (**right**) images obtained 24 hours after the intravenous administration of 6.2 mCi of In-111 octreotide. Multiple areas of increased accumulation of the radiotracer in the liver are seen with central areas of decreased activity compatible with necrosis. Normal excretion of radiotracer is seen in the bowel and bladder.

◆ DIFFERENTIAL DIAGNOSIS

◆ **Neuroendocrine tumor metastatic to the liver:** This is the likely diagnosis because of the increased accumulation of In-111 octreotide in the focal masses in the liver.

◆ **Metastatic colon cancer:** This diagnosis is unlikely because In-111 octreotide does not accumulate in metastatic colon cancer.

◆ **Pheochromocytoma:** This is an unlikely consideration because neither the meta-iodobenzylguanidine (MIBG) scan nor the In-111 octreotide scan showed abnormal accumulation in the region of the adrenal glands.

◆ **Neuroendocrine tumor metastatic to the left chest:** This diagnosis is unlikely because the accumulation in the left chest on the MIBG scan is a normal finding related to cardiac innervation.

◆ **Multicentric hepatoma:** This diagnosis is unlikely because hepatoma does not accumulate In-111 octreotide.

◆ DIAGNOSIS: Liver metastases from neuroendocrine tumor.

◆ KEY FACTS

CLINICAL

◆ Neuroendocrine tumors are derived from the amine precursor uptake and decarboxylation (APUD) system and contain secretory granules.

◆ Somatostatin, a peptide hormone consisting of 14 amino acids, has a short plasma half-life (2 to 4 minutes).

◆ Octreotide, a peptide that has eight amino acids, is an analog of somatostatin that is used therapeutically to block secretions from neuroendocrine tumors that contain somatostatin receptors.

◆ Somatostatin receptors have been demonstrated in a wide variety of tumors, including pituitary tumors, gastrinomas, insulinomas, glucagonomas, paragangliomas, medullary thyroid carcinomas, pheochromocytomas, carcinoid tumors, small cell lung cancer, neuroblastomas, meningiomas, breast cancers, lymphomas, granulomatous diseases, and the thyroid glands of patients with Graves' disease.

RADIOLOGIC

◆ Indium-111 octreotide localizes in most neuroendocrine tumors because they have somatostatin receptors.

◆ Indium-111 octreotide imaging can be used to select patients who are likely to respond to octreotide treatment.

◆ MIBG labeled with either I-131 or I-123 localizes in most neuroendocrine tumors because of the presence of a neuronal pump mechanism for norepinephrine.

◆ MIBG and In-111 octreotide demonstrate different metabolic functions, and the images in a patient may be abnormal with one radiotracer but not with the other.

◆ Iodine-131 MIBG has been used therapeutically in patients who have neuroendocrine tumors that accumulate radiotracer on diagnostic imaging.

◆ At present, there is no therapeutic analog of In-111 octreotide.

◆ SUGGESTED READING

Hanson MW, Feldman JM, Leight GS, Coleman RE. Iodine 131-labeled meta-iodobenzylguanidine scintigraphy and biochemical analyses of pheochromocytomas. Arch Intern Med 1991;151:1397–1402.

Kvols LK. Somatostatin-receptor imaging of human malignancies: A new era in the localization, staging, and treatment of tumors. Gastroenterology 1993;105:1909–1911.

Tenenbaum F, Lumbroso J, Schlumberger M, et al. Comparison of radiolabeled octreotide and meta-iodobenzylguanidine (MIBG) scintigraphy in malignant pheochromocytoma. J Nucl Med 1995;36:1–6.

HISTORY

A 28-year-old woman with a nontender, firm, palpable thyroid nodule.

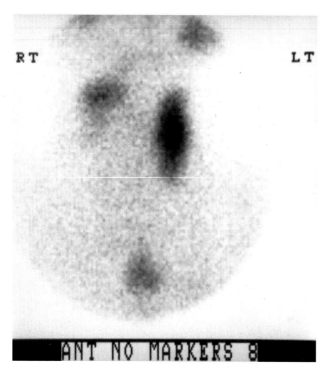

FIGURE 10-13A Anterior pinhole images of the thyroid obtained following the intravenous administration of 6 mCi of Tc-99m sodium pertechnetate. A solitary focal region of markedly decreased accumulation of radiopharmaceutical involving most of the right lobe of the thyroid is seen.

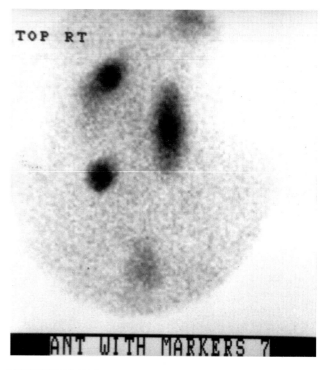

FIGURE 10-13B An image with markers on the superior and inferior margins of the palpable nodule. The focal region of decreased accumulation between the markers corresponds to the palpable nodule.

◆ DIFFERENTIAL DIAGNOSIS

◆ **Carcinoma:** Carcinoma constitutes 10% to 20% of solitary nonfunctioning nodules. The nodules are usually very firm or hard on palpation. This is the most likely diagnosis.

◆ **Functioning adenoma:** These lesions are usually firm but not hard in texture. This is an unlikely diagnosis because a functioning adenoma would be expected to accumulate Tc-99m sodium pertechnetate.

◆ **Colloid cyst:** This entity is usually soft on palpation and therefore unlikely to be the etiology in this case.

These lesions are usually well defined by sonography, but biopsy is definitive.

◆ **Chronic thyroiditis (Hashimoto's disease):** This is an unlikely diagnosis because chronic thyroiditis is usually multinodular on palpation and has a more inhomogeneous appearance on radionuclide imaging than the finding in the patient illustrated.

◆ **Hemorrhage:** Hemorrhage into an adenoma or cyst can present as a solitary nodule but is usually tender, making it an unlikely diagnosis in this patient.

◆**DIAGNOSIS: Thyroid carcinoma.**

◆**KEY FACTS**

CLINICAL

◆ Papillary carcinomas are the most common thyroid neoplasm in North America, are four times more frequent in women, and have peak incidence between ages 20 and 40 years. They metastasize primarily via the lymphatic system. Patients with papillary carcinomas have about a 90% 10-year survival rate.

◆ Follicular carcinomas comprise about 15% of thyroid carcinomas and usually occur after 40 years of age. They metastasize via hematogenous spread. Patients with follicular carcinomas have a 10-year survival rate of about 70%.

◆ Hürthle cell carcinomas are considered variants of follicular cell carcinoma, are relatively rare, and have a variable prognosis.

◆ Medullary carcinomas comprise 5% to 10% of thyroid carcinomas. About one-fifth of these patients inherit this disease as part of one of the following three syndromes: multiple endocrine neoplasia (MEN) groups 1 and 2 and a non-MEN syndrome. The familial non-MEN group has the best prognosis, followed by the familial MEN 2A, and then the nonfamilial (sporadic) form. Familial MEN 2B syndrome has the worst prognosis. Overall 10-year survival for all patients with medullary carcinoma of the thyroid is about 60%.

◆ Anaplastic carcinomas comprise about 10% of thyroid carcinomas, usually occur late in life (after the sixth decade), and have a 5-year survival for all patients with medullary carcinoma of the thyroid rate of <5%.

◆ The risk of metastasis increases with age at time of diagnosis, particularly for follicular thyroid carcinoma. In addition, recurrence and mortality rates are significantly higher after 45 years of age.

◆ External beam radiation therapy to the neck region before late adolescence increases the risk of developing either or both benign and malignant thyroid nodules.

◆ Based on autopsy series, incidental small foci of occult malignant thyroid cells are found in about 10% of patients with no prior clinical evidence of thyroid malignancy.

◆ Between 10% and 20% of solitary nonfunctioning nodules seen on radioiodine thyroid imaging studies in adults are malignant.

◆ Only 5% of thyroid nodules are hyperfunctioning and cause suppression of normal thyroid tissue. These nodules may result in toxic nodular goiter. A very small percentage (2% to 4%) of hyperfunctioning thyroid nodules have been reported to have regions of malignant neoplasia. Clinicians who treat toxic nodular goiter with radioiodine usually presume the hyperfunctioning nodule to be of benign histology.

◆ With the advent of fine-needle aspiration biopsy, large-needle aspiration biopsy, and large-needle cutting ("core") biopsy as definitive means of evaluating thyroid nodules, radionuclide imaging studies for this purpose are performed infrequently. Nonetheless, these studies can be useful in defining an autonomous functioning or hyperfunctioning thyroid nodule, which usually precludes the need for biopsy.

◆ A solitary thyroid nodule in a prepubescent child has a higher likelihood of being malignant than that in an adult.

◆ Initial reports suggested that the presence of a diffuse toxic goiter offered protection from developing a thyroid malignancy. However, it has subsequently been shown that the likelihood of a solitary nonfunctioning thyroid nodule being malignant does not differ in patients with diffuse toxic goiter and patients who are euthyroid.

RADIOLOGIC

◆ The radiopharmaceutical tracer of choice for thyroid imaging is I-123 sodium iodide. Tc-99m sodium pertechnetate, which is less expensive and readily available, is an acceptable alternative. I-131 sodium iodide can be used when I-123 sodium iodide is not available or in patients who are suspected of having a substernal thyroid.

◆ Thyroid gland palpation at the time of imaging is mandatory and allows the examiner to outline the thyroid nodule or superimpose a radionuclide point source marker in the region of the nodule.

◆ The hypertrapping nodule on Tc-99m sodium pertechnetate images is usually hyperfunctioning on radioiodine images. However, there is an approximately 10% frequency of hypertrapping nodules on a Tc-99m sodium pertechnetate study that are hypo- to nonfunctioning on radioiodine thyroid images (so-called discordant nodules). Even less frequent are instances in which a nontrapping thyroid nodule on a Tc-99m sodium pertechnetate study is seen to be a functioning nodule on radioiodine imaging.

◆ An acronym for the differential diagnosis of solitary nonfunctioning thyroid nodules is CATCH PALLM: Carcinoma, Adenoma, Thyroiditis, Colloid cyst, Hemorrhage, Parathyroid adenoma, Abscess, Lymph node, Lymphoma, and Metastasis.

◆**SUGGESTED READING**

Ashcraft MW, Van Herle AJ. Management of thyroid nodules. Parts I and II. Head Neck Surg 1981;3:216–230, 297–322.

Livadas D, Psarras A, Koutras DA. Malignant cold nodules in hyperthyroidism. Br J Surg 1976;63:726–728.

Ridgeway EC. Clinical Evaluation of Solitary Thyroid Nodules. In LE Braverman, RD Utiger (eds), Werner and Ingbar's The Thyroid (6th ed). Philadelphia: Lippincott, 1991;1197–1203.

HISTORY

A 26-year-old woman has partial complex seizures that are refractory to anticonvulsants. The seizures are preceded by an aura of a feeling of fear, followed by staring and oral automatic movements. An interictal F-18 FDG positron emission tomography (PET) brain scan is performed for seizure focus localization before temporal lobectomy.

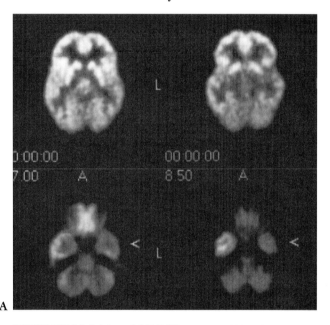

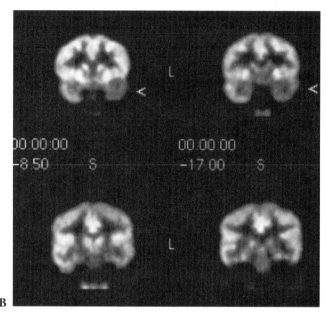

FIGURES 10-14A and 10-14B Transverse (**A**) and coronal (**B**) F-18 fluorodeoxyglucose positron emission tomography images through the temporal lobes. Marked F-18 fluorodeoxyglucose hypometabolism is seen in the left temporal lobe (arrows).

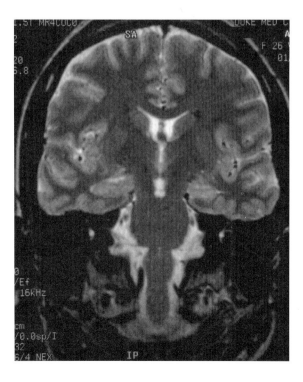

FIGURE 10-14C Coronal T2-weighted MRI through the temporal lobes. The left hippocampus is decreased in size and has slightly increased signal.

◆ DIFFERENTIAL DIAGNOSIS

◆ **Low-grade tumor:** A low-grade tumor with associated edema can have diminished F-18 FDG uptake. The loss of hippocampal volume, rather than a mass lesion, on the MR image makes this diagnosis unlikely.

◆ **Radiation necrosis:** Tissue necrosis following radiation therapy can have diminished F-18 FDG uptake, but the absence of a brain tumor or prior radiation therapy excludes this diagnosis.

◆ **Ictal seizure focus:** After F-18 FDG injection at the time of a seizure, increased radiotracer uptake would be expected rather than the decreased uptake seen in the case presented, making this diagnosis incorrect.

◆ **Interictal seizure focus:** When F-18 FDG is injected at a point when the patient is between seizures (i.e., interictally), the uptake of radiotracer in the dormant seizure focus is diminished. This choice, therefore, is the most likely diagnosis.

◆ **Infarction:** Infarcted brain tissue can have diminished F-18 FDG uptake. The clinical history and the fact that the abnormality is confined to the hippocampus on the MR image make this diagnosis unlikely.

◆ DIAGNOSIS: Interictal seizure focus.

◆ KEY FACTS

CLINICAL

◆ Complex partial seizures (psychomotor or temporal lobe seizures) are frequently preceded by an aura manifested by hallucinations, illusions, affective changes, or aberrations of cognition, and often are accompanied by complex movements. These auras are characteristic of a seizure focus in certain regions of the temporal lobe or limbic system.

◆ Most complex partial seizures are due to epileptiform activity in the temporal lobes (especially the hippocampus or amygdala), but they can also originate from mesial parasagittal or orbital frontal regions.

◆ The surface electroencephalogram (EEG) can be normal in patients with complex partial seizures. Depth electrode placement may be required to define the seizure focus by EEG criteria more accurately.

◆ Complex partial seizures can progress to generalized major motor (grand mal) seizures, manifested by loss of consciousness and tonic/clonic movements.

RADIOLOGIC

◆ F-18 FDG is a positron-emitting radiopharmaceutical with a half-life of 110 minutes that functions as an analog of glucose. It accumulates in viable cells in proportion to the individual cellular consumption of glucose.

◆ F-18 FDG imaging of the central nervous system is optimally performed at approximately 30 minutes following the injection of radiotracer. During the 30-minute delay, the patient should be unstimulated—i.e., kept in a quiet, dimly lit environment with only background noise.

◆ In the evaluation of patients for a seizure focus, an EEG should be acquired during the 30-minute uptake phase of F-18 FDG to document the presence or absence of seizure activity that may not be apparent clinically during this interval.

◆ Metabolic imaging with F-18 FDG of patients with seizures can show functional abnormalities even when MRI studies and histologic specimens obtained from the temporal lobe fail to show an abnormality.

◆ F-18 FDG imaging is more useful for localization of a seizure focus in patients with suspected temporal lobe seizures than in those with a suspected extratemporal lobe origin of seizure activity.

◆ Single-photon emission computed tomography (SPECT) brain perfusion imaging performed in the ictal and interictal states has an accuracy similar to F-18 FDG PET in localizing the seizure focus.

◆ High-resolution MRI of the hippocampus also has an accuracy similar to F-18 FDG PET in localization of the seizure site.

◆ SUGGESTED READING

Engel J Jr, Henry TR, Risinger MW, et al. Presurgical evaluation for partial epilepsy: Relative contributions of chronic depth-electrode recordings versus FDG-PET and scalp-sphenoidal ictal EEG. Neurology 1990;40:1670–1677.

Radtke RA, Hanson MW, Hoffman JM, et al. Temporal lobe hypometabolism on PET: Predictor of seizure control after temporal lobectomy. Neurology 1993;43:1088–1092.

Radtke RA, Hanson MW, Hoffman JM, et al. Positron emission tomography: Comparison of clinical utility in temporal lobe and extra-temporal epilepsy. J Epilepsy 1994;7:27–33.

CASE 15

R. Edward Coleman

HISTORY

A 54-year-old man referred for evaluation of dyspnea on exertion. Exercise (Figure 10-15A) and redistribution (Figure 10-15B) Tl-201 images are obtained.

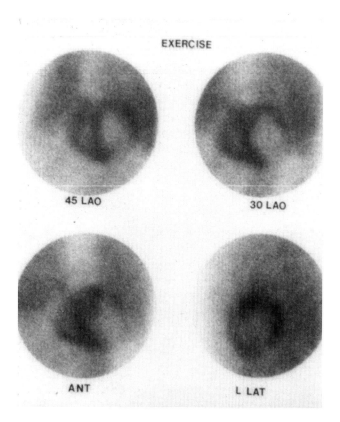

FIGURE 10-15A Tl-201 images obtained immediately after exercise. A large perfusion defect involving the anterior, posterolateral, apical, and inferior myocardium is seen. Increased accumulation of tracer is present in the right ventricular myocardium. The left ventricular cavity is dilated. Abnormal accumulation of tracer in the lungs is also seen.

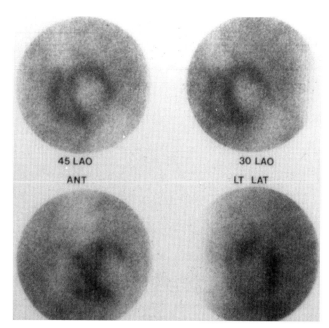

FIGURE 10-15B Tl-201 images obtained 4 hours after radio-tracer administration. No significant change is seen in distribution of Tl-201 in myocardium or in the defect. Increased accumulation in the right ventricular myocardium is again seen. The left ventricular cavity is again noted to be dilated. The abnormal accumulation of tracer in the lungs has diminished markedly.

◆ DIFFERENTIAL DIAGNOSIS

- **Myocardial ischemia:** The lack of normalization of the perfusion defects makes this diagnosis unlikely.
- **Myocardial infarction:** The perfusion abnormalities at exercise without normalization on redistribution makes this diagnosis the most likely.
- **Nonischemic cardiomyopathy:** The presence of large perfusion defects makes this diagnosis unlikely.
- **Valvular heart disease:** The presence of large perfusion defects makes this diagnosis unlikely.
- **Normal study with attenuation of inferolateral myocardium:** The extent of the perfusion abnormality, the dilated ventricle, and accumulation of radiotracer in the lungs on the images obtained after exercise make this diagnosis unlikely.

◆ DIAGNOSIS: Myocardial infarction.

◆ KEY FACTS

CLINICAL

- Approximately 5 million adults in the United States have symptomatic coronary artery disease. One and one-half million people have an acute myocardial infarction each year. Coronary artery disease accounts for 25% of deaths from all causes.
- Myocardial ischemia occurs when coronary artery blood flow is inadequate to meet the metabolic requirements of the myocardium. Myocardial infarction occurs when the myocardial blood flow to a segment of the myocardium is <0.1 ml/min/g of tissue (normal flow is 0.5 to 1.0 ml/min/g of tissue).
- The normal end diastolic volume of the left ventricle is approximately 150 ml. When the ejection fraction decreases from a normal value of >50% to <50% (such

as can occur with myocardial infarction), the ventricle dilates to maintain an adequate stroke volume and cardiac output.

- With exercise, transient ischemia that causes ventricular failure can result in an increase in ventricular cavity size and an increased left ventricular end diastolic pressure. The transient increase in left ventricular end diastolic pressure results in a transient pulmonary edema, and thereby increased pulmonary radiotracer accumulation.

RADIOLOGIC

- The Tl-201 images in the case presented above show a large fixed defect in myocardial perfusion, abnormal Tl-201 accumulation in the lungs on the postexercise images, and prominent right ventricular Tl-201 accumulation on both sets of images. These findings are typical of myocardial infarction with exercise-induced left ventricular failure causing transient Tl-201 lung accumulation. Lung accumulation on a Tl-201 study is definitely abnormal if the lungs are clearly outlined on the images. Regions of interest can be obtained in the left lung adjacent to the anterior wall and in the myocardium. A ratio of lung counts to myocardial counts >0.5 is indicative of abnormal lung accumulation and left ventricular dysfunction.
- The prominent right ventricular accumulation in the case shown above is diagnostic of right ventricular hypertrophy.

◆ SUGGESTED READING

Bonow RO, Dilsizian V. Thallium-201 for assessment of myocardial viability. Semin Nucl Med 1991; 21:230–241.

Palmer EL, Scott JA, Strauss HW. Practical Nuclear Medicine. Philadelphia: Saunders, 1992;71–120.

Verani MS. Tl-201 myocardial perfusion imaging. Curr Opin Radiol 1991;3:797–809.

HISTORY

A 59-year-old man with diabetes, hypertension, and hyperlipidemia presents with dyspnea on exertion and peripheral edema. The patient has no history of prior myocardial infarction. Cardiac catheterization (not shown) reveals normal coronary arteries but diminished left ventrivular ejection fraction (LVEF). He is referred for a multiple gated acquisition (MUGA) study.

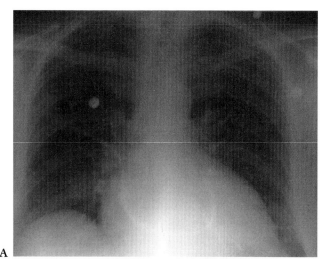

A

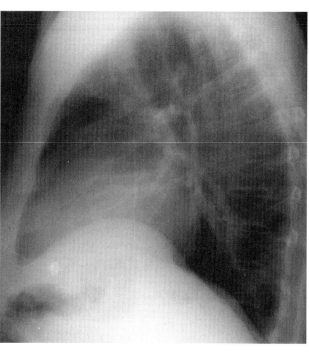

B

FIGURES 10-16A and 10-16B Posteroanterior (**A**) and lateral (**B**) chest radiographs. Marked cardiomegaly is present without findings of pulmonary edema.

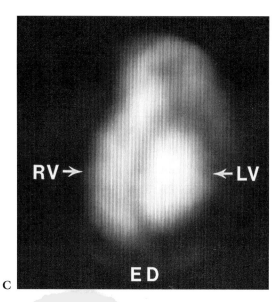

C

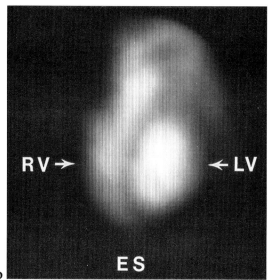

D

FIG   0-16D Forty-five degree left anterior oblique MUGA at end diastole (**C**) and end systole (**D**). Markedly dilated
          d volumes in diastole and systole. Global hypokinesis of the left ventricle is seen. The left ventricular ejection frac-
            and that of the right ventricle (RVEF) at 20%.

◆ DIFFERENTIAL DIAGNOSIS

◆ **Left ventricular aneurysm:** The ventricular abnormalities in the case illustrated are diffuse, rather than focal, as would be expected with an aneurysm.

◆ **Restrictive cardiomyopathy:** Typical findings of restrictive cardiomyopathy are mild cardiac enlargement and a left ventricle that has preserved systolic function but is resistant to diastolic filling. In the case illustrated, however, a dilated left ventricle with poor systolic function is seen, making this an incorrect diagnosis.

◆ **Myocardial infarction:** A focal abnormality, typically involving the left ventricle, would be expected with infarction, rather than the diffuse dysfunction involving both ventricles in the case illustrated.

◆ **Dilated (congestive) cardiomyopathy:** Dilated cardiomyopathy produces varying degrees of cardiac enlargement (as seen in Figures 10-16A and 10-16B), left ventricular dilatation, increased left ventricular volume, global patterns of abnormal contractility, and a diminished LVEF (as seen in Figures 10-16C and 10-16D). This diagnosis the most likely one for the case illustrated.

◆ **Hypertrophic cardiomyopathy:** Hypertrophic cardiomyopathy can produce mild to moderate cardiac enlargement, but it is usually associated with vigorous left ventricular contractility and septal thickness that is increased out of proportion to the thickness of the left ventricular free wall. The absence of these findings in the case shown above makes this diagnosis unlikely.

◆ DIAGNOSIS: Dilated (congestive) cardiomyopathy.

◆ KEY FACTS

CLINICAL

◆ Dilated cardiomyopathy is most commonly seen in middle-aged men but can occur at any age.

◆ Infectious, metabolic, and toxic causes are the most common etiologies of dilated cardiomyopathy. Known specific causes include alcohol, Adriamycin, cyclophosphamide, neuromuscular disease (muscular dystrophies), and pregnancy. However, a definite etiology cannot be discerned in many cases.

◆ Histologic examination of the myocardium in dilated cardiomyopathy reveals extensive regions of perivascular and interstitial fibrosis accompanied by mild necrosis and cellular infiltration.

◆ Patients with dilated cardiomyopathy present with symptoms of left- or right-sided congestive heart failure—e.g., fatigue, peripheral edema, dyspnea on exertion, orthopnea, paroxysmal nocturnal dyspnea, and palpations. Vague chest discomfort can occur, but typical angina pectoris is uncommon and, when present, implies the presence of concomitant coronary artery disease.

◆ Most patients with dilated cardiomyopathy have progressive clinical deterioration. The disease is often fatal within 2 years of symptom onset, especially for older (>55 years old) patients. Progressive congestive heart failure and ventricular arrhythmias are the most common causes of death.

RADIOLOGIC

◆ The gated blood pool study is widely accepted as an accurate imaging technique for evaluation of left ventricular function and is often used for assessment of congestive heart failure, effects of cardiotoxic drugs, left ventricular function following cardiac surgery, and effects of exercise on left ventricular function in patients with suspected coronary artery disease.

◆ A gated blood pool study can be performed using either Tc-99m sodium pertechnetate-labeled autologous red blood cells (the preferred technique) or Tc-99m–labeled human serum albumin.

◆ The best septal view is one that allows separation of the ventricles, facilitating determination of both the LVEF and the right ventricular ejection fraction (RVEF). This view is typically a 45-degree left anterior oblique projection (Figures 10-16C and 10-16D above).

◆ Correct determination of background activity (usually 30% to 60% of left ventricular end diastolic counts) is critical in calculating an accurate LVEF. Overestimation of background activity falsely elevates the LVEF, while underestimation of background activity falsely decreases the LVEF.

◆ Calculation of the RVEF on a gated blood pool study is less accurate than LVEF calculation. This fact is primarily due to the contribution of activity from the right atrium into the right ventricular region of interest and the uncertainty of the location of the pulmonic valve. Because of the larger volume of the right ventricle, the accepted normal RVEF is generally 5% to 10% less than the normal LVEF.

◆ SUGGESTED READING

Borges-Neto S, Coleman RE. Radionuclide ventricular function analysis. Radiol Clin North Am 1993;31:817–830.

Friesinger GC. Accuracy of radionuclide ventriculography for estimation of left ventricular volume changes and end-systolic pressure-volume relationships. J Am Coll Cardiol 1985;6:1064–1072.

Kronenberg MW, Parrish MD, Jenkins DW, et al. Cardiac blood pool imaging. II: Applications in noncoronary heart disease. J Nucl Med 1990;31:10–22.

CASE 17

Robert R. Reiman, Jr., and
R. Edward Coleman

HISTORY

A 27-year-old woman being treated for gestational trophoblastic disease with a 36-hour history of severe, intermittent, left pleuritic chest pain.

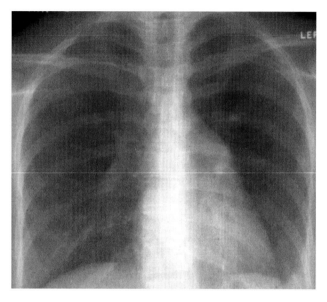

FIGURE 10-17A Posteroanterior chest radiograph shows no parenchymal abnormalities, normal pulmonary arteries, and a small, left pleural effusion.

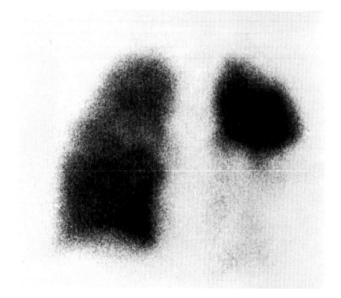

FIGURE 10-17B Tc-99m macroaggregated albumin perfusion study performed in the anterior projection shows multiple segmental defects involving both lungs, with the largest involving most of the lower left lung zone. A Xe-133 ventilation study (not shown) was normal.

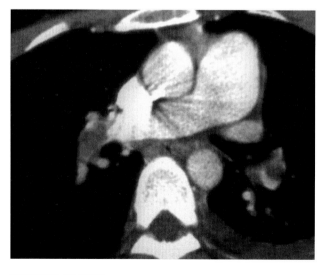

FIGURE 10-17C Contrast-enhanced helical CT scan of the chest shows filling defects in the left lower lobe and right interlobar pulmonary arteries.

◆ DIFFERENTIAL DIAGNOSIS

◆ **Pulmonary artery obstruction by extrinsic mass:** A focal area of ventilation-perfusion ($\dot{V}/\dot{Q}$) mismatch can result from compression by a hilar or mediastinal mass. The presence of multiple bilateral mismatched $\dot{V}/\dot{Q}$ abnormalities makes this diagnosis unlikely. Furthermore, no extrinsic mass is seen compressing the pulmonary arteries on the CT scan.

◆ **Radiation therapy port:** The presence of multiple perfusion defects that correspond to vascular segments makes this diagnosis incorrect.

◆ **Vasculitis:** The multiple segmental $\dot{V}/\dot{Q}$ mismatches and the presence of emboli on the CT scan make this diagnosis unlikely.

◆ **Pulmonary embolism (PE):** The multiple segmental perfusion defects in areas that are normal on the ventilation study and the chest radiograph make this diagnosis the most likely. The diagnosis is confirmed by the presence of thromboemboli that are seen on the contrast-enhanced CT scan.

◆ **Multiple peripheral pulmonary arterial stenoses:** The presence of emboli on the CT scan makes this an incorrect diagnosis.

◆ DIAGNOSIS: Pulmonary embolism.

◆ KEY FACTS

CLINICAL

◆ Risk factors for PE include advanced age, immobilization, history of previous PE, concurrent malignancy (usually adenocarcinoma), and hereditary causes of a hypercoagulable state—e.g., factor S deficiency.

◆ The presence of abnormal blood gas findings, the typical history of pleuritic chest pain, shortness of breath, and characteristic electrocardiogram changes can be helpful in raising a strong suspicion of the diagnosis. However, because some of these features are often not present, imaging studies, in particular $\dot{V}/\dot{Q}$ scans and pulmonary angiography, are important in helping to establish the diagnosis firmly.

RADIOLOGIC

◆ The chest radiograph is frequently normal in patients with PE. Atelectasis, a small pleural effusion, and elevated hemidiaphragm are nonspecific radiographic findings that are seen in many patients with PE.

◆ The high probability pattern—i.e., two or more perfusion abnormalities without matching ventilatory abnormalities—is most often caused by PE. Some entities—e.g., vasculitis—can produce a pattern of $\dot{V}/\dot{Q}$ mismatch simulating the high probability pattern, but these entities often result in a more heterogeneous pattern than seen in the case illustrated above.

◆ The low-probability pattern includes: (1) defects surrounded by normal lung (stripe sign), (2) corresponding defects and large pleural effusion, (3) nonsegmental perfusion defects, (4) corresponding defects and opacity in the upper or middle lung zones, (5) a perfusion defect with a substantially larger radiographic abnormality, (6) matched ventilation and perfusion abnormalities with a normal radiograph, and (7) more than three small perfusion defects.

◆ The intermediate probability pattern includes (1) one moderate to two large perfusion defects without corresponding ventilation of radiographic abnormalities, (2) corresponding ventilation, perfusion, and parenchymal abnormalities in the lower lung zones, and (3) corresponding defects and small pleural effusion.

◆ The very low probability category consists of three or fewer small defects. The normal category consists of no perfusion abnormalities.

◆ The gold standard examination for the diagnosis of PE is pulmonary angiography. However, MRI and helical CT can identify patients who have proximal thromboemboli and also serve to exclude pulmonary artery compression as a cause of $\dot{V}/\dot{Q}$ mismatch.

◆ SUGGESTED READING

Gottschalk A, Sostman HD, Coleman RE, et al. Ventilation-perfusion scintigraphy in the PIOPED study. Part II. Evaluation of the scintigraphic criteria and interpretations. J Nucl Med 1993;34: 1119–1126.

Grist TM, Sostman HD, MacFall JR, et al. Pulmonary angiography using MRI: Initial clinical experience. Radiology 1993;189: 528–530.

Worsley DF, Alavi A. Comprehensive analysis of the results of the PIOPED study. J Nucl Med 1995;36:2380–2387.

HISTORY

A 67-year-old man with pain and swelling in both knees 3 years after left upper lobe resection and radiation therapy for adenocarcinoma of the lung.

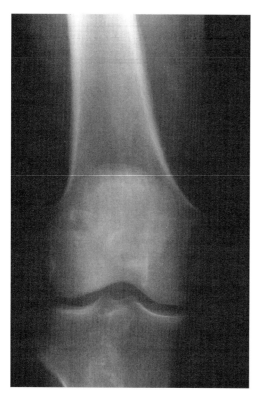

FIGURE 10-18A Frontal radiograph of the right knee. A thin layer of smooth periosteal new bone formation is seen along the distal femur, involving both the metaphysis and distal diaphysis.

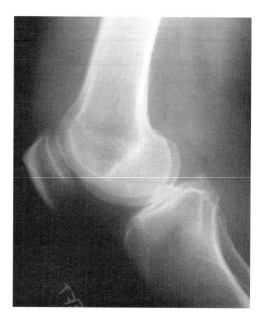

FIGURE 10-18B Lateral radiograph of the left knee. The periosteal reaction is seen best along the anterior femoral cortex. There is mild soft-tissue fullness in the suprapatellar area, consistent with a joint effusion.

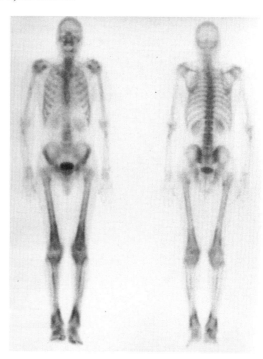

FIGURE 10-18C Whole body bone scintigraphy, anterior (**left**) and posterior (**right**) views. Symmetrically increased radiotracer uptake is seen in a cortical distribution ("tram track" pattern) within the long bones of both lower extremities. The uptake is most increased in the metaphyseal regions at the knees and ankles but also involves the diaphyses.

◆ DIFFERENTIAL DIAGNOSIS

◆ **Primary hypertrophic osteoarthropathy (pachyder-moperiostosis):** This is a rare, familial, autosomal dominant disorder that occurs predominantly in men. However, the periostitis appears shaggy, irregular, and commonly involves epiphyses, unlike the findings in this case, making this an unlikely diagnosis.

◆ **Vascular insufficiency:** The distribution of periostitis in vascular insufficiency is similar to that seen in the case under discussion, but the appearance is typically more thick and undulating.

◆ **Thyroid acropachy:** The typical periostitis of thyroid acropachy appears solid and spiculated, not smooth (as in the case illustrated), and primarily involves the diaphyses of metacarpals and phalanges (and not the long bones, as in Figure 10-18A).

◆ **Fluorosis:** Solid, undulating periosteal thickening (periostitis deformans) in the appendicular skeleton, somewhat similar to that in the present case, can occur in fluorosis. However, osteosclerosis of the axial skeleton, the most striking feature in fluorosis, is absent in the case illustrated.

◆ **Secondary hypertrophic osteoarthropathy (HOA):** HOA is the best diagnosis because of the metaphyseal and diaphyseal involvement, soft-tissue swelling, joint pain, and history of lung cancer.

◆ DIAGNOSIS: Hypertrophic osteoarthropathy (secondary to a previously undiagnosed recurrence of lung adenocarcinoma).

◆ KEY FACTS

CLINICAL

◆ HOA can be secondary to a wide variety of conditions, including pulmonary (bronchogenic carcinoma, lymphoma, abscess, bronchiectasis, cystic fibrosis, metastasis, emphysema), pleural (mesothelioma, fibroma), cardiovascular (cyanotic congenital heart disease, infected vascular grafts), and gastrointestinal (inflammatory disorders, portal or biliary cirrhosis, biliary atresia, polyposis, neoplasms) etiologies.

◆ The pathogenesis is unknown, but neurogenic mechanisms, increased blood flow, and chemical mediators have been implicated.

◆ Articular findings occur in about 40% of patients with HOA. Joint pain and swelling can be the presenting complaint. Joint effusions are common.

◆ Digital clubbing is a frequent, but nonspecific, finding.

◆ Treatment of the underlying lesion (e.g., thoracotomy, chemotherapy, or radiotherapy for lung carcinoma) is often followed by rapid clinical improvement of symptoms related to HOA.

◆ There is anecdotal evidence that regrowth of a previously treated neoplasm causing HOA is associated with worsening HOA. In the case illustrated, appearance of HOA was the first indication of a recurrence of lung carcinoma.

RADIOLOGIC

◆ Bone scintigraphy is a highly sensitive method for detecting HOA. The scintigraphic findings appear before radiographic abnormalities, correspond to clinical signs and symptoms, and regress with therapy.

◆ The "tram track" or "parallel stripe" sign is due to diffuse cortical radiotracer uptake in the metaphyses and diaphyses of tubular bones that results from periosteal new bone formation.

◆ HOA findings are typically bilateral and symmetric and primarily involve the appendicular skeleton. Less common sites include the clavicles, scapulae, pelvis, digits, and facial bones.

◆ Increased periarticular radiotracer uptake in HOA often indicates associated synovitis.

◆ Plain film appearance of periostitis in HOA is variable. Findings include (1) simple periosteal elevation; (2) smooth laminated ("onion-skin") periostitis; (3) irregular, wavy, or solid periostitis; and (4) cortical thickening.

◆ The periostitis of HOA begins in the diaphyses, then later involves the metaphyses and sometimes tendinous insertions.

◆ Digital clubbing can manifest as soft-tissue swelling, with or without focal tuftal resorption or hypertrophy.

◆ The soft-tissue swelling, periarticular osteoporosis, and joint effusions of HOA can mimic rheumatoid arthritis. However, the joint space narrowing and erosions seen in rheumatoid arthritis are not present in HOA.

◆ SUGGESTED READING

Pineda CJ, Sartoris DJ, Clopton P, Resnick D. Periostitis in hypertrophic osteoarthropathy: Relationship to disease duration. AJR Am J Roentgenol 1987;148:773–778.

Resnick D. Bone and Joint Imaging. Philadelphia: Saunders, 1989;1237–1246.

HISTORY

A 31-year-old man with left side neck swelling found to have enlarged lymph nodes on physical examination.

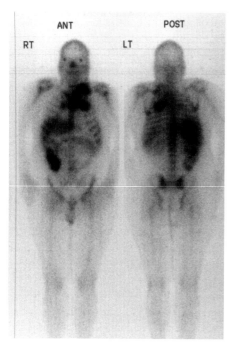 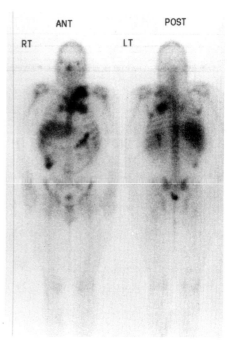

FIGURES 10-19A and 10-19B Anterior (**left**) and posterior (**right**) whole body images obtained 48 hours (**A**) and 96 hours (**B**) after the administration of 10 mCi of Ga-67 citrate. Abnormal Ga-67 accumulations are noted in the hilar regions bilaterally and in the mediastinum and left supraclavicular region. Marked radiotracer activity is also seen in the right abdomen on (**A**), which decreases on (**B**), suggesting that the radiotracer accumulation is in the bowel.

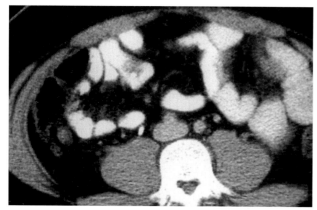

FIGURE 10-19C Noncontrast abdominal CT at the level of the Ga-67 accumulation in the right abdomen. No abdominal lymphadenopathy or visceral abnormality is seen, further evidence that the abdominal radiotracer seen in 10-19A is in bowel.

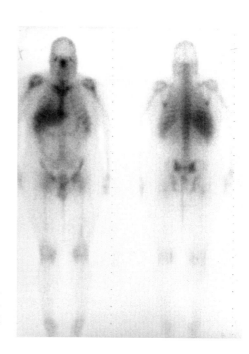

FIGURE 10-19D▶ Repeat study performed 6 months after starting chemotherapy. Anterior (**left**) and posterior (**right**) whole body images obtained 72 hours after Ga-67 citrate administration. Marked improvement has occurred, with no abnormal accumulation noted.

◆ DIFFERENTIAL DIAGNOSIS

- **Sarcoidosis:** This diagnosis is unlikely because of the absence of salivary and lacrimal gland radiotracer accumulation.
- **Hodgkin's lymphoma:** This diagnosis is the best consideration because the abnormal radiotracer accumulation is limited to the thorax, particularly the hilum and supraclavicular regions.
- **Non-Hodgkin's lymphoma:** This diagnosis is unlikely because the abnormal radiotracer accumulation is limited to the chest and supraclavicular region.
- **Opportunistic infection:** This diagnosis is unlikely because abnormal radiotracer activity diffused throughout the lung parenchyma (as is typically seen in infection with *Pneumocystis carinii* pneumonia) would be expected.
- **Abdominal abscess:** An abdominal process, such as an abscess, is unlikely because, as noted above, the radiotracer activity in the right abdomen has changed (decreased) in the 96-hour study, indicating that it is due to normal colonic activity.

◆ DIAGNOSIS: Hodgkin's lymphoma.

◆ KEY FACTS

CLINICAL

- Hodgkin's lymphoma has a bimodal age distribution, with one peak around age 20 years and a second peak at age >50 years.
- The most common mode of presentation is a painless mass in the neck. Constitutional symptoms include fever, weight loss, night sweats, and generalized pruritus.
- Pain in an involved lymph node following alcohol ingestion is an uncommon symptom that is nonetheless rather characteristic.
- An important clinical feature is the tendency of Hodgkin's lymphoma to arise within one lymph node area and spread to contiguous lymph nodes. However, late in the course of the disease, vascular invasion can lead to hematogenous dissemination.

- Hodgkin's disease should be distinguished pathologically from other malignant lymphomas.
- Patients with stages I-A and II-A disease have 10-year survival rates >80%.
- Patients with disseminated disease (III-B, IV) have a 5-year survival rate of 50% to 60%.
- Patients who relapse after chemotherapy may be cured with autologous bone marrow transplantation.

RADIOLOGIC

- Ga-67 imaging is an effective means of detecting nodal and visceral involvement in Hodgkin's and non-Hodgkin's lymphoma. Sensitivity and specificity of gallium imaging in Hodgkin's lymphoma is on the order of 90%. The sensitivity of gallium imaging is improved by the use of SPECT imaging.
- Abdominal lesions <2 cm in diameter are difficult to detect with gallium imaging. Lesions in the liver or spleen are also difficult to identify because they can be obscured against the background of normal radiotracer accumulation in these organs.
- The utility of the gallium study is enhanced when used in a serial fashion to monitor the course of the disease and results of therapy. Recurrence of tumor is frequently associated with return of gallium uptake. Loss of gallium uptake following treatment (particularly radiation therapy) is associated with tumor ablation. Irradiation of tumor may lead to transient or permanent nonuptake of gallium by the tumor.
- CT is more sensitive than gallium scans for detection of subtle mediastinal involvement, but it is less accurate after therapy. The gallium scan is particularly useful to distinguish residual tumor from post-treatment fibrosis.

◆ SUGGESTED READING

Front D, Ben Haim S, Israel O, et al. Lymphoma: Predictive value of Ga-67 scintigraphy after treatment. Radiology 1992;182: 359–363.

Kaplan WD. Residual mass and negative gallium scintigraphy in treated lymphoma: When is the gallium scan really negative? J Nucl Med 1990;31:369–371.

Scott AM, Larson SM. Tumor imaging and therapy. Radiol Clin North Am 1993;31:859–879.

CASE *20* *Robert H. Wilkinson, Jr.*

HISTORY

A 56-year-old woman with a history of left hand laceration and tendon repair to the left fourth and fifth digits. Several months later she developed pain and a burning sensation in her left hand and fingers.

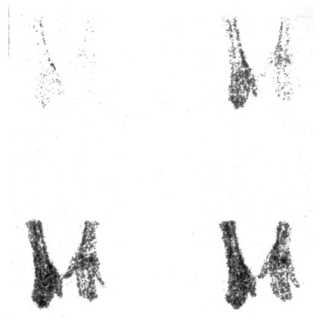

FIGURE 10-20A Dynamic perfusion images of the wrists and hands. The patient's left hand is to the reader's left. Earlier and greater perfusion to the left wrist and hand is seen compared to the right wrist and hand.

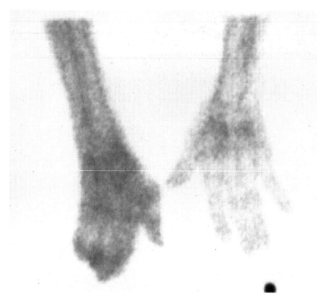

FIGURE 10-20B Immediate blood pool image of wrists and hands. A marker source is distal to the fingers of the right hand. Generalized greater radiotracer accumulation in the left wrist and hand is seen compared to the right wrist and hand.

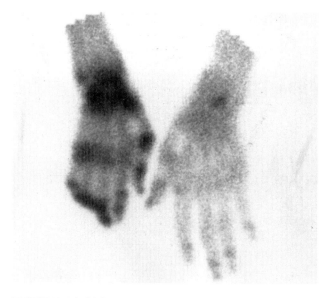

FIGURE 10-20C Delayed image of wrists and hands. Diffusely increased radiotracer accumulation is seen in the left wrist and hand in a periarticular distribution.

◆ DIFFERENTIAL DIAGNOSIS

- **Reflex sympathetic dystrophy syndrome (RSDS):** This diagnosis is the most likely because of the clinical history of trauma, physical findings of pain and dysesthesias, and the abnormal three-phase bone scan.
- **Acute arthritis:** This entity can produce the three-phase bone scan findings seen in the case illustrated, but the periarticular radiotracer uptake pattern is usually less uniform.
- **Extremity immobilization:** This entity can produce the bone scan findings shown above but is not associated with the dysesthesias present in this patient.
- **Fracture:** A recent fracture of the wrist or hand can produce increased radiotracer activity on all three phases of the bone scan, but a focal abnormality, rather than the diffuse pattern seen in the case illustrated, should be present at the site of the fracture.
- **Osteomyelitis:** The same argument against a diagnosis of fracture applies to osteomyelitis—although all three phases of the bone scan can be abnormal, a focal lesion, rather than a diffuse pattern, should be seen.

◆ DIAGNOSIS: Reflex sympathetic dystrophy.

◆ KEY FACTS

CLINICAL

- The RSDS complex consists of upper or lower extremity swelling, hyperesthesia, burning dysesthesias, hyperhidrosis, and trophic changes to the skin and bone. It occurs in both children and in adults.
- The RSDS complex refers to a spectrum of clinical abnormalities, which includes variations such as causalgia (with or without evidence of peripheral nerve injury), shoulder-hand syndrome, and Sudek's atrophy of bone. Not all of the clinical manifestations of RSDS are readily encompassed by one unifying pathophysiologic concept.
- RSDS may be classified clinically as acute, dystrophic, or atrophic.
- The diagnosis of RSDS is based primarily on clinical criteria. Differential neural blockade is probably the most reliable diagnostic test. Supportive evidence can also come from findings on radiographs and radionuclide bone imaging.

- Clinically defined nerve damage and minor soft-tissue trauma can both result in RSDS (minor causalgia).
- Therapy is based on reducing or eliminating the clinical manifestations of sympathetic hyperactivity. Varying degrees of success have been achieved using different techniques, including surgery.

RADIOLOGIC

- Typical findings on the three-phase bone imaging study include (1) generalized increased radiotracer perfusion on the first phase, (2) diffusely increased radiotracer with some periarticular radiotracer accumulation on the second phase, and (3) marked periarticular radiotracer uptake in the affected extremity distally (foot or hand).
- The three-phase bone scan is reported to have a sensitivity of 60% to 96% and specificity of 92% to 97%.
- Occasionally, a pattern of decreased radiotracer accumulation, both generalized and periarticular, is seen on the three-phase study. This pattern occurs more often in children.
- Three scintigraphic stages of RSDS have been described. In the first stage (up to 20 weeks), the typical three-phase bone scan findings outlined above are seen. In the second stage (20 to 60 weeks postonset), normal first- and second-phase scans are seen, but increased radiotracer in the third phase is found. The third stage (60 to 100 weeks postonset) is marked by reduced radiotracer accumulation in the first two phases, but the third phase appears normal.
- Some investigators report having encountered only the typical findings of increased radiotracer on all three phases in adults.

◆ SUGGESTED READING

Demangeat JL, Constantinesco A, Brunot B, et al. Three-phase bone scanning in reflex sympathetic dystrophy of the hand. J Nucl Med 1988;29:26–32.

Holder LE, Cole LA, Myerson MS. Reflex sympathetic dystrophy in the foot: Clinical and scintigraphic criteria. Radiology 1992;184:531–535.

Holder LE, Mackinnon SE. Reflex sympathetic dystrophy in the hands: Clinical and scintigraphic criteria. Radiology 1984;152:517–521.

Schwartzman RJ, McLellan TL. Reflex sympathetic dystrophy. A review. Arch Neurol 1987;44:555–561.

CASE 21

R. Edward Coleman

HISTORY

A 69-year-old man with recurrent hypercalcemia after previous parathyroidectomy for hyperparathyroidism. Physical examination is normal.

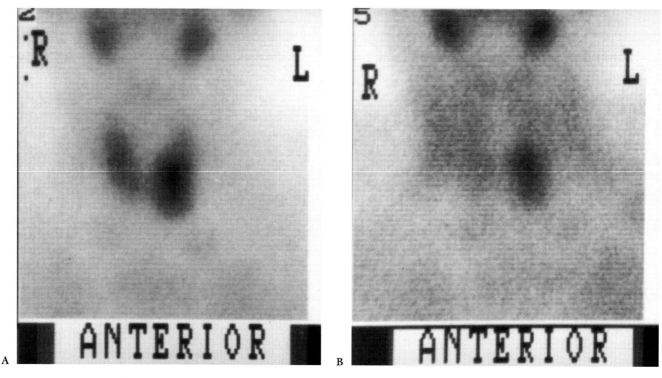

FIGURES 10-21A and 10-21B Anterior image of the neck obtained 10 minutes (**A**) and 2 hours (**B**) after the intravenous administration of 20 mCi of Tc-99m sestamibi. (**A**) shows normal accumulation of the tracer in the thyroid and salivary glands. The radioactivity has cleared from the right thyroid gland in (**B**), but radioactivity persists in the region of the inferior pole of the left thyroid gland.

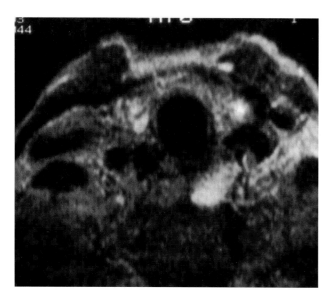

FIGURE 10-21C T2-weighted MRI of the neck. A 1.5 × 1.0 cm area of increased signal is seen posterior to the left lobe of the thyroid gland.

◆ DIFFERENTIAL DIAGNOSIS

◆ **Parathyroid hyperplasia:** This is an unlikely diagnosis because only a single abnormality is present. Multiple foci of tracer activity would be expected with parathyroid hyperplasia.

◆ **Thyroid cancer:** The absence of a palpable mass on physical examination, elevated serum calcium level, and normal image obtained 10 minutes after radiopharmaceutical administration make this diagnosis unlikely.

◆ **Thyroid adenoma:** The history of hypercalcemia makes this diagnosis less likely. Furthermore, the abnormality on the MR image is not located within the thyroid gland but is posterior to it.

◆ **Metastatic disease to a supraclavicular node:** The lack of a history of a primary malignancy and absence of other abnormalities on the MRI study make this diagnosis unlikely, although it is not excluded. However, the history of hypercalcemia in association with the neck lesion is best explained by an alternative diagnosis—namely, parathyroid adenoma.

◆ **Parathyroid adenoma:** The presence of a single, focal abnormality on the Tc-99m sestamibi image in a patient with hypercalcemia makes parathyroid adenoma the most likely diagnosis.

◆ DIAGNOSIS: Parathyroid adenoma.

◆ KEY FACTS

CLINICAL

◆ Hyperparathyroidism is the result of increased parathormone production. Two types of hyperparathyroidism are recognized: primary and secondary.

◆ Primary hyperparathyroidism is due to endogenous hypersecretion of parathormone, which is caused by an adenoma (usually a solitary lesion) in 80% of cases, hyperplasia (usually of all four glands) in 10% to 15% of cases, and parathyroid carcinoma in about 5% of cases.

◆ Secondary hyperparathyroidism results from hypocalcemia causing stimulation of the parathyroid glands and increased parathormone production. It is usually secondary to renal failure but can be seen in malabsorption and renal tubular disorders.

◆ Tertiary hyperparathyroidism occurs when one or more glands hypertrophy due to secondary hyperparathyroidism and then function autonomously.

◆ Symptomatic patients with hyperparathyroidism and radiologic or metabolic disturbance should be treated by surgery.

◆ Persistent hypercalcemia after surgery for hyperparathyroidism occurs in 3% to 10% of cases and results from failure to remove all hyperfunctioning glands.

◆ The combination of radionuclide imaging and new parathormone assays that can be performed very quickly (<15 minutes) and, hence, intraoperatively, permit decreased operative time and help in identifying all hyperfunctioning tissue, allowing total resection of all hyperfunctioning glands.

RADIOLOGIC

◆ The double-phase Tc-99m sestamibi study consists of early (10 to 20 minutes after radiopharmaceutical administration) and delayed (2 to 3 hours) imaging. It is very accurate in the localization of hyperfunctioning parathyroid tissue.

◆ The double-phase technique is based on the more rapid tracer clearance from normal thyroid than from abnormal parathyroid tissue.

◆ Tc-99m sestamibi is more accurate in localizing abnormal parathyroid tissue than other radionuclide techniques, sonography, CT, and MRI, which are also used for this purpose.

◆ The detection rate of abnormal parathyroid tissue depends on gland size. Adenomas are generally larger than hyperplastic glands (frequently >500 mg) and thus more accurately detected.

◆ Tc-99m sestamibi is very accurate in detecting ectopic parathyroid glands that cause hyperparathyroidism, but the abnormality must be in the field of view of the study. Parallel-hole, high-resolution collimation is used to ensure that the neck and upper chest are in the field of view.

◆ Thyroid adenomas, thyroid carcinomas, and lymph nodes involved with sarcoid have been reported to cause false-positive results on Tc-99m sestamibi imaging studies for parathyroid adenoma evaluation.

◆ SUGGESTED READING

Coakley AJ. Parathyroid imaging. Nucl Med Comm 1995;16:522–533.

Irvin GL, Prudhomme DL, Deriso GT, et al. A new approach to parathyroidectomy. Ann Surg 1994;219:574–581.

Lee VS, Wilkinson RH, Leight GS, et al. Hyperparathyroidism in high-risk surgical patients: Evaluation with double-phase technetium-99m sestamibi imaging. Radiology 1995;197:627–633.

HISTORY

A 61-year-old woman with coronary artery disease, congestive heart failure, severe peripheral vascular disease, hypertension, and a creatinine level of 2.8 mg/dl.

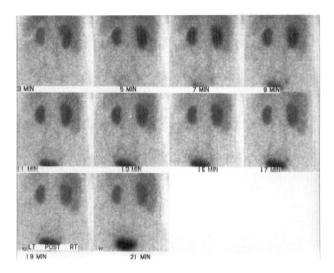

FIGURE 10-22A Baseline posterior images of the abdomen obtained after the administration of 1 mCi of Tc-99m MAG3. Asymmetric parenchymal radiotracer uptake is seen on the immediate image with less uptake in the left kidney than in the right kidney. The left kidney is smaller than the right. No evidence for obstruction to drainage is seen within either kidney. The image obtained at 21 minutes shows less cortical activity bilaterally than the image obtained at 5 minutes.

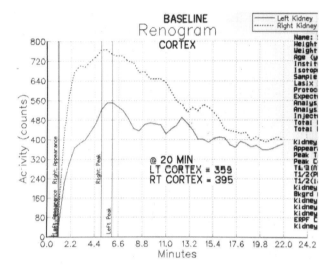

FIGURE 10-22B Baseline time activity curves from the right and left renal cortex. A slight delay in peak cortical activity is seen, more pronounced for the left kidney. The residual cortical activity is 48% for the right kidney and 65% for the left.

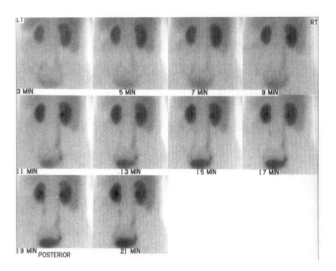

FIGURE 10-22C Posterior images of the abdomen obtained after intravenous administration of 2.5 mg of enalaprilat, followed by 9 mCi of Tc-99m MAG3. Asymmetry of the kidneys is again noted. Progressive radiotracer accumulation is seen within the left renal cortex, as well as significant residual activity within the right renal cortex.

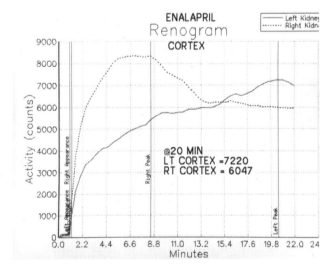

FIGURE 10-22D Time activity curves from the right and left renal cortex after the administration of enalaprilat. The right cortical renogram has significant residual radiotracer activity at the end of 21 minutes, with 61% retention from the peak and a 13% increase from the baseline study. The left cortical renogram shows an ascending pattern with a 35% increase from baseline.

◆ DIFFERENTIAL DIAGNOSIS

◆ **High-grade obstruction:** This diagnosis is unlikely because the baseline study does not show a rising baseline renogram, as would be expected with high-grade obstruction.

◆ **Acute tubular necrosis:** This diagnosis is very unlikely because of lack of a history of an appropriate precipitating event (e.g., an episode of hypotension) and because acute tubular necrosis would be expected to affect both kidneys in a symmetric fashion.

◆ **Unilateral renal artery stenosis:** This is not the appropriate diagnosis because the function of both kidneys (rather than one kidney) worsened after administration of angiotension-converting enzyme inhibitor.

◆ **Bilateral renal artery stenoses:** This is the best diagnosis because the function of both kidneys decreased following enalaprilat administration. The findings in the left kidney are characteristic for severe renal artery stenosis—there is a change from an ascending/descending pattern on the baseline cortical renogram to an ascending pattern after enalaprilat administration. The pattern in the right kidney, however, is also abnormal, with a prolonged cortical phase, significant residual tubular radiotracer activity relative to peak, and a 13% increase from the baseline study (which exceeds 10% from baseline, thereby meeting criteria for renal artery stenosis).

◆ **Chronic renal disease not causing hypertension:** This diagnosis is unlikely because of the abnormal response to the angiotension converting enzyme inhibitor.

◆ **DIAGNOSIS: Bilateral renal artery stenoses (75% right kidney and 99% left kidney).**

◆ KEY FACTS

CLINICAL

◆ Renal artery stenosis is a common cause of secondary hypertension and is present in 1% to 4% of hypertensive patients. It predominantly occurs in whites.

◆ Renovascular hypertension is produced by excessive renin release, which itself results from a decrease in renal perfusion.

◆ Fibromuscular hyperplasia is the etiology in 30% of patients who have renovascular hypertension (being more common in women) and is the predominant cause of renovascular hypertension in adults <40 years. In 70% of cases, renovascular hypertension results from atherosclerotic stenosis.

◆ The following clinical features increase the likelihood that hypertension is secondary to renal artery stenosis:

1. Onset at age <20 and >50 years of age
2. Abdominal bruit
3. Atherosclerotic disease at other sites
4. Abrupt deterioration of renal function after the administration of angiotensin-converting enzyme inhibitors

◆ Some patients may be managed clinically if renal function does not deteriorate.

◆ The use of angiotensin-converting enzyme inhibitors has improved the success rate of medical therapy. However, patients with bilateral renal artery stenosis develop marked hypotension and deterioration of renal function after administration of these agents.

◆ Surgical treatment is generally successful, but percutaneous transluminal angioplasty is now the preferred approach for fibromuscular hyperplasia and discrete atherosclerotic lesions.

RADIOLOGIC

◆ Angiography is the gold standard diagnostic procedure for determining renal artery stenosis but has a number of drawbacks: (1) it is an invasive procedure, and (2) it provides an anatomic definition of the arterial luminal diameter but not the physiologic significance of a stenosis—i.e., that hypertension is on a renovascular basis. Renal vein renin determination is also an invasive procedure and has not proved to be accurate in the diagnosis.

◆ Urography and conventional radionuclide scintigraphy have an unacceptably high rate of false-negative and false-positive results in the diagnosis of renovascular hypertension. Doppler ultrasonography also has variable sensitivity and specificity in diagnosis of renovascular hypertension.

◆ Response of hypertension to renal artery angioplasty cannot be predicted from degree of arterial stenosis alone but must be combined with provocative tests such as scintigraphy following administration of angiotensin-converting enzyme. Some patients with mild stenosis but positive angiotensin-converting enzyme inhibitor scintigraphy have substantial reduction in hypertension following angioplasty, whereas patients with severe stenoses but negative scintigraphic studies do not generally respond to revascularization.

◆ SUGGESTED READING

Blaufox MD. Procedures of choice in renal nuclear medicine. J Nucl Med 1991;32:1301–1309.

Dunnick NR, Sfakianakis GN. Screening for renovascular hypertension. Radiol Clin North Am 1991;29:497–510.

Sfakianakis GN, Bourgoignie JJ, Georgiou M, Guerra JJ Jr. Diagnosis of renovascular hypertension with ACE inhibition scintigraphy. Radiol Clin North Am 1993;4:831–848.

CASE 23

Michael W. Hanson

HISTORY

A 76-year-old man with a transient episode of chest pain on returning to bed after voiding during the night and an episode of unexplained syncope. He is referred for exercise stress testing and myocardial perfusion imaging.

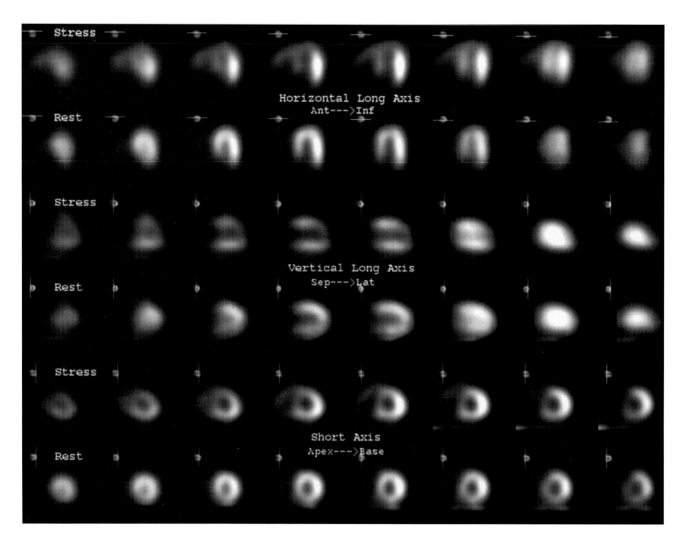

FIGURE 10-23 Stress Tc-99m sestamibi (rows 1, 3, and 5) and rest Tl-201 (rows 2, 4, and 6) myocardial perfusion images. The axes are noted on the images. The rest Tl-201 myocardial perfusion images (rows 2, 4, and 6) show normal homogeneous radiotracer uptake throughout the 1myocardium. No perfusion defects are seen on the rest images. The stress Tc-99m sestamibi myocardial perfusion images (rows 1, 3, and 5) show a segmental region of diminished perfusion involving the low anterior, anteroapical, and interventricular septal areas.

DIFFERENTIAL DIAGNOSIS

- **Myocardial infarction:** Myocardial infarction would not be expected to have normal homogeneous radiotracer uptake on the resting Tl-201 study, making this diagnosis incorrect.
- **Myocardial ischemia:** The development of a stress-induced perfusion defect that is not present on the resting perfusion image is the typical finding in myocardial ischemia. The findings in this case are most consistent with this diagnosis.
- **Attenuation artifact:** Most often a problem in obese women, this artifact should be seen on both the rest and stress images. It usually involves the lower anterior wall and the antero-apex region. The defect seen in the case presented is larger than that typically seen due to attenuation artifact. Furthermore, attenuation artifact would not be expected to involve the septum, as in the present case.
- **Artifact from left bundle branch block:** This electrocardiographic abnormality can create a reversible perfusion defect, but it most often involves primarily the interventricular septum and is not as extensive as the defect presented in this case.
- **Artifact from patient motion on the stress image:** Motion artifact can create apparent perfusion defects that usually, though not exclusively, occur in the apex. This diagnosis is incorrect because the defect seen in the case presented is much more extensive than that expected from patient motion. In general, review of the raw data in a cine mode can often identify patient motion of a degree sufficient to create apparent perfusion defects.

DIAGNOSIS: Stress-induced myocardial ischemia in the vascular territory of the left anterior descending coronary artery.

KEY FACTS

CLINICAL

- The symptoms, pain location and radiation patterns, and precipitating factors of angina pectoris due to myocardial ischemia can be variable. If the clinical index of suspicion is sufficiently high—i.e., a >10% probability that the patient has significant coronary artery disease—further evaluation is indicated.

- The episode of unexplained syncope in this patient is worrisome because it may have been related to transient myocardial ischemia and a potentially fatal arrhythmia.
- Based on this patient's presentation and perfusion images, the diagnosis is significant coronary artery disease, which was documented at cardiac catheterization.
- Prevention of myocardial infarction and left ventricular damage is a primary objective for the treatment of this patient.

RADIOLOGIC

- The scintigraphic findings in the case presented are the typical pattern seen with stress-induced myocardial ischemia. A perfusion defect following stress testing that is not seen on the resting image indicates segmental myocardial ischemia. The perfusion defect is secondary to altered blood flow during coronary artery dilatation that occurs in response to physical (e.g., exercise) or pharmacologic (e.g., dipyridamole or dobutamine) stress testing.
- A fixed defect at rest and stress can be caused by either myocardial infarction or artifact due to attenuation of photons by surrounding soft tissue or noncardiac structures.
- Myocardial perfusion imaging can be performed with Tl-201 alone, Tc-99m sestamibi alone, or as above, with a combination of the two agents. The dual isotope technique combines the advantage of Tl-201 (the preferred single-photon radiopharmaceutical for identifying viable myocardium) and the advantage of Tc-99m sestamibi (superior image quality following stress). The dual isotope technique also decreases overall imaging time.

SUGGESTED READING

Berman DS, Kiat HS, Van Train KF, et al. Myocardial perfusion imaging with technetium-99m sestamibi: Comparative analysis of available imaging protocols. J Nucl Med 1994;35:681–688.

Kiat H, Germano G, Friedman J, et al. Comparative feasibility of separate or simultaneous rest thallium-201/stress technetium-99m sestamibi dual-isotope myocardial perfusion SPECT. J Nucl Med 1994;35:542–548.

Maddahi J, Rodrigues E, Berman DS, et al. State-of-the-art myocardial perfusion imaging. Cardiol Clin 1994;12:199–222.

Wackers FJT. Artifacts in planar and SPECT myocardial perfusion imaging. Am J Card Imag 1992;6:42–58.

Wackers FJT. The maze of myocardial perfusion imaging protocols in 1994. J Nucl Cardiol 1994;1:180–188.

HISTORY

A 15-year-old boy with a 2-week history of severe lower back pain (worse on the right) that had its onset while the patient was playing tennis. Mild point tenderness is present at L4–L5, primarily on the right side.

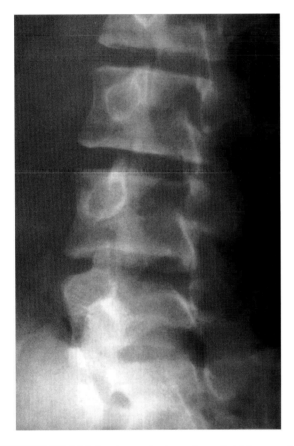

FIGURE 10-24A Lumbosacral spine radiograph (right posterior oblique view). No abnormalities are seen on the plain radiograph.

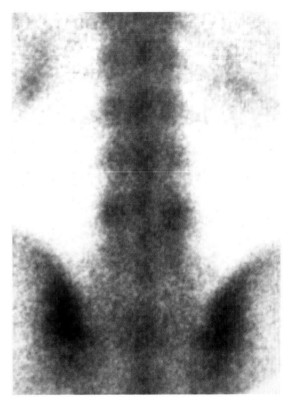

FIGURE 10-24B Posterior planar bone scan image. Radiotracer uptake is slightly more prominent at L4 than in the other lumbar vertebrae. The abnormality is bilateral but more marked on the right.

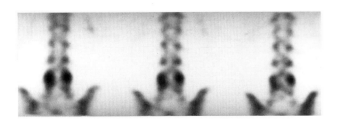

FIGURE 10-24C Coronal single-photon emission CT bone scan images. Prominent abnormal radiotracer uptake is clearly defined, bilaterally, at L4 (right greater than left) in the posterior elements.

FIGURE 10-24D Transverse single-photon emission CT bone at the L4 level. Bilateral foci of abnormal radiotracer uptake are seen (right greater than left). The transverse projection further localizes the abnormal radiotracer to the region of the pars interarticularis.

◆ DIFFERENTIAL DIAGNOSIS

◆ **Mechanical low back pain:** This entity occurs secondary to mechanical strain on paraspinal and spinal ligaments, muscles, and facet joints. Clinical findings can mimic skeletal trauma. Imaging studies are typically normal. The abnormal bone scan in the case illustrated therefore excludes this diagnosis as the sole explanation of symptoms. Instead, it indicates the presence of skeletal pathology.

◆ **Herniated lumbar disk:** Symptoms and signs can make distinction of this diagnosis from other causes of low back pain difficult. CT/myelography or MRI would be needed to confirm this diagnosis. However, the bone scan would be expected to be negative, unlike the study in the case illustrated. Furthermore, the location of abnormality in the posterior elements on the bone scan makes this diagnosis unlikely.

◆ **Stress fracture of the lamina:** This entity has typically been reported in runners with low back pain. The plain radiographs can be entirely normal. However, an abnormal accumulation of radiotracer would be expected to be seen in the lamina, rather than in the pars interarticularis (as shown in Figure 10-24D), making lamina fracture unlikely.

◆ **Pars interarticularis stress fracture (spondylolysis):** This entity is commonly seen in athletes with low back pain. Radiographs are commonly normal but bone scan, which is more sensitive, typically shows abnormal radiotracer uptake in the region of the one or both pars interarticularis. The localization of abnormal radiotracer uptake on the SPECT bone scan in the case illustrated makes this the most likely diagnosis.

◆ **Tumor or infection:** The bone scan findings are nonspecific. However, tumor or infection in the case illustrated would be unlikely to cause the small, focal, bilateral abnormalities shown.

◆ DIAGNOSIS: Bilateral stress fractures of the pars interarticularis.

◆ KEY FACTS

CLINICAL

◆ Spondylolysis refers to a break in bone continuity that results from a defect in the junction between the superior and inferior processus articularis.

◆ Spondylolysis is present in approximately 7% of individuals and as many as 50% of athletes who have low back pain.

◆ Spondylolysis is more commonly seen in gymnasts, football linemen, and weight lifters, and it is likely due to repeated hyperflexion and hyperextension of the lumbar spine.

◆ Spondylolysis is usually treated by conservative means (e.g., bracing and restricted activity).

◆ Spondylolysis is one of three principal causes of spondylolisthesis, a condition characterized by the forward (or occasionally, backward) displacement of a vertebra relative to the next lowest vertebra.

RADIOLOGIC

◆ Bone scintigraphy is a more sensitive indicator of acute stress injury than plain radiography; radiographic changes may not be seen acutely even when the bone scan is abnormal.

◆ Radionuclide bone scanning can help to determine the chronicity of fractures seen on plain radiographs. Acute fractures have increased radiotracer activity, and chronic fractures have decreased radiotracer activity.

◆ SPECT bone imaging offers an advantage over planar scintigraphic imaging by avoiding the superimposition of bony structures that is present on planar imaging. Image contrast is improved by SPECT imaging, often allowing abnormalities to be more confidently localized by SPECT than by planar imaging.

◆ SUGGESTED READING

Collier BD, Johnson RP, Carrera GF, et al. Painful spondylolysis or spondylolisthesis studied by radiology and single-photon emission computed tomography. Radiology 1985;54:207–211.

Holder LE. Bone scintigraphy in skeletal trauma. Radiol Clin North Am 1993;31:739–781.

Pecina MM, Bojanic I. Overuse Injuries of the Musculoskeletal System. Boca Raton, FL: CRC, 1993;89–120.

Pennell RG, Maurer AH, Bonakdarpour A. Stress injuries of the pars interarticularis: Radiologic classification and indications for scintigraphy. AJR Am J Roentgenol 1985;145:763–766.

Rogers LF. Radiology of Skeletal Trauma (2nd ed). New York: Churchill Livingstone, 1992;565–572.

CASE 25

Michael W. Hanson

HISTORY

A 37-year-old man with severe three-vessel coronary artery disease, prior myocardial infarction, and percutaneous transluminal coronary angioplasty presents with chest pain and cardiac enzyme elevation compatible with recurrent myocardial infarction. A multigated cardiac blood pool study showed a dilated left ventricle, multiple segmental wall motion abnormalities, and an left ventricular ejection fraction (LVEF) of 14%. He is referred for a Tl-201 myocardial perfusion study for assessment of myocardial viability.

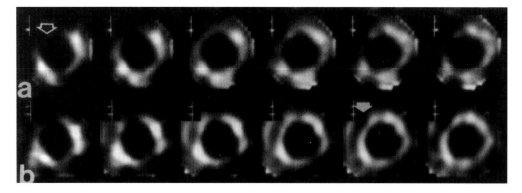

FIGURE 10-25 Short axis images from a Tl-201 study performed at rest **(top row, a)** and after 4-hour redistribution **(bottom row, b)**. The left ventricle is dilated. Markedly diminished radiotracer uptake is seen in the low anterior wall, low anteroseptum (open arrow), and anterior and inferior apex on the rest study which does not change at 4 or 24 hours, consistent with infarcted, nonviable myocardium. The mid and basilar anteroseptum has diminished radiotracer at rest that improves at 4 hours (closed arrow), consistent with ischemic, viable myocardium. The anterolateral and posterolateral walls contain viable myocardium.

◆ DIFFERENTIAL DIAGNOSIS

◆ **Normal myocardium:** This diagnosis is unlikely because of the segmental changes over time in a pattern consistent with either infarcted, nonviable myocardium or ischemic, viable myocardium.

◆ **Hypertrophic cardiomyopathy:** The marked dilatation of the left ventricle with segmentally heterogeneous distribution of radiotracer makes this diagnosis unlikely.

◆ **Ischemic cardiomyopathy:** The distribution of Tl-201 is heterogeneous, with segmental areas of diminished Tl-201 uptake on the immediate image that improves over time (indicating viable myocardium) and areas of markedly diminished Tl-201 uptake that do not change over time (indicating nonviable myocardium). These findings, in conjunction with the prior cardiac catheterization findings, make this the most likely diagnosis.

◆ **Idiopathic dilated cardiomyopathy:** The left ventricle in this case is dilated, which can be seen in idiopathic dilated cardiomyopathy. However, the myocardial perfusion is more heterogeneous in this study than is typically seen in idiopathic cardiomyopathy, making this diagnosis unlikely.

◆ DIAGNOSIS: Ischemic cardiomyopathy with areas of ischemic, viable myocardium.

◆ KEY FACTS

CLINICAL

◆ The term *stunned myocardium* is used to refer to transiently dysfunctional myocardium (i.e., myocardium having impaired contractility) that is reversible after restoration of coronary artery blood flow. Stunned myocardium is seen in several settings, including (1) after an acute episode of myocardial ischemia (e.g., an episode of angina pectoris), and (2) after acute coronary artery occlusion reversed by thrombolytic therapy.

◆ The term *hibernating myocardium* is used to refer to longstanding (potentially reversible) dysfunctional myocardium in the resting basal state. Hibernating myocardium is seen with chronic myocardial ischemia from prolonged periods of reduction in coronary artery blood flow (i.e., in the setting of chronic coronary artery disease). This impaired myocardial contractility is reversible after restoration of coronary artery perfusion.

◆ An accurate, noninvasive determination of viable (i.e., stunned or hibernating) myocardium is important for identification of myocardial segments that will benefit most from revascularization procedures.

◆ In patients with unexplained congestive heart failure, severely depressed LVEF, and no history of angina pectoris or myocardial infarction, it is important to distinguish ischemic from idiopathic left ventricular dysfunction so that appropriate therapy can be started.

◆ Myocardial viability studies in patients with known severe multivessel coronary artery disease and left ventricular dysfunction can help to decide which revascularization procedure (i.e., complete revascularization with bypass surgery or limited revascularization with coronary angioplasty) should be performed.

RADIOLOGIC

◆ Myocardium can be confidently assumed to be viable if there is normal contractility on imaging studies that are used to assess wall motion (e.g., MUGA, first-pass radionuclide angiography, contrast ventriculography, or echocardiography). However, if there is a resting wall motion abnormality, the status of myocardial viability (i.e., whether the myocardium is stunned, hibernating, or nonviable) cannot be reliably determined based on the wall motion abnormality alone. Segmental myocardial viability can, however, be assessed reliably using Tl-201 myocardial perfusion imaging by either a rest-redistribution method or a stress-reinjection method.

◆ An alternative imaging technique for assessment of myocardial viability is positron emission tomography (PET) using F-18 FDG, viewed by some investigators as the preferred imaging technique. Viable myocardium takes up this radiotracer, while nonviable myocardium does not take it up. Limitations include availability, cost, the need to regulate plasma glucose levels to optimize F-18 FDG uptake, and regional heterogeneity of F-18 FDG uptake that can occur even in normal subjects.

◆ Same-day rest/stress myocardial perfusion imaging with Tc-99m sestamibi is another technique for assessment of myocardial viability in patients with chronic coronary artery disease and left ventricular dysfunction. However, in comparison to Tl-201 redistribution or reinjection and F-18 FDG PET, it underestimates the extent of viable myocardium.

◆ SUGGESTED READING

Dilsizian V, Arrighi JA, Diodati JG, et al. Myocardial viability in patients with chronic coronary artery disease. Comparison of Tc-99m sestamibi with thallium reinjection and F-18 fluorodeoxyglucose. Circulation 1994;89:578–587.

Dilsizian V, Bonow RO. Current diagnostic techniques of assessing myocardial viability in patients with hibernating and stunned myocardium. Circulation 1993;87:1–20.

Schelbert HR. Metabolic imaging to assess myocardial viability. J Nucl Med 1994;35(Suppl):8S–14S.

INDEX